T0290046

# Respiratory Infections, Vaccines and Treatment

# Respiratory Infections, Vaccines and Treatment

Editor: Piers Corbyn

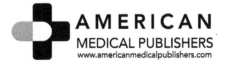

AMERICAN
MEDICAL PUBLISHERS
www.americanmedicalpublishers.com

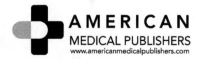

Cataloging-in-Publication Data

Respiratory infections, vaccines and treatment / edited by Piers Corbyn.
        p. cm.
Includes bibliographical references and index.
ISBN 979-8-88740-437-0
1. Respiratory infections. 2. Respiratory organs--Diseases--Vaccination.
3. Respiratory organs--Diseases--Treatment. 4. Respiratory infections--Vaccination.
5. Respiratory infections--Treatment. I. Corbyn, Piers.
RC740 .R47 2023
616.2--dc23

American Medical Publishers,
41 Flatbush Avenue,
1st Floor, New York,
NY 11217, USA

ISBN 979-8-88740-437-0 (Hardback)

# Contents

# Preface

Humans can breathe due to the presence of the respiratory system which comprises nose, throat, larynx, trachea, bronchi, and lungs. Respiratory tract infections (RTIs), commonly called respiratory infections, occur when the parts of the body that are involved in breathing such as sinuses, throat, airways and lungs are infected. The underlying cause of RTIs may be viral or bacterial infections. Symptoms of the RTIs include cough, throwing-up phlegm, sneezing, stuffy or runny nose, sore throat, headaches, muscle aches, breathlessness, tight chest, fever, and a general feeling of being unwell. They can be diagnosed using physical examination, lung X-ray, lung CT scan, lung function test, nasal swab test, throat swab test and sputum test. The treatment of the RTI depends on its cause. The RTIs caused by viruses clear up by themselves and do not require antibiotics. However, the treatment for RTIs caused by bacteria involves the usage of antibiotics. The risk and severity of respiratory infections such as seasonal and pandemic influenza, COVID-19, pertussis, pneumococcal infection, tuberculosis (TB), etc. can be reduced by conducting immunization or vaccination drives. This book discusses the fundamentals and advanced studies on the vaccines and treatment of respiratory infections. It presents researches and studies performed by experts across the globe. The book will serve as a valuable source of reference for students, researchers and medical practitioners.

Significant researches are present in this book. Intensive efforts have been employed by authors to make this book an outstanding discourse. This book contains the enlightening chapters which have been written on the basis of significant researches done by the experts.

Finally, I would also like to thank all the members involved in this book for being a team and meeting all the deadlines for the submission of their respective works. I would also like to thank my friends and family for being supportive in my efforts.

**Editor**

# Intranasal Vaccination with Lipoproteins Confers Protection Against Pneumococcal Colonisation

Franziska Voß[1], Thomas P. Kohler[1], Tanja Meyer[2], Mohammed R. Abdullah[1],
Fred J. van Opzeeland[3], Malek Saleh[1], Stephan Michalik[2], Saskia van Selm[3],
Frank Schmidt[2,4], Marien I. de Jonge[3] and Sven Hammerschmidt[1]*

[1] Department of Molecular Genetics and Infection Biology, Center for Functional Genomics of Microbes, Interfaculty Institute of Genetics and Functional Genomics, University of Greifswald, Greifswald, Germany, [2] Department of Functional Genomics, Center for Functional Genomics of Microbes, Interfaculty Institute of Genetics and Functional Genomics, University Medicine Greifswald, Greifswald, Germany, [3] Section Pediatric Infectious Diseases, Laboratory of Medical Immunology, Radboud Center for Infectious Diseases, Radboud Institute for Molecular Life Sciences, Radboud University Medical Center, Nijmegen, Netherlands, [4] ZIK-FunGene, Department of Functional Genomics, Interfaculty Institute for Genetics and Functional Genomics, University Medicine Greifswald, Greifswald, Germany

*Correspondence:
Sven Hammerschmidt
sven.hammerschmidt@
uni-greifswald.de

Streptococcus pneumoniae is endowed with a variety of surface-exposed proteins representing putative vaccine candidates. Lipoproteins are covalently anchored to the cell membrane and highly conserved among pneumococcal serotypes. Here, we evaluated these lipoproteins for their immunogenicity and protective potential against pneumococcal colonisation. A multiplex-based immunoproteomics approach revealed the immunogenicity of selected lipoproteins. High antibody titres were measured in sera from mice immunised with the lipoproteins MetQ, PnrA, PsaA, and DacB. An analysis of convalescent patient sera confirmed the immunogenicity of these lipoproteins. Examining the surface localisation and accessibility of the lipoproteins using flow cytometry indicated that PnrA and DacB were highly abundant on the surface of the bacteria. Mice were immunised intranasally with PnrA, DacB, and MetQ using cholera toxin subunit B (CTB) as an adjuvant, followed by an intranasal challenge with S. pneumoniae D39. PnrA protected the mice from pneumococcal colonisation. For the immunisation with DacB and MetQ, a trend in reducing the bacterial load could be observed, although this effect was not statistically significant. The reduction in bacterial colonisation was correlated with the increased production of antigen-specific IL-17A in the nasal cavity. Immunisation induced high systemic IgG levels with a predominance for the IgG1 isotype, except for DacB, where IgG levels were substantially lower compared to MetQ and PnrA. Our results indicate that lipoproteins are interesting targets for future vaccine strategies as they are highly conserved, abundant, and immunogenic.

Keywords: Streptococcus pneumoniae, lipoprotein, immunogenicity, colonization, protection

## INTRODUCTION

Streptococcus pneumoniae continues to be a major cause of life-threatening invasive diseases such as pneumonia, sepsis and meningitis, especially in young children, the elderly and immunodeficient people (1). Two different types of vaccines are currently recommended by the World Health Organization (WHO) for the prevention of pneumococcal infections: the 23-valent polysaccharide vaccine (PPV23) and the pneumococcal conjugate vaccines PCV7, PCV10, and PCV13 (2). Despite their proven efficacy (3, 4), these vaccines have some important limitations, including restricted serotype coverage, which may facilitate replacement by non-vaccine serotypes, and high manufacturing costs (5–7). It is therefore vital to develop a new generation of vaccines, which can provide serotype-independent protection against pneumococcal infections, while being affordable for developing countries.

The pneumococcal cell-surface is decorated with a variety of proteins, which are exposed to the extracellular milieu of the host and are therefore the most promising targets for future protein-based vaccines. Consequently, pneumococcal surface proteins have been extensively studied over the last two decades, with the majority being characterised as virulence factors. Promising vaccine candidates, including PspA (Pneumococcal surface protein), PhtD (Pneumococcal histidine triad), PcpA (Pneumococcal choline-binding protein), PcsB (Pneumococcal cell wall separation protein), and StkP (serine/threonine protein kinase), have already been shown to be safe and immunogenic in clinical trials (8).

In this study, we particularly focussed on the lipoproteins, which are embedded in the pneumococcal cell membrane via a covalently anchored lipid moiety. Lipoproteins are highly conserved, and many of them influence pneumococcal fitness and virulence (9–14). Some studies have indicated the protective potential of lipoproteins against pneumococcal infections, with the well-characterised lipoprotein pneumococcal surface antigen A (PsaA), a manganese substrate-binding protein, being particularly in the research spotlight. PsaA is expressed by all serotypes of S. pneumoniae and is known to bind to human E-cadherin, thereby acting as an adhesin (15–19). Moreover, PsaA is highly immunogenic, as shown by the increased antibody responses that have been described as a result of pneumococcal exposure in children (20–22). Using intranasal challenge models in mice, PsaA has been shown to protect against pneumococcal carriage, demonstrated by reduced bacterial loads in the nasopharynx (23). A multivalent recombinant subunit protein vaccine containing PsaA, StkP, and PcsB was tested in a phase I trial (IC47, Intercell AG, Austria, NCT00873431) and shown to be safe and immunogenic (24, 25), resulting in the induction of protective antibodies against all three proteins. Besides PsaA, two other lipoproteins, SP_0148 and SP_2108, have emerged as promising vaccine candidates. Following intranasal immunisation, these proteins, which function as substrate-binding proteins for ABC transporters, showed protective efficacy in a mouse model of colonisation, which correlated with the observed elevation in IL-17A levels and depended on Toll-like receptor 2 signalling (26). Recently, Genocea Biosciences tested the GEN-004 vaccine (SP_0148, SP_2108 and SP_1912) using a human challenge model. Although the differences were not statistically significant, there was a trend in reducing carriage acquisition by 18–36% vs. the placebo (27), supporting the further development of GEN-004 and indicating the high potential of lipoproteins as components of a protein-based vaccine.

We therefore focused in our study on pneumococcal lipoproteins, aiming to identify new and promising candidates for a protein-based and serotype-independent vaccine. We analysed the immunogenicity of our candidates in mouse immunisation studies and by screening convalescent patient sera, while also assessing their abundance on the surface of pneumococci. It is essential that the antibodies raised by immunisation can recognise and bind to accessible surface proteins. Three lipoproteins were identified as the most promising candidates based on their high levels of conservation, their immunogenicity and their abundance on the pneumococcal cell-surface: the L,D-carboxypeptidase DacB (9), the methionine-binding protein MetQ (12), and the nucleoside-binding protein PnrA (11). DacB is a cell wall hydrolase and therefore essential for pneumococcal peptidoglycan turnover and the preservation of cell shape (9). MetQ and PnrA are substrate-binding lipoprotein components of the ABC transporters responsible for methionine or nucleoside uptake, respectively, from the extracellular space (11, 12). Pneumococcal mutants lacking these lipoproteins were previously shown to have significantly attenuated virulence in either systemic or pulmonary mouse infection models, although there is contradictory information regarding the role of MetQ in causing systemic infection in mice (9, 11, 12, 28, 29).

In our study, intranasal vaccination with these lipoproteins resulted in a reduced bacterial load in the nasal cavity, which correlated with increased nasal IL-17A levels. Humoral immune responses were characterised by high serum levels of IgG1 and substantial IgG2 levels, with the exception of the DacB vaccination. Our findings demonstrate the high potential of DacB and PnrA in particular for use in a future protein-based pneumococcal vaccine.

## MATERIALS AND METHODS
### Ethics Statement
All animal experiments were conducted in accordance with the guidelines of the ethics committee at the University of Greifswald, the German regulations of the Society for Laboratory Animal Science (GV-SOLAS) and the European Health Law of the Federation of Laboratory Animal Science Associations (FELASA). All experiments were approved by the Landesamt für Landwirtschaft, Lebensmittelsicherheit und Fischerei Mecklenburg-Vorpommern (LALLF M-V, Rostock, Germany) and the LALLF M-V ethical board (LALLF M-V permit no. 7221.3-1-061/17). All efforts were made to minimise the discomfort of the animals and ensure the highest ethical standards.

## Bacterial Strains, Culture Conditions, and Pneumococcal Mutant Construction
Streptococcus pneumoniae wild-type and isogenic deletion mutants (Table 1) were grown on Columbia blood agar plates (Oxoid) supplemented with the appropriate antibiotics (50 μg/ml kanamycin, 5 μg/ml erythromycin or 10 μg/ml trimethoprim) and cultivated to mid-log phase ($A_{600} = 0.35$–$0.40$) in THY containing 36.4% Todd-Hewitt broth (Roth) and 0.5% yeast extract (Roth) at 37°C and in 5% $CO_2$. Escherichia coli strains were cultured on solid Luria-Bertani

(LB) medium plates or in liquid LB medium (Roth) to mid-log phase ($A_{600}$ = 0.8) on an environmental shaker in the presence of kanamycin (50 µg/ml), ampicillin (100 µg/ml), and/or erythromycin (250 µg/ml) at 30°C. To generate the $\Delta metQ$ (sp_0149), $\Delta sp\_0191$, $\Delta pnrA$ (sp_0845), $\Delta sp\_0899$, and $\Delta adcAII$ (sp_1002) mutants, the loci of the respective genes and their upstream and downstream flanking sequences were amplified from S. pneumoniae TIGR4 genomic DNA using PCR and the primer pairs listed in **Table 2**. Following the manufacturer's instructions, the PCR products were directly cloned into pGEM®-T Easy vectors (Promega, Madison, WI, USA) and transformed into E. coli DH5α competent cells. The recombinant plasmids p559, p560, p576, p573, and p572 harbouring the desired DNA inserts were purified and used as templates for inverse PCR reactions with the primer pairs listed in **Table 2**. The deleted sequences were replaced with the ermB resistance gene, which was amplified from plasmid pE89 using PCR with the primer pair ermB_105/ermB_106 (**Table 2**). These recombinant plasmids were used to transform pneumococci, as described previously (35). The non-encapsulated pneumococcal mutants D39ΔpsaA, D39ΔpspA, D39ΔppmA, and D39ΔslrA were generated by transformation with the recombinant plasmid p873, in which the capsule gene locus is replaced by the aphA3 resistance gene.

## Heterologous Expression, Purification of Recombinant Proteins, and Production of Polyclonal Antisera

The N-terminally His$_6$-tagged proteins used in this study were either described previously (**Table 2**) or were generated by cloning the PCR products of the target genes metQ, sp_0191, pnrA, sp_0899, and adcAII, without their signal sequences, into the pTP1 expression vector (10). PCR reactions were performed using S. pneumoniae TIGR4 chromosomal DNA as a template and the primer pairs listed in **Table 2**. The primers contained restriction sites (NheI/SacI, NheI/HindIII, or NdeI/HindIII), which were used to ligate the fragments into similarly digested expression vectors. The resulting plasmids (**Table 1**) were transformed into competent E. coli BL21 (DE3). For protein production, the recombinant E. coli BL21 (DE3) were cultured in LB, supplemented with kanamycin (50 µg/ml) or ampicillin (100 µg/ml), to an $A_{600}$ of 0.6–0.8 at 30°C. Protein expression was induced with 1 mM IPTG (isopropyl-β-D-1-thiogalactopyranoside; Hartenstein, Wuerzburg, Germany) and the cells were cultured for another 3 h. The resulting His$_6$-tagged proteins were purified using affinity chromatography in a His Trap™ HP Ni-NTA column (1 ml; GE Healthcare, Chicago, IL, USA) on the ÄKTA Purifier liquid chromatography system (GE Healthcare), following the manufacturer's instructions. Purified proteins were dialysed (12–14 kDa molecular weight cut off) against phosphate-buffered saline (PBS; pH 7.4). The absorbance of the proteins was determined at $A_{280}$ using a NanoDrop® ND-1000 (Thermo Fisher Scientific, Waltham, MA, USA) to calculate the protein concentrations while considering the extinction coefficients and molecular weights. After sodium dodecyl sulphate polyacrylamide gel electrophoresis (SDS-PAGE), the

purity of the proteins was analysed using silver staining and immunoblotting (**Figure 1**) with an anti-Penta-His-tag mouse antibody (Qiagen, Hilden, Germany). The recombinant proteins were used in intraperitoneal immunisations using Imject™ Alum as an adjuvant (Thermo Fisher Scientific). Six- to eight-week-old female CD-1 mice (Charles River Laboratories, Sulzfeld, Germany) were vaccinated by intraperitoneal injection with 100 µl of a 1:1 emulsion containing 20 µg recombinant protein and the adjuvant. The mice received vaccine boosters at days 14 and 28 and were bled after 6 weeks. Serum samples were taken before each immunisation step (pre-immune, priming, 1st boost) and 2 weeks after the third immunisation (post-immune) and stored at −20°C until use.

## Purification of Polyclonal IgG and Immunoblotting

Polyclonal IgGs were purified from the generated antisera using protein A-sepharose chromatography. Protein A sepharose CL-4B columns (GE Healthcare), stored in 20% ethanol at 4°C, were equilibrated in binding buffer (50 mM Tris-HCl, pH 7.0). After mixing the antisera with one volume of binding buffer, the mixture was applied to the column and incubated for 15 min at room temperature (RT). The column was washed with binding buffer until the absorption measured using a NanoDrop® ND-1000 dropped below $A_{280}$ = 0.05. The elution was performed using 1-ml aliquots of elution buffer (100 mM glycine, pH 3.0) collected in 50 µl phosphate buffer (50 mM $K_2HPO_4$, pH 8.5). The IgG concentration of each sample was determined by measuring the absorption at $A_{280}$ using a NanoDrop® ND-1000. Immunoblots were carried out to analyse the specificity of the purified polyclonal IgGs. After the SDS-PAGE-mediated separation of bacterial lysates from late exponential growth phase cells, the proteins were transferred onto a nitrocellulose membrane using semidry blotting (Bio-Rad Laboratories, Hercules, CA, USA). The membrane was blocked with 5% skim milk (in Tris-buffered saline (TBS), Roth) overnight at 4°C. Following an incubation with mouse polyclonal IgGs (1:1,000 in blocking buffer) recognising lipoproteins or rabbit anti-enolase serum (1:25,000 in blocking buffer) for 1 h at RT, the membrane was washed three times with washing buffer (TBS, 0.05% Tween® 20). A secondary antibody, goat anti-mouse IgG (Dianova, Hamburg, Germany; 1:5,000) or goat anti-rabbit IgG (Dianova; 1:5,000) horseradish peroxidase conjugate was used for 1 h at RT, then washed three times with washing buffer. Finally, antibody binding was detected using an enhanced chemiluminescence reaction (luminol and p-coumaric acid, Roth).

## Antibody Titration of Polyclonal IgGs Using Enzyme-Linked Immunosorbent Assays (ELISAs) and the Flow Cytometric Analysis of Surface Abundance

The antibody titres of polyclonal IgGs were determined using ELISAs. Microtiter plates (96-well, PolySorp®, Nunc, Thermo Fisher Scientific) were coated with equimolar amounts of pneumococcal proteins (30 pmol/well) overnight at 4°C. The

**TABLE 1 |** Strain and plasmid list.

| Strain/plasmid | Serotype and relevant genotype | Resistance* | Source or reference |
|---|---|---|---|
| ***Streptococcus pneumoniae*** | | | |
| SP257 (D39) | 2 | None | NCTC7466 |
| PN111 | D39Δ*cps* | Km$^r$ | (30, 31) |
| PN282 | D39Δ*cps* Δ*adcAII* (*spd_0888*) | Km$^r$, Erm$^r$ | This work |
| PN279 | D39Δ*cps* Δ*dacB* (*spd_0549*) | Km$^r$, Erm$^r$ | (9) |
| PN253 | D39Δ*cps* Δ*etrx1* (*spd_0572*) | Km$^r$, Erm$^r$ | (10) |
| PN281 | D39Δ*cps* Δ*etrx2* (*spd_0886*) | Km$^r$, Erm$^r$ | (10) |
| PN238 | D39Δ*cps* Δ*metQ* (*spd_0151*) | Km$^r$, Erm$^r$ | This work |
| PN732 | D39Δ*cps* Δ*ppmA* (*spd_0868*) | Km$^r$, Trm$^r$ | This work |
| PN280 | D39Δ*cps* Δ*pnrA* (*spd_0739*) | Km$^r$, Erm$^r$ | This work |
| PN301 | D39Δ*cps* Δ*psaA* (*spd_1463*) | Km$^r$, Erm$^r$ | This work |
| PN733 | D39Δ*cps* Δ*slrA* (*spd_0672*) | Km$^r$, Erm$^r$ | This work |
| PN241 | D39Δ*cps* Δ*spd_0179* | Km$^r$, Erm$^r$ | This work |
| PN312 | D39Δ*cps* Δ*spd_0792* | Km$^r$, Erm$^r$ | This work |
| PN735 | D39Δ*cps* Δ*pspA* (*spd_0126*) | Km$^r$, Erm$^r$ | This work |
| PN278 | D39Δ*adcAII* (*spd_0888*) | Erm$^r$ | This work |
| PN275 | D39Δ*dacB* (*spd_0549*) | Erm$^r$ | (9) |
| PN246 | D39Δ*etrx1* (*spd_0572*) | Erm$^r$ | (10) |
| PN277 | D39Δ*etrx2* (*spd_0886*) | Erm$^r$ | (10) |
| PN311 | D39Δ*metQ* (*spd_0151*) | Erm$^r$ | This work |
| PN093 | D39Δ*ppmA* (*spd_0868*) | Trm$^r$ | (32) |
| PN276 | D39Δ*pnrA* (*spd_0739*) | Erm$^r$ | This work |
| PN172 | D39Δ*psaA* (*spd_1463*) | Erm$^r$ | (13) |
| PN095 | D39Δ*slrA* (*spd_0672*) | Erm$^r$ | (32) |
| PN243 | D39Δ*spd_0179* | Erm$^r$ | This work |
| PN251 | D39Δ*spd_0792* | Erm$^r$ | This work |
| PN031 | D39Δ*pspA* (*spd_0126*) | Erm$^r$ | (33) |
| ***Escherichia coli*** | | | |
| DH5α | Δ*(lac)U169, endA1, gyrA46, hsdR17, Φ80Δ(lacZ)M15, recA1, relA1, supE44, thi-1* | None | Bethesda Research Labs, Gaithersburg, U.S. |
| BL21(DE3) | *E. coli* B, F- *dcm ompT hsdS gal* λ(DE3), T7 polymerase gene under control of the lacUV5 promoter | None | Novagen, Merck KGaA, Darmstadt, Germany |
| **Plasmids** | | | |
| pGEM®-T easy | TA cloning vector for PCR products | Ap$^r$ | Madison, U.S. |
| p89 | pCR2.1Topo with erythromycin (*ermB*) cassette | Ap$^r$, Km$^r$, Erm$^r$ | (34) |
| p873 | pGXT with capsule locus replaced by *aphA3* gene resistance cassette, flanking genes *dex* ,and *aliA* | Ap$^r$, Km$^r$ | (10) |
| p572 | pGEM-T derivative with *sp_1002* (*adcAII*) 5′ and 3′ flanking region for mutagenesis | Ap$^r$ | This work |
| p598 | pGEM-T derivative with *sp_1002* (*adcAII*) interrupted by *ermB* gene resistance cassette | Ap$^r$, Erm$^r$ | This work |
| p559 | pGEM-T derivative with *sp_0149* (*metQ*) 5′ and 3′ flanking region for mutagenesis | Ap$^r$ | (28) |
| p563 | pGEM-T derivative with *sp_0149* (*metQ*) interrupted by *ermB* gene resistance cassette | Ap$^r$, Erm$^r$ | (28) |
| p576 | pGEM-T derivative with *sp_0845* (*pnrA*) 5′ and 3′ flanking region for mutagenesis | Ap$^r$ | This work |
| p646 | pGEM-T derivative with *sp_0845* (*pnrA*) interrupted by *ermB* gene resistance cassette | Ap$^r$, Erm$^r$ | This work |
| p560 | pGEM-T derivative with *sp_0191* (*spd_0179*) 5′ and 3′ flanking region for mutagenesis | Ap$^r$ | This work |
| p565 | pGEM-T derivative with *sp_0191* (*spd_0179*) interrupted by *ermB* gene resistance cassette | Ap$^r$, Erm$^r$ | This work |
| p573 | pGEM-T derivative with *sp_0899* (*spd_0792*) 5′ and 3′ flanking region for mutagenesis | Ap$^r$ | This work |

*(Continued)*

**TABLE 1 |** Continued

| Strain/plasmid | Serotype and relevant genotype | Resistance* | Source or reference |
| --- | --- | --- | --- |
| p577 | pGEM-T derivative with sp_0899 (spd_0792) interrupted by ermB gene resistance cassette | Ap$^r$, Erm$^r$ | This work |
| pTP1 | pET28 expression vector, N-terminal His-tag, TEV protease cleavage site, induction by IPTG | Km$^r$, Erm$^r$ | (10) |
| p648 | pTP1 with TIGR4 sp_1002 (adcAII) for protein production and mice immunisation | Km$^r$ | This work |
| p652 | pTP1 with TIGR4 sp_0629 (dacB) for protein production and mice immunisation | Km$^r$ | (9) |
| p629 | pTP1 with TIGR4 sp_0659 (etrx1) for protein production and mice immunisation | Km$^r$ | (10) |
| p651 | pTP1 with TIGR4 sp_1000 (etrx2) for protein production and mice immunisation | Km$^r$ | (10) |
| P732 | pTP1 with TIGR4 sp_0149 (metQ) for protein production and mice immunisation | Km$^r$ | This work |
| p264 | pET11a with R6 spr0884 (ppmA) for protein production and mice immunisation | Km$^r$ | (32) |
| p649 | pTP1 with TIGR4 sp_0845 (pnrA) for protein production and mice immunisation | Km$^r$ | This work |
| p653 | pTP1 with TIGR4 sp_1650 (psaA) for protein production and mice immunisation | Km$^r$ | This work |
| p263 | pET11a with R6 spr0679 (slrA) for protein production and mice immunisation | Km$^r$ | (32) |
| p628 | pTP1 with TIGR4 sp_0191 (spd_0179) for protein production and mice immunisation | Km$^r$ | This work |
| p631 | pTP1 with TIGR4 sp_0899 (spd_0792) for protein production and mice immunisation | Km$^r$ | This work |
| p105 | pQE30 with PspA (aa 32-289) without choline-binding domain | Ap$^r$ | (33, 68) |

*Km$^r$, Kanamycin; Erm$^r$, Erythromycin; Ap$^r$, Ampicillin; Trm$^r$, Trimethoprim.

plates were washed three times with washing buffer (PBS, pH 7.4, 0.05% Tween® 20) and blocked with blocking buffer (PBS, 0.1% Tween® 20 supplemented with 2% bovine serum albumin) for 1 h at RT. The wells were washed and incubated for 1 h at RT with polyclonal IgGs in serial dilutions ranging from 1:750 to 1:24,000 in blocking buffer. Antibody binding was detected using goat anti-mouse IgG coupled to horseradish peroxidase (1:1,000, Jackson ImmunoResearch Laboratories, Inc., Ely, UK) as the secondary antibody (1 h incubation at RT). For the detection, 0.03% $H_2O_2$ and o-phenylenediamine dihydrochloride (OPD, Agilent Technologies, Santa Clara, CA, USA) at a final concentration of 0.67 mg/ml were used in a colorimetric reaction, which was stopped by adding 2M $H_2SO_4$. The absorbance of each sample was measured at $A_{492}$ using the FLUOstar Omega Microplate Reader (BMG Labtech, Ortenberg, Germany). This resulted in hyperbolic titration curves ($y = \frac{Bmax \cdot x}{Kd+x}$, Bmax, maximal binding; Kd, concentration for half the maximal binding), which were used to calculate the relative IgG concentrations. The absorbance was therefore set to $A_{492} = 0.3$ (y) in the linear dynamic range and the IgG concentrations (x) were calculated and denoted as the 1× end concentration in the flow cytometry. The polyclonal IgGs with equal contents of IgGs specific to the lipoproteins were therefore applied to enable the comparison of surface abundances.

For flow cytometry, S. pneumoniae wild-type D39, its capsule-deficient derivative (D39Δcps) and the isogenic mutants were cultured in 30 ml THY to $A_{600}$ 0.35–0.4. The bacteria were

washed with PBS, then resuspended in 1 ml of PBS. To detect the proteins on the surface of the pneumococci, $2 \times 10^8$ bacteria were incubated with mouse polyclonal IgG (1×, 5×, 10×, 20×, and 50× end concentration in PBS) for 45 min at 4°C. The bacteria were washed with PBS and stained using secondary antibody goat anti-mouse IgG Alexa-Fluor-488 conjugate (1:1,000; Thermo Fisher Scientific). After another 45-min incubation at 4°C, the bacteria were washed with PBS and fixed with 1% paraformaldehyde overnight at 4°C. The flow cytometry was conducted using a FACSCalibur™ (BD Biosciences, Heidelberg, Germany), and the CellQuestPro Software 6.0 (BD Biosciences) was used for data acquisition. The data were analysed using Flowing Software 2.5.1 (by Perttu Terho, Turku Centre for Biotechnology). The bacteria were detected and gated as described previously (36).

## Intranasal Immunisation and Pneumococcal Challenge of Mice

Seven-week-old female C57BL/6 mice ($n = 12$; Charles River Laboratories) were intranasally immunised three times at 2-week intervals under anaesthesia (50 mg ketamine and 5 mg xylazine per kg mouse weight). The 10 μl vaccine contained 5 μg recombinant DacB, MetQ, PnrA, or PspA proteins in combination with 4 μg cholera toxin subunit B (CTB; Sigma-Aldrich, St. Louis, MO, USA) in PBS. Control mice were mock-treated with an equivalent volume of PBS and adjuvant. Three weeks after the last vaccination, the mice were infected with

**TABLE 2 |** Primer list.

| Primer use | Primer | Sequence (5′-3′)* |
|---|---|---|
| **INSERTION-DELETION MUTAGENESIS** | | |
| Amplification of *sp_1002* + 5′ and 3′ flanking region | adcAll_427 | 5′-CTACTA<u>GAATTC</u>GATGATGCCGTTGCCTTT-3′ |
| | adcAll_430 | 5′-TTCCAAG<u>CTGCAG</u>ATCCCTGCTTCCCATTCC-3′ |
| Inverse PCR of *sp_1002* + 5′ and 3′ flanking region (pGEM-T Easy) | adcAll_429 | 5′-CTCACTG<u>AAGCTT</u>GACCCACAAAATGACAAGACC-3′ |
| | adcAll_428 | 5′-ATCATCG<u>AAGCTT</u>CCCCCAAGCACAAAAGAA-3′ |
| Amplification of *sp_0149* + 5′ and 3′ flanking region | metQ_382 | 5′-CTACTACTA<u>GAATTC</u>ATGCTGAACACACGGACAAC-3′ |
| | metQ_385 | 5′-AACCTTCCAAG<u>CTGCAG</u>CCGCTCCCTCCATGATAAAG-3′ |
| Inverse PCR of *sp_0149* + 5′ and 3′ flanking region (pGEM-T Easy) | metQ_384 | 5′-ACTCACTCACTG<u>AAGCTT</u>ATCGCAGCTTACCACACAGA-3′ |
| | metQ_383 | 5′-ATCATCATCATCG<u>AAGCTT</u>AGCCAAACCTGCGACTGTAG-3′ |
| Amplification of *sp_0845* + 5′ and 3′ flanking region | pnrA_415 | 5′-CTACTA<u>GAATTC</u>AAAAAGCTGGGGCTGAC-3′ |
| | pnrA_418 | 5′-CCAAG<u>CTGCAG</u>CGGTCAGAAACTGCTCGAAT-3′ |
| Inverse PCR of *sp_0845* + 5′ and 3′ flanking region (pGEM-T Easy) | pnrA_417 | 5′-CTCACTG<u>CTCGAG</u>TGGAAGCGTAAAAGTTCCTGA-3′ |
| | pnrA_416 | 5′-ATCATC<u>GGTACC</u>GAGCGGTTACCACATGCAG-3′ |
| Amplification of *sp_0191* + 5′ and 3′ flanking region | sp_0191_392 | 5′-CTACTACTA<u>GAATTC</u>ATGTAGCGAAAGGGGTAGG-3′ |
| | sp_0191_395 | 5′-AACCTTCCAAG<u>CTGCAG</u>CTTTGCTCCGTAGGCTTGAC-3′ |
| Inverse PCR of *sp_0191* + 5′ and 3′ flanking region (pGEM-T Easy) | sp_0191_394 | 5′-ACTCACTCACTG<u>AAGCTT</u>ATGGCGGACAGAACAATAG-3′ |
| | sp_0191_393 | 5′-ATCATCATCATCG<u>AAGCTT</u>AACCAACCAGGACAAAAAGG-3′ |
| Amplification of *sp_0899* + 5′ and 3′ flanking region | sp_0899_419 | 5′-CTACTA<u>GAATTC</u>CCTTGTCTGGGTGGTTCC-3′ |
| | sp_0899_422 | 5′-CCAAG<u>CTGCAG</u>TGGGACTAGCGCCAGAA-3′ |
| Inverse PCR of *sp_0899* + 5′ and 3′ flanking region (pGEM-T Easy) | sp_0899_421 | 5′-CTCACTGC<u>TCGAG</u>GCGAGGGACTGGCTAA-3′ |
| | sp_0899_420 | 5′-ATCATC<u>GGTACC</u>CAAGCAGCCAAGCCTAAAA-3′ |
| **ANTIBIOTIC CASSETTE AMPLIFICATION** | | |
| Erythromycin (*ermB*) | ermB_105 | 5′-GATGATGATGATCCCG<u>GGGTACCAAGCTTGAATTC</u>ACGGTTCGTGTTCGTGCTG-3′ |
| | ermB_106 | 5′-AGTGAGTGAGTCCCGGGC<u>TCGAGAAGCTTGAATTC</u>GTAGGCGCTAGGGACCTC-3′ |
| **RECOMBINANT PROTEIN PRODUCTION** | | |
| *sp_0899* (TIGR4) | sp_0899_463 | 5′-GCGCG<u>GCTAGC</u>CAACAACAACATGCTACTTC-3′ |
| | sp_0899_464 | 5′-GGCC<u>GAGCTC</u>TTAAAGTTTAACCCACTTATC-3′ |
| *sp_1002* (TIGR4; *adcAll*) | adcAll_451 | 5′-GGGCG<u>GCTAGC</u>GGTCAAAAGGAAAGTCAGAC-3′ |
| | adcAll_452 | 5′-GCGGCC<u>AAGCTT</u>ACTTTAATTCTTCTGCTAG-3′ |
| *sp_0149* (TIGR4; *metQ*) | metQ_410 | 5′-AAAG<u>CATATG</u>AGCGGCGAAAACCTGTATTTTCAGGGCGCTAGCGGAAACTCAGAAAAGAAAGC-3′ |
| | metQ_391 | 5′-CCAACCTTCC<u>AAGCTT</u>ACCAAACTGGTTGATCC-3′ |
| *sp_0845* (TIGR4; *pnrA*) | pnrA_449 | 5′-AAGC<u>GCTAGC</u>GGTAACCGCTCTTCTCGTA-3′ |
| | pnrA_450 | 5′-GGGGC<u>AAGCTT</u>ATTTTTCAGGAACTTTTACGC-3′ |
| *sp_1650* (TIGR4; *psaA*) | psaA_488 | 5′-GCGC<u>GCTAGC</u>GGAAAAAAAGATAC-3′ |
| | psaA_489 | 5′-GCGC<u>AAGCTT</u>ATTTTGCCAATCCTTCAG-3′ |
| *sp_0191* (TIGR4) | sp_0191_392 | 5′-TATTTTCAGGGC<u>GCTAGC</u>GGACAGAAAAAAGAAACTGG-3′ |
| | sp_0191_393 | 5′-CCAACCTTCC<u>AAGCTT</u>ATTGTTCTGTCGCGCCATTTG-3′ |

*Restriction sites used for cloning are underlined.*

10 µl PBS containing $3.4 \times 10^6$ CFU of *S. pneumoniae* D39. Three days after the bacterial challenge, the mice were euthanised and their blood and nasal tissues were harvested. Nasal tissue was homogenised in 1 ml PBS using a T10 basic blender (IKA, Staufen, Germany), and serially diluted samples were plated on blood agar (Oxoid) to quantify the recovered bacteria (log CFU/ml). Serum samples were taken before each immunisation step (pre-immune, priming, 1st boost), 2 weeks after the third immunisation (post-immune) and after the challenge with pneumococci. They were stored at −20°C until use.

## Detection of Local IL-17A in the Nasopharyngeal-Associated Lymphoid Tissue (NALT)

Cytokine production in mouse nasal samples was determined using a bead-based immunoassay (Bio-Rad Laboratories),

according to manufacturer's instructions. The assay was performed using the Bio-Plex Pro™ Reagent Kit, the Bio-Plex Pro™ mouse cytokine IL-17A set and the Bio-Plex Pro™ mouse cytokine standard group I, 23-Plex. The concentrations were calculated using Graph Pad Prism 5.

## Local and Systemic Antibody and Isotype Levels

Local IgG and IgA levels in the nasal tissue and the systemic total levels of IgG, IgG1, and IgG2a/IgG2c isotype were determined in the post-immune (Alum immunisation) or post-challenge sera (CTB immunisation) using an ELISA. PolySorp® Microtiter plates (96-well, Nunc, Thermo Fisher Scientific) were coated with equimolar amounts of pneumococcal proteins (3 pmol/well) and stored overnight at 4°C. The plates were washed and blocked as described above, then the wells were incubated with samples diluted in blocking buffer for 1 h at 37°C. The IgA and IgG levels in the nasal tissue samples were detected using 1:2 and 1:10 dilutions, respectively. Post-immune (immunisation only) and post-challenge sera (immunisation and challenge) were serially diluted ranging from 1:100 to 1:60,000 or 1:50 to 1:10,000, respectively. The plates were washed and incubated for 1 h at RT with horseradish peroxidase coupled with rabbit anti-mouse total IgG (Jackson ImmunoResearch Laboratories, Inc.), rabbit anti-mouse IgG1 (Sigma-Aldrich), goat anti-mouse IgG2a (Sigma-Aldrich), goat anti-mouse IgG2c (Abcam, Cambridge, UK), or goat anti-mouse IgA antibody (Sigma-Aldrich). The protection study using CTB as an adjuvant was carried out in C57BL/6 mice, which express IgG2c instead of IgG2a due to a gene replacement (37). These mice were therefore isotyped for IgG2c rather than the IgG2a used for the CD-1 mice. Detection was performed as described above. The antibody titre of each serum specimen was denoted as the $\log_{10}$ of its reciprocal dilution of the serum giving twice the average absorbance of the sera derived from the PBS-treated group.

## Monitoring of Antibody Titres Directed Against Pneumococcal Lipoproteins Using a FLEXMAP 3D® Analysis

The bead-based flow cytometric technique FLEXMAP 3D® (Luminex Corporation) was applied to simultaneously quantify the antibodies directed against the 12 pneumococcal surface proteins. This analysis was carried out as described recently (38), using the same commercially available reagents and instruments. Purified $His_6$-tagged proteins were covalently coupled to 6.25 × $10^5$ fluorescent FLEXMAP 3D® MagPlex® beads. The beads were protected from light throughout the workflow to avoid photo bleaching, and all incubation steps were carried out under agitation (900 rpm). After three washes with 100 mM monobasic sodium phosphate (activation buffer, pH 6.2) using a magnetic 96-well separator, the carboxyl groups on the surface of the beads were activated for 20 min by a resuspension in activation buffer (5 mg/ml each of EDC and sulpho-NHS). The activated beads were washed three times with coupling buffer [50 mmol/l 2-($N$-morpholino)ethanesulphonic acid, pH 5.0] followed by a 2-h incubation with 125 μl recombinant *S. pneumoniae* protein solution (100 μg/ml). The coupled beads were washed three times with washing buffer (PBS, 0.05% (v/v) Tween® 20, pH 7.4) and adjusted to a concentration of 125 beads per μl using blocking-storage buffer (1% (w/v) bovine serum albumin and 0.05% (v/v) ProClin™ 300 in PBS, pH 7.4). The beads were stored at 4°C until use. A coupling control was applied to validate the coupling efficiency. A master mix of sonicated coupled beads was prepared by diluting the beads 1:50 in bead buffer [50% (v/v) blocking-storage buffer and 50% (v/v) LowCross-Buffer® (LCB)]. After incubation with the anti-Penta-His tag mouse antibody (final concentration 10 μg/ml) for 45 min, the beads were washed three times with washing buffer and stained for 30 min using R-phycoerythrin (RPE)-conjugated goat anti-mouse IgG (final concentration 5 μg/ml). After another washing procedure, the beads were resuspended in 100 μl xMAP® Sheath Fluid and measured in the Luminex® FLEXMAP 3D® system with the

following instrumental setup: sample size 80 μl, sample timeout 60 s, bead count 10,000, and gate settings 7,500–15,000 under standard PMT (Photomultiplier tube) settings.

A multiplex immunoassay was used to compare differences in the amounts of anti-pneumococcal antibodies in serum samples obtained from 22 patients convalescent from pneumococcal infections. Convalescent-phase sera were kindly provided by Gregor Zysk, University of Düsseldorf, Germany (39). The infections included pneumonia ($n = 6$), meningitis ($n = 7$), sepsis ($n = 4$), and unknown clinical outcomes ($n = 5$), which were all caused by different pneumococcal serotypes. In addition, post-immune sera (2 weeks after the third immunisation) were obtained from CD-1 mice ($n = 6$) intraperitoneally immunised with Imject™ Alum or C57BL/6 mice intranasally immunised with CTB as an adjuvant, and were analysed to determine their antibody titres for the indicated proteins.

For the multiplex assay, serum samples were serially diluted (1:50, 1:500, 1:1,000, 1:10,000, 1:25,000, 1:50,000 and 1:100,000) in assay buffer (90% (v/v) bead buffer and 10% (v/v) *E. coli* BL21 lysate) and incubated for 20 min at RT to block unspecific binding. A bead master mix was prepared with a bead count of 1,000 per well. A 50-μl aliquot of the diluted sample was added to the beads and incubated overnight at 4°C, after which the beads were washed three times with 100 μl washing buffer. The beads were incubated with 50 μl RPE-conjugated goat anti-human IgG (final concentration 5 μg/ml) or 50 μl RPE-conjugated goat anti-mouse IgG (final concentration 5 μg/ml) for 1 h at RT. After three washes with 100 μl washing buffer, the beads were resuspended in 100 μl xMAP® Sheath Fluid (Invitrogen™) and measured in the Luminex® FLEXMAP 3D® system using the following instrumental setup: sample size 80 μl, sample timeout 60 s, bead count 100, and gate settings 7,500–15,000 under standard PMT.

The data were analysed as described recently (38). Following Clark's theory interaction model, the titration curves were used to determine the percentage of the half-maximal MFI (mean fluorescence intensity) for the respective coupling control. The MFI was multiplied with the reciprocal serum dilution corresponding to the half-maximal MFI. The resulting MFI values reflect the antigen binding intensity of antibodies contained in each serum sample. Calculations were performed using R (package 3.0.1) or GraphPad Prism version 5.0 (GraphPad Software).

## Statistical Analysis

All statistical analyses were performed using GraphPad Prism version 5.0 (GraphPad Software). The one-way ANOVA Kruskal-Wallis test with Dunn's post-test was used to compare multiple groups, while a Mann-Whitney $U$-test was used to compare two groups in the analysis of the protection efficacy and IL-17A levels in the nasal tissues or local/systemic humoral immune responses.

## RESULTS

## Selection and Purification of Pneumococcal Lipoproteins

A previous *in silico* analysis of the pneumococcal genome (*S. pneumoniae* strain D39) predicted more than 100 surface-associated or secreted proteins, including 37 lipoproteins (40). We selected 11 of these lipoproteins based on the following criteria: (i) confirmed member of the lipoprotein cluster (40), (ii) expressed in pneumococci (11, 17, 40), and (iii) high levels of conservation (>85%, **Table 3**). The selected lipoproteins included the four substrate-binding proteins AdcAII, MetQ, PnrA, and PsaA, which are components of ABC transporters responsible for the uptake of zinc(II), methionine, nucleosides and manganese(II), respectively. We also selected the following non-ABC transporter lipoproteins: (i) the thioredoxins Etrx1 and Etrx2, which are involved in pneumococcal resistance to oxidative stress, (ii) the L,D-carboxypeptidase DacB, (iii) and the peptidyl-prolyl cis/trans isomerases putative proteinase maturation protein A (PpmA) and streptococcal lipoprotein rotamase A (SlrA). PpmA and SlrA have a role in the folding or activation of the surface-exposed proteins. The two other candidate lipoproteins, SP_0191 and SP_0899, are so far uncharacterised lipoproteins. With the exception of the uncharacterised lipoproteins SP_0191 and SP_0899, previous studies using *in vivo* mouse models have demonstrated that the selected lipoproteins are involved in virulence (9–11, 14, 28, 32, 41, 42). It can therefore be hypothesised that blocking these antigens, for example through the use of specific antibodies, may lead to the attenuation of virulence and thus confer protection. The lipoprotein-encoding genes were therefore cloned into a pTP1 vector (10) and plasmids were transformed into *E. coli* BL21 for protein expression. The recombinant proteins were purified using affinity chromatography, and their quality and purity was confirmed using the silver staining of an SDS-gel and immunoblotting (**Figure 1**). All lipoproteins were shown to be stable in solution, and no degradation was observed.

## Antigen-Specific Polyclonal IgGs and the Surface Abundance of Pneumococcal Lipoproteins

Mice were intraperitoneally immunised with the heterologously expressed lipoproteins to generate antigen-specific antisera. Purified polyclonal IgGs were used for immunoblot analyses, which were performed using the whole-cell lysates of non-encapsulated *S. pneumoniae* D39 and its isogenic lipoprotein-deficient mutants. The immunoblots demonstrated that the anti-lipoprotein IgGs are highly specific; the protein bands were only detected in wild-type pneumococci but not in the corresponding isogenic mutants (**Figure 2A**). Furthermore, under *in vitro* growth conditions, the protein levels were highly variable, with Etrx1, Etrx2, and SP_0899 showing the lowest levels and PnrA, PsaA, and MetQ the highest levels of expression.

The recognition of pneumococci by the immune system is vital for the host to clear these pathogens. The binding of antigen-specific antibodies depends on the expression, abundance and accessibility of antigens. In order to analyse the surface abundance and accessibility of the selected lipoproteins, we determined the relative antibody titres in mice following immunisation. For this purpose, the recombinant lipoproteins were immobilised in equimolar amounts and incubated with

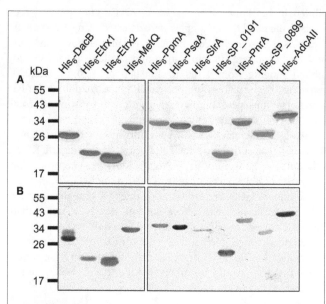

**FIGURE 1** | Pneumococcal lipoproteins heterologously expressed *in E. coli*. A 1-μg aliquot of heterologously expressed pneumococcal lipoproteins was separated using SDS-PAGE and the proteins were detected using silver staining **(A)** or with immunoblotting using a monoclonal mouse anti-Penta-His$_6$ antibody and alkaline phosphatase-conjugated goat anti-mouse IgG **(B)**.

serial dilutions of the polyclonal IgGs, and the initial IgG concentrations were calculated from the resulting hyperbolic titration curves. The highest IgG titres were measured for MetQ, AdcAII, and PspA, while the lowest titres were observed for Etrx1, Etrx2, and SP_0191 (**Figure 2B**). *S. pneumoniae* D39 and the non-encapsulated mutant D39Δ*cps* were incubated with increasing concentrations of polyclonal IgGs (1×, 5×, 10×, 20×, and 50×) to elucidate the abundance of the 11 selected lipoproteins on the pneumococcal surface using flow cytometry. The initial IgG concentrations calculated in the antibody titration study (**Figure 2B**), enabled the application of comparable amounts of lipoprotein-specific IgGs in the flow cytometric analysis. We used anti-PspA IgG as a positive control, as it is already known that the choline-binding protein PspA is highly abundant on the surface of these bacteria (43). Overall, the antigen-specific IgGs bound in a dose-dependent manner to the surface of pneumococci (**Figure 2C**, **Table S1**). Our data confirm that PspA is probably one of the most abundant pneumococcal surface proteins (**Figure 2C**, **Table S1**). When using the highest anti-PspA antibody concentrations, over 80% of the fluorescent pneumococci were detectable. Of our tested lipoproteins, PnrA, PpmA, DacB, SP_0191, and SlrA showed the highest surface abundance, with up to 60% positive fluorescent events, while PsaA and MetQ had lower levels, with approximately 40% of fluorescent pneumococci detectable. The lowest surface abundance was observed for thioredoxins Etrx1 and Etrx2, the putative lipoprotein SP_0899, and the zinc transport system binding protein AdcAII, the latter two of which were almost undetectable. Some of the tested proteins were also accessible for antibody binding when covered by the capsular polysaccharide. DacB, PpmA, SlrA, and MetQ

**TABLE 3 |** Sequence homology of selected lipoproteins among different pneumococcal strains based on protein sequences from *S. pneumoniae* TIGR4.

| S. p. strain | AdcAII | DacB | Etrx1 | Etrx2 | MetQ | PnrA | PpmA | PsaA | SlrA | SP0191 | SP0899 |
|---|---|---|---|---|---|---|---|---|---|---|---|
| TIGR4 | 100.00 | 100.00 | 100.00 | 100.00 | 100.00 | 100.00 | 100.00 | 100.00 | 100.00 | 100.00 | 100.00 |
| D39 | 100.00 | 99.16 | 99.47 | 98.92 | 99.30 | 98.29 | 99.68 | 99.68 | 99.25 | 98.94 | 99.31 |
| P1031 | 99.02 | 98.32 | 99.47 | 98.38 | 99.30 | 98.86 | 99.36 | 99.68 | 98.88 | 100.00 | 99.31 |
| G54 | 99.02 | 96.64 | 100.00 | 98.92 | 98.24 | 98.57 | 93.15 | 99.35 | 99.25 | 100.00 | 98.97 |
| Hungary19A | 99.67 | 89.92 | 100.00 | 98.92 | 99.30 | 98.86 | 99.68 | 99.35 | 98.88 | 98.41 | 98.62 |
| 70585 | 99.34 | 89.08 | 99.47 | 100.00 | 99.65 | 98.86 | 100.00 | 99.68 | 99.25 | 100.00 | 99.31 |
| JJA | 100.00 | 86.97 | 100.00 | 100.00 | 99.65 | 98.57 | 99.68 | 96.76 | 99.63 | 100.00 | 98.89 |
| Taiwan19F | 100.00 | 86.97 | 100.00 | 100.00 | 99.65 | 98.57 | 99.68 | 99.68 | 99.25 | 98.94 | 99.31 |

could be detected in the presence of the capsule (**Figure 2D, Table S2**). However, as expected, the binding capacity was strongly diminished and the positive fluorescent events dropped to 20–30%. Strikingly, the capsule does not block antibody binding to PspA, confirming its exposure and accessibility for antibodies (43). To confirm that IgG binding to *S. pneumoniae* was antigen-specific, mutants deficient for the lipoproteins were incubated with the corresponding polyclonal IgGs. We detected only minor non-specific IgG binding for some of the lipoproteins, indicating that the generated antibodies were overall antigen-specific (**Figure S1**).

## PnrA, DacB, MetQ, and PsaA Are Highly Immunogenic

The immunogenicity of the selected lipoproteins was investigated using multiplex immunoassay technology. Two different types of sera were analysed: (i) convalescent patient sera and (ii) antisera from mice intraperitoneally immunised with pneumococcal antigens using Alum as the adjuvant (**Figure 3**). Recombinant proteins covalently coupled to fluorescent MagPlex® beads were incubated with serial dilutions of human or mouse sera. Measurements of convalescent patient sera revealed the highest IgG levels for PsaA and PnrA, which were both comparable to those of the positive control, PspA (**Figure 3A**). DacB, PpmA, and Etrx1 IgG levels were also high, although they were an order of magnitude lower than those for PsaA. The titres of antibodies for Etrx2, AdcAII, MetQ, SP_0191, SP_0899, and SlrA were comparatively low in randomly selected convalescent sera. The final antibody titres of mouse sera obtained 2 weeks after the third and final immunisation ranged from $2.9 \times 10^6$ AU (α-PspA) to $1.8 \times 10^8$ AU (α-PsaA), and were at least three orders of magnitude higher than the titres of the pre-immune sera. The highest antibody titres were measured for PsaA, MetQ, AdcAII, and DacB. The second boost did not substantially increase the antibody titres, which were on average only 2.5-fold higher than the levels measured after the first booster immunisation. Notably, the changes in antibody titres for MetQ and DacB were highly similar when compared between individual mice. However, the antibody titres for the majority of the other lipoproteins varied substantially. In conclusion, lipoproteins such as DacB, MetQ, and PnrA represent promising candidates for the development of a robustly effective and reliable vaccination.

## Intranasal Vaccination With DacB, MetQ, or PnrA Reduces Pneumococcal Load in the Nasal Cavity

Based on the previous screenings, three lipoproteins DacB, PnrA, and MetQ were selected to assess whether their use in an intranasal vaccination would confer protection against pneumococcal colonisation. Mice were intranasally immunised with the protein candidates in combination with CTB as an adjuvant, and received two booster immunisations. PspA was included as a positive control, while PBS mock-treated mice were used as a negative control. Three weeks after the final vaccination, the mice were intranasally infected with a non-lethal dose of $3.4 \times 10^6$ *S. pneumoniae* D39. Three days post-infection, mice were euthanised and live pneumococci were recovered from their nasal tissues. Consistent with previous studies, an intranasal vaccination with PspA induced the strongest reduction (263-fold) of bacterial load in the nasal cavity when comparing the bacterial load to mock-treated mice (**Figure 4A**). PnrA also showed strong efficacy, causing a 58-fold reduction in the number of *S. pneumoniae* in the nasopharynx. Of the mice, which received the PnrA immunisation, 50% had almost completely cleared the pneumococci within 3 days post-infection. Immunisation with DacB and MetQ showed a trend in reducing the bacterial load. However, reduction was only 14- or 4-fold, respectively, and not statistically significant.

## Protective Immunity Correlates With Increased Intranasal IL-17A Levels

Immunity to *S. pneumoniae* infection was shown to be dependent on the induction of IL-17A-secreting CD4[+] T cells, leading to the recruitment of neutrophils to enable the clearance of the pneumococci (44–46). To determine the role of IL-17A in our protection studies, we quantified the levels of this cytokine in the nasal tissues of mice immunised with DacB, MetQ, or PnrA 3 days after infection. Significantly increased IL-17A levels were identified in the DacB- and PnrA-immunised mice in comparison with the negative control, both reaching IL17A levels comparable to mice immunised with PspA (**Figure 4B**). Importantly, production of nasopharyngeal IL-17A significantly correlated with the level of protective immunity induced by the pneumococcal lipoproteins ($\rho = -0.3916$; $p = 0.002$), which was indicated by a Spearman correlation test (**Figure S2**). These

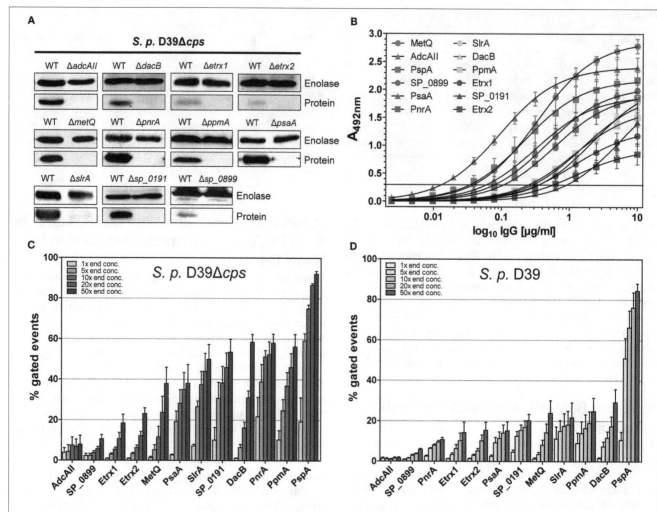

**FIGURE 2 |** Pneumococcal lipoproteins are highly abundant on the pneumococcal surface. **(A)** In immunoblots, the specificity of antisera derived from intraperitoneal immunisations of CD-1 mice ($n = 6$) with recombinant lipoproteins was assessed. Therefore, the wild-type strain *S. pneumoniae* D39$\Delta$cps and the corresponding isogenic lipoprotein deficient mutants ($2 \times 10^8$ bacteria per lane) were used. Enolase was detected with a rabbit anti-enolase serum and served as a loading control. **(B)** IgG antibody titrations were performed by incubating equimolar amounts of recombinant proteins with serial dilutions of isolated polyclonal IgGs. Detection was carried out using a peroxidase-coupled goat anti-mouse IgG followed by incubation with OPD as a substrate and absorbance was measured at 492 nm. Titrations were performed at least three times and the error bars represent the SEM. **(C,D)** Using the equation for the hyperbolic regression curve ($y [Abs] = \frac{Bmax \cdot x}{Kd+x}$, Bmax, maximal binding; Kd, concentration for half maximal binding) an initial IgG concentration was calculated in the linear dynamic range. The polyclonal IgGs with equal contents of IgG specific for each lipoprotein were therefore applied to enable the comparison of their surface abundances. In a flow cytometric approach, D39$\Delta$cps **(C)** and D39 **(D)** were incubated with the appropriate calculated concentration of IgG and concentrations 5-, 10-, 20-, and 50-fold greater to analyse the surface abundance of the selected lipoproteins. Antibody binding was detected using a goat anti-mouse Alexa Fluor® 488-coupled secondary antibody. The percentage of positive gated events is depicted in the graphs, thereby indicating the proportion of wild-type bacteria positive for the binding of the respective anti-lipoprotein IgGs. The mean values of at least three independent experiments are shown, with error bars corresponding to SEM.

results confirm the important role of IL-17A in protecting against pneumococcal colonisation.

## Intranasal Immunisation Only Partially Induces Local and Systemic Antigen-Specific Antibodies

Humoral immune responses following intranasal immunisation with recombinant lipoproteins were investigated by analysis of antibody kinetics in post-immune antisera and the local antibody titres in nasal tissues harvested 3 days after infection with pneumococci. As shown in **Figure 5A**, intranasal immunisation

with recombinant MetQ, PnrA, and PspA induced strong systemic antigen-specific antibody responses in all tested mice. However, a substantial systemic IgG response for recombinant DacB was only detected in one of the six mice. Three days after infection, we analysed the local humoral immune responses in the nasal tissues of all mice used in the model of colonisation ($n = 12$) to elucidate whether lipoprotein-specific immunoglobulins are present in the nasal cavity, which might contribute to protection (**Figures 5B,C**). MetQ and PspA were found to be potent immunogens when administered intranasally, as demonstrated by the resulting high local titres of IgG, while the local IgG response for PnrA was significantly lower

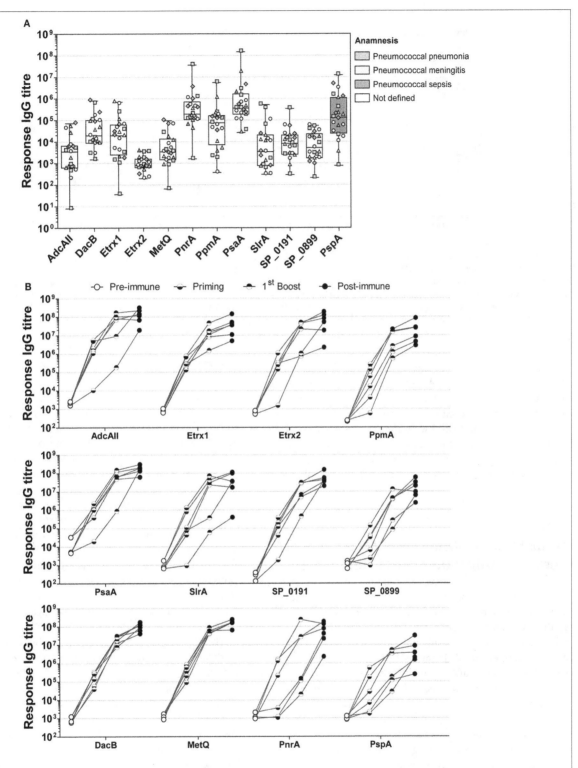

**FIGURE 3 |** Analysis of convalescent patient sera and mouse sera derived from intraperitoneal immunisations indicate the high immunogenicity of PnrA, DacB, and MetQ. **(A)** A total of 22 antisera from convalescent patients who suffered from pneumococcal infections such as pneumonia ($n = 6$), meningitis ($n = 7$), sepsis ($n = 4$), and unknown clinical outcomes ($n = 5$) caused by different pneumococcal serotypes were analysed to compare their levels of anti-lipoprotein antibodies. Each symbol represents a single antiserum, while the different colours indicate the clinical outcome of every patient. **(B)** The immunogenicity of the lipoproteins was further demonstrated by analysing the antibody kinetics of intraperitoneally immunised CD-1 mice ($n = 6$). The mice received three vaccinations with 20 µg antigen and Alum as the adjuvant, with a 2-week interval between treatments. Before each treatment and 2 weeks after the final immunisation, antisera were collected to enable the determination of the antibody kinetics. Each individual mouse is depicted in the graphs. All serum samples were serially diluted and measured using the FLEXMAP 3D® system. Response values reflect the levels of antigen-specific IgG for the 11 tested lipoproteins and the positive control PspA.

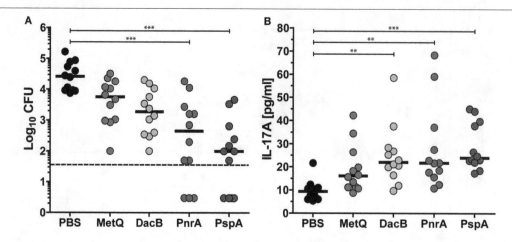

**FIGURE 4 |** Intranasal vaccinations with the lipoproteins MetQ, DacB or PnrA reduce pneumococcal colonisation and increase local IL-17A levels. Bacterial recovery of *S. pneumoniae* D39 from nasal tissue **(A)** and nasopharyngeal IL-17A levels **(B)** 3 days after the intranasal challenge of C57BL/6 mice ($n = 12$) with $3.4 \times 10^6$ CFU. Each mouse received three intranasal immunisations with 5 $\mu$g of one of the four recombinant proteins, MetQ, DacB, PnrA, or PspA, in combination with 4 $\mu$g CTB in 2-week intervals. The data were statistically analysed using a Kruskal Wallis test accompanied by Dunn's multiple comparison post-test, with all conditions compared to control mice that received an intranasal treatment with PBS and CTB. Symbols indicate individual mice, bars represent the group median, and the dotted line indicates the lower limit of detection. $^{**}p < 0.01$; $^{***}p < 0.001$.

(**Figure 5B**). The local IgG response for DacB was substantially lower than MetQ and PspA, which was consistent with the antibody kinetics. Intranasal immunisation with PspA or MetQ induced considerable levels of local antigen-specific IgA, whereas nasal IgA for PnrA and DacB were almost too low to be detected (**Figure 5C**). Taken together, these data suggest that local and serum antigen-specific antibody responses might not perfectly correlate with protection *in vivo*, as was especially shown for PnrA and DacB.

## Immunisations With DacB, MetQ, or PnrA Predominantly Induce IgG1 Responses

To shed light on the type of immune response induced by the intraperitoneal or intranasal vaccinations with our candidate proteins in combination with Alum or CTB as the adjuvant, respectively, we determined the IgG1 and IgG2a/IgG2c levels in post-immune sera (**Figure 6**). Overall, intraperitoneal immunisation with the lipoproteins DacB, MetQ and PnrA elicited higher total IgG responses than intranasal immunisation (**Figures 6A,C**). Immunising mice either intranasally or intraperitoneally with the four pneumococcal antigens predominantly led to high IgG1 and lower but still substantial levels of IgG2, suggesting a Th2-biased response (**Figures 6B,D**). The intranasal immunisation with DacB resulted in a remarkably high IgG1/IgG2 ratio and a very weak humoral immune response overall (**Figure 6B**). In summary, intranasal immunisation with the lipoproteins DacB, MetQ, and PnrA reduced pneumococcal colonisation, and the level of protection correlated with IL-17A levels. However, immunisation only partially induced local and systemic antigen-specific antibody responses.

## DISCUSSION

Pneumococcal colonisation of the upper respiratory tract is a prerequisite for invasive disease (47). Higher colonisation rates facilitate the transmission of this opportunistic pathogen from host to host, enabling pneumococci to spread within a population, as was shown in influenza A co-infection mouse models (48). Protein-based vaccines should therefore include one or more antigens that reduce nasopharyngeal colonisation to prevent infectious diseases and the shedding of pneumococci. In order to elicit serotype-independent protection, conserved pneumococcal surface proteins are of special interest. Previous studies have already shown that PsaA, a highly conserved manganese-binding lipoprotein, provides cross-protection in a mouse model of colonisation following intranasal immunisation (23). Here, we selected 11 pneumococcal lipoproteins with high sequence homology (>85%) and investigated their potential for use as subunits of such a vaccine.

The expression and surface accessibility of potential vaccine candidates is important for the host immune system to recognise and counteract the dissemination of pneumococci to normally sterile body sites. Under *in vitro* growth conditions in a rich medium, the highest surface abundance of lipoproteins was observed for PpmA, PnrA, and DacB, while AdcAII and the thioredoxins Etrx1 and Etrx2 were detected at a substantially lower abundance. The highest surface abundance was shown for the choline-binding protein PspA, a major virulence factor of pneumococci known to be highly immunogenic and abundant on the surface (43, 49). The pneumococcal capsular polysaccharide (CPS) is known to mask surface-exposed antigens, thereby blocking opsonisation by inhibiting antibody binding and consequently limiting pathogen uptake by professional phagocytes. Indeed, we also indicate that the detection of surface-localised lipoproteins was decreased

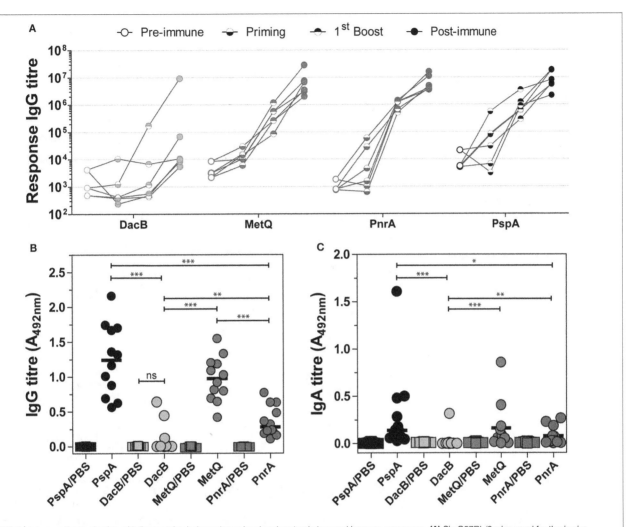

**FIGURE 5 |** Intranasal immunisation with lipoproteins induces lower local and systemic humoral immune responses. **(A)** Six C57BL/6 mice used for the *in vivo* colonisation model were randomly selected for the analysis of their antibody kinetics following an intranasal immunisation with the lipoproteins MetQ, DacB, and PnrA. The mice received three doses with 5 μg antigen and 4 μg CTB as the adjuvant in 2-week intervals. Before each treatment and 2 weeks after the third immunisation, antisera were collected to determine the antibody kinetics. The data from each individual mouse are depicted for every protein. Antisera were serially diluted and measured using the FLEXMAP 3D® system. The response values reflect the levels of antigen-specific IgG. **(B,C)** Three weeks after the final immunisation, the mice were challenged with *S. pneumoniae* D39 ($3.4 \times 10^6$ CFU) and 3 days after infection their nasal tissues were harvested, homogenised and analysed for local antigen-specific IgG **(B)** and IgA **(C)** using ELISA. The IgG and IgA levels were determined using a 1:10 or 1:2 dilution of the nasal homogenate, respectively. The data were statistically analysed using a Mann-Whitney *U*-test. Symbols represent individual mice ($n = 12$) and the bars represent the group median. *$p < 0.05$; **$p < 0.01$; ***$p < 0.001$.

when using the encapsulated strain D39, while the CPS only marginally diminished antibody binding to PspA, consistent with the findings of previous studies (43). The presence of the CPS could not completely inhibit antibody binding to the surface-exposed lipoproteins, however, as indicated by the dose-dependent increase of fluorescence intensities in the flow cytometric analysis. In previous studies, the iron uptake ABC transporter lipoproteins PiaA and PiuA and the nucleoside-binding lipoprotein PnrA were shown to be surface accessible. Indeed, antigen-specific antibodies bound to encapsulated pneumococci, but cross-reactivity to heterologous strains was only demonstrated for the PnrA-specific antibodies, suggesting that PnrA is conserved across pneumococcal serotypes (11, 50).

It was previously reported that anti-PsaA and anti-PpmA failed to detect PsaA and PpmA on the surface of different pneumococcal strains (49), in contrast to our findings. The differences in the accessibilities of the analysed lipoproteins could be due to the variable capsular structures and expression levels, their localisation in the cell wall, and especially the different levels of expression for each lipoprotein gene. The latter point must be seriously evaluated when searching for a new protein-based vaccine, because several studies have shown that pneumococcal gene expression is highly dependent on the strain and the host compartment in which the pneumococci reside (51–55).

To evaluate the humoral immune responses induced by the selected pneumococcal lipoproteins, a multiplex bead-based

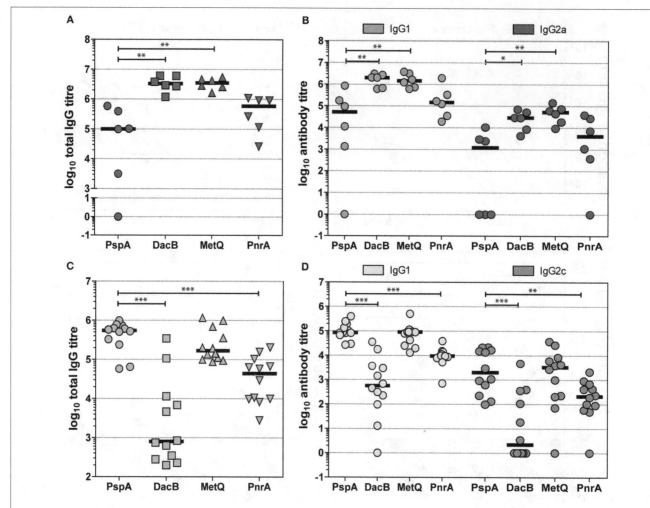

**FIGURE 6 |** Intraperitoneal and intranasal immunisations with DacB, MetQ, or PnrA predominantly induce IgG1 responses. Antigen-specific total IgG, IgG1, and IgG2 titres were monitored using an ELISA in either post-immune sera following an intraperitoneal immunisation with Alum as the adjuvant **(A,B)** or in post-challenge sera obtained after intranasal immunisation with CTB as the adjuvant followed by an intranasal challenge with *S. pneumoniae* D39 **(C,D)**. Antibody titres of each serum specimen are denoted as the log$_{10}$ of the reciprocal dilution of the serum giving twice the average absorbance of the sera derived from the PBS-treated group. The data were statistically analysed using a Mann-Whitney *U*-test. Symbols represent individual mice (*n* = 6 for Alum group, *n* = 12 for CTB group) and bars represent the group median. *$p < 0.05$; **$p < 0.01$; ***$p < 0.001$.

immunoassay was performed. Our analysis of convalescent patient sera revealed high antibody titres for the lipoproteins PsaA, PnrA, PpmA, and DacB. Therefore, we concluded that these lipoproteins are immunogenic during natural infections. PspA elicited an exceptionally high humoral immune response, as also reported previously (36, 56). We further investigated the immunogenicity of the selected lipoproteins in an immunisation study using intraperitoneally vaccinated mice. High endpoint antibody titres were measured for PsaA, DacB, PnrA, MetQ, and AdcAII. Immunisation with DacB and MetQ was particularly effective, rapidly increasing the antibody titres in all mice. In most cases the first booster immunisation was sufficient to elicit high antibody responses, suggesting that a two-dose immunisation strategy may be sufficient for accomplishing an optimal humoral immune response. Taken together, these data show that pneumococcal lipoproteins are generally highly immunogenic.

Lipoproteins are able to elicit humoral immune responses during natural pneumococcal colonisation or infections, as shown for PsaA, PnrA, and DacB (20–22, 56, 57), and may also be used in immunisation to induce a substantial immune response. These findings are strongly supported by several other studies using different lipoproteins as vaccine antigens, including PsaA, PnrA, PiuA, and PiaA (11, 23, 58).

As mentioned above, colonisation is the first step towards the establishment of pneumococcal infections Hence, protection against colonisation is a crucial aspect of pneumococcal vaccine development. Based on the surface abundances, accessibility and immunogenicity of the lipoproteins, we selected DacB, MetQ, and PnrA for the assessment of their protective potential in a mouse model of colonisation. Subcutaneous immunisation with PnrA was previously shown to induce protective immunity against an intraperitoneal challenge with heterologous *S. pneumoniae* strains (11). In the present work, we further confirmed the potential of PnrA as a component of protein-based subunit vaccines. Its use in the intranasal immunisation of mice significantly decreased the bacterial loads in the nasal cavity. Immunization with DacB and MetQ only tended to reduce bacterial load in the nasal cavity to an insignificant extent. Basavanna et al. indicated that systemic vaccination with MetQ does not extend the survival or result in differences in the progression of fatal infections. Based on a transcriptome analysis, they reasoned that this lack of protection might be due to the low expression of *metQ* in infection-related niches (12). This might be the critical factor causing the comparatively low protective effect of MetQ immunisation against pneumococcal colonisation in our study.

The pro-inflammatory cytokine IL-17, among others secreted by Th17 cells, is essential for recruitment and activation of macrophages and neutrophils to the nasopharynx, a process critical for clearing pneumococci from the host (59). Th17-mediated immunity is essential for protection against pneumococcal colonisation, as CD4$^+$ T cell-derived IL-17, but not IFNγ or IL-4, is required for the clearance of colonisation (46). Furthermore, intranasal immunisation with pneumococcal whole-cell antigens or a subunit-protein vaccine was found to provide IL-17-mediated, but antibody-independent, protection (45). Here, we monitored that the nasal tissues of mice vaccinated with DacB, PnrA, and PspA showed significantly increased IL-17A levels 3 days after infection with pneumococci that correlated with protection. These elevated local IL-17A concentrations probably result from recall responses of immunization-induced memory towards these antigens. Accordingly, the immunisation of mice with MetQ, which caused the lowest reduction in bacterial load, provoked only a slight increase in IL-17A levels. Consistent with our results, strong correlations between high IL-17A levels and protection against colonisation have been reported in previous studies, where increased *ex vivo* IL-17A was predictive of *in vivo* nasal IL-17A levels following vaccination and, furthermore, was an indicator of protective efficacy (60, 61).

CTB is a potent adjuvant with various immunomodulatory functions, which are mainly attributed to its ability to bind to monosialotetrahexosylganglioside (GM1). GM1 is broadly distributed in a variety of cell types, including the epithelial cells of the gut and antigen-presenting cells, macrophages, dendritic cells, and B cells. Therefore, CTB can enhance the immune responses to bystander antigens, a phenomenon indicated by the production of effective antigen-specific antibodies at the mucosal surfaces (62–65). Immunity to pathogens at mucosal surfaces is especially driven by antigen-specific secretory IgA (sIgA), which acts as an inhibitor of adherence and inflammation and is able to neutralise viruses, toxins and enzymes (66–70). Here, we showed that intranasal immunisation with PspA plus CTB had the strongest effect on the reduction of pneumococcal load in the nasal cavity. We could only detect considerable local IgA levels in a few mice immunised with PspA and CTB, although they were still significantly higher than those found for DacB and PnrA. In contrast, substantial amounts of nasal IgG were detected for PspA and MetQ, though significantly less DacB- and PnrA-specific

local IgG was identified. After either intranasal immunisation with CTB followed by a challenge with *S. pneumoniae* D39 or intraperitoneal immunisation with Alum as the adjuvant, the systemic humoral immune responses varied depending on the antigen and route of immunisation. Overall, they were characterised by a predominance for IgG1 and substantial IgG2a/IgG2c production, suggesting a primary Th2 response, which is consistent with previous studies and was attributed to the use of Alum as adjuvant (63, 71, 72). While intraperitoneal immunisation with DacB and Alum as an adjuvant led to a strong systemic antibody response, the intranasal administration of DacB in combination with CTB induced only marginal levels of IgG production. The opposite was observed for PspA, where intranasal immunisation provoked higher antibody titres compared with the intraperitoneal administration. It is unclear why PspA is a potent immunogen when administered in combination with CTB via the nasal route but less immunogenic in a systemic vaccination using Alum as an adjuvant; however, our results are in accordance with a previous study using a different mouse strain and a slightly different immunisation protocol (73). It has been reported that the efficient induction of an immune response depends on the adjuvant, the route of immunisation and the immunogenicity of the antigen itself (74, 75). Both Alum and CTB represent potent adjuvants, as the antibody titres for at least two proteins in our vaccinations were highly elevated. This further indicates that, in principle, our tested lipoproteins are immunogenic, a fact supported by the analysis of convalescent patient sera. It therefore seems likely that the route of immunisation has a profound role on the magnitude of the immune response. In a vaccination study where rats were immunised with three structurally different types of pneumococcal polysaccharide (PPS-3, PPS-4, and PPS-14) using four immunisation routes, remarkable differences were observed in both the magnitude of the immune response and the distribution of the isotypes (76). The authors concluded that, besides the route of immunisation, the structural features of the pneumococcal polysaccharides have a pivotal influence on the elicited immune response. Likewise, structural differences of the proteins could be one of the reasons for the varying immune responses *in vivo*. Although intranasal vaccination with DacB could not induce high levels of antigen-specific antibody production, it had a drastic effect on the reduction of pneumococcal colonisation accompanied by elevated local levels of IL-17. This suggests that protection is rather characterised by a cellular immune response mediated by local antigen-specific CD4$^+$ memory T cells than by a humoral immune response. Accordingly, in a previous study it was shown that protection against pneumococcal colonisation by intranasal immunisation with three pneumococcal proteins (PspC, PsaA, and PdT) was dependent on CD4$^+$ T cells but independent of antibodies (45). It therefore remains unclear whether local or systemic antibody responses, especially towards DacB, result in the protective effect in the mouse model of colonisation following intranasal immunisation.

In conclusion, we showed that vaccination of mice with a monovalent protein-based vaccine containing the lipoprotein PnrA impairs nasopharyngeal colonisation by pneumococci after intranasal challenge with *S. pneumoniae* D39. There was a possible protective effect for DacB and MetQ as vaccine candidates, although it was less pronounced and not significant. The lipoproteins evaluated here are highly conserved among pneumococcal serotypes, abundant on the pneumococcal surface, and immunogenic. These properties mean they are promising protein antigens for a next-generation subunit vaccine for the reduction of pneumococcal colonisation, which could be accompanied by a decline in the transmission of pneumococcal infections. Future studies are required to elucidate the mechanisms of protective immunity induced by these lipoproteins and to identify the optimal route of immunisation and appropriate adjuvant.

## AUTHOR CONTRIBUTIONS

FV, MdJ, and SH conceived and designed the experiments. FV, TK, TM, FvO, MA, MS, and SvS performed the experiments. FV, TM, SM, FS, and SH analysed the data. FV, MdJ, and SH wrote the manuscript.

## FUNDING

This work was supported by a grant from the Deutsche Forschungsgemeinschaft (DFG GRK 1870; Bacterial Respiratory Infections to SH) and the Bundesministerium für Bildung und Forschung (BMBF-ZIK FunGene to FS and BMBF- Zwanzig20—InfectControl 2020—project VacoME-FKZ 03ZZ0816A to SH).

## ACKNOWLEDGMENTS

We gratefully acknowledge Sarah Jose (Radboud in'to Languages, Radboud University, Nijmegen, The Netherlands) for critically reading and correcting our manuscript. This study is part of the Ph.D. thesis of FV.

## REFERENCES

1. Song JY, Nahm MH, Moseley MA. Clinical implications of pneumococcal serotypes: invasive disease potential, clinical presentations, and antibiotic resistance. *J Korean Med Sci.* (2013) 28:4–15. doi: 10.3346/jkms.2013.28.1.4
2. WHO. Pneumococcal vaccines WHO position paper—2012. *Wkly Epidemiol Rec.* (2012) 87:129–44. doi: 10.1016/j.vaccine.2012.04.093
3. Whitney CG, Farley MM, Hadler J, Harrison LH, Bennett NM, Lynfield R, et al. Decline in invasive pneumococcal disease after the introduction of protein-polysaccharide conjugate vaccine. *N Engl J Med.* (2003) 348:1737–46. doi: 10.1056/NEJMoa022823
4. Ruckinger S, van der Linden M, Reinert RR, von Kries R. Efficacy of 7-valent pneumococcal conjugate vaccination in Germany: an analysis using the indirect cohort method. *Vaccine* (2010) 28:5012–6. doi: 10.1016/j.vaccine.2010.05.021
5. van Hoek AJ, Andrews N, Waight PA, George R, Miller E. Effect of serotype on focus and mortality of invasive pneumococcal disease: coverage of different vaccines and insight into non-vaccine serotypes. *PLoS ONE* (2012) 7:e39150. doi: 10.1371/journal.pone.0039150
6. Weinberger DM, Malley R, Lipsitch M. Serotype replacement in disease after pneumococcal vaccination. *Lancet* (2011) 378:1962–73. doi: 10.1016/S0140-6736(10)62225-8
7. Jauneikaite E, Tocheva AS, Jefferies JM, Gladstone RA, Faust SN, Christodoulides M, et al. Current methods for capsular typing of *Streptococcus pneumoniae*. *J Microbiol Methods* (2015) 113:41–9. doi: 10.1016/j.mimet.2015.03.006
8. Pichichero ME, Khan MN, Xu Q. Next generation protein based *Streptococcus pneumoniae* vaccines. *Hum Vaccines Immunotherapeut.* (2016) 12:194–205. doi: 10.1080/21645515.2015.1052198
9. Abdullah MR, Gutierrez-Fernandez J, Pribyl T, Gisch N, Saleh M, Rohde M, et al. Structure of the pneumococcal l,d-carboxypeptidase DacB and pathophysiological effects of disabled cell wall hydrolases DacA and DacB. *Mol Microbiol.* (2014) 93:1183–206. doi: 10.1111/mmi.12729
10. Saleh M, Bartual SG, Abdullah MR, Jensch I, Asmat TM, Petruschka L, et al. Molecular architecture of *Streptococcus pneumoniae* surface thioredoxin-fold lipoproteins crucial for extracellular oxidative stress resistance and maintenance of virulence. *EMBO Mol Med.* (2013) 5:1852–70. doi: 10.1002/emmm.201202435
11. Saxena S, Khan N, Dehinwal R, Kumar A, Sehgal D. Conserved surface accessible nucleoside ABC transporter component SP0845 is essential for

pneumococcal virulence and confers protection *in vivo*. *PLoS ONE* (2015) 10:e0118154. doi: 10.1371/journal.pone.0118154
12. Basavanna S, Chimalapati S, Maqbool A, Rubbo B, Yuste J, Wilson RJ, et al. The effects of methionine acquisition and synthesis on *Streptococcus pneumoniae* growth and virulence. *PLoS ONE* (2013) 8:e49638. doi: 10.1371/journal.pone.0049638
13. Berry AM, Paton JC. Sequence heterogeneity of PsaA, a 37-kilodalton putative adhesin essential for virulence of *Streptococcus pneumoniae*. *Infect Immun.* (1996) 64:5255–62.
14. McAllister LJ, Tseng HJ, Ogunniyi AD, Jennings MP, McEwan AG, Paton JC. Molecular analysis of the psa permease complex of *Streptococcus pneumoniae*. *Mol Microbiol.* (2004) 53:889–901. doi: 10.1111/j.1365-2958.2004.04164.x
15. Lawrence MC, Pilling PA, Epa VC, Berry AM, Ogunniyi AD, Paton JC. The crystal structure of pneumococcal surface antigen PsaA reveals a metal-binding site and a novel structure for a putative ABC-type binding protein. *Structure* (1998) 6:1553–61. doi: 10.1016/S0969-2126(98)00153-1
16. Dintilhac A, Alloing G, Granadel C, Claverys JP. Competence and virulence of *Streptococcus pneumoniae*: Adc and PsaA mutants exhibit a requirement for Zn and Mn resulting from inactivation of putative ABC metal permeases. *Mol Microbiol.* (1997) 25:727–39. doi: 10.1046/j.1365-2958.1997.5111879.x
17. Sampson JS, Furlow Z, Whitney AM, Williams D, Facklam R, Carlone GM. Limited diversity of *Streptococcus pneumoniae* psaA among pneumococcal vaccine serotypes. *Infect Immun.* (1997) 65:1967–71.
18. Anderton JM, Rajam G, Romero-Steiner S, Summer S, Kowalczyk AP, Carlone GM, et al. E-cadherin is a receptor for the common protein pneumococcal surface adhesin A (PsaA) of *Streptococcus pneumoniae*. *Microbial Pathogen.* (2007) 42:225–36. doi: 10.1016/j.micpath.2007.02.003
19. Morrison KE, Lake D, Crook J, Carlone GM, Ades E, Facklam R, et al. Confirmation of psaA in all 90 serotypes of *Streptococcus pneumoniae* by PCR and potential of this assay for identification and diagnosis. *J Clin Microbiol.* (2000) 38:434–7.
20. Rapola S, Jantti V, Haikala R, Syrjanen R, Carlone GM, Sampson JS, et al. Natural development of antibodies to pneumococcal surface protein A, pneumococcal surface adhesin A, and pneumolysin in relation to pneumococcal carriage and acute otitis media. *J Infect Dis.* (2000) 182:1146–52. doi: 10.1086/315822
21. Simell B, Korkeila M, Pursiainen H, Kilpi TM, Kayhty H. Pneumococcal carriage and otitis media induce salivary antibodies to pneumococcal surface adhesin a, pneumolysin, and pneumococcal surface protein a in children. *J Infect Dis.* (2001) 183:887–96. doi: 10.1086/319246

22. Laine C, Mwangi T, Thompson CM, Obiero J, Lipsitch M, Scott JA. Age-specific immunoglobulin g (IgG) and IgA to pneumococcal protein antigens in a population in coastal kenya. *Infect. Immun.* (2004) 72:3331–5. doi: 10.1128/IAI.72.6.3331-3335.2004

23. Briles DE, Hollingshead S, Brooks-Walter A, Nabors GS, Ferguson L, Schilling M, et al. The potential to use PspA and other pneumococcal proteins to elicit protection against pneumococcal infection. *Vaccine* (2000) 18:1707–11. doi: 10.1016/S0264-410X(99)00511-3

24. Miyaji EN, Oliveira ML, Carvalho E, Ho PL. Serotype-independent pneumococcal vaccines. *Cell Mol Life Sci.* (2013) 70:3303–26. doi: 10.1007/s00018-012-1234-8

25. Schmid P, Selak S, Keller M, Luhan B, Magyarics Z, Seidel S, et al. Th17/Th1 biased immunity to the pneumococcal proteins PcsB, StkP and PsaA in adults of different age. *Vaccine* (2011) 29:3982–9. doi: 10.1016/j.vaccine.2011.03.081

26. Moffitt K, Skoberne M, Howard A, Gavrilescu LC, Gierahn T, Munzer S, et al. Toll-like receptor 2-dependent protection against pneumococcal carriage by immunization with lipidated pneumococcal proteins. *Infect Immun.* (2014) 82:2079–86. doi: 10.1128/IAI.01632-13

27. Skoberne M, Ferreira DM, Hetherington S, Fitzgerald R, Gordon SB. "Pneumococcal protein vaccine GEN-004 reduces experimental human pneumococcal carriage in healthy adults," In: *International Symposium on Pneumococci and Pneumococcal Diseases* (Glasgow) (2016).

28. Saleh M, Abdullah MR, Schulz C, Kohler T, Pribyl T, Jensch I, et al. Following in real time the impact of pneumococcal virulence factors in an acute mouse pneumonia model using bioluminescent bacteria. *J Visual Exp.* (2014) 84:e51174. doi: 10.3791/51174

29. Basavanna S, Khandavilli S, Yuste J, Cohen JM, Hosie AH, Webb AJ, et al. Screening of *Streptococcus pneumoniae* ABC transporter mutants demonstrates that LivJHMGF, a branched-chain amino acid ABC transporter, is necessary for disease pathogenesis. *Infect Immun.* (2009) 77:3412–23. doi: 10.1128/IAI.01543-08

30. Rennemeier C, Hammerschmidt S, Niemann S, Inamura S, Zahringer U, Kehrel BE. Thrombospondin-1 promotes cellular adherence of gram-positive pathogens via recognition of peptidoglycan. *FASEB J.* (2007) 21:3118–32. doi: 10.1096/fj.06-7992com

31. Pearce BJ, Iannelli F, Pozzi G. Construction of new unencapsulated (rough) strains of *Streptococcus pneumoniae*. *Res Microbiol.* (2002) 153:243–7. doi: 10.1016/S0923-2508(02)01312-8

32. Hermans PW, Adrian PV, Albert C, Estevao S, Hoogenboezem T, Luijendijk IH, et al. The streptococcal lipoprotein rotamase A (SlrA) is a functional peptidyl-prolyl isomerase involved in pneumococcal colonization. *J Biol Chem.* (2006) 281:968–76. doi: 10.1074/jbc.M510014200

33. Hammerschmidt S, Bethe G, Remane PH, Chhatwal GS. Identification of pneumococcal surface protein A as a lactoferrin-binding protein of *Streptococcus pneumoniae*. *Infect Immun.* (1999) 67:1683–7.

34. Hammerschmidt S, Tillig MP, Wolff S, Vaerman JP, Chhatwal GS. Species-specific binding of human secretory component to SpsA protein of *Streptococcus pneumoniae* via a hexapeptide motif. *Mol Microbiol.* (2000) 36:726–36. doi: 10.1046/j.1365-2958.2000.01897.x

35. Hammerschmidt S, Talay SR, Brandtzaeg P, Chhatwal GS. SpsA, a novel pneumococcal surface protein with specific binding to secretory immunoglobulin A and secretory component. *Mol Microbiol.* (1997) 25:1113–24. doi: 10.1046/j.1365-2958.1997.5391899.x

36. Jensch I, Gamez G, Rothe M, Ebert S, Fulde M, Somplatzki D, et al. PavB is a surface-exposed adhesin of *Streptococcus pneumoniae* contributing to nasopharyngeal colonization and airways infections. *Mol Microbiol.* (2010) 77:22–43. doi: 10.1111/j.1365-2958.2010.07189.x

37. Martin RM, Brady JL, Lew AM. The need for IgG2c specific antiserum when isotyping antibodies from C57BL/6 and NOD mice. *J Immunol Methods* (1998) 212:187–92. doi: 10.1016/S0022-1759(98)00015-5

38. Schmidt F, Meyer T, Sundaramoorthy N, Michalik S, Surmann K, Depke M, et al. Characterization of human and *Staphylococcus aureus* proteins in respiratory mucosa by in vivo- and immunoproteomics. *J Proteomics* (2017) 155:31–9. doi: 10.1016/j.jprot.2017.01.008

39. Zysk G, Bongaerts RJ, ten Thoren E, Bethe G, Hakenbeck R, Heinz HP. Detection of 23 immunogenic pneumococcal proteins using convalescent-phase serum. *Infect Immun.* (2000) 68:3740–3. doi: 10.1128/IAI.68.6.3740-3743.2000

40. Pribyl T, Moche M, Dreisbach A, Bijlsma JJ, Saleh M, Abdullah MR, et al. Influence of impaired lipoprotein biogenesis on surface and exoproteome of *Streptococcus pneumoniae. J Proteome Res.* (2014) 13:650–67. doi: 10.1021/pr400768v

41. Plumptre CD, Eijkelkamp BA, Morey JR, Behr F, Counago RM, Ogunniyi AD, et al. AdcA and AdcAII employ distinct zinc acquisition mechanisms and contribute additively to zinc homeostasis in *Streptococcus pneumoniae. Mol Microbiol.* (2014) 91:834–51. doi: 10.1111/mmi.12504

42. Cron LE, Bootsma HJ, Noske N, Burghout P, Hammerschmidt S, Hermans PW. Surface-associated lipoprotein PpmA of *Streptococcus pneumoniae* is involved in colonization in a strain-specific manner. *Microbiology* (2009) 155 (Pt 7):2401–10. doi: 10.1099/mic.0.026765-0

43. Daniels CC, Briles TC, Mirza S, Hakansson AP, Briles DE. Capsule does not block antibody binding to PspA, a surface virulence protein of *Streptococcus pneumoniae. Microbial Pathogen.* (2006) 40:228–33. doi: 10.1016/j.micpath.2006.01.007

44. Malley R, Trzcinski K, Srivastava A, Thompson CM, Anderson PW, Lipsitch M. CD4+ T cells mediate antibody-independent acquired immunity to pneumococcal colonization. *Proc Natl Acad Sci USA.* (2005) 102:4848–53. doi: 10.1073/pnas.0501254102

45. Basset A, Thompson CM, Hollingshead SK, Briles DE, Ades EW, Lipsitch M, et al. Antibody-independent, CD4+ T-cell-dependent protection against pneumococcal colonization elicited by intranasal immunization with purified pneumococcal proteins. *Infect Immun.* (2007) 75:5460–4. doi: 10.1128/IAI.00773-07

46. Lu YJ, Gross J, Bogaert D, Finn A, Bagrade L, Zhang Q, et al. Interleukin-17A mediates acquired immunity to pneumococcal colonization. *PLoS Pathog.* (2008) 4:e1000159. doi: 10.1371/journal.ppat.1000159

47. Bogaert D, De Groot R, Hermans PW. *Streptococcus pneumoniae* colonisation: the key to pneumococcal disease. *Lancet Infect Dis.* (2004) 4:144–54. doi: 10.1016/S1473-3099(04)00938-7

48. Zafar MA, Kono M, Wang Y, Zangari T, Weiser JN. Infant Mouse Model for the Study of Shedding and Transmission during *Streptococcus pneumoniae* Monoinfection. *Infect Immun.* (2016) 84:2714–22. doi: 10.1128/IAI.00416-16

49. Gor DO, Ding X, Briles DE, Jacobs MR, Greenspan NS. Relationship between surface accessibility for PpmA, PsaA, and PspA and antibody-mediated immunity to systemic infection by *Streptococcus pneumoniae. Infect Immun.* (2005) 73:1304–12. doi: 10.1128/IAI.73.3.1304-1312.2005

50. Jomaa M, Yuste J, Paton JC, Jones C, Dougan G, Brown JS. Antibodies to the iron uptake ABC transporter lipoproteins PiaA and PiuA promote opsonophagocytosis of *Streptococcus pneumoniae. Infect Immun.* (2005) 73:6852–9. doi: 10.1128/IAI.73.10.6852-6859.2005

51. Mahdi LK, Ogunniyi AD, LeMessurier KS, Paton JC. Pneumococcal virulence gene expression and host cytokine profiles during pathogenesis of invasive disease. *Infect Immun.* (2008) 76:646–57. doi: 10.1128/IAI.01161-07

52. Ogunniyi AD, Giammarinaro P, Paton JC. The genes encoding virulence-associated proteins and the capsule of *Streptococcus pneumoniae* are upregulated and differentially expressed in vivo. *Microbiology* (2002) 148 (Pt 7):2045–53. doi: 10.1099/00221287-148-7-2045

53. Orihuela CJ, Radin JN, Sublett JE, Gao G, Kaushal D, Tuomanen EI. Microarray analysis of pneumococcal gene expression during invasive disease. *Infect Immun.* (2004) 72:5582–96. doi: 10.1128/IAI.72.10.5582-5596.2004

54. Mahdi LK, Wang H, Van der Hoek MB, Paton JC, Ogunniyi AD. Identification of a novel pneumococcal vaccine antigen preferentially expressed during meningitis in mice. *J Clin Invest.* (2012) 122:2208–20. doi: 10.1172/JCI45850

55. Mahdi LK, Van der Hoek MB, Ebrahimie E, Paton JC, Ogunniyi AD. Characterization of pneumococcal genes involved in bloodstream invasion in a mouse model. *PLoS ONE* (2015) 10:e0141816. doi: 10.1371/journal.pone.0141816

56. Croucher NJ, Campo JJ, Le TQ, Liang X, Bentley SD, Hanage WP, et al. Diverse evolutionary patterns of pneumococcal antigens identified by pangenome-wide immunological screening. *Proc Natl Acad Sci USA.* (2017) 114:E357–66. doi: 10.1073/pnas.1613937114

57. Jimenez-Munguia I, van Wamel WJ, Olaya-Abril A, Garcia-Cabrera E, Rodriguez-Ortega MJ, Obando I. Proteomics-driven design of a multiplex bead-based platform to assess natural IgG antibodies to pneumococcal protein antigens in children. *J Proteomics* (2015) 126:228–33. doi: 10.1016/j.jprot.2015.06.011

58. Brown JS, Ogunniyi AD, Woodrow MC, Holden DW, Paton JC. Immunization with components of two iron uptake ABC transporters protects mice against systemic *Streptococcus pneumoniae* infection. *Infect Immun.* (2001) 69:6702–6. doi: 10.1128/IAI.69.11.6702-6706.2001

59. Marques JM, Rial A, Munoz N, Pellay FX, Van Maele L, Leger H, et al. Protection against *Streptococcus pneumoniae* serotype 1 acute infection shows a signature of Th17- and IFN-gamma-mediated immunity. *Immunobiology* (2012) 217:420–9. doi: 10.1016/j.imbio.2011.10.012

60. Moffitt KL, Gierahn TM, Lu YJ, Gouveia P, Alderson M, Flechtner JB, et al. T(H)17-based vaccine design for prevention of *Streptococcus pneumoniae* colonization. *Cell Host Microbe* (2011) 9:158–65. doi: 10.1016/j.chom.2011.01.007

61. Kuipers K, Jong WSP, van der Gaast-de Jongh CE, Houben D, van Opzeeland F, Simonetti E, et al. Th17-mediated cross protection against pneumococcal carriage by vaccination with a variable antigen. *Infect Immun.* (2017) 85:e00281–17. doi: 10.1128/IAI.00281-17

62. Stratmann T. Cholera toxin subunit B as adjuvant—An accelerator in protective immunity and a break in autoimmunity. *Vaccines* (2015) 3:579–96. doi: 10.3390/vaccines3030579

63. Wiedinger K, Pinho D, Bitsaktsis C. Utilization of cholera toxin B as a mucosal adjuvant elicits antibody-mediated protection against *S. pneumoniae* infection in mice. *Therapeut Adv Vaccines* (2017) 5:15–24. doi: 10.1177/2051013617691041

64. Li J, Arevalo MT, Chen Y, Posadas O, Smith JA, Zeng M. Intranasal immunization with influenza antigens conjugated with cholera toxin subunit B stimulates broad spectrum immunity against influenza viruses. *Hum Vaccines Immunotherapeut.* (2014) 10:1211–20. doi: 10.4161/hv.28407

65. Habets MN, van Selm S, van Opzeeland FJ, Simonetti E, Hermans PWM, de Jonge MI, et al. Role of antibodies and IL17-mediated immunity in protection against pneumococcal otitis media. *Vaccine* (2016) 34:5968–74. doi: 10.1016/j.vaccine.2016.09.057

66. Pilette C, Ouadrhiri Y, Godding V, Vaerman JP, Sibille Y. Lung mucosal immunity: immunoglobulin-A revisited. *Eur Resp J.* (2001) 18:571–88. doi: 10.1183/09031936.01.00228801

67. Svanborg-Eden C, Svennerholm AM. Secretory immunoglobulin A and G antibodies prevent adhesion of *Escherichia coli* to human urinary tract epithelial cells. *Infect Immun.* (1978) 22:790–7.

68. Johnson S, Sypura WD, Gerding DN, Ewing SL, Janoff EN. Selective neutralization of a bacterial enterotoxin by serum immunoglobulin A in response to mucosal disease. *Infect Immun.* (1995) 63:3166–73.

69. Mazanec MB, Kaetzel CS, Lamm ME, Fletcher D, Nedrud JG. Intracellular neutralization of virus by immunoglobulin A antibodies. *Proc Natl Acad Sci USA.* (1992) 89:6901–5. doi: 10.1073/pnas.89.15.6901

70. Underdown BJ, Schiff JM. Immunoglobulin A: strategic defense initiative at the mucosal surface. *Ann Rev Immunol.* (1986) 4:389–417. doi: 10.1146/annurev.iy.04.040186.002133

71. Brewer JM, Conacher M, Hunter CA, Mohrs M, Brombacher F, Alexander J. Aluminium hydroxide adjuvant initiates strong antigen-specific Th2 responses in the absence of IL-4- or IL-13-mediated signaling. *J Immunol.* (1999) 163:6448–54.

72. Gupta RK. Aluminum compounds as vaccine adjuvants. *Adv Drug Deliv Rev.* (1998) 32:155–72. doi: 10.1016/S0169-409X(98)00008-8

73. Coats MT, Benjamin WH, Hollingshead SK, Briles DE. Antibodies to the pneumococcal surface protein A, PspA, can be produced in splenectomized and can protect splenectomized mice from infection with *Streptococcus pneumoniae*. *Vaccine* (2005) 23:4257–62. doi: 10.1016/j.vaccine.2005.03.039

74. Mozdzanowska K, Zharikova D, Cudic M, Otvos L, Gerhard W. Roles of adjuvant and route of vaccination in antibody response and protection engendered by a synthetic matrix protein 2-based influenza A virus vaccine in the mouse. *Virol J.* (2007) 4:118. doi: 10.1186/1743-422X-4-118

75. Debache K, Guionaud C, Alaeddine F, Hemphill A. Intraperitoneal and intra-nasal vaccination of mice with three distinct recombinant *Neospora caninum* antigens results in differential effects with regard to protection against experimental challenge with *Neospora caninum* tachyzoites. *Parasitology* (2010) 137:229–40. doi: 10.1017/S0031182009991259

76. van den Dobbelsteen GP, Brunekreef K, Sminia T, van Rees EP. Effect of mucosal and systemic immunization with pneumococcal polysaccharide type 3, 4 and 14 in the rat. *Scandinavian J Immunol.* (1992) 36:661–9.

# 2

# Utilization of Staphylococcal Immune Evasion Protein Sbi as a Novel Vaccine Adjuvant

Yi Yang[1†], Catherine R. Back[1†], Melissa A. Gräwert[2], Ayla A. Wahid[1], Harriet Denton[3], Rebecca Kildani[3], Joshua Paulin[3], Kristin Wörner[4], Wolgang Kaiser[4], Dmitri I. Svergun[2], Asel Sartbaeva[5], Andrew G. Watts[6], Kevin J. Marchbank[3*] and Jean M. H. van den Elsen[1*]

[1] Department of Biology and Biochemistry, University of Bath, Bath, United Kingdom, [2] Hamburg Unit, European Molecular Biology Laboratory, Deutsches Elektronen-Synchrotron, Hamburg, Germany, [3] Institute of Cellular Medicine, Newcastle University, Newcastle-upon-Tyne, United Kingdom, [4] Dynamic Biosensors GmbH, Martinsried, Germany, [5] Department of Chemistry, University of Bath, Bath, United Kingdom, [6] Department of Pharmacy and Pharmacology, University of Bath, Bath, United Kingdom

*Correspondence:
Kevin J. Marchbank
kevin.marchbank@ncl.ac.uk
Jean M. H. van den Elsen
j.m.h.v.elsen@bath.ac.uk

† These authors have contributed equally to this work

Co-ligation of the B cell antigen receptor with complement receptor 2 on B-cells via a C3d-opsonised antigen complex significantly lowers the threshold required for B cell activation. Consequently, fusions of antigens with C3d polymers have shown great potential in vaccine design. However, these linear arrays of C3d multimers do not mimic the natural opsonisation of antigens with C3d. Here we investigate the potential of using the unique complement activating characteristics of Staphylococcal immune-evasion protein Sbi to develop a pro-vaccine approach that spontaneously coats antigens with C3 degradation products in a natural way. We show that Sbi rapidly triggers the alternative complement pathway through recruitment of complement regulators, forming tripartite complexes that act as competitive antagonists of factor H, resulting in enhanced complement consumption. These functional results are corroborated by the structure of the complement activating Sbi-III-IV:C3d:FHR-1 complex. Finally, we demonstrate that Sbi, fused with *Mycobacterium tuberculosis* antigen Ag85b, causes efficient opsonisation with C3 fragments, thereby enhancing the immune response significantly beyond that of Ag85b alone, providing proof of concept for our pro-vaccine approach.

Keywords: vaccine, adjuvant, complement, immune evasion, *Staphycoccus aureus*

## INTRODUCTION

Opsonisation of an antigen with C3d(g), the final degradation product of complement component C3, results in the co-ligation of the B cell antigen receptor and complement receptor 2 (CR2) on B cells, thereby instigating a profound molecular adjuvant effect, i.e., this co-ligation of receptor complexes lowers the threshold of antigen required for B cell activation by up to 10,000 fold (1–3). Furthermore, as CR2 is also expressed highly on follicular dendritic cells (FDCs) (4) the presence of C3d(g) on the antigen allows it to be trafficked onto and trapped at the surface of these cells (5). This provides an essential depot of antigen to support the germinal center reaction and maintain the ongoing immune response including the generation of high affinity antibodies and memory B-cells (3, 4, 6). B cells can also have an important role as antigen presenting cells (APCs) (7, 8) and have been shown to contribute to T-helper cell priming (9, 10) and therefore, antigen-C3d-CR2 interactions play a key role in humoral immunity (5). Additionally, C3d activation of T helper cells has also been described in a CR2 independent manner (11), underlining the importance of C3d opsonisation in stimulating the immune system to respond.

Not surprisingly, this functionality led to the idea that recombinant versions of C3d would make an ideal natural adjuvant and to the subsequent design of linear polymers of human C3d (12). Indeed, these linear arrays of C3d multimers (3-mer to 20-mer) when fused directly to an antigen can act as potent activators of human B-cells. However, they do not mimic the natural opsonisation of antigens by C3d at a molecular level and do not always enhance immune responses (13). After activation of C3, C3b attaches directly to the antigen surface via the reactive thioester on the convex face of the protein's thioester domain (TED). In the presence of complement regulators [factor I (FI) and its co-factors, such as factor H (FH) and CR1] this is rapidly converted to iC3b and then to C3d, exposing the concave CR2 binding site of the TED fragment away from the antigen surface (14). It is likely that multiple iC3b/C3d molecules attach to complex antigens/pathogen surfaces during the initial activation phases of complement, creating high-avidity binding sites for complement fragment receptors.

In the last two decades, structural biology has helped to unveil many of the molecular aspects that are crucial for the activation and regulation of the complement system. Most notable are the crystal structures of the central complement component activation states, native C3 (15), activated C3b, and inactive C3c (16). The structure of C3b in complex with factors B and D (17) subsequently revealed a detailed view of the alternative pathway C3 convertase assembly and its activation, leading to the amplified cleavage of C3 molecules that result in opsonisation, and clearance of microbial pathogens, and host debris. The covalent attachment of C3b to surfaces does not discriminate between self or non-self surfaces and requires tight regulation to protect host surfaces. Structures of C3b in complex with FH domains 1–4 (18) and domains 19–20 (19, 20) provided insights into protection of host cells (21) and demonstrated how factor H-related proteins (FHRs) function as competitive antagonists of FH, modulating complement activation and providing improved discrimination of self and non-self surfaces (22). The subsequent structure of the complex of C3b, $FH_{1-4}$, and regulator factor I (23) improved our understanding in the proteolytic cleavage of C3b to the late-stage opsonins iC3b or C3dg and provided the basis for the regulator-dependent differences in processing and immune recognition of opsonized material.

Here we investigate the potential to harness the unique complement-stimulatory characteristics of *Staphylococcus aureus* immunomodulator Sbi to develop "pro-vaccines." Sbi components would trigger natural complement activation in the host and coat antigen surfaces with complement component C3 degradation products, thereby enhancing the degree of immunogenicity of target antigens. Research from our lab previously revealed that Sbi contains two domains (III and IV), which bind to the central complement component C3 and cause futile fluid phase consumption

of this component (24). Therefore, these two domains of Sbi offer the potential to not only coat an antigen with the natural adjuvant C3d, but also to generate anaphylatoxins and the full range of C3 opsonins. Such an approach has the clear potential to activate many immune cells unlike recombinant C3d fragment-based adjuvants of the past, that, due to the restricted expression pattern of CR2, were largely focused to B cells. Furthermore, the direct activation of complement close to the target antigen (with the associated anaphylatoxin generation) may be critical for generating appropriate inflammatory immune responses, both humoral and cellular; needed to immunize against complex pathogenic targets.

In this study we first investigate the molecular mode of action of Sbi-III-IV and evaluate the importance of the tripartite complex formation between Sbi, C3d, and complement regulators factor H (FH) or factor H-related proteins (FHRs) for complement activation. Based on these findings, we then tested whether our pro-vaccine strategy would be successful by using *Mycobacterium tuberculosis* antigen 85b (Ag85b) as a model antigen in a fusion construct containing Sbi domains III and IV. We show that this Sbi-Ag85b conjugate is opsonized by C3 degradation products in serum, and when administered to mice, leads to an enhanced immune response *in vivo,* but only in mice that possess C3 and complement receptor 1 and 2, demonstrating proof of concept for this adjuvant compound.

# RESULTS

## Sbi-III-IV Triggers C3 Consumption via Activation of the Alternative Complement Pathway, Forming a Covalent Adduct With C3b

To investigate the molecular details of the C3 futile consumption caused by Sbi, a protein construct consisting of domains III and IV (Sbi-III-IV) was incubated with normal human serum (NHS) and analyzed using western blotting. As seen previously (24), we found that Sbi-III-IV-induced C3 consumption results in the deposition of metastable C3b molecules onto serum proteins, causing the formation of high molecular weight C3b covalent adduct species with serum proteins (**Figure 1A**). Immuno-blotting analyses using a polyclonal anti-Sbi antibody (**Figure 1B**) reveals that a small fraction of Sbi-III-IV molecule also forms a covalent adduct with a nascent C3b molecule that is subsequently converted into a smaller Sbi-iC3b adduct as a result of proteolytic processing by serum proteases. In addition, we show that Sbi-III-IV-induced C3 consumption coincides with the release of the C3a anaphylatoxin fragment (**Figure 1C**), and the proteolytic activation of factor B (FB) (**Figure 1D**), confirming the alternative complement pathway as the driving force behind this process. Pre-incubation of serum with Sbi-III-IV results in the loss of serum hemolytic ability caused by the futile consumption of fluid C3 (**Figure 1E**). Without pre-incubation, the Sbi-III-IV construct does not

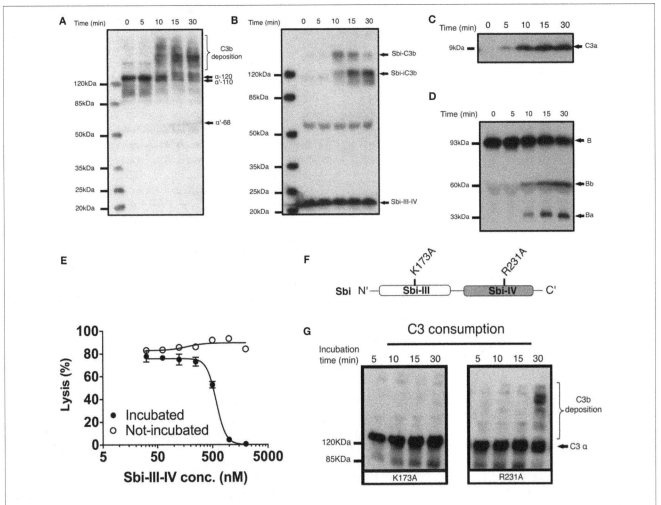

FIGURE 1 | Sbi-III-IV induces C3 futile consumption via the alternative complement pathway and thereby causes C3b adduct formation and C3a anaphylatoxin production. (A) C3 activation and C3b deposition in NHS after incubation with 10 μM Sbi-III-IV, visualized using anti-C3d western blot analysis. C3b adducts formed with serum proteins are indicated. Positions of α-120 (C3) α'110 (C3b) and α'-68 (iC3b) are indicated. The 10 min lag-time in C3 activation we observe in the presence of excess Sbi-III-IV (10 μM) correlates with the delay reported in the natural C3 "tick-over" process, required for supplying the critical enzymatic component for the initial fluid phase Alternative Pathway (AP) C3 convertase. (B) Sbi-C3b adduct formation, visualized with anti-Sbi western blot. These adducts migrate at higher than expected molecular weights (Sbi-α'110: ~160 kDa and Sbi-α'68: ~120 kDa, with expected molecular weights of 125 and 83 kDa, respectively) which is caused by the high pI of the Sbi-III-IV construct (pI = 9.3). Sbi-III-IV has a molecular weight of 14.8 kDa, but migrates to ~22 kDa in SDS-polyacrylamide gel due to the positively charged electrophoresis buffer. (C) C3a anaphylatoxin production, followed using anti-C3a western blot analysis (showing only the low molecular weight region). (D) FB cleavage, monitored by anti-FB western blot analysis. (E) Concentration dependent Sbi-III-IV induced C3 consumption, studied by a rabbit erythrocytes haemolytic assay. Rabbit erythrocytes were exposed to normal human serum pre-incubated with Sbi-III-IV (incubated, closed circles) and normal human serum with Sbi-III-IV added at the start of the experiment (not incubated, open circles). (F) Schematic representation of the relative positions of point mutations that display the most profound functional defects, K173A and R231A. (G) C3 consumption profiles of Sbi-III-IV mutants K173A and R231A. For (B–E) and (G), one representative blot of three independent experiments was shown. For (E), four independent measurements of two experiments were shown. The mean and SD for each measurement were calculated for all datasets. Curves were fitted using non-linear variable slope (four parameters) function in GraphPad Prism.

protect rabbit erythrocytes from lysis in NHS under AP conditions.

## Sbi Domain III Residue K173 Is Essential for Complement Consumption

In order to gain understanding of the individual roles of Sbi domains III and IV in AP activation, a systematic site-directed mutagenesis approach was used, mainly focusing on charged and polar amino acids (for details see **Table S1** and **Figure S1**).

Functional screening of these mutants identified K173, located within Sbi domain III (**Figure 1F**), as an essential contributor to triggering C3 consumption. Sbi mutant K173A shows no complement activation after 30 min incubation with human serum, demonstrating a comparable complement activation defect to the previously identified C3d binding mutant R231A (24, 25) (**Figures 1F,G**), located in Sbi domain IV. Assessment of the C3d binding affinity, using *switch*SENSE (**Table 1** and **Figure S2A**), shows that contrary to R231A the C3d binding capacity of K173A is unaffected, indicating it is essential for the role for domain III in the futile consumption of C3.

**TABLE 1** | Sbi-III-IV:C3d interaction affinity determined by *switch*SENSE.

| | $K_d$ (nM) | $k_{ON}$ ($M^{-1}S^{-1}$) | $k_{OFF}$ ($S^{-1}$) |
|---|---|---|---|
| WT:C3d | $5.0 \pm 0.8$ | $5.9 \pm 1.0 \times 10^5$ | $3.0 \pm 0.1 \times 10^{-3}$ |
| K173A:C3d | $5.8 \pm 1.2$ | $5.3 \pm 0.9 \times 10^5$ | $3.0 \pm 0.4 \times 10^{-3}$ |
| R231:C3d | No binding | | |

**TABLE 2** | Sbi-III-IV:C3d complex hydrodynamic diameter determined by *switch*SENSE.

| | $D_H$ (nm) of Sbi-III-IV | $D_H$ (nm) of Sbi:C3d complex |
|---|---|---|
| WT | $4.3 \pm 0.1$ | $6.6 \pm 0.2$ |
| K173A | $3.8 \pm 0.3$ | $5.0 \pm 0.3$ |
| R231A | $4.7 \pm 0.3$ | No binding |

Interestingly, our *switch*SENSE analyses of the C3d binding characteristics also shows a reduced hydrodynamic diameter for K173A compared to WT and the C3d impaired binding mutant R231A, indication that this mutation in domain III results in a more compact Sbi:C3d complex (**Table 2** and **Figure S2B**). A more detailed structural analysis of these conformational changes follows below.

## Sbi-III-IV Enhances Binding of FH or FHRs to C3 Breakdown Products

In a previous study, we reported that Sbi-III-IV binds C3 isoforms in combination with the C-terminal part of FH ($FH_{19-20}$), forming tripartite complexes (26). Many FHRs share SCR modules with high $FH_{19-20}$ sequence identity (22) particularly FHR-1 which has been demonstrated to have significant complement dysregulation potential (21). Thus, we investigated the potential role for Sbi-III-IV in mediating the formation of tripartite complexes with C3 fragments and FHR-1, FHR-2, or FHR-5.

On a C3b opsonised surface plasmon resonance (SPR) sensor chip, the presence of wild-type Sbi-III-IV clearly enhanced the binding of FH, FHR-1, FHR-2, FHR-5 as well as $FH_{19-20}$ (at fixed concentrations of 100, 12.5, 20, 25, and 20 nM, respectively) to the surface in a concentration dependent manner (**Figure 2A**). However, in the case of the K173A mutant, tripartite complex formation with FH or FHR-1, 2, 5, or $FH_{19-20}$ is significantly impaired, showing decreased binding and more rapid dissociation compared to WT Sbi-III-IV (**Figures 2B,C**). We also co-injected Sbi-III-IV with FH or FHR-1, flowing opsonized iC3b or amine-coupled C3d(g) across the surface. On these surfaces, the fold-changes in FH (or FHR-1) binding levels were also enhanced even at reduced Sbi-III-IV concentration (**Figures S3A-D**).

## Sbi-III-IV Acts as a Competitive Antagonist of FH via the Recruitment of FHRs

Our SPR data, described above, show that Sbi-III-IV enables FH or FHR-1, 2 and 5 binding to the C3 activation fragment C3b and late-stage proteolytic fragments iC3b and C3d(g). To

further our understanding of the mechanism of FH or FHR recruitment and the contribution of these tripartite complexes to AP complement activation, we used a rabbit erythrocyte haemolytic assay. In the presence of Sbi-III-IV and endogenous FH (and FHRs), in NHS, addition of recombinant FHR-1 or FHR-2 resulted in significantly enhanced C3 consumption (**Figure 3A**), as evidenced by the reduction in erythrocyte lysis in a concentration dependent manner. In the absence of Sbi-III-IV only baseline C3 consumption was observed. Although FHR-5 alone can reduce erythrocyte lysis in a concentration dependent manner, as described previously (27), in the presence of Sbi-III-IV C3 consumption by FHR-5 is clearly enhanced (**Figure 3B**). As predicted, the results in **Figure 3C** indicate that the observed reduction in erythrocyte lysis caused by C3 fluid phase consumption, in the case of FHR1 and likely the remaining FHRs, is mediated by the C-terminal SCR domains of the protein rather than the N-terminal domains.

Whilst our SPR and rabbit erythrocyte assay clearly indicate that *in vitro* Sbi-III-IV can recruit FHRs in tripartite complexes with C3b and thereby enhance fluid phase complement consumption, it has to be taken into account that the physiological molar concentrations of FHR-1, 2, and 5 are 13–164 fold less than that of FH (21, 28). To further investigate the potential competitive binding between FH and the FHRs in Sbi-III-IV mediated tripartite complexes, we used an ELISA-based assay where we applied FH (25 nM) and Sbi-III-IV [1 μM, in the presence of a concentration range of FHRs (9.3–150 nM)] onto a C3b coated plate. Subsequently, we assessed the percentage of FH bound using monoclonal antibody OX-24. **Figure 3D** shows that FHR-1 can compete with FH to bind C3b, decreasing the percentage of residual FH bound to C3b from ~70% at the lowest FHR-1 concentration to ~30% at the highest concentration. In the presence of Sbi-III-IV WT this effect is dramatically increased with only ~25% residual FH bound at the lowest FHR-1 concentration, reducing to ~0% at the highest FHR-1 concentration (**Figure 3E**). These results clearly indicate that Sbi-III-IV can preferentially recruit FHR-1 to form a tripartite complex with C3b. Similarly, enhancement of recruitment was observed with FHR-5 and fragment $FH_{19-20}$ but only weakly with FHR-2. Although unable to activate complement, Sbi-III-IV mutant K173A is still able to compete for the binding of FHR-1 in the presence of FH, but its ability to enhance binding of FHR-2 and FHR-5 to C3b is clearly affected (**Figure 3F**).

To assess the potential AP de-regulatory roles of the Sbi-III-IV mediated tripartite complexes we subjected them to a novel C3 convertase decay acceleration activity (DAA) assay and a fluid phase C3b co-factor activity (CFA) assay (29, 30). We demonstrated that in absence of Sbi, FHR-1 failed to antagonize FH efficiently and show a difference in the level of C3 convertase formation (**Figure 3G**). Co-injection of FHR-1 and −5 shows reduced C3 convertase formation, which is in accordance with the results from a previous study (31). However, the presence of Sbi (2 μM) potentiates the FH antagonizing effect of FHR-1, and to a lesser extent that of FHR-5, at a physiologically relevant concentration ratio (FH 2,000 nM: FHR-1 200 nM: FHR-5 20 nM), resulting in increased C3 convertase formation on a C3b surface (**Figure 3H**). The

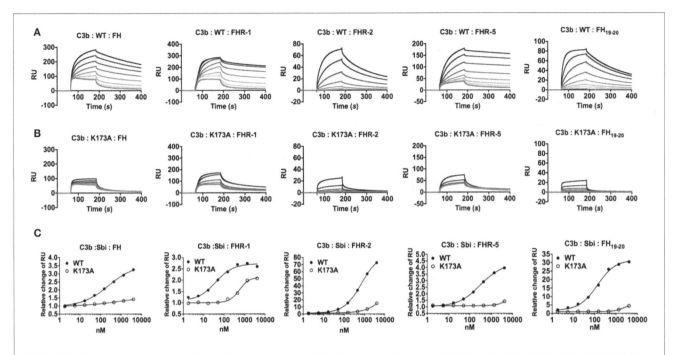

**FIGURE 2 |** Surface plasmon resonance analyses of tripartite complexes. A triply diluted concentration series (4,050 to 1.8 nM) of **(A)** WT or **(B)** K173A Sbi-III-IV were co-injected with plasma purified FH, recombinant FHR-1, FHR-2, FHR-5, or $FH_{19-20}$. The red response curves were indicative of binding experiment in the absence of Sbi. The co-injection experiments of a fixed analyte concentration in combination with increasing Sbi concentration were depicted by increasingly dark lines. **(C)** Relative changes of Sbi-III-IV mediated FH (or FHR) binding to C3b. By subtracting the co-injection sensorgram (i.e., Sbi+FH) with the corresponding Sbi binding dataset **(Figure S3)**, the changes in FH (or FHRs) binding was deduced **(Figure S3)**. Changes in FH (or FHRs) binding were expressed as the relative change, derived from dividing the Sbi mediated binding by the FH (or FHR) only control, using the response-difference values at the equilibrated binding point (173.5 s). Each sensorgram is representative of two experiments. Relative change curves were fitted using non-linear variable slope (four parameters) function in GraphPad Prism.

baseline C3b breakdown rate was acquired in the presence of FH (0.160 μM) and FI (0.017 μM), and subsequent measurements were performed in the presence of FHR alone (0.32 μM) and in combination with Sbi-III-IV (1 μM). As shown in **Figure 3I** and **Figure S3F**, the presence of FHR-1, 2 or 5 increases the C3b fluid phase half-life to different degrees, with FHR-5 showing the largest increase in half-life. Most interestingly, the C3b half-life could be further extended by the addition of Sbi-III-IV.

## The Sbi-III-IV:C3d:FHR-1 Tripartite Complex Forms a Dimer in Solution

To investigate the structural characteristics of the Sbi-III-IV:C3d:FHR1 tripartite complex, we used small angle X-ray scattering (SAXS). The scattering profile collected at an equimolar mixing ratio is shown in **Figure 4** in log plot (a) as well as Kratky plot (b). The featureless descend in the log plot and the plateau in the latter is characteristic for scattering of particles that are, at least partially, disordered.

The SAXS data and the overall parameters obtained (**Table S2**) suggest that the complex is largely dimeric but rather flexible in solution. Quantitative flexibility analysis was performed using the ensemble optimisation method EOM (32), which fits the experimental data using scattering computed from conformational ensembles. Models with randomized linkers were generated based on the known structures of $FHR-1_{1-2}$

[3zd2, (21)]; $FH_{18-20}$ [3sw0, (33)], containing the equivalent of $FHR-1_3$; $FH_{19-20}$:C3d complex [2xqw, (20)], corresponding with $FHR-1_{4-5}$; and the Sbi-IV:C3d complex [2wy8, (34)]. To account for the dimerisation, P2 symmetry was applied, using the $FHR-1_{1-2}$ dimer interface as seen in the crystal structure (3zd2). The distributions of the overall parameters in the selected structures compared with those of the original pool (**Figure 4C**) suggests that the complex is rather flexible with a slight preference for extended structures in solution. The subset of most typical models (and the volume percentage of their contribution) shown in **Figure 4C** indicate that in addition to the expected contact sites with C3d, Sbi-III domain appears to also interact with FHR-1, corroborating the functional results described above. **Figure 4D** shows a schematic representation of the dimeric Sbi-III-IV:C3d:FHR-1 complex observed in solution.

## K173A Restricts the Conformational Freedom of Sbi Domain III

To examine the possible structural effects of the K173A substitution in Sbi domain III, SAXS data was collected on the Sbi-III-IV(K173A):C3d complex, and compared to the wild-type Sbi-III-IV:C3d complex published previously (34). The experimental scattering pattern collected at 240 μM (~12 mg/ml) is presented in **Figure 4E** and the structural parameters derived from this data are given in **Table S2**. The estimated

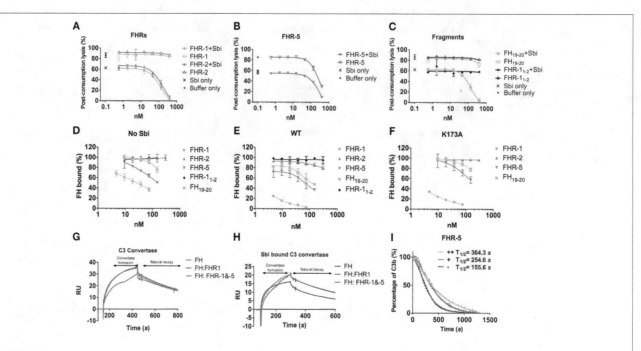

**FIGURE 3 |** Functional characterization of tripartite complexes in complement AP regulation. NHS was incubated with Sbi-III-IV, in combination with specified reagents or just buffer, the consumption of AP activity was indicated by the protection of rabbit red blood cell from lysis. **(A)** Pre-incubation of recombinant FHR-1 or −2 with the presence or absence of Sbi-III-IV. **(B)** Pre-incubation of recombinant FHR-5 in the presence or absence of Sbi-III-IV. **(C)** Pre-incubation of recombinant FH$_{19-20}$ or FHR-1$_{1-2}$ in the presence or absence of Sbi-III-IV. Using an ELISA assay, the ability of FHR-1,−2,−5, FH$_{19-20}$, or FHR-1$_{1-2}$ to modulate FH binding to a C3b coated surface was studied in the absence **(D)** or presence of WT Sbi-III-IV **(E)**, or K173A Sbi-III-IV **(F)**. C3 convertase formation in the absence **(G)** or presence of Sbi-III-IV **(H)** was assessed by flowing factor B (500 nM) and factor D (100 nM) in the presence of FH (2,000 nM) or FH +FHR-1 (2,000 and 200 nM) or FH+FHR-1&-5 (2,000, 200 and 20 nM) across a surface amine coupled with 500 RU C3b. To form Sbi bound C3 convertase, experiments were conducted in addition of 2,000 nM of Sbi-III-IV. Detailed experimental and data processing procedures are provided in Materials and Methods and **Figure S3E**. **(I)** Percentage of intact C3b derived from continuous recording of ANS fluorescence changes between 465 and 475 nm spectrum. Baseline C3b breakdown curve (−) was recorded in the presence of FH and FI, interference caused by the addition of FHR-5 (+) or FHR-5 in combination of Sbi (++) was also examined. The data for FHR-1 and FHR-2 are presented in **Figure 3F**. Normalized data was depicted in solid lines, simulated breakdown curves were shown as dotted-lines. Each curve represents the mean value of three independent experiments. For **(A–F)**, the mean and standard deviation for each measurement was calculated; For **(G–H)**, each sensorgram is representative of two experiments. For **(I)**, simulated breakdown curves were fitted using one phase exponential decay function in GraphPad Prism.

molecular mass (MM) of the solute agrees within the errors with the values predicted for a 1:1 complex (∼15 + 35 kDa). At lower concentration a decrease in the MM estimates is observed which suggests that the complex slowly begins to dissociate. The previously described wild-type Sbi-III-IV:C3d data on the other hand, suggests that at higher concentrations, higher oligomeric species are present, thus, for the comparison here, data collected at 0.6 mg/ml is shown. The faster descend of the wild-type data, which translates to a larger Rg, suggests that rearrangements of the flexible N-terminus lead to a more elongated particle (Rg wild-type = 32.8 Å) as compared to K173A mutant (Rg K173A = 30.6 Å). This is in strong agreement with the *switch*SENSE analysis of the C3d binding characteristics, which show a reduced hydrodynamic diameter for K173A compared to WT (**Table 2**).

The *ab initio* low resolution models of the complex reconstructed from the highest concentration data using DAMMIF (35) showed a large cone shaped molecule with a volume of 124 nm³ (**Figure 4F**). The resolution of the reconstruction is estimated to be 29 ± 2 Å (36). The large base of the cone can accommodate the crystal structure of

Sbi-IV:C3d complex (2wy8) (34). The extra space at the tip of the cone would be sufficient to harbor the 60 N-terminal residues comprising the Sbi-III domain. A more detailed modeling was conducted with the program Coral (37), utilizing the available high-resolution model of Sbi-IV:C3d and allowing for 60 additional beads to be added that mimic the missing Sbi-III domain. Twenty independent Coral runs were performed which all yielded models with a more or less structured N-terminal region, suggesting that Sbi-III-IV(K173A) in complex with C3d is conformationally restricted compared to wild-type Sbi-III-IV. This is further supported by the narrow distributions obtained with EOM (**Figure S4B**). Surprisingly, whilst repeating these analyses using a proposed alternative binding mode of the Sbi-IV:C3d complex (represented by 2wy7), where Sbi-IV is seen bound at the convex face of C3d, the $\chi^2$ value is greatly improved (**Figure S4C**). With this modeling approach a similar restricted conformation is observed for the N-terminus of Sbi-III-IV(K173A). Further studies are currently being conducted to further investigate the potential physiological relevance of this alternative Sbi-IV:C3d binding mode.

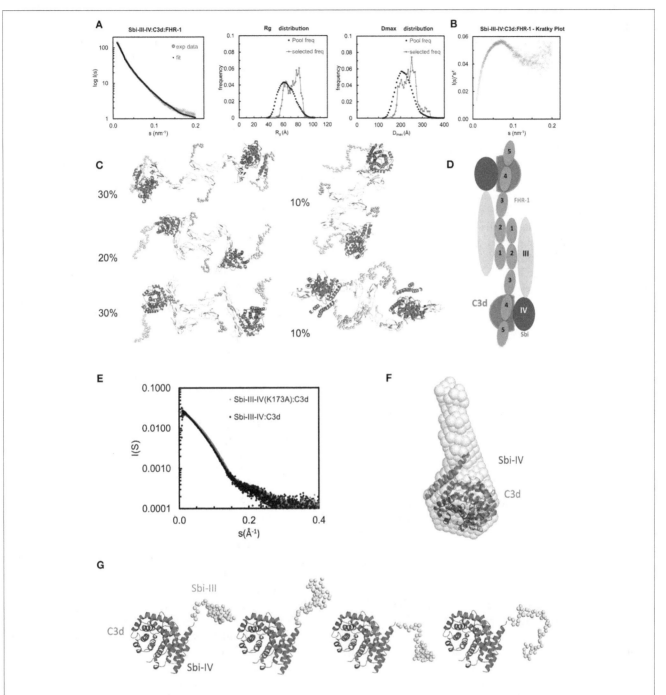

**FIGURE 4 |** Structural analysis of the Sbi-III-IV:C3d:FHR-1 tripartite complex. SAXS solution structure analysis and EOM modeling of the Sbi-III-IV:C3d:FHR-1 tripartite complex: **(A)** Left panel, fit of the selected ensemble of conformers to the experimental scattering. Radius of gyration (Rg, middle panel), particle maximum dimension (Dmax, right panel), and distribution histograms of the selected conformers vs. the pool. **(B)** Kratky plot of the tripartite complex. **(C)** Examples of rigid body models of the selected conformers corresponding to the histogram peaks. The volume fraction of each species is indicated. The relative positions of C3d, Sbi-III-IV, and FHR-1 in the dimeric tripartite complex are indicated, with C3d in red, Sbi-IV in dark blue, Sbi-III in turquoise and FHR-1 in orange. **(D)** Schematic representation of the dimeric Sbi-III-IV:C3d:FHR-1 tripartite complex. **(E)** Comparison of the solutions structure of wild-type Sbi-III-IV:C3d and mutated version Sbi-III-IV(K173A):C3d of the dual complex. Radius of gyration (Rg), particle maximum dimension (Dmax), and distribution histograms of the selected conformers vs. the pool are shown in **Figure S4A**. **(F)** Ab initio shape reconstruction shown as gray spheres in comparison to the partial crystal structure Sbi-IV:C3d (2wy8). **(G)** Examples of rigid body models. Complete set of models as well as flexibility assessment is presented in **Figure S5**. C3d in shown red, Sbi-IV in dark blue, and Sbi-III in turquoise.

## A Fusion Construct of Sbi-III-IV With *M. tuberculosis* Ag85b Activates the AP

To test the potential of Sbi-III-IV to induce C3d opsonisation in a vaccine setting, a recombinant construct was designed whereby Sbi-III-IV is fused to *Mycobacterium* protein Ag85b (**Figure 5A**, and detailed in **Figure S5A**). Based on the SAXS structure of the Sbi-III-IV:C3d:FHR-1 tripartite complex, revealing the importance of a flexible and extended conformation of Sbi domain III, we decided to attach Ag85b at the C-terminus of Sbi domain IV and included a long flexible linker between Sbi-IV and Ag85b to ensure accessibility and flexibility of the functional domains. Expressed and purified fusion protein was subsequently structurally and functionally characterized.

Circular dichroism analysis of the Sbi-III-IV-Ag85b fusion indicates that the protein construct is folded and that the secondary structural elements of both parent proteins have been preserved (**Figure S5B**). SAXS data obtained for the fusion protein demonstrate that both the Ag85b domain as well as Sbi-IV domain are accessible (**Figure 5B** and **Figure S5C**).

Functional activity of the Sbi-III-IV-Ag85b fusion construct was assessed using an AP complement activity assays (WIESLAB, Euro Diagnostica), showing strong C3 depletion activity (**Figure S5D**), whilst Ag85b on its own showed no complement activating properties. These results confirm that the complement activating properties of Sbi III-IV are not impaired as part of the fusion construct. The western blot analyses presented in **Figure 5C** and **Figure S5E** confirm these results, showing both C3 activation and opsonisation by the Sbi-III-IV-Ag85b fusion construct when incubated with NHS. Interestingly, C3 activation, and consumption occur more rapidly with the fusion construct when compared to Sbi-III-IV (**Figures 1A,B**) under the same conditions. Whilst Sbi-III-IV shows opsonisation with a single molecule of C3b (**Figure 1B**), the Sbi-III-IV-Ag85b fusion is opsonized by 2 molecules of C3b that over time degrade to iC3b and C3d (**Figure 5C** and **Figure S5E**). Interestingly, opsonisation of Ag85b with C3 fragments also occurs when co-incubated with Sbi-III-IV in NHS.

## Sbi-III-IV Acts as an Adjuvant in Mice When Immunized With Ag85b

Based on the ability of Sbi-III-IV to activate complement [**Figures 1B,C** (human serum) and **Figure 6A** (mouse serum)] and opsonise Ag85b with complement C3 break down fragments (**Figure 5C**), we expected that this new fusion protein when injected into mice would elicit a greater immune response to the Sbi-III-IV-Ag85b fusion protein than Ag85b administered alone (in PBS). Indeed, wild-type C57bl/6 mice immunized I.P. (or I.V., data not shown) with Sbi-III-IV-Ag85b generated a >4 fold increase in immune response initially and following the boost when compared to Ag85b alone (**Figure 6B**). Furthermore, when mice were immunized with a mixture of Sbi-III-IV and Ag85b (not fused together), this also resulted in a significantly improved immune response, corroborating the role of C3 fragment opsonisation of the antigen in this process (see **Figure S5E**). Subsequent, studies using C3$^{-/-}$ and Cr2$^{-/-}$ mice clearly demonstrated that C3 and C3 breakdown fragment

receptors (CR1 and CR2) were essential for this "adjuvant" function, respectively (**Figure 6C**). Overall, these data clearly suggest that complement AP dysregulation function of the Sbi-III-IV domain can be harnessed to improve immune responses through the coating of antigens with C3 breakdown fragments.

## DISCUSSION

Previous work from our group (24) revealed that *Staphylococcus aureus* immunomodulator Sbi binds complement component C3 within the thioester domain of C3 or the C3dg portion of the molecule and resulted in futile consumption of C3 via uncontrolled activation of the AP. In this study, we endeavored to both understand the mechanism of action of Sbi-III-IV and harness it; in order to develop pro-vaccines which would trigger natural complement activation and thereby coat antigen surfaces with complement component C3 degradation products, generate anaphylatoxins at the site of immunization and strongly enhance the immunogenicity of antigens (**Figure 6D**).

The seminal studies by Pepys (38), using C3 activating/depleting agents including cobra venom factor and Zymosan, clearly demonstrated intact C3 function was important for the T-dependent response (38). A molecular mechanism explaining this effect was established by Fearon and Carter (39) supported by studies in both C3 (40) and *Cr2* (complement receptor type I and II) knock-out mice (41). Dempsey et al. exploited these findings and established that multiple copies of C3d, in a linear trimer, could enhance antigen-specific responses up to 10,000 fold (3). However, the initial potential of trimeric C3d, as a highly potent molecular adjuvant, has not been realized and the reason(s) for this remain(s) unclear. One possible explanation is that the artificial linear trimer structure fails to represent naturally opsonised antigen, and consequently does not provide sufficient CR cross-linking or additional inflammatory signals for the B cell (or APC) activation threshold to be reached. One possible approach to overcome this is attaching more C3d to test antigens, but that approach is also limited (42). In the light of these and other findings (11, 13, 43), we considered that with understanding of the mode of action of Sbi-III-IV we might be able to develop a new complement activation based immune adjuvant.

The first clue to a mechanism for Sbi's ability to rapidly activate the AP came from monitoring Sbi-III-IV treated NHS in a time course using anti-C3 and anti-Sbi immuno-blotting. Here, we demonstrated that metastable C3b not only attaches covalently to serum proteins but also to Sbi-III-IV itself; as a transacylation target (**Figure 1**). This makes sense in the respect that Sbi's affinity to C3 obviously places it in close proximity to the site of complement turnover and we speculate that C3b deposited on Sbi-III-IV could help extend the fluid phase half-life of C3b, preventing FH, and FI from binding and inactivating as normal, perhaps similar to covalent adducts of C3b with IgG (44, 45).

However, as we have shown previously, Sbi-III-IV also interacts with complement regulators FH and FHR-1, in addition to binding C3b and its degradation products, thereby forming

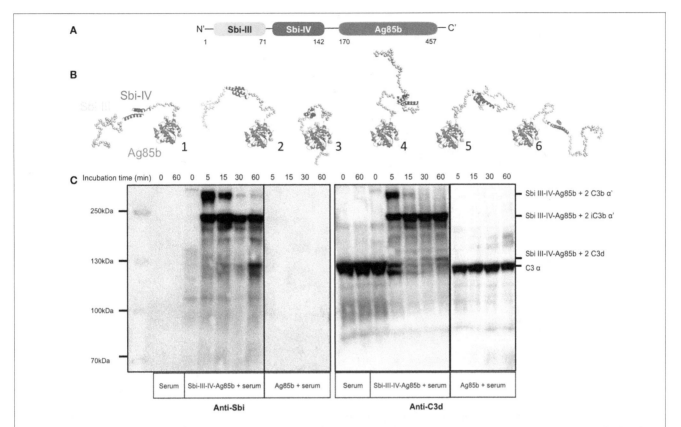

**FIGURE 5** | Structural and functional analysis of the Sbi-III-IV-Ag85b fusion protein. **(A)** Schematic structure of the Sbi-III-IV-Ag85b fusion protein (see details of the construct in **Figure S5**). **(B)** SAXS analysis of the fusion protein indicates a monomeric molecule with a radius of gyration of $R_g = 3.7$ nm and maximum particle size of $D_{max} = 15$ nm. The various molecular mass estimation range from 44 to 51 kDa and are comparable with a predicted monomer mass of 50 kDa. The 10 independent *ab initio* models obtained with DAMMIF are similar to each other, and according to the $\chi^2$ values that estimate the goodness of the fit, the final structures fit well with the experiment. More detailed modeling with Coral and EOM show that the flexibility of the missing structural information is restricted. **(C)** C3 activation and C3-fragment deposition in NHS after incubation with Sbi-III-IV-Ag85b (100 μM) or Ag85b (100 μM), visualized using anti-Sbi and anti-C3d western blot analysis. Resultant higher molecular weight bands with Sbi III-IV-Ag85b were identified as Sbi-III-IV-Ag85b with two covalently attached C3b α' chains; Sbi-III-IV-Ag85b with two iC3b α'-68 chains and Sbi-III-IV-Ag85b with two C3d molecules. Ag85b alone is unable to activate C3 as indicated by the presence of an intact C3 α-chain.

tripartite complexes (26). We next investigated whether Sbi-III-IV acts as a competitive antagonist of FH via the recruitment of FHR-1 and −5 into tripartite complexes and that FHR-1 can effectively displace FH from the tripartite complex. To this end, data from our systematic site-directed mutagenesis screen brought to light several Sbi mutants with complement activation defects (**Figure 1** and **Figure S1**). For instance, we demonstrated that an alanine substitution in Sbi domain III at position 173 resulted in a dramatic reduction in C3 consumption activity (**Figure 1G**). Notably, although a similar effect was observed with a previously identified mutation in domain IV with impaired C3d binding (R231A), K173A showed only slightly impaired C3d binding capacity (**Table 1**) suggesting a different mechanism. We therefore postulated that the K173A mutant would be ideal to elucidate the structural and functional role of Sbi domain III in the activation of complement and found that K173 in Sbi domain III was crucial for the recruitment of FHR-5 and that the K173A mutation only slightly affects FHR-1 binding (**Figures 2, 3**). These findings implicate a direct role of Sbi domain III in the tripartite complex formation with these FHRs and that this

likely occurs via interactions with the C-terminal SCR domains that share sequence identity with $FH_{19-20}$. We confirm this by showing that increasing concentrations of recombinant FHR-1, FHR-2, FHR-5, and $FH_{19-20}$ in serum indeed potentiate Sbi-III-IV mediated C3 consumption, whilst the N-terminal SCRs ($FHR-1_{1-2}$) fail to do this (**Figure 3**).

We also observed that Sbi greatly enhances the binding of FHRs to C3b, thereby antagonizing FH activity, as shown by the C3 convertase decay accelerating activity (DAA) assay (**Figures 3G,H**). These results imply that the FHR-1 or FHR-5 containing tripartite complexes can protect the AP C3 convertase, aiding the consumption of C3. These findings further enhance the notion that the FHR family has diversified AP de-regulatory functions, where FHR-1 seems more efficient in counteracting the DAA of FH, whilst in contrast FHR-5 potently antagonizes the cofactor activity (CA) of FH. The observed Sbi-III-IV mediated shift in the complement regulatory balance toward C3 activation could potentially be further enhanced by the formation of homo/heterodimeric forms of FHR-1 with itself and with other FHRs (FHR-2 and FHR-5) (12). These data

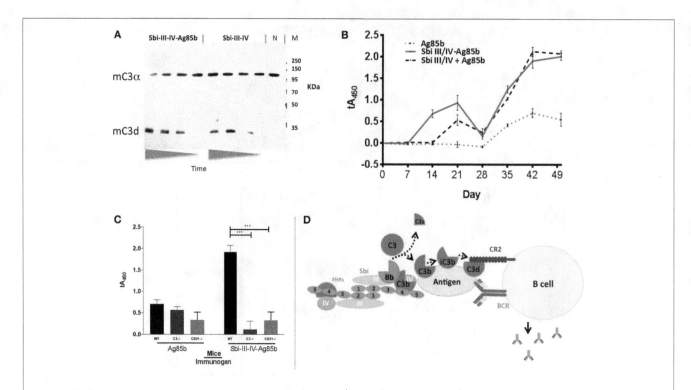

**FIGURE 6 |** Sbi-III-IV is an effective adjuvant in mice. **(A)** Freshly prepared CD21$^{-/-}$ mouse serum was mixed with Sbi-III-IV-Ag85b or just Sbi-III-IV. The reaction was stopped at various time points (0, 30, 60, 120 min). Western blot was developed with rabbit anti-C3 at 1/1000 and goat anti-rabbit at 1/2000. C3d is shown as confirmation that C3 has been activated and broken down. (N) is $Cr2^{-/-}$ serum incubated for 120 min with saline. **(B)** C57Bl/6 mice (groups of 6) where immunized intraperitoneally with either 2.7 μg Sbi-III-IV-Ag85b protein, 2 μg Ag85b, or 0.7 μg Sbi-III-IV plus 2 μg Ag85b in 150 mM NaCl solution, followed by weekly bleed and boosted (day 28) before terminal bleed at day 49. Serum IgG reactivity to Ag85b was measured over time by ELISA. Sera was diluted 1/50 and the mean absorbance ± SEM of each mouse group is shown. All data has been normalized to the day 0 average of all WT mice. **(C)** The previous experiment was repeated in C57Bl/6 mice deficient of C3 (C3$^{-/-}$)and complement receptor type I and 2 ($Cr2^{-/-}$). Data is representative of at least 2 repeats (***$P < 0.001$, Student's $T$-test, GraphPad Prism). **(D)** Schematic representation of the dimeric Sbi-III-IV:C3d:FHR-1 solution structure providing a nidus for AP C3 convertase generation that overwhelms local complement regulators, leading to the opsonisation of the nearby antigen surface by C3 break-down products that help facilitate the co-ligation of the B cell antigen receptor (BCR) with complement receptor 2 (CR2) thereby lowering the threshold for B cell activation.

link to an ongoing evolutionary "arms race" where FH was initially hijacked by *S. aureus* to protect it from complement (46) and then FHRs (devoid of intrinsic complement regulatory activity) were evolved/deployed by the host to compete with FH on that surface and restore complement opsonisation of the pathogen (22). Perhaps the release/secretion of Sbi from *S. aureus* is a more recent event in this arms race with the host, which takes the C3b/C3 convertase binding potential away from the bacterial surface and leads to local rapid fluid phase consumption of complement, i.e., local decomplementation and bacterial survival/propagation. Our understanding of the role and complexity of FHRs in immune evasion strategies is still in its infancy (46), but this study underlines the potency of another strategy in this process.

Using FHR-1 as a "model" dimerization domain containing FHR, structural analysis of the Sbi-III-IV:C3d:FHR-1 tripartite complex, using SAXS, indeed suggests the formation of a dimer mediated by FHR-1 domain 1 and 2 and provides details of the role of the extended unfolded nature of domain III in the binding of FHR-1 (**Figure 4**). The molecular basis of the preferential binding of FHR-1 over FH cannot easily be explained on the

basis of differences in amino acid sequence between the two complement regulators, since their C3d binding regions (SCR 4–5 of FHR-1 and SCR 19–20 of FH) share 99% sequence identity. However, our SAXS analyses, and binding studies using C3d(g) or iC3b as ligands (**Figures 3, 4**), indicate that the C-terminal regions of FHR proteins are readily exposed, unlike those of FH that exist in a "latent" conformation with the C-terminal part of the protein folded back and partially blocked (47–50). The dimeric physiological state of FHR-1 and the other FHRs tested in this study is also likely to enhance their ability, due to increased avidity, to assemble a tripartite complex.

Analysis of the hydrodynamic volume of the Sbi-III-IV:C3d complex using *switch*SENSE highlighted a significant contraction of the normally extended conformation Sbi-III-IV structure (34) caused by the K173A substitution in domain III (**Table 2**). SAXS analysis confirms these findings, showing a partially kinked N-terminal structure of domain III in K173A with reduced conformational freedom (**Figures 4E–G**). The contraction of the Sbi-III-IV structure caused by the K173A substitution suggests that the normally flexible and extended conformation of domain III plays an important role in the recruitment of FHRs, especially

FHR-5 into the tripartite complex after the initial interaction between Sbi-IV and C3b. Previous structural analyses of the Sbi's domain III, using NMR, revealed that this domain is indeed natively unfolded (51).

Based on the structural and functional information described here we decided to construct a Sbi-III-IV-Ag85b fusion construct that could be used to test its effect on the immune response against this model antigen *in vivo*. We chose *Mycobacterium tuberculosis* Ag85b, a fibronectin-binding protein with mycolyltransferase activity (52), because it is known to be immunogenic and previously suggested as a vaccine candidate (53). Indeed, there is evidence that Ag85b can elicit both humoral and cellular immune reactions in patients with TB, but there is conflicting evidence of its efficacy as a vaccine (54, 55), suggesting adjuvants may improve its overall immunogenicity. This target also gives scope to allow further testing in animal models of disease (56). Structural analysis, using Circular Dichroism and SAXS confirmed that secondary structural elements of both parent proteins have been preserved in the fusion protein construct and that the crucial functional Sbi domains are accessible for interactions with complement (**Figure 5** and **Figure S5**). We also show that the Sbi-III-IV-Ag85b fusion construct can induce AP activation and is opsonized with C3 breakdown products (**Figure 5C**).

With AP activation in human and mouse serum confirmed (**Figures 5, 6**), we opted to use straightforward immune response, IgG titer, analysis to demonstrate the potential of Sbi-III-IV to trigger complement *in vivo* and act as a vaccine adjuvant in a mouse model, in a similar manner to many previous studies (57). Our data herein firstly indicates that Sbi-III-IV can activate mouse complement in an analogous manner to that of the human complement system. This obviously allows direct analysis of these pro-vaccine compounds in both mouse and human model systems (a huge advantage to previous C3d based adjuvants) (13), indeed Sbi-III-IV has acted as a C3 activator in all species tested thus far (data not shown). As predicted from the *in vitro* work, the opsonisation of fusion proteins or co-immunized antigen by mouse complement breakdown fragments results in a significant increase in the immunogenicity of Ag85b, with increased IgG titres noted in the presence of fused or co-immunized Ag85b (**Figure 6**). The adjuvant function both increased the intensity of the response and the rate of the response when compared to Ag85b immunized alone. We will need to further explore the potency of this response to that of common adjuvants and with a mix of target antigens to fully assess the utility of Sbi-III-IV as a universal vaccine adjuvant. For instance, comparison of the action of Sbi-III-IV to the Glaxo-Smith-Kline's adjuvant systems, particularly AS01 (58), or to MF59 (59) may be of key interest and recent approaches may provide ideal pre-clinical model systems to facilitate this (60, 61) before progression to clinical studies. This is because our data provides evidence of a 4-fold increase in humoral response whilst AS01 has been demonstrated to have a much more significant effect of T cell effector function (58). The work is ongoing but the data herein demonstrate the initial proof of concept.

In summary, we have demonstrated that Sbi-III-IV triggers consumption of complement component C3 via activation of the alternative complement pathway, by acting as a competitive antagonist of FH via the recruitment of FHRs into dimeric tripartite complexes that can protect C3b bound to Sbi (**Figure 6D**). It is likely this provides a stable nidus for alternative pathway mediated C3 convertase generation, i.e., local fluid phase C3bBb generation that overwhelms any local complement regulators, providing the potential for bystander lysis, or opsonisation of surfaces. Our ability to harness this potential, targeting complement opsonisation to the surface of an antigen (in this case from *Mycobacterium*) and therefore use Sbi-III-IV as a vaccine adjuvant clearly demonstrates Sbi-III-IV has great potential for use with a range of antigens across multiple species, including humans, although more work remains to make that a reality.

## MATERIALS AND METHODS
### Proteins, Antibodies, and Sera

Factor H (FH), C3b, factor B (FB), factor D (FD), factor I (FI), properdin (FP), FI-depleted serum, goat anti-human C3 polyserum, and goat anti-human FB polyserum were purchased from Complement Technologies (Tyler, TX). FHR-$1_{1-2}$, FHR-1, $-2$, and $-5$ used in the tripartite complex reconstruction and binding competition assay were produced using Chinese Hamster ovary cell culture [as previously described Nichols et al. (62)]. Horse radish peroxidase (HRP)-conjugated rabbit anti-goat immunoglobulin polyserum and HRP-conjugated Streptavidin were acquired from Sigma Aldrich. HRP-conjugated goat anti-rabbit immunoglobulin G (Thermo Fisher, catalog no. 815-968-0747), HRP-conjugated rabbit anti-mouse immunoglobulin G (Thermo Fisher, catalog no. 31452) and biotin-conjugated FH monoclonal antibody OX24 (catalog no. MA5-17735) were purchased from Thermo Fisher Scientific. The goat anti-human FH polyclonal serum (catalog no. 341276-1 ml) that was previously used to detect human FH and FHR-1 was purchased from Merck Millipore. Human C3 was purified from mixed pool citrated human plasma (TCS Bioscience, PR100) using polyethylene glycol 4,000 precipitation, anion, and cation exchange chromatography as previously described (63). A pET15b-C3d construct was acquired from Prof. David E. Isenman and transformed into *Escherichia coli* (*E. coli*) stain BL21 (DE3), recombinant C3d was then expressed, and purified using a previously described protocol (64). Lyophilized normal human serum (NHS) was purchased from Euro Diagnostica (catalog no. PC300). Additional proteins and antibodies are described in the specific experimental section.

### Sbi-III-IV Constructs

The expression and purification of the N-terminally 6×His tagged recombinant Sbi-III-IV from a pQE30:*sbi-III-IV* construct were described previously (24).

## Sbi-III-IV Mutagenesis

Mutations in the Sbi-III-IV sequence were introduced using the QuikChange II XL site-directed mutagenesis kit (Agilent Technologies), the primers used are listed in **Table S1**. The mutated pQE30:*sbi-III-IV* plasmids were sequenced to confirm the success of the mutagenesis. SDS-PAGE profiles of all the Sbi-III-IV mutant proteins used in this study are shown in **Figure S1**.

## Sbi-III-IV Induced C3 Consumption Assay

Lyophilized NHS was re-suspended in chilled $dH_2O$ to a 2× concentration. Equal volumes of 2×NHS and Sbi (10 μM) were combined. Sbi treated sera were then incubated in a thermocycler at 37°C for 30 min. Treated serum samples were collected at time intervals, 0.5 μl of serum was loaded on an SDS-PAGE gel analyzed under reducing condition. The proteins were Western blotted, and the blots were probed with anti-C3d, anti-Sbi, anti-C3a or anti-factor B antibodies.

A hemolytic assay was modified from a previously published procedure (65) to measure Sbi induced consumption of C3. Briefly, rabbit erythrocytes (TCS Bioscience) were resuspended in GVB buffer (5 mM veronal, 145 mM NaCl, 10 μM EDTA, 0.1 % (w/v) gelatin) by washing three times via centrifugation at 600 g for 6 min. The concentration of rabbit red cells to be used in each experiment was determined by adding a stock of 5 μl of erythrocytes to 245 μl of water to give complete lysis and then re-adjusting cell concentration until an optical density reading of 0.7 ($A_{405}$) was reached. Lysis experiments were conducted in two steps, first, 15 μl of NHS, 5 μl of Mg$^+$-EGTA (70 mM MgCl$_2$, and 100 mM EGTA), 20 μl of protein in E2 buffer was mixed and pre-incubated at 37°C for 30 min. Subsequently, 5 μl of rabbit erythrocyte was added and incubated for an additional 30 min at 37°C. At the end of the incubation, 150 μl of quenching buffer (GVB supplemented with 10 mM EDTA) was added. The cells were pelleted by centrifugation at 1,500g for 10 min, and absorbance ($A_{405}$) of 100 μl of supernatant measured. Post-consumption lysis percentage was calculated as 100×(($A_{405}$ test sample-$A_{405}$ 0% control)/($A_{405}$ 100%-$A_{405}$ 0% control)).

## *In vitro* Complement Activation Assay in Mouse Serum

Mouse serum was collected from male $Cr2^{-/-}$ mice by cardiac puncture and allowed to clot fully on ice for 4 h followed by separation of serum by centrifugation at 2,000 g in a refrigerated centrifuge. Serum was then mixed with Sbi-III-IV or Sbi-III-IV-Ag85b, ensuring that the amount of Sbi-III-IV in each preparation was equivalent. The reaction was stopped at 0, 30, 60, and 120 min, by the addition of reducing sample buffer, boiled for 5 min and analyzed on a 10% SDS-PAGE gel. After transfer to nitrocellulose the blots were probed with Rabbit anti-C3d (1/1000, DAKO, A0063) and Goat anti-Rabbit-HRPO (1/2000, 111-035-046-JIR, Stratech), developed with ECL substrate (Pierce), and exposed to X-Ray film for 2 min.

## Binding Kinetics and Hydrodynamic Diameter Analysis

A *switch*SENSE DRX 2,400 instrument (Dynamic Biosensors) was used to characterize the binding kinetics and protein size changes based on *switch*SENSE technology (66, 67). Purified Sbi-III-IV-cys, K173A, R231A, and their ligand C3d were sent to Dynamic Biosensor's protein analyzing facility for binding kinetic and hydrodynamic diameter analysis. In the case of a protein binding event, based on the real-time measurements of the switching dynamics in a range of ligand concentrations, binding rate constants ($k_{ON}$ and $k_{OFF}$) and dissociation constants ($K_D$) can be analyzed (67). Alternatively, under saturated binding conditions, the switching dynamic of the protein (or protein complex) can be compared with the switching dynamics of bare DNA and with a biophysical model with which the size of the immobilized protein (or protein complex) can be determined. For determination of Sbi-III-IV:C3d binding kinetic parameters, 130, 100, 70, and 40 nM of C3d were applied sequentially onto the Sbi-III-IV immobilized microchip. All Sbi:C3d complexes' hydrodynamic diameters were estimated at a C3d concentration of 130 nM.

## Fluorometric C3b Breakdown Assay

Fluorometric C3b breakdown assay was performed using a black 96 well microplate (Thermofisher, M33089) in a TECAN Spark 20 M temperature-controlled fluorescence plate reader. Excitation was at 386 nm and emission was recorded at 475 nm with a 20 nm bandwidth. The control C3b breakdown rate, performed in PBS, contained 100 μl of 1 μM C3b, 160 nM FH, 17 nM of FI and 10 μM ANS, and was scanned every 5 s for 15 min. To study the interruption of C3b breakdown, 32 nM of FHR was either added alone or in combination with 1 μM of Sbi-III-IV. Data were collected at 25°C, normalized by Excel using the equation "Percentage of C3b=(($F_X$-($F_{15min}$))/($F_{15min}$-$F_{0min}$))*100" and plotted by Graphpad Prism.

## Small Angle X-ray Scattering Analysis

Synchrotron radiation X-ray scattering from solutions of the Sbi-III-IV:C3d:FHR-1 tripartite complex, the Sbi-III-IV(K173A):C3d complex, and the Sbi-III-IV-Ag85b fusion protein were collected at the EMBL P12 beamline of the storage ring PETRA III (DESY, Hamburg, Germany). Images were collected using a photon counting Pilatus-2M detector and a sample to detector distance of 3.1 m and a wavelength (λ) of 0.12 nm covering the range of momentum transfer (s) $0.1 < s < 4.5$ nm$^{-1}$; with s=4πsinθ/λ. Different solute concentrations were measured using a continuous flow cell capillary. To monitor radiation damage, 20 successive 50 ms exposures were compared and frames displaying significant alterations were discarded. The data were normalized to intensity of the transmitted beam and radially averaged; the scattering of the buffer was subtracted, and the different curves were scaled for solute concentration. The forward scattering I(0), the radius of gyration (Rg) along with the probability distribution of the particle [p(r)] and the maximal dimension ($D_{max}$) were computed using the automated SAXS data analysis pipeline SASFLOW (68).

For the Sbi-III-IV-Ag85b fusion protein data quality was improved with SEC-SAXS mode and the parallel analysis of light scattering data in a similar manner as described in Gräwert et al. (69). Frames comprising solely the monomeric version of the fusion protein were averaged and used for further processing after background subtraction.

The molecular masses (MM) were evaluated by comparison of the forward scattering with that from a reference solution of BSA and based on the Porod volumes of the constructs. With SAXS, the former estimation of MM is within an error of 10%, provided the sample and standard concentrate are determined accurately. DAMMIF was used to compute the *ab initio* shape models. For this, 10 independent models fitting the experimental scattering curves were generated and compared to each other. More detailed modeling was obtained with Coral. Here, existing partial crystal structure of the Sbi-IV:C3d complex was extended with 60 additional beads placed at the N-terminus of Sbi-IV to mimic the missing Sbi-III domain. Here too, 10 independent runs were performed, and the degree of variation addressed. Further analysis of the flexibility of the samples was addressed with Ensemble Optimization Method (EOM). For this, ensembles of models with variable conformations are selected from a pool of randomly generated models such that the scattering from the ensemble fits the experimental data, and the distributions of the overall parameters (e.g., $D_{max}$) in the selected pool are compared to the original pool.

The proteins in the Sbi-III-IV:C3d:FHR-1 tripartite complex were combined 1:1:1 at a concentration of $45\,\mu M$. The Sbi-III-IV(K173A):C3d complex were formed at a 1:1 ratio at $240\,\mu M$ (12 mg/ml). PDB structure 2wy8 (Sbi-IV:C3d complex) was used to model the complex using and compared with SAXS data previously recorded (34). The Sbi-III-IV-Ag85b fusion protein was provided at 29, 72, and $145\,\mu M$ concentrations (1.45, 3.6, and 7.2 mg/ml, respectively). The samples were dialysed against PBS, which was also used for background subtraction. From all samples concentration series were measured to exclude any concentration dependent alterations.

## Surface Plasmon Resonance Analysis

Tripartite complexes were analyzed by surface plasmon resonance (SPR) technology using a Biacore S200 (GE Healthcare). All experiments were conducted at 25°C on CM5 chips, using HBST (10 mM HEPES, 150 mM NaCl, and 0.005% Tween 20, pH 7.4) as running buffer, which was optionally supplemented with 1 mM of $MgCl_2$ ($HBST^+$) to be compatible with AP amplification condition. On the chip surface 800 RU of C3b was opsonized via AP C3 convertase through a method described before (70, 71). The iC3b surface was produced by injecting of repetitive cycles of FH and FI across a C3b opsonized surface, the completeness of the conversion was confirmed by the inability of FB binding. A separate chip surface was made by amine coupling 600 RU of recombinant C3d (CompTech, USA). In all SPR experiments, response differences were derived using the signal from a flow cell to subtract the parallel reading from a reference flow cell that blocked with carbodiimide, N-hydroxysuccinimide and ethanolamine. Analytes were injected in duplicate (at $30\,\mu l/min$ for 200 s) followed by running buffer for 300 s and a regeneration phase involving injection of regeneration buffer (10 mM sodium acetate, 1 M NaCl pH 4.0) for 60 s. To analyze Sbi-III-IV binding and the assembly of tripartite complex, concentration series of Sbi-III-IV WT or K173A were flowed cross separately or co-injected with FH, FHR-1, FHR-2, FHR-5, or $FH_{19-20}$ at a fixed concentration (100, 12.5, 20, 25, or 20 nM, respectively).

The C3 convertase DAA assay was performed on a CM5 chip amine coupled with 500 RU C3b, using $HBST^+$ as running buffer throughout. A mixture of analytes for building C3 convertase were flowed across, including FB and FD in addition to various FH reagent combinations (FH or FH and FHR-1 or FH, FHR-1 and −5). The various FH reagents combinations were also flow across separately in order to derive the sensorgram for C3 convertase. To examining Sbi bound C3 convertase, $2\,\mu M$ of wild-type Sbi-III-IV was added to the mixture of analytes for building C3 convertase. The various FH reagent combinations spiked with Sbi were flowed across separately in order to derive the sensorgram for Sbi bound C3 convertase. Each injection cycle includes Injection of the C3 convertase mixture for 200–300 s, followed by running buffer for 300–400 s and two consecutive 60 s regeneration phases.

## FH/FHR-1 Competition Assay

C3b was diluted in carbonate buffer (pH 9.5) and coated on to wells of a Nunc MaxiSorp plate ($0.25\,\mu g$/well) for 16 h at 4°C. The wells were blocked with PBST (PBS with 0.1% Tween 20) supplemented with and 2% BSA for 1 h at 37°C, and then washed with PBST buffer. Doubly diluted concentration series (9-600 nM) of FHRs, $FH_{19-20}$, $FHR-1_{1-2}$ in PBST-2% BSA were then added to the wells, together with a constant concentration of FH (25 nM) and Sbi-III-IV (1,000 nM). The plate was incubated for 1 h at 37°C, then washed with PBST. Fifty microliter of monoclonal anti-FH antibody OX-24 (specific to the FH SCR domain 5) diluted with PBS-2% BSA ($0.6\,\mu g$/ml) was added to the wells and the plate incubated for a further 1 h. The wells were washed with PBST, and 50 μl sheep anti-mouse IgG (1:5000 dilution in PBST-2% BSA) was added to the wells for 1 h at 37°C. The wells were washed again and the conjugate was detected using TMB ELISA substrate solution, which was added to the wells for 5 min. The color reaction was stopped by 10% $H_2SO_4$ and the plate was read at $A_{450}$ using a plate reader.

## Design and Purification of the Sbi-III-IV-Ag85b Fusion Construct

The DNA sequence coding for Sbi-III-IV ($sbi_{448-798}$) was fused to the 5' end of the DNA sequence for Ag85b ($ag85b_{121-975}$) via a linker region of 84 bp (**Figure S5A**). The fusion gene was commercially synthesized and ligated into the pET15b vector, containing an ampicillin resistance cassette and a T7 promoter. The pET15b:*sbi-III-IV-ag85b* plasmid was verified using sequencing, and the resulting construct encoded an N-terminally his-tagged Sbi-III-IV-Ag85b protein. *E. coli* BL21 (DE3) cells harboring the pET15b:*sbi-III-IV-ag85b* plasmid were grown in LB broth supplemented with $100\,\mu g$/ml ampicillin to an $A_{600} = 0.4$–0.6. Protein expression was induced with 0.5 mM IPTG and by incubating the cells at 17°C for 16 h. Bacteria were harvested, lysed using sonication (80% amplitude, for six 10 s bursts) in the presence of protease inhibitor cocktail (set VII-Calbiochem, Merck), and the protein initially purified using nickel-affinity chromatography (His-Trap column, GE Healthcare) with a gradient of 0–0.5 M imidazole in 50 mM Tris, 150 mM NaCl, pH 7.4. It was further purified using size-exclusion chromatography (Hi-Load 16/60 Superdex

S200 column, GE Healthcare) equilibrated in 20 mM Tris, 150 mM NaCl, pH 7.4. Fractions containing protein were pooled and concentrated. Protein concentration was measured at $A_{280}$.

## Analysis of Sbi-III-IV-Ag85b Fusion Protein AP Complement Activity

Alternative pathway (AP) activity of Sbi III-IV-Ag85b-treated NHS samples was analyzed using the ELISA-based WIESLAB® (Euro Diagnostica) complement system AP assay. Sbi-III-IV-Ag85b was mixed with normal human serum (NHS) at a 1:1 volume ratio and incubated for 30 min at 37°C in a thermal cycler. Treated serum was then diluted with AP diluent (blocking the activation of the other two complement pathways) by 1 in 20. From this point the manufacturer's instructions were followed. A blank (AP diluent), positive control (NHS) and negative control (heat-inactivated NHS) were also recorded. Complement activation was converted to residual AP activity (%) using the equation: (sample - negative control)/(positive control - negative control) × 100.

## Analysis of C3 Fragment Deposition on Sbi-III-IV-Ag85b Fusion Protein

The method used is similar to that described for WT Sbi-III-IV. Lyophilised NHS (Euro Diagnostica) was re-suspended in chilled $dH_2O$. Sbi-III-IV-Ag85b (100 μM) was mixed with NHS in a 1:1 ratio, and incubated for 1 h at 37°C in a thermocycler. Samples were taken at regular intervals (0, 5, 15, 30, and 60 min), and separated by SDS-PAGE followed by Western blot analysis using either rabbit anti-Sbi (1.5:5000 dilution), rabbit anti-C3d (1.5:5000 dilution) or mouse anti-Ag85b (1:1000 dilution) polyclonal antibodies and detected using HRP-conjugated secondary antibodies (1:2500 goat anti rabbit or 1:1000 goat anti mouse). NHS-only was used as a negative control.

## Measurement of Immune Response to Sbi-III-IV-Ag85b Fusion Protein

Eight week old male C57bl/6 mice (wild-type, $C3^{-/-}$ and $Cr2^{-/-}$) were bled by tail vein venesection at day−2. Mice were then immunized at day 0 with molar equivalent doses of Ag85b alone (2 μg, a sub-optimal dose without adjuvant or boost, data not shown), Sbi-III-IV-Ag85b (fusion protein), Sbi-III-IV alone or a mixture of Sbi-III-IV and Ag85b, as appropriate. Mice were then bled weekly thereafter and plasma stored at −80°C until required for batch analysis. Mice were boosted at day 28 and sacrificed at day 42.

For analysis of IgG response to Ag85b by ELISA, 96 well plates (NUNC maxisorb) were coated with 1 μg/ml Ag85b (Abcam, UK) or 1.35 μg/ml Sbi-III-IV-Ag85b in carbonate buffer at 50 μl per well and incubated at 4°C for 16 h. Plates were washed with 0.01% PBS-Tween and a 1% BSA blocking solution was applied for 1 h at 20°C. Serum samples were diluted to 1/50 or 1/100 in 0.01% PBS-Tween, added at 50 μl per well and incubated for 1 h at 20°C. Plates were washed and secondary antibody (sheep anti mouse IgG-HRPO, 515-035-071-JIR, Stratech, UK) was added at 1/100 dilution, 50 μl per well and incubated for 1 h at 20°C. TMB substrate (50 μl per well) was added and allowed to develop for 6 min. The reaction was stopped by the addition of 100 μl 10% $H_2SO_4$ per well and plates were read at $A_{450}$. A mouse monoclonal anti-Ag85b (Abcam, ab43019) used as a positive control. The mean absorbance ± SEM of each mouse group is shown. Data for each mouse, at time 0, has been normalized to the day 0 average reactivity to Ag85b in all mice screened.

# AUTHOR CONTRIBUTIONS

JvdE, AGW, and KM conceived the idea of the project. YY, KM, and JvdE designed the experiments. YY, CB, AAW, RK, and JP performed and analyzed the experiments. KW and WK conducted and analyzed the *switch*SENSE experiments. MG and DS conducted SAXS experiments and oversaw the structural analysis. RK, HD, JP, and KM conducted the *in vivo* experiments. AS and AGW significantly contributed to the discussions about the overall project. YY, CB, KM, and JvdE wrote and edited the manuscript, with significant contributions from AAW, MG, and DS.

# ACKNOWLEDGMENTS

This research was funded by the Biotechnology and Biological Sciences Research Council (BBSRC Follow On Fund BB/N022165/1, awarded to JvdE and KM). AAW was supported by a Ph.D. scholarship granted Raoul and Catherine Hughes and the University of Bath Alumni. KM, HD, and RW were also supported by the MRC and Newcastle University's Confidence in Concept funding. AS thanks the Royal Society URF and Alumni Fund at the University of Bath for funding. MG was supported by the EMBL interdisciplinary Postdoc Programme under Marie Curie COFUND Actions as well as the Horizon 2020 programme of the European Union, iNEXT (H2020 Grant # 653706).

# REFERENCES

1. Green TD, Newton BR, Rota PA, Xu Y, Robinson HL, Ross TM. C3d enhancement of neutralizing antibodies to measles hemagglutinin. *Vaccine* (2001) 20:242–8. doi: 10.1016/S0264-410X(01)00266-3

2. Ross GD. Regulation of the adhesion versus cytotoxic functions of the Mac-1/CR3/alphaMbeta2-integrin glycoprotein. *Crit Rev Immunol.* (2000) 20:197–222. doi: 10.1615/CritRevImmunol.v20.i3.20

3. Dempsey PW, Allison ME, Akkaraju S, Goodnow CC, Fearon DT. C3d of complement as a molecular adjuvant: bridging innate and acquired immunity. *Science* (1996) 271:348–50. doi: 10.1126/science.271.5247.348

4. Fang Y, Xu C, Fu YX, Holers VM, Molina H. Expression of complement receptors 1 and 2 on follicular dendritic cells is necessary for the generation of a strong antigen-specific IgG response. *J Immunol.* (1998) 160:5273–9.

5. Carroll MC, Isenman DE. Regulation of humoral immunity by complement. *Immunity* (2012) 37:199–207. doi: 10.1016/j.immuni.2012.08.002

6. Roozendaal R, Carroll MC. Complement receptors CD21 and CD35 in humoral immunity. *Immunol Rev.* (2007) 219:157–66. doi: 10.1111/j.1600-065X.2007.00556.x

7. Popi AF, Longo-Maugeri IM, Mariano M. An overview of B-1 cells as antigen-presenting cells. *Front Immunol.* (2016) 7:138. doi: 10.3389/fimmu.2016.00138

8. Chan OT, Madaio MP, Shlomchik MJ. B cells are required for lupus nephritis in the polygenic, Fas-intact MRL model of systemic autoimmunity. *J Immunol.* (1999) 163:3592–6.

9. Ron Y, De Baetselier P, Gordon J, Feldman M, Segal S. Defective induction of antigen-reactive proliferating T cells in B cell-deprived mice. *Eur J Immunol.* (1981) 11:964–8. doi: 10.1002/eji.1830111203

10. Ron Y, De Baetselier P, Tzehoval E, Gordon J, Feldman M, Segal S. Defective induction of antigen-reactive proliferating T cells in B cell-deprived mice. II. Anti-mu treatment affects the initiation and recruitment of T cells. *Eur J Immunol.* (1983) 13:167–71. doi: 10.1002/eji.1830130214

11. De Groot AS, Ross TM, Levitz L, Messitt TJ, Tassone R, Boyle CM, et al. C3d adjuvant effects are mediated through the activation of C3d-specific autoreactive T cells. *Immunol Cell Biol.* (2015) 93:189–97. doi: 10.1038/icb.2014.89

12. Carter RH, Fearon DT. Polymeric C3dg primes human B lymphocytes for proliferation induced by anti-IgJ. *Immunol M.* (1989) 143:1755–60.

13. He YG, Pappworth IY, Rossbach A, Paulin J, Mavimba T, Hayes C, et al. A novel C3d-containing oligomeric vaccine provides insight into the viability of testing human C3d-based vaccines in mice. *Immunobiology* (2018) 223:125–34. doi: 10.1016/j.imbio.2017.10.002

14. van den Elsen JM, Isenman DE. A crystal structure of the complex between human complement receptor 2 and its ligand C3d. *Science* (2011) 332:608–11. doi: 10.1126/science.1201954

15. Janssen BJ, Huizinga EG, Raaijmakers HC, Roos A, Daha MR, Nilsson-Ekdahl K, et al. Structures of complement component C3 provide insights into the function and evolution of immunity. *Nature* (2005) 437:505–11. doi: 10.1038/nature04005

16. Janssen BJ, Christodoulidou A, McCarthy A, Lambris JD, Gros P. Structure of C3b reveals conformational changes that underlie complement activity. *Nature* (2006) 444:213–6. doi: 10.1038/nature05172

17. Forneris F, Ricklin D, Wu J, Tzekou A, Wallace RS, Lambris JD, et al. Structures of C3b in complex with factors B and D give insight into complement convertase formation. *Science* (2010) 330:1816–20. doi: 10.1126/science.1195821

18. Wu J, Wu YQ, Ricklin D, Janssen BJ, Lambris JD, Gros P. Structure of complement fragment C3b-factor H and implications for host protection by complement regulators. *Nat Immunol.* (2009) 10:728–33. doi: 10.1038/ni.1755

19. Morgan HP, Schmidt CQ, Guariento M, Blaum BS, Gillespie D, Herbert AP, et al. Structural basis for engagement by complement factor H of C3b on a self surface. *Nat Struct Mol Biol.* (2011) 18:463–70. doi: 10.1038/nsmb.2018

20. Kajander T, Lehtinen MJ, Hyvärinen S, Bhattacharjee A, Leung E, Isenman DE, et al. Dual interaction of factor H with C3d and glycosaminoglycans in host-nonhost discrimination by complement. *Proc Natl Acad Sci USA* (2011) 108:2897–902. doi: 10.1073/pnas.1017087108

21. Goicoechea de Jorge E, Caesar JJ, Malik TH, Patel M, Colledge M, Johnson S, et al. Dimerization of complement factor H-related proteins modulates complement activation *in vivo*. *Proc Natl Acad Sci USA* (2013) 110:4685–90. doi: 10.1073/pnas.1219260110

22. Józsi M, Tortajada A, Uzonyi B, Goicoechea de Jorge E, Rodríguez de Córdoba S. Factor H-related proteins determine complement-activating surfaces. *Trends Immunol.* (2015) 36:374–84. doi: 10.1016/j.it.2015.04.008

23. Xue X, Wu J, Ricklin D, Forneris F, Di Crescenzio P, Schmidt CQ, et al. Regulator-dependent mechanisms of C3b processing by factor I allow differentiation of immune responses. *Nat Struct Mol Biol.* (2017) 24:643–51. doi: 10.1038/nsmb.3427

24. Burman JD, Leung E, Atkins KL, O'Seaghdha MN, Lango L, Bernadó P, et al. Interaction of human complement with Sbi, a staphylococcal immunoglobulin-binding protein indications of a novel mechanism of complement evasion by Staphylococcus aureus. *J Biol Chem.* (2008) 283:17579–93. doi: 10.1074/jbc.M800265200

25. Smith EJ, Corrigan RM, van der Sluis T, Gründling A, Speziale P, Geoghegan JA, et al. The immune evasion protein Sbi of Staphylococcus aureus occurs both extracellularly and anchored to the cell envelope by binding lipoteichoic acid. *Mol Microbiol.* (2012) 83:789–804. doi: 10.1111/j.1365-2958.2011.07966.x

26. Haupt K, Reuter M, van den Elsen J, Burman J, Hälbich S, Richter J, et al. The Staphylococcus aureus Protein Sbi acts as a complement inhibitor and forms a tripartite complex with host complement factor H, and C3b. *Plos Pathogens* (2008) 4:e1000250. doi: 10.1371/journal.ppat.1000250

27. Csincsi ÁI, Kopp A, Zöldi M, Bánlaki Z, Uzonyi B, Hebecker M, et al. Factor H-related protein 5 interacts with pentraxin 3 and the extracellular matrix and modulates complement activation. *J Immunol.* (2015) 194:4963–73. doi: 10.4049/jimmunol.1403121

28. van Beek AE, Pouw RB, Brouwer MC, van Mierlo G, Geissler J, Ooijevaar-de Heer P, et al. Factor H-Related (FHR)-1 and FHR-2 Form Homo- and Heterodimers, while FHR-5 circulates only as homodimer in human plasma. *Front Immunol.* (2017) 8:1328. doi: 10.3389/fimmu.2017.01328

29. Isenman DE, Kells DI, Cooper NR, Müller-Eberhard HJ, Pangburn MK. Nucleophilic modification of human complement protein C3: correlation of conformational changes with acquisition of C3b-like functional properties. *Biochemistry* (1981) 20:4458–67. doi: 10.1021/bi00518a034

30. Pangburn MK, Muller-Eberhard HJ. Kinetic and thermodynamic analysis of the control of C3b by the complement regulatory proteins factors H and Biochemistry I. *Biochemistry* (1983) 22:178–85. doi: 10.1021/bi00270a026

31. McRae JL, Duthy TG, Griggs KM, Ormsby RJ, Cowan PJ, Cromer BA, et al. Human factor H-related protein 5 has cofactor activity, inhibits C3 convertase activity, binds heparin and C-reactive protein, and associates with lipoprotein. *J Immunol.* (2005) 174:6250–6. doi: 10.4049/jimmunol.174.10.6250

32. Tria G, Mertens HD, Kachala M, Svergun DI. Advanced ensemble modelling of flexible macromolecules using X-ray solution scattering. *IUCrJ* (2015) 2(Pt 2):207–17. doi: 10.1107/S205225251500202X

33. Morgan HP, Mertens HD, Guariento M, Schmidt CQ, Soares DC, Svergun DI, et al. Structural analysis of the C-terminal region (modules 18-20) of complement regulator factor H (FH). *PLoS ONE* (2012) 7:e32187. doi: 10.1371/journal.pone.0032187

34. Clark EA, Crennell S, Upadhyay A, Zozulya AV, Mackay JD, Svergun DI, et al. A structural basis for Staphylococcal complement subversion: X-ray structure of the complement-binding domain of Staphylococcus aureus

protein Sbi in complex with ligand C3d. *Mol Immunol.* (2011) 48:452–62. doi: 10.1016/j.molimm.2010.09.017

35. Franke D, Svergun DI. DAMMIF, a program for rapid ab-initio shape determination in small-angle scattering. *J Appl Crystallogr.* (2009) 42:342–6. doi: 10.1107/S0021889809000338

36. Tuukkanen AT, Kleywegt GJ, Svergun DI. Resolution of ab initio shapes determined from small-angle scattering. *IUCrJ* (2016) 3(Pt 6):440–7. doi: 10.1107/S2052252516016018

37. Petoukhov MV, Franke D, Shkumatov AV, Tria G, Kikhney AG, Gajda M, et al. New developments in the ATSAS program package for small-angle scattering data analysis. *J Appl Crystallogr.* (2012) 45:342–50. doi: 10.1107/S0021889812007662

38. Pepys MB. Role of complement in induction of antibody production *in vivo.* Effect of cobra factor and other C3-reactive agents on thymus-dependent and thymus-independent antibody responses. *J Exp Med.* (1974) 140:126–45. doi: 10.1084/jem.140.1.126

39. Fearon DT, Carter RH. The CD19/CR2/TAPA-1 complex of B lymphocytes: linking natural to acquired immunity. *Annu Rev Immunol.* (1995) 13:127–49. doi: 10.1146/annurev.iy.13.040195.001015

40. Wessels MR, Butko P, Ma M, Warren HB, Lage AL, Carroll MC. Studies of group B streptococcal infection in mice deficient in complement component C3 or C4 demonstrate an essential role for complement in both innate and acquired immunity. *Proc Natl Acad Sci USA* (1995) 92:11490–4. doi: 10.1073/pnas.92.25.11490

41. Ahearn JM, Fischer MB, Croix D, Goerg S, Ma M, Xia J, et al. Disruption of the Cr2 locus results in a reduction in B-1a cells and in an impaired B cell response to T-dependent antigen. *Immunity* (1996) 4:251–62. doi: 10.1016/S1074-7613(00)80433-1

42. Lee Y, Haas KM, Gor DO, Ding X, Karp DR, Greenspan NS, et al. Complement component C3d-antigen complexes can either augment or inhibit B lymphocyte activation and humoral immunity in mice depending on the degree of CD21/CD19 complex engagement. *J Immunol.* (2005) 175:8011–23. doi: 10.4049/jimmunol.175.12.8011

43. Suradhat S, Braun RP, Lewis PJ, Babiuk LA, van Drunen Littel-van den Hurk S, Griebel PJ, et al. Fusion of C3d molecule with bovine rotavirus VP7 or bovine herpesvirus type 1 glycoprotein D inhibits immune responses following DNA immunization. *Vet Immunol Immunopathol.* (2001) 83:79–92. doi: 10.1016/S0165-2427(01)00369-5

44. Fries LF, Gaither TA, Hammer CH, Frank MM. C3b covalently bound to IgG demonstrates a reduced rate of inactivation by factors H and I. *J Exp Med.* (1984) 160:1640–55. doi: 10.1084/jem.160.6.1640

45. Lutz HU, Jelezarova E. Complement amplification revisited. *Mol Immunol.* (2006) 43:2–12. doi: 10.1016/j.molimm.2005.06.020

46. Jozsi M. Factor H family proteins in complement evasion of microorganisms. *Front Immunol.* (2017) 8:571. doi: 10.3389/fimmu.2017.00571

47. Aslam M, Perkins SJ. Folded-back solution structure of monomeric factor H of human complement by synchrotron X-ray and neutron scattering, analytical ultracentrifugation and constrained molecular modelling. *J Mol Biol.* (2001) 309:1117–38. doi: 10.1006/jmbi.2001.4720

48. Oppermann M, Manuelian T, Józsi M, Brandt E, Jokiranta TS, Heinen S, et al. The C-terminus of complement regulator Factor H mediates target recognition: evidence for a compact conformation of the native protein. *Clin Exp Immunol.* (2006) 144:342–52. doi: 10.1111/j.1365-2249.2006.03071.x

49. Okemefuna AI, Gilbert HE, Griggs KM, Ormsby RJ, Gordon DL, Perkins SJ. The regulatory SCR-1/5 and cell surface-binding SCR-16/20 fragments of factor H reveal partially folded-back solution structures and different self-associative properties. *J Mol Biol.* (2008) 375:80–101. doi: 10.1016/j.jmb.2007.09.026

50. Makou E, Herbert AP, Barlow PN. Functional anatomy of complement factor H. *Biochemistry* (2013) 52:3949–62. doi: 10.1021/bi4003452

51. Upadhyay A, Burman JD, Clark EA, Leung E, Isenman DE, van den Elsen JM, et al. Structure-function analysis of the C3 binding region of staphylococcus aureus immune subversion protein Sbi. *J Biol Chem.* (2008) 283:22113–20. doi: 10.1074/jbc.M802636200

52. Belisle JT, Vissa VD, Sievert T, Takayama K, Brennan PJ, Besra GS. Role of the major antigen of *Mycobacterium tuberculosis* in cell wall biogenesis. *Science* (1997) 276:1420–2. doi: 10.1126/science.276.5317.1420

53. Palma C, Iona E, Giannoni F, Pardini M, Brunori L, Orefici G, et al. The Ag85B protein of *Mycobacterium tuberculosis* may turn a protective immune response induced by Ag85B-DNA vaccine into a potent but non-protective Th1 immune response in mice. *Cell Microbiol.* (2007) 9:1455–65. doi: 10.1111/j.1462-5822.2007.00884.x

54. Weinrich Olsen A, van Pinxteren LA, Meng Okkels L, Birk Rasmussen P, Andersen P. Protection of mice with a tuberculosis subunit vaccine based on a fusion protein of antigen 85b and esat-6. *Infect Immun.* (2001) 69:2773–8. doi: 10.1128/IAI.69.5.2773-2778.2001

55. Olsen AW, Williams A, Okkels LM, Hatch G, Andersen P. Protective effect of a tuberculosis subunit vaccine based on a fusion of antigen 85B and ESAT-6 in the aerosol guinea pig model. *Infect Immun.* (2004) 72:6148–50. doi: 10.1128/IAI.72.10.6148-6150.2004

56. Horwitz MA, Lee BW, Dillon BJ, Harth G. Protective immunity against tuberculosis induced by vaccination with major extracellular proteins of *Mycobacterium tuberculosis. Proc Natl Acad Sci USA* (1995) 92:1530–4. doi: 10.1073/pnas.92.5.1530

57. Toapanta FR, Ross TM. Complement-mediated activation of the adaptive immune responses: role of C3d in linking the innate and adaptive immunity. *Immunol Res.* (2006) 36:197–210. doi: 10.1385/IR:36:1:197

58. Montoya J, Solon JA, Cunanan SR, Acosta L, Bollaerts A, Moris P, et al. A randomized, controlled dose-finding Phase II study of the M72/AS01 candidate tuberculosis vaccine in healthy PPD-positive adults. *J Clin Immunol.* (2013) 33:1360–75. doi: 10.1007/s10875-013-9949-3

59. Seo YB, Choi WS, Lee J, Song JY, Cheong HJ, Kim WJ. Comparison of the immunogenicity and safety of the conventional subunit, MF59-adjuvanted, and intradermal influenza vaccines in the elderly. *Clin Vaccine Immunol.* (2014) 21:989–96. doi: 10.1128/CVI.00615-13

60. Kirkling ME, Cytlak U, Lau CM, Lewis KL, Resteu A, Khodadadi-Jamayran A, et al. Notch signaling facilitates invitro generation of cross-presenting classical dendritic cells. *Cell Rep.* (2018) 23:3658–72.e6. doi: 10.1016/j.celrep.2018.05.068

61. Cytlak U, Resteu A, Bogaert D, Kuehn HS, Altmann T, Gennery A, et al. Ikaros family zinc finger 1 regulates dendritic cell development and function in humans. *Nat Commun.* (2018) 9:1239. doi: 10.1038/s41467-018-02977-8

62. Nichols EM, Barbour TD, Pappworth IY, Wong EK, Palmer JM, Sheerin NS, et al. An extended mini-complement factor H molecule ameliorates experimental C3 glomerulopathy. *Kidney Int.* (2015) 88:1314–22. doi: 10.1038/ki.2015.233

63. Alsenz J, Avila D, Huemer HP, Esparza I, Becherer JD, Kinoshita T, et al. Phylogeny of the third component of complement, C3: analysis of the conservation of human CR1, CR2, H, and B binding sites, concanavalin A binding sites, and thiolester bond in the C3 from different species. *Dev Compar Immunol.* (1992) 16:63–76. doi: 10.1016/0145-305X(92)90052-E

64. Nagar B, Jones RG, Diefenbach RJ, Isenman DE, Rini JM. X-ray crystal structure of C3d: a C3 fragment and ligand for complement receptor 2. *Science* (1998) 280:1277–81. doi: 10.1126/science.280.5367.1277

65. Kerr H, Wong E, Makou E, Yang Y, Marchbank K, Kavanagh D, et al. Disease-linked mutations in factor H reveal pivotal role of cofactor activity in self-surface-selective regulation of complement activation. *J Biol Chem.* (2017) 292:13345–60. doi: 10.1074/jbc.M117.795088

66. Langer A, Hampel PA, Kaiser W, Knezevic J, Welte T, Villa V, et al. Protein analysis by time-resolved measurements with an electro-switchable DNA chip. *Nat Commun.* (2013) 4:1–8. doi: 10.1038/ncomms3099

67. Knezevic J, Langer A, Hampel PA, Kaiser W, Strasser R, Rant U. Quantitation of affinity, avidity, and binding kinetics of protein analytes with

a dynamically switchable biosurface. *J Am Chem Soc.* (2012) 134:15225–8. doi: 10.1021/ja3061276

68. Franke D, Kikhney AG, Svergun DI. Automated acquisition and analysis of small angle X-ray scattering data. *Nucl Inst Methods Phys Res Sect Acceler Spectrom Detect.* (2012) 689:52–9. doi: 10.1016/j.nima.2012.06.008

69. Gräwert MA, Franke D, Jeffries CM, Blanchet CE, Ruskule D, Kuhle K, et al. Automated pipeline for purification, biophysical and X-Ray analysis of biomacromolecular solutions. *Sci Rep.* (2015) 5:10734. doi: 10.1038/srep10734

70. Yang Y, Denton H, Davies OR, Smith-Jackson K, Kerr H, Herbert AP, et al. An Engineered complement factor H construct for treatment of C3 glomerulopathy. *J Am Soc Nephrol.* (2018) 29:1649–61. doi: 10.1681/ASN.2017091006

71. Harris CL, Abbott RJ, Smith RA, Morgan BP, Lea SM. Molecular dissection of interactions between components of the alternative pathway of complement and decay accelerating factor (CD55). *J Biol Chem.* (2005) 280:2569–78. doi: 10.1074/jbc.M410179200

# 3

# Repurposing of Drugs as Novel Influenza Inhibitors from Clinical Gene Expression Infection Signatures

Andrés Pizzorno [1,2†], Olivier Terrier [1*†], Claire Nicolas de Lamballerie [1,3], Thomas Julien [1,4], Blandine Padey [1,4], Aurélien Traversier [1], Magali Roche [3], Marie-Eve Hamelin [2], Chantal Rhéaume [2], Séverine Croze [5], Vanessa Escuret [1,6], Julien Poissy [7], Bruno Lina [1,6], Catherine Legras-Lachuer [3,8], Julien Textoris [9,10], Guy Boivin [2] and Manuel Rosa-Calatrava [1,4*]

[1] Virologie et Pathologie Humaine—VirPath Team, Centre International de Recherche en Infectiologie, INSERM U1111, CNRS UMR5308, ENS Lyon, Université Claude Bernard Lyon 1, Université de Lyon, Lyon, France, [2] Research Center in Infectious Diseases of the CHU de Quebec and Laval University, Quebec City, QC, Canada, [3] Viroscan3D SAS, Lyon, France, [4] VirNext, Faculté de Médecine RTH Laennec, Université Claude Bernard Lyon 1, Université de Lyon, Lyon, France, [5] ProfileXpert, SFR-Est, CNRS UMR-S3453, INSERM US7, Université Claude Bernard Lyon 1, Université de Lyon, Lyon, France, [6] Laboratoire de Virologie, Centre National de Référence des virus Influenza Sud, Institut des Agents Infectieux, Groupement Hospitalier Nord, Hospices Civils de Lyon, Lyon, France, [7] Pôle de Réanimation, Hôpital Roger Salengro, Centre Hospitalier Régional et Universitaire de Lille, Université de Lille 2, Lille, France, [8] Ecologie Microbienne, UMR CNRS 5557, USC INRA 1364, Université Claude Bernard Lyon 1, Université de Lyon, Villeurbanne, France, [9] Service d'Anesthésie et de Réanimation, Hôpital Edouard Herriot, Hospices Civils de Lyon, Lyon, France, [10] Pathophysiology of Injury-Induced Immunosuppression (PI3), EA 7426 Hospices Civils de Lyon, bioMérieux, Université Claude Bernard Lyon 1, Hôpital Edouard Herriot, Lyon, France

*Correspondence:
Olivier Terrier
olivier.terrier@univ-lyon1.fr
Manuel Rosa-Calatrava
manuel.rosa-calatrava@univ-lyon1.fr

† These authors have contributed equally to this work

Influenza virus infections remain a major and recurrent public health burden. The intrinsic ever-evolving nature of this virus, the suboptimal efficacy of current influenza inactivated vaccines, as well as the emergence of resistance against a limited antiviral arsenal, highlight the critical need for novel therapeutic approaches. In this context, the aim of this study was to develop and validate an innovative strategy for drug repurposing as host-targeted inhibitors of influenza viruses and the rapid evaluation of the most promising candidates in Phase II clinical trials. We exploited in vivo global transcriptomic signatures of infection directly obtained from a patient cohort to determine a shortlist of already marketed drugs with newly identified, host-targeted inhibitory properties against influenza virus. The antiviral potential of selected repurposing candidates was further evaluated in vitro, in vivo, and ex vivo. Our strategy allowed the selection of a shortlist of 35 high potential candidates out of a rationalized computational screening of 1,309 FDA-approved bioactive molecules, 31 of which were validated for their significant in vitro antiviral activity. Our in vivo and ex vivo results highlight diltiazem, a calcium channel blocker currently used in the treatment of hypertension, as a promising option for the treatment of influenza infections. Additionally, transcriptomic signature analysis further revealed the so far undescribed capacity of diltiazem to modulate the expression of specific genes related to the host antiviral response and cholesterol metabolism. Finally, combination treatment with diltiazem and virus-targeted oseltamivir neuraminidase inhibitor further increased antiviral efficacy, prompting rapid authorization for the initiation of a Phase II clinical trial. This original, host-targeted, drug repurposing strategy constitutes an effective and highly reactive process for the rapid identification of novel anti-infectious drugs, with potential major implications for the management of antimicrobial resistance and the rapid response to future epidemic or pandemic (re)emerging diseases for which we are still disarmed.

Keywords: influenza viruses, antivirals, inhibitors of viral infection, transcriptome, host targeting, drug repurposing

# INTRODUCTION

Besides their well-known pandemic potential, annual outbreaks caused by influenza viruses account for several million respiratory infections and 250,000 to 500,000 deaths worldwide (1). This global high morbidity and mortality of influenza infections represents a major and recurrent public health threat with high economic burden. In this context, the suboptimal vaccine coverage and efficacy, coupled with recurrent events of viral resistance against a very limited antiviral portfolio, emphasize an urgent need for innovative treatment strategies presenting fewer obstacles for their clinical use (2).

For decades, the strategy for antiviral development was mostly based on serial screenings of hundreds of thousands of molecules to identify "hits" and "leads" that target specific viral determinants, a quite costly and time-consuming process. However, the dramatic reduction in successful candidate identification over time (3), along with a concomitant increase of regulatory complexity to implement clinical trials, have fostered rising interest in novel strategies. Indeed, new approaches, focused on targeting the host instead of the virus, as well as on marketed drug repurposing for new antiviral indications (3–5) have been recently proposed in the context of global health emergencies posed by Ebola (6) and Zika (7) viruses. Such innovative strategies are strongly supported by a shift of paradigms in drug discovery, from "one-drug-one-target" to "one-drug-multiple-targets" (8). In that sense, different *in silico* approaches based on structural bioinformatic studies (9, 10), systems biology approaches (11), and host gene expression analyses (12) have been applied to decipher multi-purpose effects of many US Food and Drug Administration (FDA)-approved drugs. Additionally, as successfully demonstrated in antiretroviral therapy (13), targeting host instead of viral determinants may confer a broad-spectrum antiviral efficacy, and also reduce the risk of emergence of drug resistance against influenza viruses (14). As a result, the last decade has witnessed several host-directed experimental approaches against influenza infections, notably nitazoxanide, DAS181 or acetylsalicylic acid (15–17).

In line with this emerging trend, we previously postulated that host global gene expression profiling can be considered as a "fingerprint" or signature of any specific cell state, including during infection or drug treatment, and hypothesized that the screening of databases for compounds that counteract virogenomic signatures could enable rapid identification of effective antivirals (18). Based on this previous proof-of-concept obtained from *in vitro* gene expression profiles, we further improved our strategy by analyzing paired upper respiratory tract clinical samples collected during the acute infection and after recovery from a cohort of influenza A(H1N1)pdm09-infected patients and determined their respective transcriptomic signatures. We then performed an *in silico* drug screening using Connectivity Map (CMAP), the Broad Institute's publicly available database of more than 7,000 drug-associated gene expression profiles (19, 20), and identified a list of candidate bioactive molecules with signatures anti-correlated with those of the patient's acute infection state (**Figure 1A**). The potential antiviral properties of selected FDA-approved molecules were firstly validated *in vitro*, and the most effective compounds were further compared to oseltamivir for the treatment of influenza A(H1N1)pdm09 virus infections in both C57BL/6 mice and 3D reconstituted human airway epithelia. Altogether, our results highlight diltiazem, a calcium channel blocker with so far undescribed capacity to stimulate the epithelial antiviral defense, as a promising repurposed host-targeted inhibitor of influenza infection. Moreover, our results plead in favor of the combination of diltiazem with the virus-targeted antiviral oseltamivir for the improvement of current anti-influenza therapy, and possibly decreasing the risk of antiviral resistance. This study confirms the feasibility and interest of integrating clinical virogenomic and chemogenomic inputs as part of a drug repurposing strategy to accelerate bedside-to-bench and bench-to-bedside drug development.

# MATERIALS AND METHODS

## Ethics Approval and Consent to Participate

Adult patients were recruited by general practitioners in the context of a previously published randomized clinical trial Escuret et al. (21) (ClinicalTrials.gov identifier NCT00830323) and all of them provided written informed consent. The study protocol was approved by the Lyon Ethics Committee (Comité de Protection des Personnes Lyon B) on September 9th, 2009 and conducted in accordance with the Declaration of Helsinki.

All animal procedures were approved by the Institutional Animal Care Committee of the Center Hospitalier Universitaire de Québec (CPAC protocol authorization #2012-068-3) according to the guidelines of the Canadian Council on Animal Care.

## Clinical Samples

A previously published randomized clinical trial (ClinicalTrials.gov identifier NCT00830323) was conducted in Lyon and Paris (France) during the peak circulation of the influenza A(H1N1)pdm09 virus, with the aim to assess the efficacy of oseltamivir-zanamivir combination therapy compared with oseltamivir monotherapy (21). Briefly, patients tested positive for influenza A infection by the QuickVue rapid antigen kit (Quidel) were randomized in one of the two treatment

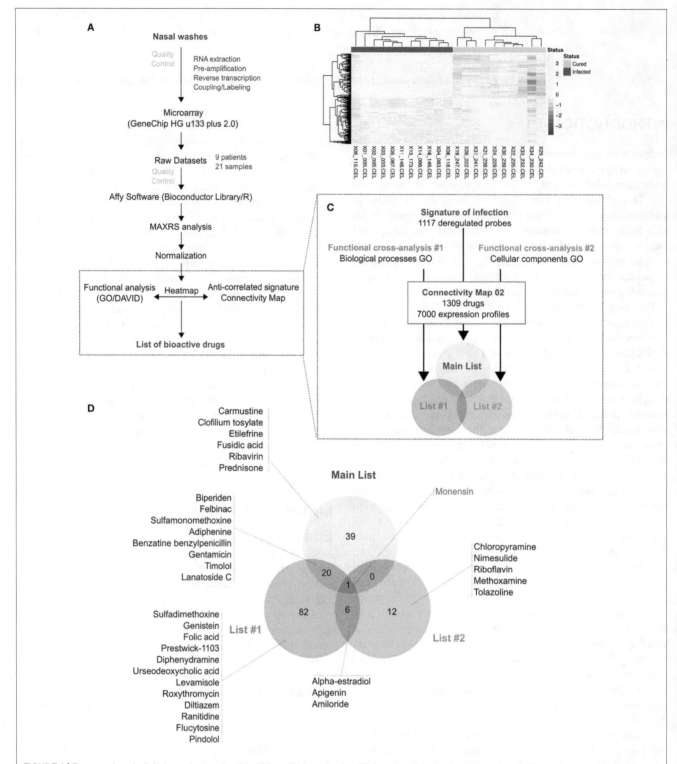

**FIGURE 1 |** From nasal wash clinical samples to a shortlist of 35 candidate molecules. **(A)** Overview of the *in silico* strategy used in this study. A detailed description of the strategy is described in the Online Methods section. **(B)** Hierarchical clustering and heatmap of the 1,117 most differentially deregulated genes between "infected" (red) and "cured" (light green) samples. Raw median centered expression levels are color coded from blue to yellow. Dendrograms indicate the correlation between clinical samples (columns) or genes (rows). **(C)** Functional cross-analysis of candidate molecules obtained from Connectivity Map (CMAP). Three lists of candidate molecules were obtained using different set of genes in order to introduce functional bias and add more biological significance to this first screening: a Main List based on the complete list of differentially expressed genes, and two other lists (List #1 and #2) based on subsets of genes belonging to significantly enriched Gene Ontology (GO) terms. **(D)** Venn Diagram comparing the total 160 molecules obtained from the three lists described in **(C)**, with monensin as the only common molecule. Only the candidates selected for *in vitro* screening and validation are depicted.

groups and nasal wash specimens were collected within 2 h of the first visit and every 24 h until 96 h after treatment initiation. Nasal swabs were also performed on days 5 and 7. In voluntary patients, an optional supplementary nasal wash was performed at least 3 months after influenza infection (recovery phase). H1N1 subtype was further confirmed by PCR. For nine of these patients, transcriptomic data were obtained from paired samples collected during influenza infection without treatment and in the recovery phase.

## Sample Processing, RNA Preparation and Hybridization

Nasal wash samples were collected in RNAlater® Stabilization Solution (Thermo Fisher Scientific). Total RNA was extracted using RNeasy Micro kit (Qiagen) following the manufacturer's instructions. RNA quality was assessed using a Bioanalyzer2100 (Agilent technologies, Inc, Palo Alto, CA, USA). To account for samples having low amount and/or partially degraded RNA (RNA Integrity Numbers between 1 and 8), we applied two types of corrections: (i) cRNA labeling was performed after a linear amplification protocol, as previously described (22) and (ii) raw signals obtained after hybridization of labeled cRNA on microarray and data acquisition were processed using the MAXRS algorithm (23). Labeled cRNA were hybridized on Affymetrix HG-U133plus2 microarrays according to manufacturer's instructions in a GeneChip® Hybridization Oven 640 (Affymetrix) and microarrays were subsequently scanned in an Affymetrix 3000 7G scanner.

## Data Normalization and MAXRS Computational Analysis

The MAXRS algorithm (23) is particularly suited to gene expression analysis under low hybridization conditions. Briefly, this method takes advantage of the specific design of Affymetrix probe sets, which are composed of an average of 11 different probes that target the same locus, and is based on the observation that for most of the probe sets the same probe shows the highest fluorescence intensity in almost all arrays. For each microarray ($m = 1..M$) and for each probeset ($t = 1..T$), fluorescence intensity values on microarray m of all probes ($p = 1..P_t$) belonging to the probeset t are sorted in increasing order. These ranks are denoted as $r_{mtp}$. Then, we calculated across all microarrays the rank sum ($RS_{tp}$) for each probeset t for each probe p belonging to the probeset t. Finally, for each probeset t, we kept the three probes p with the highest $RS_{tp}$. The mean intensity of these three probes is attributed to the probeset t. As it is common practice with many modern pre-processing algorithms, and because of the low global fluorescence signal intensity, mismatched probes were excluded from MAXRS analysis.

After pre-processing the raw dataset with the MAXRS algorithm, a normalization step was performed using Tukey median-polish algorithm (24). Differential expression was assessed by applying a Student t-test for each probeset, and multiple testing was corrected using the Benjamini-Hochberg algorithm in the qvalue library (25). For further downstream analysis, genes were selected according to two criteria: (i) absolute fold change >2, and (ii) corrected p-value < 0.05. Data were generated according to the Minimum Information About a Microarray Experiment guidelines and deposited in the National Center for Biotechnology Information's Gene Expression Omnibus (GEO) (26) under accession number GSE93731.

## Functional Analysis

Functional enrichment analysis was performed on a selection of differentially-expressed genes with DAVID tools (27), using the Gene Ontology (GO) (28). To further select genes for the CMAP query, we selected 6 Biological Process (BP) terms (GO_BP: GO:0009615-response to virus; GO:0006955-immune response; GO:0042981-regulation of apoptosis; GO:0006952-defense response; GO:0009611-response to wounding; GO:0042127-regulation of cell proliferation) that shared >90% of genes with all significantly enriched GO_BP terms, and 3 relevant Cellular Component terms (GO_CC: GO:0031225-anchored to membrane; GO:0005829-cytosol; GO:0005654-nucleoplasm). To visualize and compare the different lists of compounds, Venn diagrams were obtained using the webtool developed by Dr. Van de Peer's Lab at Ghent University (http://bioinformatics.psb.ugent.be/webtools/Venn/).

## Cells and Viruses

Human lung epithelial A549 cells (ATCC CCL-185) were maintained in Dulbecco's modified Eagle's medium (DMEM) supplemented with 10% fœtal calf serum and supplemented with 2 mM L-glutamine (Sigma Aldrich), penicillin (100 U/mL), and streptomycin (100 μg/mL) (Lonza), maintained at 37°C and 5% $CO_2$. MucilAir® human airway epithelia (HAE) were obtained from Epithelix SARL (Geneva, Switzerland) and maintained in air-liquid interphase with specific MucilAir® Culture Medium in Costar Transwell inserts (Corning, NY, USA) according to the manufacturer's instructions.

Influenza viruses A/Lyon/969/09 and A/Quebec/144147/09 were produced in MDCK (ATCC CCL-34) cells in EMEM supplemented with 2 mM L-glutamine (Sigma Aldrich), penicillin (100 U/mL), streptomycin (100 μg/mL) (Lonza) and 1 μg/mL trypsin. Viral titers in plaque forming units (PFU/ml) and tissue culture infectious dose 50% (TCID50/mL) were determined in MDCK cells as previously described (29, 30).

## Viral Growth Assays

For viral growth assays in the presence of molecules, A549 cells were seeded 24 h in advance in multi-well 6 plates at $1.8 \times 10^5$ cells/well. Three treatment protocols were evaluated. (1) In pre-treatment protocol, cells were washed with DMEM and then incubated with different concentrations of candidate molecules diluted in DMEM supplemented with 2 mM L-glutamine (Sigma Aldrich), penicillin (100 U/mL), streptomycin (100 μg/mL) (Lonza) and 0.5 μg/mL trypsin. Six hours after treatment, cells were washed and then infected with A/Lyon/969/09 (H1N1)pdm09 virus at a multiplicity of infection (MOI) of 0.1. (2) In pre-treatment plus post-treatment protocol, cells were initially treated and infected in the same conditions as explained above. One hour after viral infection, a second identical dose of candidate molecules in supplemented DMEM was added. (3) In post-treatment protocol, cells without pre-treatment were infected in the conditions described and treatments with candidate molecules at the indicated concentrations were initiated 24 h p.i. In all cases, supernatants were collected at 48 h p.i. and stored at $-80°C$ for TCID50/ml viral titration.

## Viability and Cytotoxicity Assays

Cell viability was measured using the CellTiter 96® AQueous One Solution Cell Proliferation Assay (MTS, Promega). A549 cells were seeded into 96-well plates and treated with different concentrations of molecules or solvents. Cells were incubated at 37°C and 5% $CO_2$ and then harvested at different timepoints, following the same scheme as in viral growth assays. Results were presented as a ratio of control values obtained with solvents. Treatment-related toxicity in HAE was measured using the Cytotoxicity Detection Kit$^{PLUS}$ (LDH, Roche) according to the manufacturer's instructions. Briefly, duplicate 100 μL-aliquots of basolateral medium from treated and control HAEs were incubated in the dark (room temperature, 30 min) with 100 μL of lactate dehydrogenase (LDH) reagent in 96-well plates. After incubation, "stop solution" was added and the absorbance was measured in a conventional microplate ELISA reader. The photometer was set up for dual readings to determine non-specific background at 750 nm, and absorbance was measured at 490 nm. Percent cytotoxicity was calculated as indicated by the manufacturer, using mock-treated and 1% triton-treated epithelia as "low" and "high" controls, respectively. Percent viability is presented as 100–percent cytotoxicity.

## Mouse Model of Viral Infection

All protocols were carried out in seven to 9-weeks old female C57BL/6N mice (Charles River, QC, Canada). Animals were randomized in groups of 15 according to their weight to ensure comparable median values on each group, and then housed in micro-isolator cages (5 animals per cage) in a biosafety 2 controlled environment (22°C, 40% humidity, 12:12 h photoperiods), with *ad libitum* access to food and water.

On day 0, mice were lightly anesthetized with inhaled 3% isoflurane/oxygen, and then infected by intranasal (i.n.) instillation of influenza A/Quebec/144147/09 (H1N1)pdm09 virus in 30 μl of saline, as specified in each case. Control animals were mock-infected with 30 μl of saline. Candidate molecules were evaluated in two different treatment protocols: (i) treatments were started on the same day of infection (day 0, 6 h prior to infection), or (ii) treatments were started 24 h after infection (day 1). Regardless of treatment initiation time, all treatments were performed *per os* (150-μl gavage) once daily for 5 consecutive days (5 drug administrations in total). Mortality, body weight and clinical signs such as lethargy and ruffled fur were daily monitored on 10 animals/group for a total of 14 days. Animals were euthanized if they reached the humane endpoint of >20% weight loss. The remaining 5 animals/group were euthanized on day 5 p.i. to measure lung viral titers (LVTs).

Vehicle (saline) or oseltamivir were used as placebo and positive treatment control, respectively. The oseltamivir dose (10 mg/kg/day) was adjusted to confer ~50% protection in the selected experimental conditions and is considered a good correlate of half the normal dose of 150 mg/day given to humans (31). The doses of repurposed candidate molecules were selected to be in the non-toxic range for mouse studies, according to published preclinical data for their first therapeutic indication. To validate this choice in our specific model, potential drug toxicity was evaluated in mock-infected animals treated with the same regimens as virus-infected mice.

## Pulmonary Viral Titers

In order to evaluate the effect of different treatments on viral replication, 5 animals per group were euthanized on day 5 p.i. and lungs were removed aseptically. Mice were randomly selected from the 3 cages of each group to minimize cage-related bias. Lungs were homogenized in 1 ml of PBS using a bead mill homogenizer (Tissue Lyser, Qiagen) and debris was pelleted by centrifugation (2,000 g, 5 min). Triplicate 10-fold serial dilutions of each supernatant were plated on ST6GalIMDCK cells (kindly provided by Dr. Y. Kawaoka, University of Wisconsin, Madison, WI) and titrated by plaque assays (29). The investigator was blinded to group allocation.

## Viral Infection in Reconstituted Human Airway Epithelium (HAE)

For HAE infection experiments, apical poles were gently washed with warm PBS and then infected with a 100-μL dilution of influenza A/Lyon/969/09 (H1N1)pdm09 virus in OptiMEM medium (Gibco, ThermoFisher Scientific) at a MOI of 0.1. Basolateral pole sampling as well as 150-μL OptiMEM apical washes were performed at the indicated time points, and then stored at $-80°C$ for PFU/mL and TCID50/mL viral titration. Treatments with specific dilutions of candidate molecules alone or combined with oseltamivir in MucilAir® Culture Medium were applied through basolateral poles. Control HAE were mock-treated in the same conditions with MucilAir® Culture Medium without molecules. All treatments were initiated on day 0 (5 h after viral infection) and continued once daily for 5 consecutive days (5 drug administrations in total). Variations in transepithelial electrical resistance (Δ TEER) were measured using a dedicated volt-ohm meter (EVOM2, Epithelial Volt/Ohm Meter for TEER) and expressed as Ohm/cm$^2$.

## High Throughput Sequencing and Bioinformatics Analysis

cDNA libraries were prepared from 200 ng of total RNA using the Scriptseq$^{TM}$ complete Gold kit-Low Input (SCL6EP, Epicenter), according to manufacturer's instructions. Each cDNA library was amplified and indexed with primers provided in the ScriptSeq$^{TM}$ Index PCR Primers kit (RSBC10948, Epicenter) and then sequenced as 100 bp paired-end reads. Prior to sequencing, libraries were quantified with QuBit and Bioanalyzer2100, and indexed libraries were pooled in equimolar concentrations. Sequencing was performed on an Illumina HiSeq 2500 system (Illumina, Carlsbad, CA), with a required minimum of 40 million reads sequenced per sample. Conversion and demultiplexing of reads was performed using bcl2fastq 1.8.4

(Illumina). The FastQC software (http://www.bioinformatics. babraham.ac.uk/projects/fastqc) was used for quality controls of the raw data. Reads were trimmed using the Trimmomatic (32) software, with a minimum quality threshold of Q30. Trimmed reads were pseudo-aligned to the *Homo sapiens* genome (GRCh38.p11) using the Kallisto software (33). Statistical analysis was performed in R3.3.1 with the package EdgeR 3.14.0 (34). Differential expression was calculated by comparing each condition to the mock using a linear model. The Benjamini-Hochberg procedure was used to control the false discovery rate (FDR). Transcripts with an absolute fold change >2 and a corrected $p$-value < 0.05 were considered to be differentially expressed. Enriched pathways and GO terms were assessed with DAVID 6.8 (27). For visualization purposes, a heatmap and stacked barplots were constructed in R3.3.1 on mean-weighted fold changes and association between conditions were assessed by Spearman correlation analysis.

## Statistical Analysis

All experimental assays were performed in duplicate at a minimum, and representative results are shown unless indicated otherwise. No statistical methods were used to predetermine sample size in animal studies, which were estimated according to previous studies and the known variability of the assays. No mice were excluded from post-protocol analyses, the experimental unit was an individual animal and equal variance was assumed. Kaplan-Meier survival plots were compared by Log-Rank (Mantel-Cox) test and hazard ratios (HR) were computed by the Mantel-Haenszel method. Weight loss and viral titers of all groups were compared by one-way analysis of variance (ANOVA) with Tukey's multiple comparison post-test. The testing level ($\alpha$) was 0.05. Statistical analyses were performed on all available data, using GraphPad, Prism 7.

## RESULTS

### Generation of Clinical Virogenomic Profiles

We determined *in vivo* transcriptional signatures of infection from paired nasal wash samples of nine untreated patients, collected during acute A(H1N1)pdm09 pandemic influenza infection ("infected") and at least 3 months later to ensure a recovery non-infected state ("cured") (21). The nine patients from whom transcriptomic data could be obtained constitute a representative sample of the whole studied cohort, except for the male sex ratio (**Table S1**). We combined two strategies to tackle the characteristic low RNA amount/quality of this type of clinical samples. Firstly, cRNA labeling was performed after a linear amplification of initial RNA, as previously described (35). Secondly, raw signals obtained after hybridization of labeled cRNA on microarray and data acquisition were processed using the MAXRS algorithm (23) to overcome low hybridization conditions. This approach, initially developed for the analysis of heterologous hybridizations, takes advantage of the specific design of the Affymetrix® microarray used in our study, with several probes targeting the same locus (23).

After normalization, differentially expressed genes were selected based on two criteria: (i) an absolute fold change >2, and (ii) a Benjamini-Hochberg corrected $p$-value < 0.05. We therefore identified a total of 1,117 commonly deregulated probes, with almost equal proportion of up-regulated (48.4%; $n = 541$) and down-regulated probes (51.7%; $n = 576$). Remarkably, despite considerable inter-patient variability among recovery state samples, a substantial homogenization of transcriptional profiles was observed in the context of infection, as shown in the heatmap presented in **Figure 1B** and by the median Spearman's $\rho$ correlation values for both groups (0.60 "cured" vs. 0.90 "infected"). These virogenomic signatures of infection constituted the input for the subsequent *in silico* query for the identification of candidate compounds.

## *In silico* Cross-Analysis of Chemogenomic vs. Virogenomic Clinical Profiles

We then performed an *in-silico* search for molecules that reverse the virogenomic signature of infection, using the CMAP database (Build 02) as previously described (18). CMAP is a collection of genome-wide transcriptional expression data from cultured human cells treated with bioactive small molecules. HG-U133plus2 probesets were mapped to the U133A probesets using the Ensembl BioMarts online tool (36, 37), and connectivity scores and $p$-values were obtained using the CMAP algorithm (19, 20). With the global set of 1,000 most differentially expressed genes as input (**Figure 1C**, Main List), we obtained a preliminary list of 60 candidate compounds. In parallel, we used two other subsets of genes belonging to significantly enriched Gene Ontology (GO) terms obtained from microarray analyses to introduce functional bias and add more biological significance to our first screening. Hence, by using 6 Biological Process terms (GO_BP) that shared more than 90% of genes (**Figure 1C**, Functional cross-analysis #1), a second list of 109 compound candidates was obtained. A third list of 19 compounds was obtained using 3 relevant Cellular Component terms (GO_CC) (**Figure 1C**, Functional cross-analysis #2). The comparison of the 160 compounds from the three distinct lists (12.2% of compounds of CMAP, **Table S2**) highlighted monensin as the only common compound (**Figure 1D**).

To rationally reduce the number of drug candidates, bioactive drugs were excluded if not compatible with a final use as antiviral, mostly for safety (e.g., teratogens, intercalating agents), and/or pharmacological (e.g., documented low bioavailability) reasons, based on clinical data and the PubMed/PubChem databases. Thus, the number of candidates was initially decreased to 139 and then to 110 (**Figure S1**). We subsequently determined a shortlist of 35 bioactive molecules (<3% of CMAP, **Table 1**) for *in vitro* screening, based on two main criteria: (i) molecules representative of the different pharmacological classes identified, and (ii) molecules evenly distributed in the three lists obtained after *in silico* screening (Main List, List #1 and List #2, **Figure 1D**), which comprise a panoply of documented pharmacological classes, including anti-fungal agents (e.g., monensin, flucytosine), anti-inflammatory agents (e.g., felbinac, apigenin, prednisone) and adrenergic agonists/antagonists (timolol, methoxamine,

**TABLE 1 |** Shortlist of the 35 selected molecules and their documented pharmacological classes.

| Name | Pharmacological class |
| --- | --- |
| Adiphenine | Parasympatholytics/Anticholinergics/Antispamodics |
| Alpha-estradiol* | 5 alpha-reductase inhibitors/Androgenic alopecia treatment |
| Amiloride*# | Epithelial Sodium Channel Blockers/Diuretics/Acid Sensing Ion Channel Blockers |
| Apigenin*# | Anti-Inflammatory Agents, Non- steroidal/? |
| Benzathine benzylpenicillin# | Anti-Bacterial Agents |
| Biperiden* | Antiparkinson Agents/Muscarinic Antagonists/Parasympatholytics |
| Carmustine | Antineoplastic Agents, Alkylating |
| Chloropyramine | Histamine H1 Antagonists |
| Clofilium tosylate | Anti-Arrhythmia Agents |
| Diltiazem | Antihypertensive Agents/Calcium Channel Blockers/Cardiovascular Agents/Vasodilator Agents |
| Diphenhydramine | Anesthetics, Local/Anti-Allergic Agents/Antiemetics/Histamine H1 Antagonists/Hypnotics and Sedatives |
| Etilefrine | Adrenergic beta-1 and alpha agonist/Cardiotonic/antihypotensive agent. |
| Felbinac# | Anti-Inflammatory Agents, Non-steroidal |
| Flucytosine*# | Antifungal Agents/Antimetabolites |
| Folic acid | Hematinics/Vitamin B Complex |
| Fusidic acid# | Anti-Bacterial Agents/Protein Synthesis Inhibitors |
| Genistein | Anticarcinogenic Agents/Phytoestrogens/Protein Kinase Inhibitors |
| Gentamicin# | Anti-Bacterial Agents/Protein Synthesis Inhibitors |
| Lanatoside C | Anti-Arrhythmia Agents |
| Levamisole* | Adjuvants, Immunologic/Antinematodal Agents/Antirheumatic Agents |
| Methoxamine | Adrenergic alpha-1 Receptor Agonists/Sympathomimetics/Vasoconstrictor Agents |
| Monensin*# | Antifungal Agents/Antiprotozoal Agents/Coccidiostats/Proton Ionophores/Sodium Ionophores |
| Nimesulide*# | Anti-Inflammatory Agents, Non-steroidal/Cyclooxygenase Inhibitors |
| Pindolol | Adrenergic beta-Antagonists/Antihypertensive Agents/Serotonin Antagonists/Vasodilator Agents |
| Prednisone# | Anti-Inflammatory Agents/Antineoplastic Agents, Hormonal/Glucocorticoids |
| Prestwick-1103# | Anti-Inflammatory Agents, Non-steroidal/Cyclooxygenase Inhibitors |
| Ranitidine | Anti-Ulcer Agents/Histamine H2 Antagonists |
| Ribavirin* | Antimetabolites/Antiviral Agents |
| Riboflavin* | Photosensitizing Agents/Vitamin B Complex |
| Roxithromycin# | Anti-Bacterial Agents |
| Sulfadimethoxine# | Anti-Infective Agents |
| Sulfamonomethoxine# | Anti-Infective Agents |
| Timolol* | Adrenergic beta-Antagonists/Anti-Arrhythmia Agents/Antihypertensive Agents |
| Tolazoline | Adrenergic alpha-Antagonists/Antihypertensive Agents/Vasodilator Agents |
| Ursodeoxycholic acid | Cholagogues and Choleretics |

*Shortlist of the 35 selected candidates representative of the 110 molecules obtained from the in silico screening (**Figure 1** and **Figure S1**). Documented pharmacological classes were obtained from PubChem (https://pubchem.ncbi.nlm.nih.gov). (\*) indicate molecules previously evaluated for their antiviral properties according to the literature, and numerals (#) those belonging to anti-microbial or anti-inflammatory related pharmacological classes.*

tolazoline), as represented in the Venn diagram (**Figure 1D, Table 1**). Interestingly, at least 14 (40%) molecules from our short-list belong to a pharmacological class related with anti-microbial or anti-inflammatory activities (**Table 1**, #), and 11 (31.4%) have already been reported in the literature for their antiviral properties against influenza or other viruses (**Table 1**, *), notably the nucleoside inhibitor ribavirin (38, 39) and the ionophore monensin (40).

## Inhibitory Effect of the Selected Molecules on A(H1N1)pdm09 Viral Growth *in vitro*

*In vitro* screening of the antiviral potency of the 35 selected molecules was performed in A549 human lung epithelial cells

seeded in 6-well plates. Firstly, we evaluated the impact of 6 h pre-treatment with a 10-fold drug concentration range, using the original CMAP concentration as reference. Six hours after treatment, cells were washed and infected with influenza A(H1N1)pdm09 virus at a MOI of 0.1. Viral titers in supernatants collected from treated samples at 48 h post infection (p.i.) were normalized with those measured in mock-treated controls ($>10^5$ TCID50/mL). Potential treatment-induced cell toxicity was evaluated in the same experimental conditions using the MTS assay and expressed also as the percentage of cell viability compared to non-infected controls (**Figure 2**). Based on antiviral activity and cell viability profiles obtained (**Figure 2A**, blue triangles), we defined as "inhibitors"

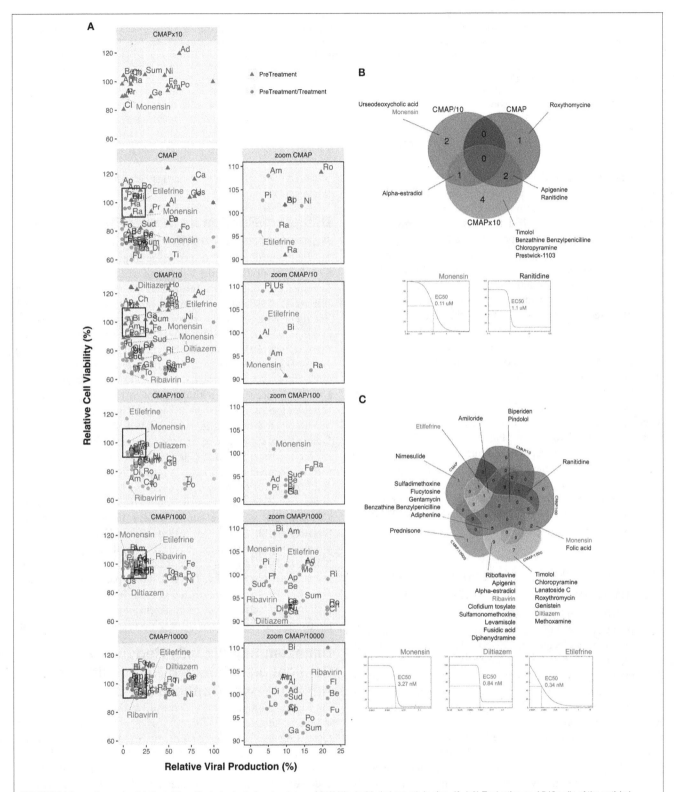

**FIGURE 2 |** Screening and validation of the effect of selected molecules on A(H1N1)pdm09 viral growth *in vitro*. (**A**, left) Evaluation on A549 cells of the antiviral potency of the 35 candidates selected by *in silico* analysis. Relative viral production (%, X axis) and relative cell viability (%, Y axis) of both pre-treatment (blue triangles) and pre-treatment/treatment (green circles) regimens were evaluated. A 10-fold drug concentration range using CMAP as reference (CMAP × 10, CMAP, CMAP/10, CMAP/100, CMAP/1,000, and CMAP/10,000) was used. CMAP × 10 was only tested in the context of pre-treatment, by anticipation of a lower efficacy of molecules in this experimental setup. All experimental assays were performed in triplicate and mean values are represented. (**A**, right) Zoom panels depicting molecules defined

*(Continued)*

compounds that fulfilled the following two criteria: (i) induce >75% reduction on viral production, and (ii) have minor impact on cell viability, with relative values in the 90–110% range (**Figure 2A**, squares in left panels and zooms in right panels). A total of 10 compounds (28.6%) matched both criteria, mainly when used at a 10-fold CMAP concentration (**Figure 2B**), yet only a limited number of them exhibited classic dose-dependent inhibition. Whenever possible, as in the case of monensin or ranitidine for example, EC50 values were calculated, which were mostly in the micromolar range (**Figure 2B**).

In a second round of screening, we tested the same 6 h pre-treatment but with serial 10-fold dilutions from the initial CMAP concentration to CMAP/10,000, followed by one additional treatment immediately after infection (**Figure 2A**, green circles in left and right panels). In these conditions, 30 compounds (85.7%) met our criteria to be considered as inhibitors of viral production (**Figure 2C**), with half of them showing a classic dose-dependent inhibition effect. Calculated EC50 values were in the nanomolar range and hence significantly lower than those calculated in the context of pre-treatment only. Dose response curves and calculated EC50 for all the 35 compounds are presented in **Figure S2** and **Table S3**, respectively.

## Efficacy of Selected Molecules for the Treatment of Influenza A(H1N1)pdm09 Virus Infection in Mice

Based on EC50 and cytoxicity data from the *in vitro* screening, we selected 8 molecules to investigate their potential as inhibitors of influenza A(H1N1)pdm09 in C57BL/6 mice. Oseltamivir, the standard antiviral for the treatment of influenza infections was used as control. All treatments were performed *per os*, starting 6 h before infection and being continued once daily for 5 consecutive days (5 drug administrations in total) (**Figure 3**). While animals treated with oseltamivir or monensin showed clinical improvement compared to the saline (placebo) group in terms of survival and weight loss (oseltamivir only), treatment with Lanatoside C, prednisolone, flucytosine, felbinac, and timolol showed no clinical benefit at the selected concentrations (**Figure S3A**). In contrast, diltiazem and etilefrine not only significantly improved survival and maximum mean weight losses (**Figures 3A,B**), but also showed at least 1-log reductions in LVTs on day 5 p.i. (**Figure 3C**). Importantly, no signs of toxicity were observed for any of the drugs at the regimens tested (**Figure S3B**).

## Diltiazem Retains Its *in vivo* Efficacy When Administered 24 h After Viral Infection

To best mimic the therapeutic setting, we next evaluated the efficacy of the same 5-day oral regimen with diltiazem or etilefrine but when initiated 24 h after viral infection (**Figure 4**). As with oseltamivir and monensin, diltiazem treatment completely prevented mortality and reduced weight loss in influenza A(H1N1)pdm09 infected mice, which otherwise showed only 50% (5/10) survival for the etilefrine and saline groups (**Figures 4A,B**). Interestingly, 1- to 1.5-log reductions in LVTs compared to the saline group were observed at day 5 in groups of mice treated with diltiazem or etilefrine (**Figure 4C**). We then used a more stringent approach by increasing the viral inoculum to evaluate the same delayed (24 h post infection) 5-day diltiazem regimen in the context of a 100% lethal A(H1N1)pdm09 infection (**Figures 4D–F**). Whereas, treatment with oseltamivir and diltiazem successfully rescued 40% (4/10) and 20% (2/10) of mice, respectively, half-dose treatment with diltiazem (45 mg/kg) rescued 30% (3/10) of mice from death, also showing significant improvement in mean weight loss (**Figures 4D,E**). Calculated hazard ratios (HR) for the saline group compared to these three treatment groups were 8.41 (CI95: 1.65–43.02), 2.85 (0.56–14.47), and 7.62 (1.49–38.96), respectively. Noteworthy, LVTs at day 5 p.i. were comparable among all treated and untreated groups (**Figure 4F**), suggesting mainly a protective effect of diltiazem toward severe influenza infection rather than a direct role in decreasing viral production.

## Diltiazem Significantly Reduces Viral Replication in Infected Reconstituted Human Airway Epithelia (HAE)

To further complement *in vivo* data, we characterized the inhibitory properties of diltiazem using a biologically relevant reconstituted airway epithelium model, derived from human primary bronchial cells (MucilAir®, Epithelix). HAE were infected with influenza A(H1N1)pdm09 at a MOI of 0.1, and treatments on the basolateral medium were initiated 5 h p.i. and continued once daily for 5 consecutive days. Viral replication at the apical surface of mock-treated (MucilAir® Culture Medium without molecules) HAE peaked at 48 h p.i. (~1 × 10^8 PFU/ml) and was detectable at important levels for at least 7 days. As expected, trans-epithelial electrical resistance (TEER) values, measuring tight junction and cell

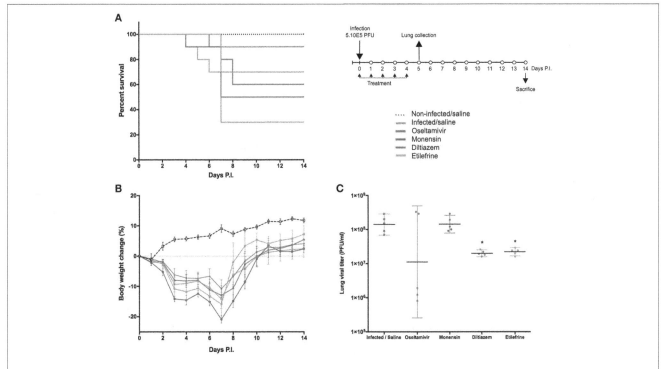

FIGURE 3 | Efficacy of oral administration of selected molecules in mice infected with influenza A(H1N1)pdm09 virus. C57BL/6N mice (n = 15/group) were intranasally inoculated with 5 × 10⁵ PFU of influenza A/Quebec/144147/09 virus on day 0 and treated by gavage with saline (gray), oseltamivir 10 mg/kg/day (red), monensin 10 mg/kg/day (blue), diltiazem 90 mg/kg/day (green), or etilefrine 3 mg/kg/day (orange). A mock-infected, saline-treated group (black dotted line, n = 6) was included as control. Treatments were initiated on day 0 (6 h before infection) and administered once daily for 5 consecutive days. (A) Survival rates (n = 10/group), (B) mean weight changes (±SEM, n = 10/group or remaining mice) and (C) median (±CI95, n = 5/group) lung viral titers on day 5 p.i. are shown. *p < 0.05, compared to the infected saline-treated group by one-way ANOVA with Tukey's post-test. Data are representative of two independent experiments.

layer integrity, sharply decreased and bottomed out at 72 h p.i. in the untreated control, correlating with the first virus detection on the basolateral medium (**Figure 5A** and **Table S6**). A similar pattern was observed in infected HAE treated with oseltamivir 0.1 μM or diltiazem 9 μM (CMAP), which conferred no significant advantage over the untreated control. Conversely, oseltamivir 1 μM and diltiazem 90 μM treatments (10-fold CMAP) strongly inhibited viral replication, delaying the peak of viral production by 24 h. Both treatments induced >3-log reductions in apical viral titers at 48 h p.i. compared to the untreated control, and >2-log reductions when comparing peak titers (48 h p.i. untreated vs. 72 h p.i. treated). Moreover, whereas oseltamivir treatment stabilized TEER during the time-course of infection, diltiazem treatment partially buffered the TEER decrease observed in the untreated control (**Figure 5A** and **Table S6**). No virus was detected on the basolateral medium for these two treated groups, and absence of treatment-induced toxicity was confirmed by measuring the release of intracellular lactate dehydrogenase (LDH). Interestingly, we observed that inhibitory and protective properties demonstrated by diltiazem were progressively reversible when basolateral medium was replaced with fresh medium without drugs. Overall, these results are in accordance and strongly support the inhibitory and protective effects of diltiazem observed *in vitro* and in mice, respectively.

## Diltiazem-Oseltamivir Combination Confers Improved Efficacy When Compared to Monotherapy in Infected HAE

We anticipated that the combination of two antiviral compounds that target different viral/cellular determinants could induce better virological and physiological responses when compared to antiviral monotherapy. We therefore evaluated the diltiazem-oseltamivir combination in the same conditions described above, notably a 5-day treatment course with treatment initiation at 5 h p.i. The diltiazem 90 μM/oseltamivir 1 μM combination conferred >3-log reduction in apical peak viral titers when compared to the untreated control, even greater than that observed with same dose monotherapy. TEER values remained stable during combined treatment, comparable to those observed with oseltamivir 1 μM monotherapy (**Figure 5B** and **Table S6**). Remarkably, although not effective as monotherapy in the low concentrations tested above, the diltiazem 9 μM/oseltamivir 0.1 μM combination contrariwise delayed the peak of viral production, significantly reduced apical viral titers, and slightly buffered TEER values compared to the untreated control (**Figure 5B** and **Table S6**). Once again, no treatment-related toxicity was observed for any of the combinations tested. These results plead in favor of the potential of diltiazem for the improvement of current anti-influenza therapy with neuraminidase inhibitors.

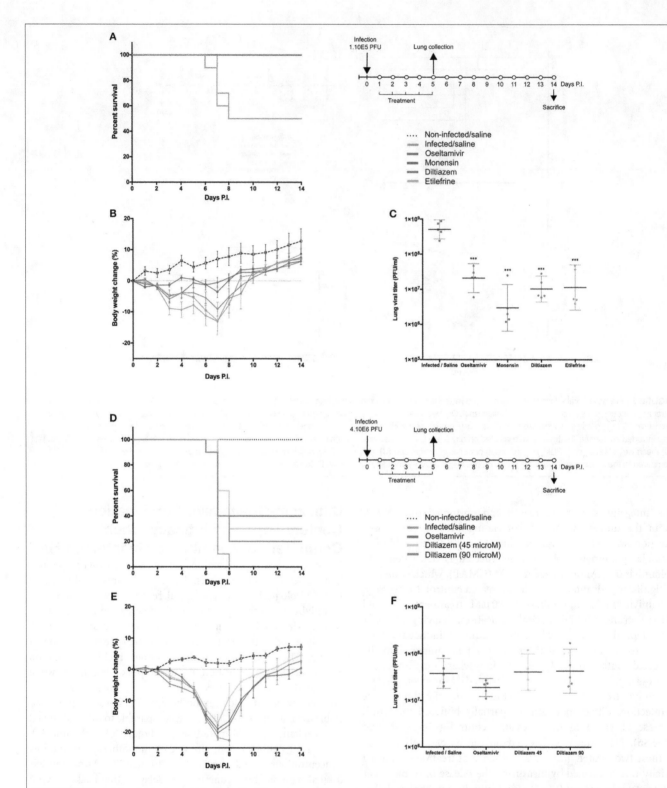

**FIGURE 4 |** Efficacy of post-infection oral treatment with diltiazem and etilefrine in mice infected with influenza A(H1N1)pdm09 virus. C57BL/6N mice ($n = 15$/group) were intranasally inoculated with $1 \times 10^5$ **(A–C)** or $4 \times 10^6$ **(D–F)** PFU of influenza A/Quebec/144147/09 virus on day 0 and treated by gavage with saline (gray), oseltamivir 10 mg/kg/day (red), monensin 10 mg/kg/day (blue, A only), diltiazem 45 mg/kg/day (light green, B only), diltiazem 90 mg/kg/day (dark green), or etilefrine 3 mg/kg/day (orange, **(A)** only). A mock-infected, saline-treated group (black dotted line, $n = 6$) was included as control. Treatments were initiated on day 1 (24 h after infection and administered once daily for 5 consecutive days. **(A,D)** Survival rates ($n = 10$/group), **(B,E)** mean weight changes ($\pm$SEM, $n = 10$/group or remaining mice), and **(C,F)** median ($\pm$CI95, $n = 5$/group) lung viral titers on day 5 p.i. are shown. ***$p < 0.001$, compared to the infected saline-treated group by one-way ANOVA with Tukey's post-test. Data are representative of two independent experiments.

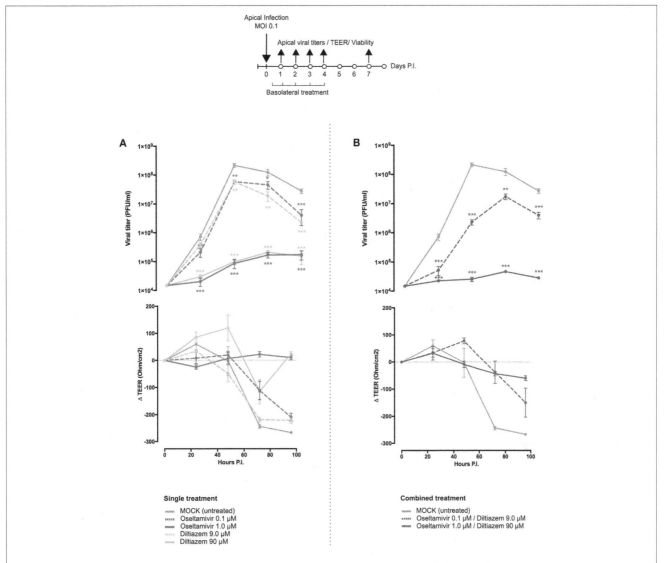

**FIGURE 5 |** Diltiazem significantly reduces viral replication in infected reconstituted human airway epithelia (HAE). Apical viral production (±SEM) and transepithelial electrical resistance (Δ TEER±SEM) in MucilAir® human airway epithelium infected on the apical pole with influenza A/Lyon/969/09 (H1N1) pdm09 virus at a MOI of 0.1 and subjected to **(A)** single or **(B)** combined treatments by the basolateral pole. Treatments with culture medium (mock, gray), oseltamivir 0.1 μM (red, dotted line), oseltamivir 1 μM (red, solid line), diltiazem 9 μM (green, dotted line), diltiazem 90 μM (green, solid line), oseltamivir 0.1 μM/diltiazem 9 μM (brown, dotted line) or oseltamivir 1 μM/diltiazem 90 μM (brown, solid line) were initiated 5 h after infection and administered once daily for 5 consecutive days. **p < 0.01 and ***p < 0.001 compared to the infected Mock-treated group by one-way ANOVA with Tukey's post-test. Data are representative of three independent experiments.

## Diltiazem Treatment Induces a Significant Reversion of the Viral Infection Signature

Since the rationale behind our approach relies on attaining antiviral activity through a drug-induced global and multi-level inversion of the infection signature, we advantageously used the MucilAir® HAE model coupled with high-throughput sequencing in order to characterize and compare the specific transcriptional signatures induced by infection and/or diltiazem treatment (**Figure 6** and **Figure S4**). HAE were mock-infected or infected with influenza A(H1N1)pdm09 virus and then mock-treated or treated in the same experimental conditions in which the antiviral effect of diltiazem has been previously validated (MOI of 0.1, 90 μM diltiazem). At 72 h p.i., cells

were lysed and total RNA was extracted. cDNA libraries were then produced, amplified, and subjected to high-throughput sequencing. Taking the mock-infected / mock-treated ("mock") as baseline, we initially performed DAVID functional gene enrichment (absolute fold change >2, Benjamini-Hochberg corrected $p < 0.05$) on the specific transcriptional signature of diltiazem with the objective of gaining insight on the putative host pathways involved in its antiviral effect. The lists of up-regulated ($n = 194$) and down-regulated ($n = 110$) transcripts in the mock-infected/diltiazem ("mock + diltiazem") condition were analyzed using DAVID 6.8 to highlight associations with specific GO terms. Although no enriched BP was identified among down-regulated transcripts, the list of up-regulated

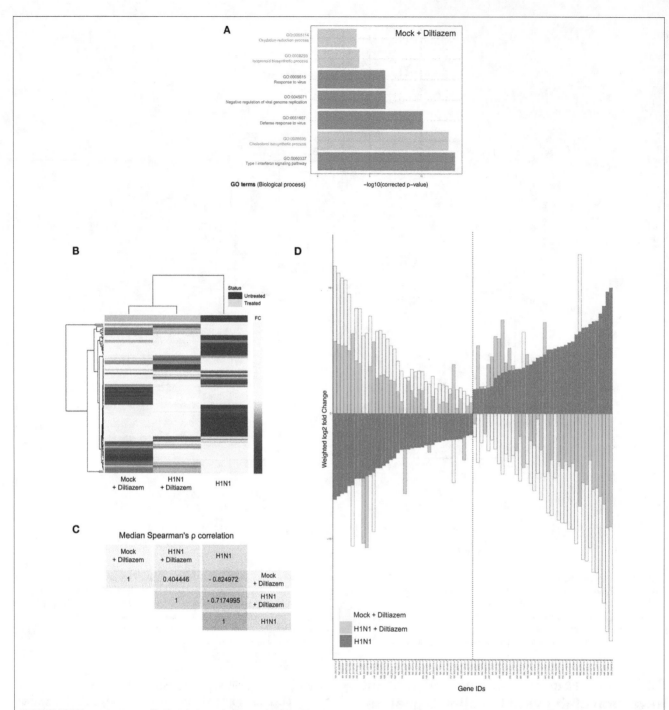

**FIGURE 6 |** Diltiazem treatment effectively induces significant reversion of the viral infection signature. **(A)** DAVID gene enrichment analysis of the diltiazem transcriptional signature. The seven most significant biological processes (BP) are presented. BP related to antiviral response and cholesterol biosynthesis/metabolism are represented in blue and green, respectively. **(B)** Hierarchical clustering and heatmap of the 118 common differentially expressed transcripts (absolute fold change >2, Benjamini-Hochberg corrected $p$-value < 0.05) between mock-infected/diltiazem ("mock + diltiazem"), infected/mock-treated ("H1N1"), or infected/diltiazem ("H1N1 + diltiazem") HAE. The mock-infected/mock-treated ("mock") condition was used as baseline. Mean-weighted fold changes are color-coded from blue to yellow. **(C)** Median Spearman ρ correlation value calculations between the 3 conditions highlighted in the heatmap. **(D)** Stacked barplot representation of the 40 most up/down-regulated transcripts highlighted in the analysis. Barplots were constructed in R3.3.1 based on mean-weighted fold changes and ordered according to H1N1 values (blue). Mock + diltiazem and H1N1 + diltiazem conditions are represented in yellow and green, respectively.

transcripts associated with diltiazem treatment highlighted 7 particularly enriched BP. While 4 of these BP (GO:0009615; GO:0045071; GO:0051607; GO:0060337) are directly linked to antiviral response/cellular response to virus, the remaining 3 (GO:0055114; GO:0008299; GO:0006695) are involved in cholesterol biosynthesis/metabolism (**Figure 6A**). We then compared the common differentially expressed transcript levels between the three infection/treatment conditions. These transcriptional signatures revealed a marked anti-correlated profile between the "mock + diltiazem" and the infected / mock-treated ("H1N1") conditions (**Figure 6B**), supported by a median Spearman's ρ correlation value of −0.82 (**Figure 6C**). Most important, the infected/diltiazem ("H1N1 + diltiazem") condition yielded ρ correlation values of 0.40 and −0.72 when compared to either "mock + diltiazem" or "H1N1," respectively, therefore confirming a partial reversion of the infection virogenomic signature during effective antiviral treatment with diltiazem (**Figure 6D** and **Figure S4**), as expected.

## DISCUSSION

The existing urge for alternative strategies to cope with the limited efficacy of currently approved antivirals for the prevention and treatment of influenza infections (2, 41, 42), mostly in the case of patients with severe influenza and acute respiratory distress syndrome (ARDS) (43, 44), represented the central driving force of this study. Here, we developed and validated for the first time an innovative approach based on clinical genomic signatures of respiratory viral infections for the rapid discovery, *in vitro, in vivo,* and *ex-vivo* evaluation, as well as the repurposing of FDA-approved drugs for their newly identified host-targeted inhibitory and protective properties against influenza infections.

Targeting host components on which viral replication depends instead of viral determinants represents a real change of paradigm in antiviral development, with pioneering results mainly observed in the context of antiretroviral therapy (13, 45). Nevertheless, and despite strong putative advantages such as the achievement of broad-spectrum antiviral efficacy and the minimization of viral drug resistance, this approach usually fails to overcome two major limiting factors of classic compound screening. Firstly, it remains target-centered *per se*, therefore leading to the identification of drugs with limited efficacy due to the complex network and high redundancy of the host cellular pathways. Secondly, the need of high-throughput screenings often entails the measurement of a very limited number of viral parameters, usually in non-physiologically and hence poorly relevant conditions and/or cellular models.

Based on our initial proof-of-concept study on the *in silico* screening of the CMAP database (19, 20) with no initial *a priori* on specific host targets (18), we moved our approach up to the clinical trial setting, by determining exploitable and more relevant virogenomic profiles directly from standard clinical samples of influenza-infected patients. Since the low amount of often degraded RNA obtained from these samples represented a major challenge, we implemented an original combination of sample preparation techniques for low input but high quality samples with data processing initially designed for expression analysis of non-model species (22, 23).

Another substantial development was the integration of several lists of candidate molecules issued from different transcriptomic signatures with enriched relevant DAVID Gene

Ontology terms, and their final selection based on their pharmacological classes and potential compatibility as antivirals. Our refined strategy allowed the selection of a shortlist of 35 high potential candidates out of a rationalized computational screening of a total of 1,309 FDA-approved bioactive molecules. This drastic positive selection step constituted a major advantage, since it enabled the implementation of relevant and integrated *in vitro, in vivo* and *ex-vivo* evaluations in a time- and cost-effective manner. Most important, the use of patient (*in vivo*) virogenomic profiles led to the identification of molecules with highly improved *in vitro* activity and significant *in vivo* antiviral efficacy as compared with compounds previously obtained from our initial study based on cell culture (*in vitro*) virogenomic profiles (18). These results truly highlight the added value of using relevant clinical virogenomic signatures to optimize the computational screening for active drugs.

Two of the molecules identified in this study with transcriptomic profiles that counteract clinical virogenomic signatures (e.g., ribavirin and monensin) have already been validated for their anti-influenza properties (38, 40), and then supported the relevance of our compound selection strategy. Nevertheless, although different modes of action have been postulated for the anti-influenza activity of the synthetic guanosine analog ribavirin (39), the exact mechanisms remain uncharacterized so far. Similarly, it has been postulated that monensin, an antibiotic isolated from *Streptomyces* spp, may have a role as a ionophore that interferes with intracellular transport of several enveloped viruses, including influenza (40). In that sense, even if we cannot rule out that some of the molecules identified *in silico* exert a direct effect on a specific pathway or cellular target, the fact that these molecules have been identified with a high anti-correlation rate in CMAP strongly supports a potential multi-target inhibitory effect, probably resulting in deep modifications of host gene expression. In fact, both monensin and ribavirin were previously reported to modulate the host cellular gene expression profile, notably through the up-regulation of the cholesterol and lipid biosynthesis genes (46) or the virus-induced ISRE signaling and antiviral ISGs genes (47), respectively.

The two most promising molecules highlighted in this study are etilefrine, an alpha and beta- adrenergic receptor agonist, currently indicated as a cardiotonic and anti-hypotensive agent (48) and mainly diltiazem, a voltage-gated Ca2+ channel antagonist that is currently used to control angina pectoris and cardiac arrhythmia (49). In addition to their strong inhibitory effect on the viral growth of circulating A(H1N1)pdm09 viruses, with *in vitro* EC50 values in the nanomolar range (**Figure 2**), both molecules also demonstrated antiviral properties against oseltamivir-resistant A(H1N1)pdm09 and prototype H3N2 and B influenza strains (**Table S4**). Interestingly, virus pre-incubation with diltiazem or etilefrine before infection did not affect final viral titers compared to PBS-incubated controls, hence suggesting that the observed antiviral effect of these molecules is not mediated by direct drug-virus interactions at early stages of viral entry (**Table S5**). Our *in vivo* results (**Figures 3, 4**), obtained without previous treatment optimization in terms of dosage or administration route, also suggest that these drugs harbor a protective role toward influenza infection, particularly in the case of diltiazem, which conferred increased survival in mice even in a model of severe influenza infection (**Figures 4D–F**). Moreover, the inhibitory and protective properties of diltiazem were validated in the reconstituted human airway epithelium model, also showing enhanced efficacy when combined with oseltamivir (**Figure 5**).

Finally, a very recent study by Fujioka and colleagues (50) confirmed the antiviral activity of diltiazem anticipated by our approach. In that study, based on the role of Ca2+ channels on the attachment of influenza viruses to the host cell, the authors discuss whether the diltiazem induced modulation of Ca2+ channel activity might not fully explain such observed antiviral activity, consistent with a multi-level (off-target) effect of diltiazem. In this context, in which not all Ca2+ channel inhibitors confer significant antiviral activity, the newly described capacity of diltiazem to partially reverse the global virogenomic signature of infection and modulate specific genes related to the host antiviral response and cholesterol metabolism (**Figures 6** and **Figure S4**) suggests a putative explanation for its inhibitory effect observed *in vitro*, *ex vivo* and in mice. Nevertheless, although RT-qPCR mRNA quantification performed on a set of genes representative of the two hubs further validated these observations (**Figure S5**), further investigations are underscored to shed light on the specific mechanisms underlying such potential multi-level mode of action of diltiazem.

Overall, the results presented here set a solid baseline for our drug repurposing strategy and for the use of diltiazem as a host-targeted antiviral in clinical practice. Moreover, the increased antiviral efficacy observed in reconstituted human airway epithelium (**Figure 5B** and **Table S6**) plead in favor of the combination of diltiazem with the virus-targeted antiviral oseltamivir for the improvement of current anti-influenza therapy, and possibly decreasing the risk of development of viral resistance. In that regard, our results prompted a French multicenter randomized clinical trial aimed at assessing the effect of diltiazem-oseltamivir bitherapy compared with standard oseltamivir monotherapy for the treatment of severe influenza infections in intensive care units, hence completing the bedside-to-bench and bench-to-bedside cycle of our innovative approach. Additionally, retrospective signature analysis of sequential respiratory samples from patients included in both study arms and stratified according to their clinical response to treatment will provide valuable data to pursue the investigations on the specific mediators of the diltiazem-related antiviral response.

This trial (FLUNEXT TRIAL PHRC #15-0442, ClinicalTrials.gov identifier NCT03212716) is currently ongoing.

Finally, our study underscores the high value of clinical specimens and the advantages of exploiting virogenomic and chemogenomic data for the successful systematic repurposing of drugs already available in our modern pharmacopeia as new effective antivirals. We propose that our approach targeting respiratory epithelial cells, the principal influenza infected cell type in the lung, could be extended to other respiratory viruses and eventually to other pathogens involved in acute infections. Importantly, drug repurposing presents several financial and regulatory advantages compared to the development of *de novo* molecules (5), which are of particular interest not only in the context of antimicrobial resistance but also against both emerging or recurrent pathogens for which we are still disarmed.

## AUTHOR CONTRIBUTIONS

AP, OT, JT, GB, and MR-C designed and coordinated the study. VE, JP, and BL acquired clinical data from the cohort. AP, OT, TJ, BP, AT, MR, M-EH, CR, CN, SC, CL-L, and JT performed experiments and provided technical support. AP, OT, MR, JP, JT, GB, and MR-C interpreted data. AP, OT, and MR-C wrote the manuscript. JT, GB, and MR-C revised the manuscript.

## ACKNOWLEDGMENTS

The authors want to thank Jacques Corbeil and Frederic Raymond (Research Center in Infectious Diseases of the CHU de Quebec and Laval University, Quebec) for their help and useful advice. This work was funded by grants from the French Ministry of Social Affairs and Health (DGOS), Institut National de la Santé et de la Recherche Médicale (INSERM), the Université Claude Bernard Lyon 1, the Région Auvergne Rhône-Alpes (CMIRA N° 14007029 and AccueilPro COOPERA N°15458 grants), and Canadian Institutes of Health Research (N° 229733 and 230187). GB is the holder of the Canada Research Chair on influenza and other respiratory viruses. Funding institutions had no participation in the design of the study, collection, analysis and interpretation of data, or in the writing of the manuscript.

## REFERENCES

1. *Influenza Facts Sheet n°211* (2014) Available online at: http://www.who.int/mediacentre/factsheets/fs211/en/ (Accessed January 20, 2016).
2. Loregian A, Mercorelli B, Nannetti G, Compagnin C, Palù G. Antiviral strategies against influenza virus: towards new therapeutic approaches. *Cell Mol Life Sci CMLS* (2014) 71:3659–83. doi: 10.1007/s00018-014-1615-2
3. Booth B, Zemmel R. Prospects for productivity. *Nat Rev Drug Discov.* (2004) 3:451–6. doi: 10.1038/nrd1384
4. Ashburn TT, Thor KB. Drug repositioning: identifying and developing new uses for existing drugs. *Nat Rev Drug Discov.* (2004) 3:673–83. doi: 10.1038/nrd1468
5. Law GL, Tisoncik-Go J, Korth MJ, Katze MG. Drug repurposing: a better approach for infectious disease drug discovery? *Curr Opin Immunol.* (2013) 25:588–92. doi: 10.1016/j.coi.2013.08.004

6. Johansen LM, DeWald LE, Shoemaker CJ, Hoffstrom BG, Lear-Rooney CM, Stossel A, et al. A screen of approved drugs and molecular probes identifies therapeutics with anti-Ebola virus activity. *Sci Transl Med.* (2015) 7:290ra89. doi: 10.1126/scitranslmed.aaa5597

7. Xu M, Lee EM, Wen Z, Cheng Y, Huang W-K, Qian X, et al. Identification of small-molecule inhibitors of Zika virus infection and induced neural cell death via a drug repurposing screen. *Nat Med.* (2016) 22:1101–7. doi: 10.1038/nm.4184

8. Naylor S, Schonfeld JM. Therapeutic drug repurposing, repositioning and rescue - Part I: Overview. *Drug Discov World* (2014) 16:49–62. Available online at: https://www.ddw-online.com/drug-discovery/p274232-therapeutic-drug-repurposing:-repositioning-and-rescue-winter-14.html

9. Keiser MJ, Setola V, Irwin JJ, Laggner C, Abbas AI, Hufeisen SJ, et al. Predicting new molecular targets for known drugs. *Nature* (2009) 462:175–81. doi: 10.1038/nature08506

10. Haupt VJ, Schroeder M. Old friends in new guise: repositioning of known drugs with structural bioinformatics. *Brief Bioinform.* (2011) 12:312–26. doi: 10.1093/bib/bbr011

11. Li Y, Agarwal P. A pathway-based view of human diseases and disease relationships. *PLoS ONE* (2009) 4:e4346. doi: 10.1371/journal.pone.0004346

12. Lussier YA, Chen JL. The emergence of genome-based drug repositioning. *Sci Transl Med.* (2011) 3:96ps35. doi: 10.1126/scitranslmed.3001512

13. Hütter G, Bodor J, Ledger S, Boyd M, Millington M, Tsie M, et al. CCR5 targeted cell therapy for HIV and prevention of viral escape. *Viruses* (2015) 7:4186–203. doi: 10.3390/v7082816

14. Ludwig S. Disruption of virus-host cell interactions and cell signaling pathways as an anti-viral approach against influenza virus infections. *Biol Chem.* (2011) 392:837–47. doi: 10.1515/BC.2011.121

15. Rossignol JF, La Frazia S, Chiappa L, Ciucci A, Santoro MG. Thiazolides, a new class of anti-influenza molecules targeting viral hemagglutinin at the post-translational level. *J Biol Chem.* (2009) 284:29798–808. doi: 10.1074/jbc.M109.029470

16. Belser JA, Lu X, Szretter KJ, Jin X, Aschenbrenner LM, Lee A, et al. DAS181, a novel sialidase fusion protein, protects mice from lethal avian influenza H5N1 virus infection. *J Infect Dis.* (2007) 196:1493–9. doi: 10.1086/522609

17. Mazur I, Wurzer WJ, Ehrhardt C, Pleschka S, Puthavathana P, Silberzahn T, et al. Acetylsalicylic acid (ASA) blocks influenza virus propagation via its NF-kappaB-inhibiting activity. *Cell Microbiol.* (2007) 9:1683–94. doi: 10.1111/j.1462-5822.2007.00902.x

18. Josset L, Textoris J, Loriod B, Ferraris O, Moules V, Lina B, et al. Gene expression signature-based screening identifies new broadly effective influenza a antivirals. *PLoS ONE* (2010) 5:e13169 doi: 10.1371/journal.pone.0013169

19. Lamb J, Crawford ED, Peck D, Modell JW, Blat IC, Wrobel MJ, et al. The Connectivity Map: using gene-expression signatures to connect small molecules, genes, and disease. *Science* (2006) 313:1929–35. doi: 10.1126/science.1132939

20. Lamb J. The Connectivity Map: a new tool for biomedical research. *Nat Rev Cancer* (2007) 7:54–60. doi: 10.1038/nrc2044

21. Escuret V, Cornu C, Boutitie F, Enouf V, Mosnier A, Bouscambert-Duchamp M, et al. Oseltamivir-zanamivir bitherapy compared to oseltamivir monotherapy in the treatment of pandemic 2009 influenza A(H1N1) virus infections. *Antiviral Res.* (2012) 96:130–7. doi: 10.1016/j.antiviral.2012.08.002

22. Khaznadar Z, Boissel N, Agaugué S, Henry G, Cheok M, Vignon M, et al. Defective NK cells in acute myeloid leukemia patients at diagnosis are associated with blast transcriptional signatures of immune evasion. *J Immunol.* (2015) 195:2580–90. doi: 10.4049/jimmunol.1500262

23. Degletagne C, Keime C, Rey B, de Dinechin M, Forcheron F, Chuchana P, et al. Transcriptome analysis in non-model species: a new method for the analysis of heterologous hybridization on microarrays. *BMC Genomics* (2010) 11:344. doi: 10.1186/1471-2164-11-344

24. Tukey J, Wilder J. *Exploratory Data Analysis.* Reading, PA: Addison-Wesley (1977).

25. Benjamini Y, Hochberg Y. Controlling the false discovery rate: a practical and powerful approach to multiple testing. *J R Stat Soc Ser B Methodol.* (1995) 57:289–300.

26. Barrett T, Edgar R. Gene expression omnibus: microarray data storage, submission, retrieval, and analysis. *Methods Enzymol.* (2006) 411:352–69. doi: 10.1016/S0076-6879(06)11019-8

27. Dennis G Jr, Sherman BT, Hosack DA, Yang J, Gao W, Lane HC, et al. DAVID: database for annotation, visualization, and integrated discovery. *Genome Biol.* (2003) 4:P3.

28. Ashburner M, Ball CA, Blake JA, Botstein D, Butler H, Cherry JM, et al. Gene ontology: tool for the unification of biology. The gene ontology consortium. *Nat Genet.* (2000) 25:25–9. doi: 10.1038/75556

29. Hatakeyama S, Sakai-Tagawa Y, Kiso M, Goto H, Kawakami C, Mitamura K, et al. Enhanced expression of an alpha2,6-linked sialic acid on MDCK cells improves isolation of human influenza viruses and evaluation of their sensitivity to a neuraminidase inhibitor. *J Clin Microbiol.* (2005) 43:4139–46. doi: 10.1128/JCM.43.8.4139-4146.2005

30. Moules V, Ferraris O, Terrier O, Giudice E, Yver M, Rolland JP, et al. In vitro characterization of naturally occurring influenza H3NA-viruses lacking the NA gene segment: toward a new mechanism of viral resistance? *Virology* (2010) 404:215–24. doi: 10.1016/j.virol.2010.04.030

31. Tsai AW, McNeil CF, Leeman JR, Bennett HB, Nti-Addae K, Huang C, et al. Novel ranking system for identifying efficacious anti-influenza virus PB2 inhibitors. *Antimicrob Agents Chemother.* (2015) 59:6007–16. doi: 10.1128/AAC.00781-15

32. Bolger AM, Lohse M, Usadel B. Trimmomatic: a flexible trimmer for Illumina sequence data. *Bioinforma Oxf Engl.* (2014) 30:2114–20. doi: 10.1093/bioinformatics/btu170

33. Bray NL, Pimentel H, Melsted P, Pachter L. Near-optimal probabilistic RNA-seq quantification. *Nat Biotechnol.* (2016) 34:525–7. doi: 10.1038/nbt.3519

34. Robinson MD, McCarthy DJ, Smyth GK. edgeR: a Bioconductor package for differential expression analysis of digital gene expression data. *Bioinforma Oxf Engl.* (2010) 26:139–40. doi: 10.1093/bioinformatics/btp616

35. Dupinay T, Nguyen A, Croze S, Barbet F, Rey C, Mavingui P, et al. Next-generation sequencing of ultra-low copy samples: from clinical FFPE samples to single-cell sequencing. *Curr Top Virol.* (2013) 10:63–83.

36. Kinsella RJ, Kähäri A, Haider S, Zamora J, Proctor G, Spudich G, et al. Ensembl BioMarts: a hub for data retrieval across taxonomic space. *Database J Biol Databases Curation* (2011) 2011:bar030. doi: 10.1093/database/bar030

37. Flicek P, Amode MR, Barrell D, Beal K, Billis K, Brent S, et al. Ensembl 2014. *Nucleic Acids Res.* (2014) 42:D749–755. doi: 10.1093/nar/gkt1196

38. Durr FE, Lindh HF. Efficacy of ribavirin against influenza virus in tissue culture and in mice. *Ann N Y Acad Sci.* (1975) 255:366–71.

39. Leyssen P, De Clercq E, Neyts J. Molecular strategies to inhibit the replication of RNA viruses. *Antiviral Res.* (2008) 78:9–25. doi: 10.1016/j.antiviral.2008.01.004

40. Alonso FV, Compans RW. Differential effect of monensin on enveloped viruses that form at distinct plasma membrane domains. *J Cell Biol.* (1981) 89:700–5.

41. Hayden F. Developing new antiviral agents for influenza treatment: what does the future hold? *Clin Infect Dis Off Publ Infect Dis Soc Am.* (2009) 48 (Suppl. 1):S3–13. doi: 10.1086/591851

42. Lee SM-Y, Yen H-L. Targeting the host or the virus: current and novel concepts for antiviral approaches against influenza virus infection. *Antiviral Res.* (2012) 96:391–404. doi: 10.1016/j.antiviral.2012.09.013

43. Koh Y. Update in acute respiratory distress syndrome. *J Intensive Care* (2014) 2:2. doi: 10.1186/2052-0492-2-2

44. Poissy J, Terrier O, Lina B, Textoris J, Rosa-Calatrava M. La modulation de la signature transcriptomique de l'hôte infecté : une nouvelle stratégie thérapeutique dans les viroses graves ? Exemple de la grippe. *Réanimation* (2016) 25:53–61. doi: 10.1007/s13546-016-1188-1

45. Lou Z, Sun Y, Rao Z. Current progress in antiviral strategies. *Trends Pharmacol Sci.* (2014) 35:86–102. doi: 10.1016/j.tips.2013.11.006

46. Dayekh K, Johnson-Obaseki S, Corsten M, Villeneuve PJ, Sekhon HS, Weberpals JI, et al. Monensin inhibits epidermal growth factor receptor trafficking and activation: synergistic cytotoxicity in

combination with EGFR inhibitors. *Mol Cancer Ther.* (2014) 13:2559–71. doi: 10.1158/1535-7163.MCT-13-1086

47. Zhang Y, Jamaluddin M, Wang S, Tian B, Garofalo RP, Casola A, et al. Ribavirin treatment up-regulates antiviral gene expression via the interferon-stimulated response element in respiratory syncytial virus-infected epithelial cells. *J Virol.* (2003) 77:5933–47. doi: 10.1128/JVI.77.10.5933-5947.2003

48. Pubchem C10H15NO2. *Etilefrine|C10H15NO2 – PubChem.* Available online at: https://pubchem.ncbi.nlm.nih.gov/compound/Etilefrine (Accessed February 3, 2017).

49. Pubchem C22H26N2O4S. *diltiazem|C22H26N2O4S - PubChem.* Available online at: https://pubchem.ncbi.nlm.nih.gov/compound/diltiazem (Accessed February 3, 2017).

50. Fujioka Y, Nishide S, Ose T, Suzuki T, Kato I, Fukuhara H, et al. A sialylated voltage-dependent Ca2+ channel binds hemagglutinin and mediates influenza a virus entry into mammalian cells. *Cell Host Microbe* (2018) 23:809–18.e5. doi: 10.1016/j.chom.2018.04.015

# 4

# Non-Specific Effects of Live Attenuated Pertussis Vaccine Against Heterologous Infectious and Inflammatory Diseases

Stéphane Cauchi[1,2,3,4,5] and Camille Locht[1,2,3,4,5]*

[1] Univ. Lille, U1019, UMR 8204, CIIL–Centre for Infection and Immunity of Lille, Lille, France, [2] CNRS UMR8204, Lille, France,
[3] Inserm U1019, Lille, France, [4] CHU Lille, Lille, France, [5] Institut Pasteur de Lille, Lille, France

**\*Correspondence:**
Camille Locht
camille.locht@pasteur-lille.fr

*Bordetella pertussis* is the agent of pertussis, also referred to as whooping cough, a disease that remains an important public health issue. Vaccine-induced immunity to pertussis wanes over time. In industrialized countries, high vaccine coverage has not prevented infection and transmission of *B. pertussis,* leading to periodic outbreaks in people of all ages. The consequence is the formation of a large source for transmission to children, who show the highest susceptibility of developing severe whooping cough and mortality. With the aim of providing protection against both disease and infection, a live attenuated pertussis vaccine, in which three toxins have been genetically inactivated or removed, is now in clinical development. This vaccine, named BPZE1, offers strong protection in mice and non-human primates. It has completed a phase I clinical trial in which safety, transient colonization of the human airway and immunogenicity could be demonstrated. In mice, BPZE1 was also found to protect against inflammation resulting from heterologous airway infections, including those caused by other *Bordetella* species, influenza virus and respiratory syncytial virus. Furthermore, the heterologous protection conferred by BPZE1 was also observed for non-infectious inflammatory diseases, such as allergic asthma, as well as for inflammatory disorders outside of the respiratory tract, such as contact dermatitis. Current studies focus on the mechanisms underlying the anti-inflammatory effects associated with nasal BPZE1 administration. Given the increasing importance of inflammatory disorders, novel preventive and therapeutic approaches are urgently needed. Therefore, live vaccines, such as BPZE1, may offer attractive solutions. It is now essential to understand the cellular and molecular mechanisms of action before translating these biological findings into new healthcare solutions.

Keywords: *Bordetella*, influenza, RSV, asthma, contact dermatitis, inflammation

## INTRODUCTION

Despite of the use of efficacious vaccines, *Bordetella pertussis* is still one of the leading causes of neonatal morbidity and mortality worldwide (1). In the 90s, acellular pertussis vaccines (aPV) have been increasingly replacing the first-generation, whole-cell vaccines (for the description of pertussis vaccines, see **Table 1**) (2, 3). In countries with high aPV vaccination coverage, the resurgence of pertussis has revealed that aPV-induced immunity decreases faster than that induced by whole-cell vaccines or by natural infection (1). Furthermore, aPV vaccination skews the immune response to a Th2 type, both in mice and in human infants (4–6). Given that immunity induced by *B. pertussis* infection decreases later than vaccine-induced immunity (7), and that newborns are capable of inducing a strong Th1 response upon infection (8), a live attenuated pertussis vaccine candidate has been developed to be administered by nasal inoculation (9). Named BPZE1, this vaccine candidate has successfully completed a phase I clinical trial in humans (10). Genetic modifications were made to remove or inactivate three major toxins, pertussis toxin (PTX), tracheal cytotoxin (TCT), and dermonecrotic toxin (DNT). A single intranasal administration of BPZE1 led to strong and prolonged B cell and Th1 T cell responses, inducing protection against challenge infection (9, 11–14). A single nasal administration of BPZE1 in infant mice was associated with stronger protection than that induced by two inoculations of aPV (9) and was lasting substantially longer (13, 14). In addition to mice, juvenile baboons were protected by a single nasal administration of BPZE1 against infection and whooping cough disease upon challenge with a highly virulent *B. pertussis* clinical isolate (15). Therefore, BPZE1 is now in further clinical development as a vaccine candidate against pertussis in adults and in neonates.

## HETEROLOGOUS PROTECTION BY BPZE1

Clinical, immunological, and epidemiological studies have shown that live vaccines can induce immunity to organisms other than those against which they were initially intended. The Bacillus Calmette-Guerin (BCG), smallpox, measles, oral polio, and yellow fever vaccines have been extensively documented to decrease disease and/or mortality from infections that are different from tuberculosis, smallpox, measles, polio, yellow fever, respectively (16). When repurposed against cancer, inflammatory and/or auto-immune disorders, promising effects have been observed for some of these vaccines (17). These heterologous non-specific effects, also termed "off-target effects," seem to be limited to live vaccines (18). Therefore, the heterologous protection by BPZE1 was also extensively investigated.

In addition to *B. pertussis*, BPZE1 protects mice also against lung infection by other *Bordetella* species, although this was not observed after vaccination with aPV (9, 12, 19). *Bordetella parapertussis* is a respiratory pathogen that causes chronic pneumonia in sheep or pertussis-like disease in humans, albeit usually less serious than pertussis caused by *B. pertussis*. A single nasal BPZE1 vaccination led to strong protection against colonization by *B. parapertussis* (9) and protection could be transferred by splenocytes but not by serum of BPZE1-vaccinated mice, whereas serum from convalescent mice was able to protect against re-challenge with *B. parapertussis*. These observations indicate that BPZE1-mediated cross-protection was cell-mediated (12). *Bordetella bronchiseptica* can infect a large variety of mammalian species, including humans, and can cause mild to severe cough. In a mouse lethal challenge model,

BPZE1 reduced both death and lung colonization induced by *B. bronchiseptica* (19). Interestingly, these protective effects depend on two distinctive mechanisms. The decrease in colony-forming units (CFUs) in the lungs relied on adaptive T-cell-mediated immunity. However, protection against mortality was primarily due to BPZE1 potent anti-inflammatory properties. Compared to non-vaccinated mice, BPZE1-vaccinated animals had reduced inflammation, neutrophil infiltration and tissue damage in the lungs upon *B. bronchiseptica* infection. Nasal vaccination with BPZE1 also primed mice for the induction or recruitment of $CD4^+CD25^+FoxP3^+$ regulatory T cells in the lungs the amounts of which strongly increased upon *B. bronchiseptica* challenge only in the BPZE1 vaccinated mice. The role of these cells in the anti-inflammatory activities of BPZE1 was evidenced by the significantly decreased protection against *B. bronchiseptica*-induced mortality when they were depleted using anti-CD25 antibodies 24 h before challenge.

The above observations suggest that the heterologous protection induced by BPZE1 against the closely related pathogens *B. parapertussis* and *B. bronchiseptica* is likely due to cross-reactive B- or T-cells. Even the anti-inflammatory protective activity against *B. bronchiseptica*-induced mortality may be mediated by cross-reactive $CD4^+CD25^+FoxP3^+$ regulatory T cells. However, heterologous protection elicited by BPZE1 has also been assessed against very distant pathogens, totally lacking any cross-reactive antigens at the B- or T-cell levels, such as highly pathogenic influenza A virus (20). A single nasal inoculation of BPZE1 decreased mortality caused by a virulent mouse-adapted Influenza A strain (20). When mice were infected with 2 $LD_{50}$ of a mouse-adapted H3N2 virus 6 or 12 weeks after a single BPZE1 vaccination, 60% of them survived the viral challenge. No protection against H3N2-induced death was observed when the vaccine was heat-inactivated, or when it was given 3 weeks prior to challenge. These data suggest that only live BPZE1 provides protection and that BPZE1-mediated protection takes several weeks to be established for a long period of time. Protection was dose-dependent and required at least $5 \times 10^6$ CFU of BPZE1 in this model. Although live BPZE1 protected against H3N2-induced death, it did not significantly reduce the viral load, demonstrating that the virus particles were not directly targeted by the protective mechanism. This observation is consistent with the lack of B- or T-cell cross-reactivity between BPZE1 and the virus. However, BPZE1 vaccination decreased lung immunopathology, decreased neutrophil and increased macrophage numbers in the bronchoalveolar lavage fluids. Furthermore, BPZE1 protected against lymphocyte depletion and reduced the inflammatory cytokine storm resulting from the viral infection, as evidenced by a decrease in IL-1β, IL-6, and GM-CSF as compared to the non-vaccinated mice upon viral challenge. Strikingly, an additional administration of BPZE1 improved survival of the influenza-infected mice and further decreased the inflammatory cytokine levels. Since this protective mechanism did not rely on adaptive immunity, these observations suggest that BPZE1 could induce trained innate immunity, which has been shown to be based on epigenetic reprogramming of monocytes (21). This may lead to transcriptional programs that rewire the intracellular immune

**TABLE 1** | Vaccine formulations against pertussis.

| Vaccine | Producer | PTX (μg) | FHA (μg) | PRN (μg) | FIM (μg) |
|---|---|---|---|---|---|
| **DTaP** | | | | | |
| Infanrix | GlaxoSmithKline | 25 | 25 | 8 | – |
| Boostrix | GlaxoSmithKline | 8 | 8 | 2.5 | – |
| Daptacel | Sanofi Pasteur | 10 | 5 | 3 | 5 |
| Adacel | Sanofi Pasteur | 2.5 | 5 | 3 | 5 |
| **DTwP** | | | | | |
| D.T.COQ/D.T.P. | Sanofi Pasteur | NA | NA | NA | NA |
| Triple Antigen | Serum Institute of India Ltd. | NA | NA | NA | NA |
| Quinvaxem | Crucell-Janssen | NA | NA | NA | NA |
| **LIVE ATTENUATED VACCINE** | | | | | |
| BPZE1 (Phase II) | ILiAD Biotechnologies | – | NA | NA | NA |

signaling of these innate immune cells but also induce a shift of cellular metabolism, thus increasing the innate immune cells' capacity to respond to stimulation. Although not yet studied, administration of BPZE1 may potentially be associated with specific epigenetic events that are known to control myeloid cell differentiation, the acquisition of myeloid identity and innate immune memory (22).

However, the mechanism of the protective anti-inflammatory effect of BPZE1 is not yet known. Although BPZE1 administration resulted in a transient increase of IL-10-producing $CD4^+$ T cells in the bronchoalveolar lavages (23), the role of IL-10 in BPZE1-mediated protection against influenza remains uncertain. TGF-ß levels did not differ between vaccinated and non-vaccinated mice. Whether $CD4^+CD25^+FoxP3^+$ regulatory T cells play a role in this model was not investigated.

Protection against viral diseases has also been demonstrated in a murine model of respiratory syncytial virus (RSV) infection (23). RSV usually does not cause death in mice but induces dose-dependent weight loss. When mice were vaccinated with BPZE1 14 days before RSV infection, the weight loss was completely abolished. Compared to the non-vaccinated mice, the viral load was reduced 2- to 3-fold in the vaccinated animals, despite the lack of cross reactivity between BPZE1 and RSV. However, this does not fully account for the protective effect against weight loss. Lymphocyte recruitment to the lungs after RSV infection was also significantly reduced in the vaccinated mice, whereas the amounts of macrophages and polymorphonuclear cells in the bronchoalveolar lavages were increased in the BPZE1-treated animals. Interestingly, neonatal vaccination with BPZE1 induced protection for a long period of time against RSV disease as a single nasal BPZE1 dose administered to 2–5-day old mice significantly decreased RSV-induced weight loss when they reached adulthood.

Interestingly, prior BPZE1 vaccination led to an increase in IL-10-producing $CD4^+$ T cells after RSV infection, whereas the numbers of IFN-γ-producing cells were reduced. This is in apparent contrast to what was reported in the influenza model, where BPZE1 treatment resulted in reduced levels of both IL-10 and IFN-γ in the bronchoalveolar lavages after viral

challenge (20). Whether this merely reflects different read-outs or timings between the two studies or whether it suggests different mechanisms of protection against the two diseases remains to be investigated. In the RSV model, the numbers of virus-induced IL-17-producing $CD4^+$ T cells were also increased by prior BPZE1 vaccination (23), while TNF-α and RANTES levels in the bronchoalveolar lavages were decreased. The role of IL-17 in BPZE1-mediated protection against RSV disease could be demonstrated by the use of blocking anti-IL-17 antibodies administered before and during challenge to the BPZE1-vaccinated mice. Administration of these antibodies reestablished the weight loss prevented by BPZE1 vaccination and prevented the recruitment of IL-10/IFN-γ double positive T cells, whereas it did not increase viral load. These data indicate that BPZE1-mediated protection against RSV disease does not merely rely on its ability to slightly decrease the viral load. IL-17 may be important for the recruitment or expansion of IL-10 producing T cells that in turn may decrease lung inflammation. The role of IL-10 in limiting RSV disease has been well documented (24, 25). However, in addition to the induction of IL-17- and of IL-10-producing T cells, BPZE1 vaccination prior to RSV challenge also induced elevated levels of $CD4^+FoxP3^+$ regulatory T cells, which have also been documented to modulate RSV disease (26). The role of these cells in BPZE1-mediated protection against RSV disease has not been investigated yet.

## PROTECTION AGAINST NON-INFECTIOUS DISEASES BY BPZE1

As BPZE1 provided protection against inflammation induced by viral infections, it was also investigated whether BPZE1 can prevent inflammation caused by non-infectious etiologies, such as allergen-induced asthma. In a murine asthma model, nasal inoculation of BPZE1 10 days before ovalbumin sensitization reduced peribronchial inflammation upon ovalbumin challenge, as compared with the non-vaccinated control group of sensitized mice (27). In contrast, nasal infection with virulent *B. pertussis* prior to ovalbumin sensitization exacerbated the pathology. This observation is in line with *B. pertussis*-caused exacerbation of asthma in humans (28) and with the recently developed notion that *B. pertussis* infection may also be an important cause of asthma in humans (29). In contrast to virulent *B. pertussis*, which exacerbated goblet cell hyperplasia and mucus secretion, nasal administration of BPZE1 reduced mucus secretion in the ovalbumin-sensitized mice and reduced bronchial hyperreactivity (27). This was paralleled by a reduced inflammatory infiltration of the airways, as evidenced by a reduced total cell number, neutrophils and especially eosinophil influx, upon aerosol ovalbumin challenge in the BPZE1-treated mice compared to the non-vaccinated mice. However, BPZE1 treatment did not decrease the ovalbumin-specific serum IgE responses, whereas infection with virulent *B. pertussis* increased the ovalbumin-specific serum IgE levels. BPZE1 administration before sensitization by ovalbumin also decreased the levels of the Th2 cytokines IL-4, IL-5, and IL-15 in the bronchoalveolar lavages, whereas it significantly increased the IFN-$\gamma$ levels. Thus, since BPZE1 vaccination had no effect on IgE production, it is tempting to hypothesize that the increased IFN-$\gamma$ production in BPZE1-vaccinated mice has antagonized Th2-driven fibrosis and remodeling of the airways through eosinophil recruitment (30).

When the mice were vaccinated with BPZE1 6 weeks before sensitization, comparable findings were reported (31), indicating that the protective effect of BPZE1 is long-lasting. Again, pre-treatment with BPZE1 protected against airway pathology, whereas pretreatment with virulent *B. pertussis* exacerbated it, even after total clearance of the *Bordetella* infection. Similarly, mucus hypersecretion induced by ovalbumin was markedly decreased in BPZE1-treated mice, as was the inflammatory cell recruitment in the lungs, especially the recruitment of eosinophils. Interestingly, in contrast to the study by Kavanagh et al. (27), BPZE1 treatment also significantly reduced total and ovalbumin-specific serum IgE responses in ovalbumin sensitized and challenged mice (31), although the reduction was <2-fold. Finally, the levels of the Th2 cytokines IL-4, IL-5, and IL-13 in the bronchoalveolar lavages were also decreased in the BPZE1-vaccinated mice, as were the levels of IL-1ß and IL-2, whereas the IFN-$\gamma$ levels did not change. Interestingly, in this model, bronchoalveolar IL-10 levels were increased in the ovalbumin-treated mice as compared to the controls, and this increase was abolished by prior BPZE1 administration. Thus, it is possible that the protective effect of BPZE1 in this model does not depend on IL-10, although this remains to be investigated. Overall, these studies show that BPZE1 is a potent immunomodulatory agent able to suppress allergic asthma in mice even several weeks after a single administration, which is different from most other anti-inflammatory agents that only provide short-term effects.

As in the asthma models described above nasal BPZE1 administration also affected serum antibody responses (31), as well as T-cell responses in the spleen (31), it is possible that its off-target effects may not be restricted to the respiratory tract. In a murine model of allergic contact dermatitis, nasal immunization with BPZE1 was indeed found to reduce dinotrochlorobenzine-induced ear swelling and inflammation of the skin (31). When mice were intranasally vaccinated twice with BPZE1 at a 4-week interval and then treated with dinitrochlorobenzene,

a significant prevention of ear swelling was observed, with decreased tissue edema, inflammatory cell infiltration and local production of pro-inflammatory cytokines. However, in contrast to the allergic asthma model, a single administration of BPZE1 did not significantly reduce ear swelling and inflammatory cell infiltration of inflammatory cells in the skin, and two doses were necessary. Two intranasal doses of BPZE1 also reduced the amounts of IL-1ß, IL-2, IL-17, IL-6, TNF-$\alpha$, and IL-4 in ear homogenates of dinotrochlorobenzine-treated mice, without affecting the levels of IL-10. Thus, intranasal BPZE1 treatment is associated with a systemic protection against inflammatory disorders both at local and at distant sites.

## POSSIBLE MECHANISMS UNDERLYING THE ANTI-INFLAMMATORY EFFECTS OF BPZE1?

Although BPZE1 is associated with potent anti-inflammatory properties, it is likely that its nasal administration initially induces mild inflammation, since it is able to induce T and B cell responses to *B. pertussis* antigens. However, this moderate inflammation appears to be well controlled and rapidly resolved. Little is known about the post-vaccination resolution of inflammation. It has been hypothesized that there is a spontaneous decay of proinflammatory signals, potentially helped by cells of the immune system. Specifically, the regulatory T cells, which are the gateway cells protecting hosts from autoimmunity (32) and which dampen the immune response back to homeostatic levels after an acute reaction (33, 34). Regulatory T cells and Th17 cells have a dynamic relationship between immunity and inflammation, as both are linked with tolerance and immunosuppression (35). Therefore, a modification of the delicate balance between subsets of regulatory T cells and effector T cells in BPZE1-treated mice may result in a short-term mild inflammatory response followed by an tolerogenic response in case of subsequent immune stimulation.

However, as of today the cellular and molecular mechanisms of the BPZE1-associated anti-inflammatory effects remain unclear. Both CD4$^+$CD25$^+$FoxP3$^+$ Treg cells and IL-10-producing CD4$^+$ T cells may depend on IL-17 and be involved in a synergistic manner (36). However, this may vary between disease models. *In vitro* studies on human dendritic cells suggest that BPZE1 can drive Th1/Th17 responses in humans (37). BPZE1-treated dendritic cells induced T lymphocytes expressing CD39/CD73 to generate adenosine using ATP as substrate, and CD38/CD203a/CD73, which can hydrolyze NAD+ to generate adenosine as well (38), and adenosine is known for its anti-inflammatory properties (39). Thus, the induction of these enzymes may result in a regulatory phenotype that may contribute to the mechanism underlying the anti-inflammatory properties of BPZE1. Interestingly, the anti-inflammatory activities of BPZE1 are neither associated with immunodeficiency, since antibody levels or antigen-specific T cell responses to viral or bacterial antigens are not changed by BPZE1 inoculation, nor with a rise in bacterial (9) or viral load (20, 23) upon heterologous infection.

Whereas, many pathogenic bacteria lead to inflammation in the host, some bacterial proteins have the ability to prevent inflammatory responses in order to increase their survival within the host. Pathogens have developed different strategies to counter inflammatory mechanisms, such as escape from the host defense, inhibition of leukocyte recruitment to an inflamed area, deactivation of anti-microbial peptides, increased stability of endogenous inflammatory inhibitors, increased expression of anti-inflammatory cytokines, and NF-κB pathway inhibition through the cleavage of p65/relA (40).

The initial encounter of pathogens with the immune system occurs in an environment often conditioned and regulated by its endogenous microbiota. Thus, it may also be possible that the anti-inflammatory effects observed after BPZE1 administration is partly driven by commensals. It is known that commensals are critical and active inducers of regulatory responses. For example, induction of regulatory T cells was proposed as one of the main mechanisms of action of probiotics—defined bacteria known to confer a health benefit to the host (41). Whether BPZE1 administration alters the endogenous microbiota has not yet been investigated.

Three virulence factors are lacking or are inactivated in BPZE1, compared to the virulent parental strain. The DNT gene is deleted in BPZE1, the PTX gene has been genetically modified, which results in an enzymatically inactive molecule, and the level of TCT has been reduced to background levels. When functionally active, these virulence factors exacerbate airway inflammatory responses during B. pertussis infection (42–44). Therefore, their loss in BPZE1 would be expected to abolish the inflammatory effects.

The lack of widespread occurrence of PTX-deficient strains in the acellular vaccine era suggests that this virulence factor is crucial for B. pertussis pathogenicity and/or transmission (45). A B. pertussis strain not producing PTX failed to induce lethality in 4-week-old young mice, and to effectively colonize the airways of infected mice (46). A U.S. B. pertussis isolate lacking both PTX and pertactin (PRN) (47) caused no disease in a non-human primate model of pertussis (45). Mice infection with high doses of PTX-deficient strains promptly resolved inflammatory airway pathology, whereas infection with isogenic PTX-producing strains significantly prolonged inflammatory events and airway pathology (42, 48). Similarly, mice infected with a PTX-producing B. pertussis strain have significantly exacerbated respiratory reflex responses after intratracheal inoculation of bradykinin, compared to mice infected with a PTX-deficient strain (49, 50). Paroxysmal coughing lasting several days in rats infected with virulent B. pertussis (51) was not observed in rats infected with a PTX-deficient strain (52). Expression of inflammatory cytokine and chemokine genes was increased in B. pertussis-infected mouse lungs, but not in mice infected with a PTX-deficient strain (42, 53). Two distinct signaling mechanisms are used by PTX to subvert cellular responses: ADP-ribosylation of the $G\alpha_{i/o}$ proteins by the A-protomer of the toxin ($G_{i/o}$ protein-dependent action) and the interaction of the B-oligomer with cell surface proteins ($G_{i/o}$ protein-independent action) (54). As BPZE1 produces enzymatically inactive PTX, it is likely that the absence of inflammation upon

BPZE1 administration is due to the inactivation of this enzymatic activity.

However, the absence of inflammatory properties does not explain the potent anti-inflammatory properties of BPZE1, which are likely due to B. pertussis factors that are yet to be discovered. The broad effects of PTX on cell signaling may interact with these unknown factors and thus mask specific immunomodulatory properties.

The adenylate cyclase toxin (ACT), still present in BPZE1, is one potential candidate. This toxin induces a fast upregulation of cellular cAMP levels, which inhibits certain antibacterial activities, such as reactive oxygen species production, phagocytosis, and oxidative burst induction in the neutrophils (55–59). During early infection, inhibition of these activities abolishes innate immune control of B. pertussis (60, 61). In epithelial cells and macrophages, ACT may promote infection by influencing the secretion of cytokines and chemokines (43). Purified ACT was shown to suppress the generation of IL-12 and TNF-α and to increase the production of IL-6 and IL-10 in human monocyte-derived dendritic cells (MDDC) and macrophages activated by lipopolysaccharide (LPS) (61–65), implying that ACT activity is associated with a down-regulation of inflammation. In human bronchial epithelial cells, it was reported that in vitro ACT activity was related to the inhibition of expression of genes coding for the proinflammatory cytokines IL-1β, TNF-α and IL-8 (66). Conversely, within 1 h of toxin addition, the activity of ACT resulted in increased expression of genes coding for IL-1α, IL-6, and IL-10. However, within 24 h after the addition of ACT, the expression levels of these genes were back to the basal state (66). Interestingly, co-incubation of ACT (10 ng/ml) and LPS led to survival signaling in MDDCs and bone-marrow-derived dendritic cells (BMDCs) (67). ACT committed TLR-stimulated dendritic cells to induce CD4$^+$CD25$^+$Foxp3$^+$T regulatory cells in vitro. In mice, ACT-deficient mutants of B. pertussis are impaired in their ability to infect, but this impairment was detectable at later time points than that seen with a PTX-deficient strain (68). These data are consistent with another study reporting that the ACT gene promoter was upregulated later than the PTX gene promoter after infection (69). Therefore, in virulent B. pertussis, PTX may act early during infection to suppress neutrophil influx and ACT may act afterwards to affect neutrophils and other cells recruited at the site of infection (68). In the absence of active PTX early activation of ACT may thus strongly inhibit inflammatory responses in BPZE1-treated hosts.

Recently, ACT was found to interact with filamentous haemagglutinin (FHA) to suppress in vitro production of a biofilm (70). An immune-regulatory role of FHA has been proposed, as microbe-specific type 1 regulatory T cell (Tr1) clones specific for FHA could be generated from the lungs of mice during acute infection by B. pertussis (71). The Tr1 clones secreted high levels of IL-10 (but not IL-4, nor IFN-γ), expressed T1/ST2 and CC chemokine receptor 5 and inhibited Th1 responses. In addition, FHA suppressed IL-12 and stimulated IL-10 generation by dendritic cells, which directed naive T cells toward the regulatory subtype. However, another recent study did not confirm the production of IL-10 by DCs upon FHA treatment (72). Nevertheless, *in vivo* systemic administration of FHA was shown to suppress pro-inflammatory cytokine and to enhance anti-inflammatory cytokine generation by innate immune cells. They suppressed (directly or indirectly) intestinal inflammation in a T cell-mediated model of colitis through the generation of regulatory T cells (73). The inhibitory role played by FHA was also observed in a *B. bronchiseptica* animal model of infection (43). A first analysis demonstrated that FHA can down-regulate the innate immune response against *B. bronchiseptica* infection, leading to lessened inflammation and longer bacterial persistence (74). In the same model, additional studies reported that without FHA, *B. bronchiseptica* triggers a Th17 response leading to fast bacterial clearance, while the wild-type strain expressing FHA caused persistent infection (58).

PRN is yet another candidate potentially endowed with anti-inflammatory properties. PRN-deficient *B. pertussis* strains induced stronger TNF-α, IL-6, IL-8, and G-CSF production when incubated with human DCs than their PRN-producing isogenic counterparts (75). Furthermore, the expression of *IRAK1/2*, *JUN* and *MAP2K3*, as well as that of *TLR1*, *TLR5*, and *TLR6* was significantly more up-regulated in human DCs when incubated with PRN-deficient *B. pertussis* than with PRN-producing *B. pertussis*. *In vivo*, infection of mice with PRN-deficient *B. pertussis* also resulted in increased serum levels of some cytokines, such as TNF-α, IL-8 G-CSF, and IL-1ß, compared to infection with PRN-producing *B. pertussis*. In the lungs of mice the genes involved in lipid release, necrosis and cell death were significantly more expressed after infection with PRN-deficient *B. pertussis* than with PRN-producing *B. pertussis*.

Obviously, many questions remain to be answered before a vaccine such as BPZE1 can be considered as a tool to prevent or treat heterologous inflammatory diseases. Whether any of these factors alone or in combination may account for the anti-inflammatory properties of BPZE1 obviously requires further studies. Monitoring immune cell recruitment over time in bronchoalveolar lavage fluids and examining gene expression profiles of each cell type after BPZE1 treatment may improve our understanding. Inactivation or suppression of additional factors in BPZE1 may also be necessary to identify the causative factors of the anti-inflammatory effects. It is also unknown how important lung colonization with live BPZE1 is, whether

BPZE1 induces dysbiosis in the respiratory tract or elsewhere, and whether this might play a role. The duration of the anti-inflammatory effect has not been explored either. It will also be important to examine whether a single mechanism is responsible for the anti-inflammatory properties in all models investigated so far, or whether different mechanisms might be at play according to the model. Finally, all evidence for heterologous protection mediated by BPZE1 has been obtained in murine models and it remains to be assessed whether BPZE1 expresses its anti-inflammatory properties also in other species, including humans. These are among the questions that should be addressed in future investigations.

## CONCLUSION

Vaccination is considered as one of the most successful and cost-effective medical interventions ever introduced (76, 77). The assumption that vaccines have non-specific effects was first reported in the 1990s at the Bandim Health Project in West Africa by Aaby et al. (78). Since then, our understanding of the immunological landscape is changing drastically. Beyond its capacity to protect against *B. pertussis* infection, the protection of BPZE1 against heterologous infections and inflammatory diseases make this live attenuated vaccine a good candidate to treat a variety of diseases associated with exacerbated inflammation. Given the generic mechanisms and robustness of innate immunity, the capacity to understand and take advantage of this very effective system supplies an attractive method to counteract infections (79). Analyzing how pathogens induce anti-inflammatory and anti-immune machineries in their hosts will lead to a better identification of the different defense weaknesses and thereby more accurately decipher the fundamental mechanisms of microbial pathogenesis (80). Given the rising rate of new infectious and inflammatory diseases and the persistence of classical infections, including pertussis, this research remains essential to consider new preventative and therapeutic strategies.

## AUTHOR CONTRIBUTIONS

All authors listed have made a substantial, direct and intellectual contribution to the work, and approved it for publication.

## REFERENCES

1. Locht C. Live pertussis vaccines: will they protect against carriage and spread of pertussis? *Clin Microbiol Infect.* (2016) 22 (Suppl. 5):S96–102. doi: 10.1016/j.cmi.2016.05.029
2. Sato Y, Kimura M, Fukumi H. Development of a pertussis component vaccine in Japan. *Lancet Lond Engl.* (1984) 1:122–6.
3. Decker MD, Edwards KM. Acellular pertussis vaccines. *Pediatr Clin North Am.* (2000) 47:309–35. doi: 10.1016/S0031-3955(05)70209-1
4. Ryan M, Murphy G, Ryan E, Nilsson L, Shackley F, Gothefors L, et al. Distinct T-cell subtypes induced with whole cell and acellular pertussis vaccines in children. *Immunology* (1998) 93:1–10.
5. Ausiello CM, Urbani F, la Sala A, Lande R, Cassone A. Vaccine- and antigen-dependent type 1 and type 2 cytokine induction after primary vaccination of

infants with whole-cell or acellular pertussis vaccines. *Infect Immun.* (1997) 65:2168–74.
6. Mascart F, Hainaut M, Peltier A, Verscheure V, Levy J, Locht C. Modulation of the infant immune responses by the first pertussis vaccine administrations. *Vaccine* (2007) 25:391–8. doi: 10.1016/j.vaccine.2006.06.046
7. Wearing HJ, Rohani P. Estimating the duration of pertussis immunity using epidemiological signatures. *PLoS Pathog.* (2009) 5:e1000647. doi: 10.1371/journal.ppat.1000647
8. Mascart F, Verscheure V, Malfroot A, Hainaut M, Piérard D, Temerman S, et al. *Bordetella pertussis* infection in 2-month-old infants promotes type 1 T cell responses. *J Immunol.* (2003) 170:1504–9. doi: 10.4049/jimmunol.170.3.1504
9. Mielcarek N, Debrie A-S, Raze D, Bertout J, Rouanet C, Younes AB, Creusy C, Engle J, Goldman WE, Locht C. Live attenuated B. pertussis as a

single-dose nasal vaccine against whooping cough. *PLoS Pathog.* (2006) 2:e65. doi: 10.1371/journal.ppat.0020065

10. Thorstensson R, Trollfors B, Al-Tawil N, Jahnmatz M, Bergström J, Ljungman M, et al. A phase I clinical study of a live attenuated *Bordetella pertussis* vaccine–BPZE1; a single centre, double-blind, placebo-controlled, dose-escalating study of BPZE1 given intranasally to healthy adult male volunteers. *PLoS ONE* (2014) 9:e83449. doi: 10.1371/journal.pone.0083449

11. Feunou PF, Ismaili J, Debrie A-S, Huot L, Hot D, Raze D, et al. Genetic stability of the live attenuated *Bordetella pertussis* vaccine candidate BPZE1. *Vaccine* (2008) 26:5722–7. doi: 10.1016/j.vaccine.2008.08.018

12. Feunou PF, Bertout J, Locht C. T- and B-cell-mediated protection induced by novel, live attenuated pertussis vaccine in mice. Cross protection against parapertussis. *PLoS ONE* (2010) 5:e10178. doi: 10.1371/journal.pone.0010178

13. Feunou PF, Kammoun H, Debrie A-S, Mielcarek N, Locht C. Long-term immunity against pertussis induced by a single nasal administration of live attenuated B. pertussis BPZE1. *Vaccine* (2010) 28:7047–53. doi: 10.1016/j.vaccine.2010.08.017

14. Skerry CM, Mahon BP. A live, attenuated *Bordetella pertussis* vaccine provides long-term protection against virulent challenge in a murine model. *Clin Vaccine Immunol.* (2011) 18:187–93. doi: 10.1128/CVI.00371-10

15. Locht C, Papin JF, Lecher S, Debrie A-S, Thalen M, Solovay K, et al. Live attenuated pertussis vaccine BPZE1 protects baboons against B. pertussis disease and infection. *J Infect Dis.* (2017) 216:117–24. doi: 10.1093/infdis/jix254

16. Saadatian-Elahi M, Aaby P, Shann F, Netea MG, Levy O, Louis J, et al. Heterologous vaccine effects. *Vaccine* (2016) 34:3923–30. doi: 10.1016/j.vaccine.2016.06.020

17. Kowalewicz-Kulbat M, Locht C. BCG and protection against inflammatory and auto-immune diseases. *Expert Rev Vaccines* (2017) 16:1–10. doi: 10.1080/14760584.2017.1333906

18. Aaby P, Mogensen SW, Rodrigues A, Benn CS. Evidence of increase in mortality after the introduction of diphtheria-tetanus-pertussis vaccine to children aged 6–35 months in Guinea-Bissau: a time for reflection? *Front Public Health* (2018) 6:79. doi: 10.3389/fpubh.2018.00079

19. Kammoun H, Feunou PF, Foligne B, Debrie A-S, Raze D, Mielcarek N, Locht C. Dual mechanism of protection by live attenuated *Bordetella pertussis* BPZE1 against Bordetella bronchiseptica in mice. *Vaccine* (2012) 30:5864–70. doi: 10.1016/j.vaccine.2012.07.005

20. Li R, Lim A, Phoon MC, Narasaraju T, Ng JKW, Poh WP, et al. Attenuated *Bordetella pertussis* protects against highly pathogenic influenza A viruses by dampening the cytokine storm. *J Virol.* (2010) 84:7105–13. doi: 10.1128/JVI.02542-09

21. Netea MG, Joosten LAB, Latz E, Mills KHG, Natoli G, Stunnenberg HG, et al. Trained immunity: a program of innate immune memory in health and disease. *Science* (2016) 352:aaf1098. doi: 10.1126/science.aaf1098

22. Álvarez-Errico D, Vento-Tormo R, Sieweke M, Ballestar E. Epigenetic control of myeloid cell differentiation, identity and function. *Nat Rev Immunol.* (2015) 15:7–17. doi: 10.1038/nri3777

23. Schnoeller C, Roux X, Sawant D, Raze D, Olszewska W, Locht C, et al. Attenuated *Bordetella pertussis* vaccine protects against respiratory syncytial virus disease via an IL-17-dependent mechanism. *Am J Respir Crit Care Med.* (2014) 189:194–202. doi: 10.1164/rccm.201307-1227OC

24. Sun J, Cardani A, Sharma AK, Laubach VE, Jack RS, Müller W, et al. Autocrine regulation of pulmonary inflammation by effector T-cell derived IL-10 during infection with respiratory syncytial virus. *PLoS Pathog.* (2011) 7:e1002173. doi: 10.1371/journal.ppat.1002173

25. Loebbermann J, Schnoeller C, Thornton H, Durant L, Sweeney NP, Schuijs M, et al. IL-10 regulates viral lung immunopathology during acute respiratory syncytial virus infection in mice. *PLoS ONE* (2012) 7:e32371. doi: 10.1371/journal.pone.0032371

26. Loebbermann J, Thornton H, Durant L, Sparwasser T, Webster KE, Sprent J, et al. Regulatory T cells expressing granzyme B play a critical role in controlling lung inflammation during acute viral infection. *Mucosal Immunol.* (2012) 5:161–72. doi: 10.1038/mi.2011.62

27. Kavanagh H, Noone C, Cahill E, English K, Locht C, Mahon BP. Attenuated *Bordetella pertussis* vaccine strain BPZE1 modulates allergen-induced immunity and prevents allergic pulmonary pathology in a murine model. *Clin Exp Allergy* (2010) 40:933–41. doi: 10.1111/j.1365-2222.2010.03459.x

28. Harju TH, Leinonen M, Nokso-Koivisto J, Korhonen T, Räty R, He Q, et al. Pathogenic bacteria and viruses in induced sputum or pharyngeal secretions of adults with stable asthma. *Thorax* (2006) 61:579–84. doi: 10.1136/thx.2005.056291

29. Rubin K, Glazer S. The pertussis hypothesis: *Bordetella pertussis* colonization in the etiology of asthma and diseases of allergic sensitization. *Med Hypotheses* (2018) 120:101–15. doi: 10.1016/j.mehy.2018.08.006

30. Cohn L, Herrick C, Niu N, Homer R, Bottomly K. IL-4 promotes airway eosinophilia by suppressing IFN-gamma production: defining a novel role for IFN-gamma in the regulation of allergic airway inflammation. *J Immunol.* (2001) 166:2760–7. doi: 10.4049/jimmunol.166.4.2760

31. Li R, Cheng C, Chong SZ, Lim ARF, Goh YF, Locht C, et al. Attenuated *Bordetella pertussis* BPZE1 protects against allergic airway inflammation and contact dermatitis in mouse models. *Allergy* (2012) 67:1250–8. doi: 10.1111/j.1398-9995.2012.02884.x

32. Fontenot JD, Gavin MA, Rudensky AY. Foxp3 programs the development and function of $CD4^+CD25^+$ regulatory T cells. *Nat Immunol.* (2003) 4:330–6. doi: 10.1038/ni904

33. Tang D-CC, Nguyen HH. The Yin-Yang arms of vaccines: disease-fighting power versus tissue-destructive inflammation. *Expert Rev Vaccines* (2014) 13:417–27. doi: 10.1586/14760584.2014.882775

34. Terhune TD, Deth RC. A role for impaired regulatory T cell function in adverse responses to aluminum adjuvant-containing vaccines in genetically susceptible individuals. *Vaccine* (2014) 32:5149–55. doi: 10.1016/j.vaccine.2014.07.052

35. Chen X, Oppenheim JJ. Th17 cells and tregs: unlikely allies. *J Leukoc Biol.* (2014) 95:723–31. doi: 10.1189/jlb.1213633

36. Locht C. Will we have new pertussis vaccines? *Vaccine* (2017) doi: 10.1016/j.vaccine.2017.11.055

37. Fedele G, Bianco M, Debrie A-S, Locht C, Ausiello CM. Attenuated *Bordetella pertussis* vaccine candidate BPZE1 promotes human dendritic cell CCL21-induced migration and drives a Th1/Th17 response. *J Immunol.* (2011) 186:5388–96. doi: 10.4049/jimmunol.1003765

38. Fedele G, Sanseverino I, D'Agostino K, Schiavoni I, Locht C, Horenstein AL, et al. Unconventional, adenosine-producing suppressor T cells induced by dendritic cells exposed to BPZE1 pertussis vaccine. *J Leukoc Biol.* (2015) 98:631–9. doi: 10.1189/jlb.3A0315-101R

39. Ohta A, Sitkovsky M. Extracellular adenosine-mediated modulation of regulatory T cells. *Front Immunol.* (2014) 5:304. doi: 10.3389/fimmu.2014.00304

40. Sun J. Pathogenic bacterial proteins and their anti-inflammatory effects in the eukaryotic host. *Anti-Inflamm Anti-Allergy Agents Med Chem.* (2009) 8:214–27. doi: 10.2174/187152309789151986

41. Belkaid Y, Hand T. Role of the microbiota in immunity and inflammation. *Cell* (2014) 157:121–41. doi: 10.1016/j.cell.2014.03.011

42. Connelly CE, Sun Y, Carbonetti NH. Pertussis toxin exacerbates and prolongs airway inflammatory responses during *Bordetella pertussis* infection. *Infect Immun.* (2012) 80:4317–32. doi: 10.1128/IAI.00808-12

43. Fedele G, Bianco M, Ausiello CM. The virulence factors of *Bordetella pertussis*: talented modulators of host immune response. *Arch Immunol Ther Exp.* (2013) 61:445–57. doi: 10.1007/s00005-013-0242-1

44. Melvin JA, Scheller EV, Miller JF, Cotter PA. *Bordetella pertussis* pathogenesis: current and future challenges. *Nat Rev Microbiol.* (2014) 12:274–88. doi: 10.1038/nrmicro3235

45. Carbonetti NH. *Bordetella pertussis*: new concepts in pathogenesis and treatment. *Curr Opin Infect Dis.* (2016) 29:287–94. doi: 10.1097/QCO.0000000000000264

46. Bouchez V, Brun D, Cantinelli T, Dore G, Njamkepo E, Guiso N. First report and detailed characterization of B. pertussis isolates not expressing pertussis toxin or pertactin. *Vaccine* (2009) 27:6034–41. doi: 10.1016/j.vaccine.2009.07.074

47. Williams MM, Sen K, Weigand MR, Skoff TH, Cunningham VA, Halse TA, et al. *Bordetella pertussis* strain lacking pertactin and pertussis toxin. *Emerg Infect Dis.* (2016) 22:319–22. doi: 10.3201/eid2202.151332

48. Khelef N, Bachelet CM, Vargaftig BB, Guiso N. Characterization of murine lung inflammation after infection with parental *Bordetella pertussis* and mutants deficient in adhesins or toxins. *Infect Immun.* (1994) 62:2893–900.

49. Carbonetti NH. Contribution of pertussis toxin to the pathogenesis of pertussis disease. *Pathog Dis.* (2015) 73:ftv073. doi: 10.1093/femspd/ftv073

50. Hewitt M, Canning BJ. Coughing precipitated by *Bordetella pertussis* infection. *Lung* (2010) 188 (Suppl. 1):S73-79. doi: 10.1007/s00408-009-9196-9

51. Hall E, Parton R, Wardlaw AC. Cough production, leucocytosis and serology of rats infected intrabronchially with *Bordetella pertussis. J Med Microbiol.* (1994) 40:205-13. doi: 10.1099/00222615-40-3-205

52. Parton R, Hall E, Wardlaw AC. Responses to *Bordetella pertussis* mutant strains and to vaccination in the coughing rat model of pertussis. *J Med Microbiol.* (1994) 40:307-12. doi: 10.1099/00222615-40-5-307

53. Andreasen C, Powell DA, Carbonetti NH. Pertussis toxin stimulates IL-17 production in response to *Bordetella pertussis* infection in mice. *PLoS ONE* (2009) 4:e7079. doi: 10.1371/journal.pone.0007079

54. Mangmool S, Kurose H. Gi/o protein-dependent and -independent actions of pertussis toxin (PTX). *Toxins* (2011) 3:884-99. doi: 10.3390/toxins3070884

55. Weingart CL, Weiss AA. *Bordetella pertussis* virulence factors affect phagocytosis by human neutrophils. *Infect Immun.* (2000) 68:1735-9. doi: 10.1128/IAI.68.3.1735-1739.2000

56. Friedman RL, Fiederlein RL, Glasser L, Galgiani JN. *Bordetella pertussis* adenylate cyclase: effects of affinity-purified adenylate cyclase on human polymorphonuclear leukocyte functions. *Infect Immun.* (1987) 55:135-40.

57. Kamanova J, Kofronova O, Masin J, Genth H, Vojtova J, Linhartova I, et al. Adenylate cyclase toxin subverts phagocyte function by RhoA inhibition and unproductive ruffling. *J Immunol.* (2008) 181:5587-97. doi: 10.4049/jimmunol.181.8.5587

58. Henderson MW, Inatsuka CS, Sheets AJ, Williams CL, Benaron DJ, Donato GM, et al. Contribution of Bordetella filamentous hemagglutinin and adenylate cyclase toxin to suppression and evasion of interleukin-17-mediated inflammation. *Infect Immun.* (2012) 80:2061-75. doi: 10.1128/IAI.00148-12

59. Eby JC, Gray MC, Hewlett EL. Cyclic AMP-mediated suppression of neutrophil extracellular trap formation and apoptosis by the *Bordetella pertussis* adenylate cyclase toxin. *Infect Immun.* (2014) 82:5256-69. doi: 10.1128/IAI.02487-14

60. Harvill ET, Cotter PA, Yuk MH, Miller JF. Probing the function of Bordetella bronchiseptica adenylate cyclase toxin by manipulating host immunity. *Infect Immun.* (1999) 67:1493-500.

61. Vojtova J, Kamanova J, Sebo P. Bordetella adenylate cyclase toxin: a swift saboteur of host defense. *Curr Opin Microbiol.* (2006) 9:69-75. doi: 10.1016/j.mib.2005.12.011

62. Bagley KC, Abdelwahab SF, Tuskan RG, Fouts TR, Lewis GK. Pertussis toxin and the adenylate cyclase toxin from *Bordetella pertussis* activate human monocyte-derived dendritic cells and dominantly inhibit cytokine production through a cAMP-dependent pathway. *J Leukoc Biol.* (2002) 72:962-9. doi: 10.1189/jlb.72.5.962

63. Boyd AP, Ross PJ, Conroy H, Mahon N, Lavelle EC, Mills KHG. *Bordetella pertussis* adenylate cyclase toxin modulates innate and adaptive immune responses: distinct roles for acylation and enzymatic activity in immunomodulation and cell death. *J Immunol.* (2005) 175:730-8. doi: 10.4049/jimmunol.175.2.730

64. Hickey FB, Brereton CF, Mills KHG. Adenylate cycalse toxin of *Bordetella pertussis* inhibits TLR-induced IRF-1 and IRF-8 activation and IL-12 production and enhances IL-10 through MAPK activation in dendritic cells. *J Leukoc Biol.* (2008) 84:234-43. doi: 10.1189/jlb.0208113

65. Ross PJ, Lavelle EC, Mills KHG, Boyd AP. Adenylate cyclase toxin from *Bordetella pertussis* synergizes with lipopolysaccharide to promote innate interleukin-10 production and enhances the induction of Th2 and regulatory T cells. *Infect Immun.* (2004) 72:1568-79. doi: 10.1128/iai.72.3.1568-1579.2004

66. Hasan S, Kulkarni NN, Asbjarnarson A, Linhartova I, Osicka R, Sebo P, et al. *Bordetella pertussis* adenylate cyclase toxin disrupts functional integrity of bronchial epithelial layers. *Infect Immun.* (2018) 86:e00445-17. doi: 10.1128/IAI.00445-17

67. Adkins I, Kamanova J, Kocourkova A, Svedova M, Tomala J, Janova H, et al. Bordetella adenylate cyclase toxin differentially modulates toll-like receptor-stimulated activation, migration and T cell stimulatory capacity of dendritic cells. *PLoS ONE* (2014) 9:e104064. doi: 10.1371/journal.pone.0104064

68. Carbonetti NH, Artamonova GV, Andreasen C, Bushar N. Pertussis toxin and adenylate cyclase toxin provide a one-two punch for establishment of *Bordetella pertussis* infection of the respiratory tract. *Infect Immun.* (2005) 73:2698-703. doi: 10.1128/IAI.73.5.2698-2703.2005

69. Veal-Carr WL, Stibitz S. Demonstration of differential virulence gene promoter activation in vivo in *Bordetella pertussis* using RIVET. *Mol Microbiol.* (2005) 55:788-98. doi: 10.1111/j.1365-2958.2004.04418.x

70. Hoffman C, Eby J, Gray M, Heath Damron F, Melvin J, Cotter P, Hewlett E. Bordetella adenylate cyclase toxin interacts with filamentous haemagglutinin to inhibit biofilm formation in vitro. *Mol Microbiol.* (2017) 103:214-28. doi: 10.1111/mmi.13551

71. McGuirk P, McCann C, Mills KHG. Pathogen-specific T regulatory 1 cells induced in the respiratory tract by a bacterial molecule that stimulates interleukin 10 production by dendritic cells: a novel strategy for evasion of protective T helper type 1 responses by *Bordetella pertussis. J Exp Med.* (2002) 195:221-31. doi: 10.1084/jem.20011288

72. Villarino Romero R, Hasan S, Faé K, Holubova J, Geurtsen J, Schwarzer M, et al. *Bordetella pertussis* filamentous hemagglutinin itself does not trigger anti-inflammatory interleukin-10 production by human dendritic cells. *Int J Med Microbiol.* (2016) 306:38-47. doi: 10.1016/j.ijmm.2015.11.003

73. Braat H, McGuirk P, Ten Kate FJW, Huibregtse I, Dunne PJ, Hommes DW, et al. Prevention of experimental colitis by parenteral administration of a pathogen-derived immunomodulatory molecule. *Gut* (2007) 56:351-7. doi: 10.1136/gut.2006.099861

74. Inatsuka CS, Julio SM, Cotter PA. Bordetella filamentous hemagglutinin plays a critical role in immunomodulation, suggesting a mechanism for host specificity. *Proc Natl Acad Sci USA.* (2005) 102:18578-83. doi: 10.1073/pnas.0507910102

75. Hovingh ES, Mariman R, Solans L, Hijdra D, Hamstra H-J, Jongerius I, et al. *Bordetella pertussis* pertactin knock-out strains reveal immunomodulatory properties of this virulence factor. *Emerg Microbes Infect.* (2018) 7:39. doi: 10.1038/s41426-018-0039-8

76. Berkley S. Improving access to vaccines through tiered pricing. *Lancet Lond Engl.* (2014) 383:2265-7. doi: 10.1016/S0140-6736(13)62424-1

77. Rappuoli R. Vaccines: science, health, longevity, and wealth. *Proc Natl Acad Sci USA.* (2014) 111:12282. doi: 10.1073/pnas.1413559111

78. Aaby P, Andersen M, Sodemann M, Jakobsen M, Gomes J, Fernandes M. Reduced childhood mortality after standard measles vaccination at 4-8 months compared with 9-11 months of age. *BMJ* (1993) 307:1308-11.

79. Finlay BB, Hancock REW. Can innate immunity be enhanced to treat microbial infections? *Nat Rev Microbiol.* (2004) 2:497-504. doi: 10.1038/nrmicro908

80. Finlay BB, McFadden G. Anti-immunology: evasion of the host immune system by bacterial and viral pathogens. *Cell* (2006) 124:767-82. doi: 10.1016/j.cell.2006.01.034

# 5

# Dual-Isotope SPECT/CT Imaging of the Tuberculosis Subunit Vaccine H56/CAF01: Induction of Strong Systemic and Mucosal IgA and T-Cell Responses in Mice upon Subcutaneous Prime and Intrapulmonary Boost Immunization

Aneesh Thakur[1]*, Cristina Rodríguez-Rodríguez[2,3], Katayoun Saatchi[2], Fabrice Rose[1], Tullio Esposito[2], Zeynab Nosrati[2], Peter Andersen[4], Dennis Christensen[4], Urs O. Häfeli[2]* and Camilla Foged[1]*

[1] Department of Pharmacy, Faculty of Health and Medical Sciences, University of Copenhagen, Copenhagen, Denmark, [2] Faculty of Pharmaceutical Sciences, The University of British Columbia, Vancouver, BC, Canada, [3] Department of Physics and Astronomy, The University of British Columbia, Vancouver, BC, Canada, [4] Department of Infectious Disease Immunology, Statens Serum Institut, Copenhagen, Denmark

*Correspondence:
Aneesh Thakur
aneesh.thakur@sund.ku.dk
Camilla Foged
camilla.foged@sund.ku.dk
Urs O. Häfeli
urs.hafeli@ubc.ca

Pulmonary tuberculosis (TB), which is caused by *Mycobacterium tuberculosis* (*Mtb*), remains a global pandemic, despite the widespread use of the parenteral live attenuated Bacillus Calmette–Guérin (BCG) vaccine during the past decades. Mucosal administration of next generation TB vaccines has great potential, but developing a safe and efficacious mucosal vaccine is challenging. Hence, understanding the *in vivo* biodistribution and pharmacokinetics of mucosal vaccines is essential for shaping the desired immune response and for optimal spatiotemporal targeting of the appropriate effector cells in the lungs. A subunit vaccine consisting of the fusion antigen H56 (Ag85B-ESAT-6-Rv2660) and the liposome-based cationic adjuvant formulation (CAF01) confers efficient protection in preclinical animal models. In this study, we devise a novel immunization strategy for the H56/CAF01 vaccine, which comply with the intrapulmonary (i.pulmon.) route of immunization. We also describe a novel dual-isotope ($^{111}$In/$^{67}$Ga) radiolabeling approach, which enables simultaneous non-invasive and longitudinal SPECT/CT imaging and quantification of H56 and CAF01 upon parenteral prime and/or i.pulmon. boost immunization. Our results demonstrate that the vaccine is distributed evenly in the lungs, and there are pronounced differences in the pharmacokinetics of H56 and CAF01. We provide convincing evidence that the H56/CAF01 vaccine is not only well-tolerated when administered to the respiratory tract, but it also induces strong lung mucosal and systemic IgA and polyfunctional Th1 and Th17 responses after parenteral prime and i.pulmon. boost immunization. The study furthermore evaluate the application of SPECT/CT imaging for the investigation of vaccine biodistribution after parenteral and i.pulmon. immunization of mice.

Keywords: H56/CAF01 vaccine, SPECT/CT imaging, dual-isotope $^{111}$In/$^{67}$Ga, pulmonary immunization, T cells, mucosal immunity, nanomedicine, drug delivery

## INTRODUCTION

*Mycobacterium tuberculosis* (*Mtb*), which is causing pulmonary tuberculosis (TB), has infected humans for thousands of years and it is estimated that about one third of the global population is latently infected with TB, which continues to infect 10 million and kill more than 1.5 million people every year (1–3). Increased multi-drug resistance and extensive drug-resistance against existing antibiotics, and the very slow progress in developing new types of antibiotics might result in even poorer prognosis in the future if novel solutions to fight TB are not found. To date, the only licensed TB vaccine remains the live attenuated Bacillus Calmette–Guérin (BCG) vaccine developed from the closely related *Mycobacterium bovis*, causing TB in cattle. The BCG vaccine is one of the most widely used vaccines ever in the world. It is effective against disseminated childhood TB, but it fails to control pulmonary TB in adolescents and adults (4, 5). Hence, there is an urgent medical need for designing novel vaccines and delivery strategies, which can effectively boost BCG-primed immune responses in adolescents and adults, and ultimately induce protective immunity against TB (6, 7).

After infection in the lungs, *Mtb* adopts a variety of immune evasion strategies, which chiefly includes suppression of an innate immune response and subsequently delaying T cell responses in the lungs by approximately 2 weeks (8). These evasion strategies enable *Mtb* to proliferate in the lungs (8–10), eventually explaining the poor efficacy of parenteral BCG vaccination in humans (8, 11). Therefore, homologous or heterologous boost immunization strategies aiming at inducing T-cell immunity in the lungs have the potential to fill this gap (6, 10, 12). Recent preclinical studies have reported induction of protective T-cell immunity in the lungs upon mucosal vaccination *via* the airways (13–18). Mucosal immunization in the lungs has been shown to activate local dendritic cells (DCs) (19) to induce antigen-specific T cells, which effectively home back to the lung parenchyma, where they control initial *Mtb* replication after infection (6, 18). However, almost all TB vaccine candidates in the global clinical pipeline

are administered parenterally (20). Subunit vaccines based on adjuvanted, recombinant TB proteins represent an attractive approach for airway mucosal vaccination (21–23). Besides, vaccine delivery in lungs through inhalation may circumvent the potential safety concerns associated with administration of gene delivery systems, live attenuated organisms, and potentially neurotoxic adjuvant molecules through the nasal route (24, 25). However, thorough safety assessment of airway mucosal vaccination is required.

Understanding the biodistribution and pharmacokinetics of injectable and mucosally administered subunit vaccines is essential (i) for shaping and orchestrating the desired immune response and (ii) for optimal spatiotemporal targeting of the appropriate populations and numbers of effector cells at the site of infection in the lungs. Molecular imaging assessment of such low-dose biological medicinal products using for example single-photon emission computerized tomography (SPECT), allows for the characterization and quantification of biological processes at the cellular and subcellular level in intact living subjects with sufficient spatial and temporal resolution (26). SPECT imaging is based on the measurement of single photons emitted by $\gamma$-emitting radionuclides, e.g., $^{99m}$Technitium, $^{111}$Indium ($^{111}$In), and $^{67}$Gallium ($^{67}$Ga). Furthermore, SPECT imaging is non-invasive and quantitative, permitting uniform and repeated measurements using a single animal subject, thus exploiting the statistical power of longitudinal studies and reducing the required number of animals. In addition, it allows for tracer multiplexing, where several isotopes of different energies can be used in the same animal. Hence, this imaging modality is an effective substitute for conventional *ex vivo* biodistribution studies, which usually require a larger number of animals assessed at multiple time points. In addition, high structural resolution can be achieved by combining the robustness of morphological/anatomical [e.g., computer tomography (CT)] and molecular imaging modalities, which is referred to as multimodality imaging, such as SPECT/CT (26–28). SPECT/CT imaging has been successfully applied in many areas of medical science, but very few reports have been published on SPECT/CT imaging-based investigations for vaccines.

The TB protein subunit vaccine H56/CAF01, which comprises the multi-stage subunit TB fusion protein H56 (Ag85B-ESAT-6-Rv2660c) co-formulated with the liposomal adjuvant referred to as cationic adjuvant formulation 01 (CAF01), has been shown to induce protective immunity before and after *Mtb* exposure in preclinical models (29, 30). H56 is currently tested in a clinical phase 2a trial with the IC31® (Valneva, Lyon, France) adjuvant (31). CAF01, which is based on the

**Abbreviations:** BCG, Bacillus Calmette–Guérin; CAF01, cationic adjuvant formulation 01; CT, computed tomography; DC, dendritic cell; DDA; dimethyldioctadecylammonium; DTPA, diethylenetriamine pentaacetic acid; Ga, gallium; ILN, inguinal lymph node; In, indium; i. pulmon., intrapulmonary; ITLC, instant thin layer chromatography; MBq, megabecquerels; MLN, mediastinal lymph node; Mtb, *Mycobacterium tuberculosis*; NOTA, 1,4,7-triazacyclononane-1,4,7-triacetic acid; PDI, polydispersity index; PLN, popliteal lymph node; Rf, retention factor; SPECT, single-photon emission computed tomography; SUV, standardized uptake value; TB, tuberculosis; TDB, trehalose-6,6'-dibehenate; TLN, tracheobronchial lymph node; VOI, volume of interest.

surfactant dimethyldioctadecylammonium (DDA) bromide and the glycolipid trehalose-6,6′-dibehenate (TDB), has been shown to deliver antigen to and activate DCs through the Toll-like receptor (TLR)-independent Syk-CARD9 pathway (32), and it induces a Th1- and Th17-biased CD4$^+$ T cell response along with a humoral immune response (33, 34). In clinical phase I trials, CAF01 has been found safe, well-tolerated and immunogenic when co-administered with a protein-based TB antigen (NCT00922363) or a cocktail of HIV-1 peptides (NCT01141205). In preclinical studies in mice, CAF01 mixed with H56 has been shown to be safe and immunogenic following intranasal prime and/or boost immunizations (22). Thus, H56/CAF01 is a safe and efficacious multi-faceted TB vaccine.

In this study, we tested for the first time mucosal application of H56/CAF01 using intrapulmonary (i.pulmon.) administration in the airways. We also report the first radiolabeling and preclinical SPECT/CT imaging of the biodistribution and pharmacokinetics of a subunit vaccine. We provide compelling evidence that mucosal administration of H56/CAF01 in the airways induces high levels of antigen-specific lung mucosal IgA and polyfunctional CD4$^+$ T-cell responses following intramuscular (i.m.) priming and i.pulmon. mucosal boost immunization. In addition, strong systemic IgA and polyfunctional CD4$^+$ T-cell responses are induced, which are comparable to the systemic responses induced upon homologous i.m. prime-boost immunization. We show successful dual-isotope radiolabeling of H56 and CAF01 with $^{111}$In and $^{67}$Ga and observe pronounced differences in the pharmacokinetics of H56 and CAF01 following i.pulmon. immunization. Hence, this study underlines the promising potential of H56/CAF01 as a vaccine candidate for airway mucosal immunization, and thus provides the basis for its further preclinical and clinical development as an inhalable and self-administrable aerosol vaccine.

## MATERIALS AND METHODS

### Materials

DDA and 18:0 1,2-distearoyl-$sn$-glycero-3-phosphoethanolamine-N-diethylenetriaminepentaacetic acid (ammonium salt) (PE-DTPA) were obtained from Avanti Polar Lipids (Alabaster, AL, USA), and TDB was purchased from Niels Clauson-Kaas A/S (Farum, Denmark). S-2-(4-Isothiocyanatobenzyl)-diethylenetriamine pentaacetic acid (p-SCN-Bn-DTPA) and 2-S-(4-Isothiocyanatobenzyl)-1,4,7-triazacyclononane-1,4,7-triacetic acid (p-SCN-Bn-NOTA) were procured from Macrocyclics (Plano, TX, USA). Recombinant H56 protein was produced in E. coli as previously described (35). It was reconstituted in 20 mM glycine buffer (pH 8.8), checked for purity and validated for residual DNA, endotoxins and bioburden following internal good manufacturing practice standards. All other chemicals and reagents were of analytical grade and were acquired from commercial suppliers.

### Preparation and Physicochemical Characterization of Vaccine Formulations

Liposomes were prepared by using the thin film method and characterized for average intensity-weighted hydrodynamic diameter ($z$-average), polydispersity index (PDI), and zeta-potential using a Malvern Zetasizer Nano-ZS (Malvern Instruments, Worcestershire, UK) by dynamic light scattering using photon correlation spectroscopy and Laser-Doppler electrophoresis, respectively, as previously described (33). Briefly, weighed amounts of DDA and TDB (5:1, w/w) were dissolved in chloroform/methanol (9:1, v/v) in a round bottom flask. The organic solvents were removed by rotary evaporation under vacuum resulting in the formation of a thin lipid film. The lipid film was washed twice with 99% (v/v) ethanol and dried overnight under vacuum to remove trace amounts of the organic solvents. On the following day, the lipid film was hydrated with 10 mM Tris buffer (pH 7.4), sonicated for 5 min using an ultrasound cleaner (Branson Ultrasonic Cleaner, Danbury, CT, USA), and heated to 60°C for 1 h in a water bath with vortexing every 10th min. In addition, the liposome dispersions were tip-sonicated 20 min after the rehydration for 20 s with a 150 W Branson tip-sonicator to reduce the particle size. The final concentration of CAF01 was 20/4 mg/mL of DDA/TDB, corresponding to a molar ratio of 89:11. The H56 solution was mixed with equal volumes of CAF01 liposome dispersions at concentrations of 5 and 10 µg/mL, respectively, and H56 was allowed to adsorb to CAF01 by incubation for 30 min at room temperature (36).

### Radiolabeling of CAF01 and H56

For radiolabeling of CAF01 liposomes, DDA and TDB were dissolved in chloroform/methanol (9:1, v/v) with 18:0 PE-DTPA (10%, w/w), and the liposome dispersions were prepared in 100 mM HEPES buffer (pH 7.0) as described above. All H56/CAF01 vaccine formulations were radiolabeled as follows: The 18:0 PE-DTPA (10% w/w) chelated CAF01 liposomes were purified using 10 kDa centrifugal filters (Amicon® Ultra 0.5 mL, Merck Life Science, Hellerup, Denmark) to remove excess chelator. For $^{111}$In-labeling, $^{111}$InCl$_3$ (55.5 MBq, 5 µL in 0.1 M HCl) was added to purified DTPA-CAF01 in HEPES buffer (175 µL, 100 mM, pH 7.0), and the reaction mixture was stirred (600 rpm) at room temperature for 1 h. Instant thin layer chromatography (ITLC) showed high labeling efficiency, and $^{111}$In-CAF01 was therefore used without further purification. The collected $^{111}$In-CAF01 dispersion was diluted to a final volume of 275 µL with HEPES buffer, and non-labeled H56 (75 µL, 1 µg/µL) was allowed to adsorb for 30 min to the liposomes before administration.

The H56 protein in 20 mM glycine buffer (pH 8.8) was buffer-exchanged into 100 mM sodium bicarbonate buffer (pH 8.3) using 10 kDa ultracentrifugal filters (Amicon® Ultra 0.5 mL, Merck Life Science) and incubated on an Eppendorf shaker for 5 h at 10°C with p-SCN-Bn-DTPA or p-SCN-Bn-NOTA, respectively, at a molar ratio of 1:5. After 5 h, unreacted DTPA or NOTA was removed by centrifugation through 30 kDa centrifugal filters (Amicon® Ultra 0.5 mL, Millipore, Ontario, Canada), washed and buffer-exchanged into 100 mM HEPES buffer (pH 7.0). For $^{111}$In-labeling, $^{111}$InCl$_3$ (148 MBq/200 µg of H56) was added to H56, and the mixture was incubated for 1 h on an Eppendorf shaker at room temperature. For $^{67}$Ga-labeling, $^{67}$GaCl$_3$ (19.5 MBq/70 µg of H56) was added to H56 and incubated for 1 h on an Eppendorf shaker at room temperature. $^{111}$In-H56 or $^{67}$Ga-H56 was diluted to 500 or 350 μL, respectively, with HEPES buffer and mixed with non-labeled or $^{111}$In-CAF01 liposomes 30 min prior to immunization.

## Radiolabeling Efficiency and Purity of $^{111}$In-H56, $^{67}$Ga-H56 and $^{111}$In-CAF01

The radiochemical purity and labeling efficiency were measured by ITLC using a Tec-Control stationary phase (Biodex Medical Systems, Shirley, NY, USA) and a 0.1 M EDTA (pH 4) mobile phase. The $^{111}$In-CAF01 and $^{111}$In-H56 or $^{67}$Ga-H56 complexes, which have larger molecular weight, would remain at the origin, while the free $^{111}$In elutes with the mobile phase at the solvent front [Retention Factor (Rf) ($^{111}$In-CAF01, $^{111}$In-H56, or $^{67}$Ga-H56) = 0, Rf (free $^{111}$In$^{3+}$ or free $^{67}$Ga$^{3+}$) = 1]. The location of the radioactivity was assessed using a Cyclone Phosphorimager and a photostimulable phosphor plate (Perkin Elmer, Waltham, MA, USA). A NanoDrop spectrophotometer (Thermo Fischer Scientific, Waltham, MA, USA) was used to assess the protein concentration [$A_{280}$ with E1% set to 20.5 L/(g·cm)] and determine the specific activity. $^{111}$In-H56 was analyzed further via 10% native- and SDS-PAGE using established protocols in the lab.

## In vivo SPECT/CT Imaging

The imaging studies, which were conducted at The University of British Columbia, were performed in accordance with the Canadian Council on Animal Care (CCAC), and the protocols were approved by the Animal Care Committee (ACC) of the University of British Columbia (A16-0150). Five-to 6-week old healthy female C57BL/6 mice were purchased from Charles River and allowed free access to food and water. In the first study, mice were allocated into four groups of three individuals. All groups were immunized s.c. (at the base of the tail toward the right) or i.pulmon. with either 10 μg cold H56 adjuvanted with $^{111}$In-CAF01 (125/25 μg DDA/TDB) or 10 μg $^{111}$In-H56 adjuvanted with cold CAF01 (125/25 μg DDA/TDB) in a total volume of 200 μL or 50 μL, respectively. In the prime-boost immunization study, mice were distributed into two groups of three. Two groups were primed s.c. with 200 μL of either 5 μg cold, unadjuvanted H56 or 5 μg cold H56 adjuvanted with cold CAF01 (250/50 μg DDA/TDB). Two weeks later, booster immunization was performed by i.pulmon. administration of either 10 μg unadjuvanted $^{67}$Ga-H56 or $^{67}$Ga-H56 adjuvanted with $^{111}$In-CAF01 (125/25 μg DDA/TDB) in a total volume of 50 μL. The i.pulmon. administration was performed using a MicroSprayer®/Syringe Assembly (MSA-250-M, Penn-Century, Inc., Wyndmoor, PA, USA) according to a previously reported method (37). In brief, mice were anesthetized by intraperitoneal (i.p.) injection of Ketamine (Ketamin, MSD Animal Health, Havneholmen, Denmark)/Xylazine (Rompun Vet, Bayer, Copenhagen, Denmark) 100/5 mg/kg, respectively, and placed on a rodent tilting work stand at a 45° angle by the upper incisors (Hallowell EMC, Pittsfield, MA, USA). For the prime-boost immunization study, anesthesia was induced with 5% isoflurane, the mice were placed on a rodent tilting intubation stand with an integrated anesthesia facemask (Kent Scientific, Torrington, CT, USA), and anesthesia was maintained

with 3% isoflurane. A cold light source with a flexible fiber-optics arm (SCHOTT AG, Mainz, Germany) was used for optimal illumination of the trachea, which appeared as a white light spot. A cotton swab was used to open the lower jaw of the mouse, and the tongue was displaced to the left with a blunted forceps. A laryngoscope (WelchAllen, NY, USA) fitted with a 41 mm intubation specula (Halowell EMC) was used with the other hand for maximal oropharyngeal exposure. After a clear view of the trachea, the laryngoscope with the specula was taken out, and 50 μL of the formulation was administered intratracheally with the MicroSprayer®/Syringe Assembly right above the carina (first bifurcation) to ensure uniform delivery into both lungs. The tip of the syringe was immediately withdrawn, and the mouse was taken off the intubation stand. During SPECT/CT imaging, the mice were anesthetized using isoflurane (1–3% for maintenance, up to 5% for induction) and oxygen from a precision vaporizer, and they received s.c. injection of Lactated Ringer's solution (0.5 mL, B. Braun, Mississauga, Canada) for hydration prior to the SPECT/CT imaging scan. The SPECT/CT imaging was performed using a VECTor/CT preclinical small animal scanner (MILabs, Utrecht, The Netherlands). The respiratory rate and body temperature of the mice were monitored continuously during the scans, and the isoflurane dose and animal anesthesia bed temperature were adjusted accordingly. All animals recovered after each scan. Mice were euthanized 144 h post-administration using $CO_2$, the blood was collected by cardiac puncture, and the tissues were isolated to quantify the biodistribution.

## SPECT/CT Parameters and Image Reconstruction

Whole-body SPECT $^{111}$In and $^{67}$Ga data were acquired using an integrated VECTor/CT preclinical scanner (MILabs) equipped with an XUHS-2 mm mouse multi-pinhole collimator. Dynamic whole-body scans were acquired in list-mode format over 40 min (10 min/frame) post-s.c. or -i.pulmon. administration to study the biodistribution of the protein and the liposomes every 10 min. Subsequently, static 40 min scans were performed for the 6 and 24 h scans, while longer imaging times of 60 and 90 min were performed at subsequent imaging time-points (96 and 144 h) after vaccine administration to increase the statistical signal and the quality of the $^{111}$In and $^{67}$Ga images. Following each SPECT acquisition, a whole-body CT scan was acquired to obtain anatomical information, and both images were registered. For the first imaging study, the $^{111}$In photopeak window was centered at 171 keV with a 20% energy window width. For assessment of the biodistribution in the prime-boost immunization study, the $^{111}$In photopeak window was centered at 20 keV with a 60% energy window width, while the $^{67}$Ga photopeak was centered at 96 keV with a 20% energy window width. For quantitative analysis, SPECT image reconstructions were carried out using the pixel-ordered subset expectation maximization (POSEM) algorithm (38), which includes resolution recovery and compensation for distance-dependent pinhole sensitivity. Further details are provided in the **Supplementary Section**.

## Biodistribution

After the last scan at day 6 (144 h), blood samples were collected by cardiac puncture, and a complete biodistribution assessment was conducted by collecting heart, liver, kidneys, lungs, lymph nodes (LNs), small intestine, bladder, muscle, site of injection, spleen, stomach, bone, trachea, and pancreas. The organs were cleaned from blood and weighed, and the radioactivity was measured using a gamma counter (Packard Cobra II autogamma counter, Perkin Elmer, Waltham, MA, USA). The calibration factor for $^{111}$In was 163631 cpm and $^{67}$Ga was 78395 cpm (instrument-specific). The total weight of the organs was used to calculate the administered dose per organ (%AD/organ).

## Immunizations

Six-to 8-week old female CB6F1 (BALB/c x C57BL/6, Scanbur, Karlslunde, Denmark) hybrid mice were acquired and acclimatized for 1 week before experimental manipulation. All experimental work related to vaccine immunogenicity was performed at University of Copenhagen and approved by the Danish National Experiment Inspectorate under permit 2016-15-0201-01026. The studies were performed in accordance with the European Community directive 86/609 for the care and use of laboratory animals. Mice were assigned to five groups of six individuals, and they were immunized three times using a dose volume of 50 µL of Tris buffer (pH 7.4) at 2-week intervals, which is in line with our previous studies showing that three immunizations are required when applying the s.c. route of administration for optimal immune stimulation (29, 39). The immune responses were evaluated 2 weeks after the final immunization. All vaccine priming was performed by i.m. administration in the right thigh muscles, while the two booster immunizations were given i.pulmon. The first group of mice was primed with saline ($n = 3$) and 5 µg unadjuvanted H56 ($n = 3$), respectively, and boosted i.pulmon. with 10 µg unadjuvanted H56. The second group (250/50 3*i.m., $n = 6$) was primed and boosted i.m. with 5 µg H56 adjuvanted with CAF01 at a dose of 250/50 µg DDA/TDB. Groups 3–5 ($n = 6$ each) were all primed i.m. with 5 µg H56 adjuvanted with CAF01 at a dose of 250/50 µg DDA/TDB. These three groups were boosted i.pulmon. with 10 µg H56 adjuvanted with CAF01 at a dose of 125/25 (125/25 i.m./2*i.pulmon.) and 250/50 (250/50 i.m./2*i.pulmon.) for groups 3 and 4, respectively, and 500/100 µg DDA/TDB (500/100 i.m./2*i.pulmon.) for group 5. CAF01 alone does not induce immunological responses (40, 41). Hence, it was not included as a control in this study. In addition, we have previously shown that there is no difference between s.c. (29) and i.m. (42) immunization with the H56/CAF01 vaccine in mice with respect to immunogenicity and protection against TB infection. Hence, we chose the i.m. route of administration for evaluation of vaccine immunogenicity.

## *In vivo* Staining

Anti-CD45.2 FITC (clone 104; BD Biosciences, Lyngby, Denmark) was diluted to 10 µg/mL in sterile PBS, and 250 µL of the diluted antibody was injected (i.v.) *via* the tail vein 3 min prior to euthanasia of the CB6F1 mice.

## Sample Collection and Cell Preparation

Blood samples were taken by cardiac puncture. Serum was isolated by allowing the blood to clot at room temperature, and the clot was removed by centrifugation at 2,000 × g for 10 min. Subsequently, serum was collected and stored at −20°C. The lungs were aseptically removed from the euthanized mice and transferred to gentleMACS C tubes (Miltenyi Biotec Norden AB, Lund, Sweden) containing 2 mL of RPMI 1640 (Sigma-Aldrich, Brøndby, Denmark), 5% (v/v) FCS (Gibco Thermo Fisher, Hvidovre, Denmark) and 0.8 mg/mL collagenase type IV (Sigma-Aldrich, St. Louis, MO, USA). They were dissociated into 1-2 mm sized pieces using the gentleMACS dissociator (Miltenyi Biotec Norden AB). After 1 h incubation at 37°C, the lung pieces were dissociated again using the gentleMACS dissociator and centrifuged at 700 × g for 5 min. The lung supernatants were collected and stored at −20°C until antibody detection. The lung cell pellets were homogenized using a cell strainer (Falcon, Durham, NC, USA) and washed twice using RPMI-1640 (Sigma-Aldrich). The spleen, the lung-draining tracheobronchial and mediastinal lymph nodes (TLNs and MLNs) and lymph nodes draining the site of i.m. injection, i.e., inguinal (ILNs) and popliteal lymph nodes (PLNs), were aseptically collected. Single-cell suspensions were obtained from the spleens and draining LNs by homogenizing the organs through a nylon mesh cell-strainer (Falcon) followed by two washings with RPMI 1640. The cells were grown in microtiter plates (Nunc, Roskilde, Denmark) containing $2 \times 10^5$ cells per well for cytokine assays, or $1 \times 10^6$ cells per well for flow cytometry in 100 µL RPMI-1640 (Sigma-Aldrich) supplemented with $5 \times 10^{-5}$ M 2-mercaptoethanol (Gibco Thermo Fisher), 1% (v/v) sodium pyruvate (Sigma-Aldrich), 1% (v/v) penicillin-streptomycin (Gibco Thermo Fisher), 1% HEPES (Gibco Thermo Fisher), and 10% (v/v) FCS (Gibco Thermo Fisher).

## Antibody Detection

Maxisorp$^{TM}$ plates (Nunc) were coated with 0.5 µg/mL of H56 solution. Serum and lung supernatants were 5-fold or 10-fold serially diluted 8-12 times from a 1:1 dilution with bicarbonate buffer. IgA, IgG1, IgG2a, IgG2b, IgG2c, and IgM were detected with HRP-conjugated secondary antibodies (**Supplementary Table S1**). 3,3′,5,5′-tetramethylbenzidine (TMB) Plus2 (Kem-En-Tec, Taastrup, Denmark) was used as substrate. Non-linear regression analysis was performed on serum O.D. values to calculate the ELISA mid-point titers, i.e., $EC_{50}$ as previously described (43).

## Cytokine Assays

For the IFN-γ and IL-17A assays, lung and spleen cells were stimulated with 2 µg/mL H56 antigen. Wells containing medium alone or 5 µg/mL concanavalin A (Sigma-Aldrich) were included as negative and positive controls, respectively. The supernatants were harvested after 72 h incubation at 37°C/5% $CO_2$, and the IFN-γ and IL-17A production were quantified by using a standard ELISA protocol. Briefly, purified rat anti-mouse IFN-γ and IL-17A (Biolegend, San Diego, CA, USA) were used as capture antibodies, and biotin-conjugated rat anti-mouse IFN-γ and IL-17A (Biolegend) were used as detection antibodies, followed by HRP-conjugated streptavidin (BD Biosciences, Kongens Lyngby, Denmark) and TMB Plus2 ready-to-use substrate (Kem-En-Tec). The enzymatic reaction was stopped at optimal color development with 0.2 M $H_2SO_4$, and the absorbance was read at a wavelength of 450 nm.

## Flow Cytometry

The isolated lung, spleen and lymph node cells were stimulated *in vitro* in media containing 1 μg/mL anti-CD28 (37.51; BD Biosciences) and 1 μg/mL anti-CD49d (9C10; BD Biosciences) without antigen, or in the presence of 2 μg/mL H56 for 1 h, followed by incubation for 5 h at 37°C in the presence of 10 μg/mL brefeldin A (Sigma-Aldrich) and 0.7 μL/mL monensin/Golgi-stop (BD Biosciences). Following overnight storage at 4°C, the cells were washed with FACS buffer [PBS containing 0.1% (w/v) sodium azide and 1% (v/v) FCS] and stained for 30 min at 4°C for surface markers using anti-CD4-APC-eF780 (RM4-5; eBioscience, San Diego, CA, USA) and anti-CD44-APC (IM7; Biolegend) mAbs. For intracellular staining, cells were washed with FACS buffer, fixed and permeabilized using the Cytofix/Cytoperm kit (BD Biosciences) and stained for 30 min at 4°C for intracellular cytokines using anti-IFN-γ-PE-Cy7 (XMG1.2; eBioscience), anti-TNF-α-PE (MP6-XT22; eBioscience), and anti-IL-17A-PerCP-Cy5.5 (eBio17B7; eBioscience). Cells were twice washed, resuspended in FACS buffer and analyzed using an LSRFortessa flow cytometer (BD Biosciences). Gates for the surface markers are based on fluorescence-minus-one controls. All flow cytometric analyses were performed using the FlowJo software v10 (Tree Star, Ashland, OR, USA).

## Statistical Analysis

GraphPad Prism software (Graphpad Software Inc, La Jolla, CA, USA) was used to perform all statistical analyses. SPECT/CT imaging-based SUVs and *ex vivo* biodistributions were compared between the groups by two-way ANOVA and multiple comparisons were performed by Sidak's post-test. Immune responses were compared between the groups by ANOVA (IFN-γ and IL-17 responses, and antibody responses measured by ELISA) or two-way ANOVA (polyfunctional T cells) at a 0.05 significance level, and pair-wise comparison was performed using Tukey's post-test. A value of $p < 0.05$ was considered significant.

## RESULTS

## Radiolabeling of CAF01 Liposomes and H56 Protein Does Not Influence Their Physicochemical Characteristics

CAF01 was prepared by using the thin film method combined with ultrasonication as previously described (44). The resulting unilamellar liposomes had an average hydrodynamic diameter of approximately $153 \pm 17$ nm, a PDI of $0.324 \pm 0.048$ (**Figure 1A**), and a zeta-potential of $63.6 \pm 11.7$ ($n = 5$, results not shown), which are in accordance with previously reported values for CAF01 prepared using the same method (44–46). The chelation with 18:0 PE-DTPA significantly decreased the size of the CAF01

liposomes (average size = $123 \pm 11$ nm, PDI = $0.270 \pm 0.021$, **Figure 1A**, zeta-potential = $69.9 \pm 8.2$, $n = 8$, results not shown). However, the subsequent radiolabeling with [111]In (average size = $149.8 \pm 36$ nm, PDI = $0.292 \pm 0.092$, **Figure 1A**, zeta-potential = $55.8 \pm 8.52$, $n = 3$, results not shown) had no effect on the physicochemical properties of CAF01 liposome dispersions as their hydrodynamic diameter, PDI and zeta-potential are maintained after radiolabeling (**Figure 1A**). The radiochemical purity and labeling efficiency of [111]In-CAF01 (**Figure 1B**), [111]In-H56 (**Figure 1C**) and [67]Ga-H56 (**Figure 1D**) were measured using ITLC. [111]In-labeling of both CAF01 and H56 using the 18:0 PE-DTPA and p-SCN-Bn-DTPA chelator, respectively, was consistently accomplished with labeling efficiencies of approximately 95% for [111]In-CAF01 (**Figure 1B**) and 80% for [67]Ga-H56 (**Figure 1C**). The average number of bound DTPA molecules was 5 per molecule lipid molecule in CAF01 and 1 per molecule of H56, and the average number of bound NOTA molecules was 1 per molecule of H56. [67]Ga-labeling of H56 using the p-SCN-Bn-NOTA chelator resulted in labeling efficiencies of ~93% (**Figure 1D**). The protein concentrations of the radiolabeled [111]In-H56 and [67]Ga-H56 were 1 and 0.9 mg/mL, respectively. Both [111]In- (**Figure 1E**) and [67]Ga-labeled H56 protein (**Figures 1F,G**) displayed their original molecular weight of 48 kDa (36) determined using SDS-PAGE, suggesting that the radiolabeling procedure did not cause any major modification of the overall size of H56. These data suggest that radiolabeling does not affect the physicochemical properties of CAF01 and H56.

## The H56/CAF01 Vaccine Remains in the Lungs Following i.pulmon. Immunization, Whereas Un-Adjuvanted H56 Rapidly Drains to the Local Lymph Nodes

First, we evaluated the biodistribution and kinetics of the H56/CAF01 vaccine upon pulmonary administration. Mice were dosed i.pulmon. with cold H56 + [111]In-CAF01 or [111]In-H56 + cold CAF01, respectively, and the vaccine biodistribution and pharmacokinetics were visualized and quantified by SPECT/CT imaging at designated time points post-injection (**Figure 2A**). On day 6, the mice were euthanized, and the remaining activity was measured in different organs using a gamma counter. The SPECT/CT images permitted precise anatomical localization of [111]In-CAF01 and [111]In-H56 in the animals (**Figures 2B,C**). The images clearly reflect pronounced differences in the pharmacokinetics of H56 and CAF01 following i.pulmon. administration, and H56 was cleared much faster from the lungs than CAF01. Initially, the vaccine (H56 and CAF01) was apparently distributed evenly in the lungs, and it remained in the lungs during the first 30 min post-injection. Administration *via* the i.pulmon. route often results in deposition of a certain dose fraction of the radiopharmaceutical in the back of the mouth, which is subsequently swallowed (47). Hence, this dose fraction will redistribute to the stomach and the upper gastrointestinal tract, as observed in the 6 h scan. By 6 h, H56 as well as CAF01 were slowly cleared from the stomach and the intestines, and continued to transit in the gut up to 24 h after dosing. The H56 protein could only be detected in the animals up to

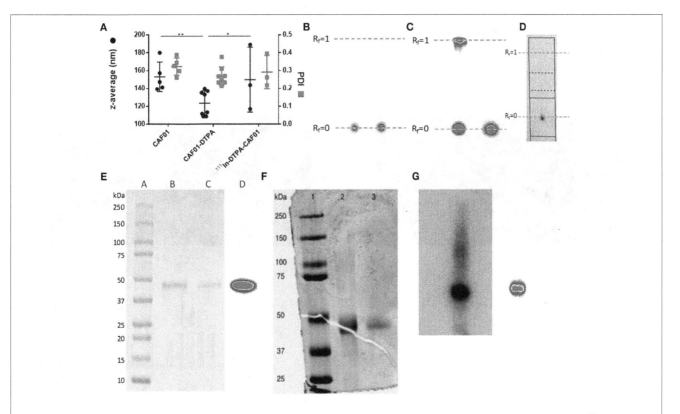

**FIGURE 1** | Physicochemical properties of radiolabeled CAF01 liposomes and H56 protein. **(A)** Chelation of DTPA and radiolabeling of CAF01 with $^{111}$In do not significantly influence the average intensity-weighted hydrodynamic diameter (z-average, circles, left axis) and polydispersity index (PDI) (squares, right axis), respectively. Statistical analysis: two-way ANOVA and Tukey's post-test. Bars represent mean values ± s.d., $n = 5$ (CAF01), $n = 8$ (CAF01-DTPA), and $n = 3$ ($^{111}$In-DTPA-CAF01). $^*p < 0.05$ and $^{**}p < 0.001$. **(B)** Instant thin layer chromatography (ITLC) analysis of $^{111}$In-DTPA-CAF01. Free $^{111}$In$^{3+}$ migrates with the solvent front ($R_f = 1.0$), whereas $^{111}$In-DTPA-CAF01 stays at the origin ($R_f = 0$). Left is $^{111}$In-DTPA-CAF01 for s.c. injection and right is $^{111}$In-DTPA-CAF01 for i.pulmon. administration. **(C)** ITLC analysis of $^{111}$In-DTPA-H56, where free $^{111}$In$^{3+}$ migrates with the solvent front ($R_f = 1.0$, left) and $^{111}$In-DTPA-H56 stays at the origin ($R_f = 0$, right). **(D)** ITLC analysis of $^{67}$Ga-NOTA-H56, where $^{67}$Ga-NOTA-H56 stays at the origin ($R_f = 0$). **(E)** SDS-PAGE analysis of $^{111}$In-labeled H56 protein. Lane A represents a protein ladder, lane B is unmodified H56 protein, lane C is $^{111}$In-DTPA-H56 protein, and lane D is $^{111}$In-DTPA-H56 protein showing the phosphorimager radioactivity signal. **(F)** SDS-PAGE analysis of $^{67}$Ga-labeled H56 protein. Lane 1 represents the protein ladder, lane 2 is NOTA-H56, and lane 3 is $^{67}$Ga-NOTA-H56 protein. **(G)** Phosphorimager radioactivity signal from $^{67}$Ga-NOTA-H56 protein.

24 h post administration (**Figure 2C**), as compared to CAF01, which remained longer in the lungs and was detectable until termination of the experiment (day 6), although with a time-dependent decline in signal intensity (**Figure 2B**). Quantification of the *in vivo* biodistribution (SUV values) supported these observations (**Figure 2D**). The activity observed in the lungs for CAF01 was relatively higher than the activity measured for H56 during the entire experiment (**Figure 2D**, upper left). Both H56 and CAF01 showed very low activity in the trachea, kidneys and bladder at the designated time-points, except at the initial 30 min, where a high activity was detected. Notably, a higher activity was also measured in the stomach 6 and 24 h post injection for H56 than for CAF01, although there was no difference in the intestinal activity at these time points (**Figure 2D**, lower right). Whole body activity was measured on day 6 after euthanizing the animals and compared to the total administered dose, and the percentage of the administered dose per organ/tissue was calculated (**Figure 2E**). The SPECT/CT image analysis corroborate with the *ex vivo* biodistribution data, which showed that the major part of the radioactive

dose was recovered in the lungs (**Figure 2E**). However, there was a statistically significant difference between the remaining activity of H56 and CAF01 in the left lung. For CAF01, a relatively low dose fraction of the radioactivity was found in the liver, kidneys and muscle. In contrast, H56 was detectable in relatively higher amounts in the liver and the kidneys, confirming a faster metabolism and elimination of H56 than CAF01. A comparatively higher activity of H56 than CAF01 was also observed in other organs, including the lung-draining LNs, which confirms the pronounced differences in the biodistribution and pharmacokinetics of H56 and CAF01.

## The Vaccine Forms a Depot Following Parenteral (s.c.) Administration

For control and comparative purposes, we examined the biodistribution of the H56/CAF01 vaccine following parenteral administration. Mice were injected s.c. with either $^{111}$In-CAF01 or $^{111}$In-H56 with cold H56 or cold CAF01, respectively, and the vaccine biodistribution was visualized and quantified by

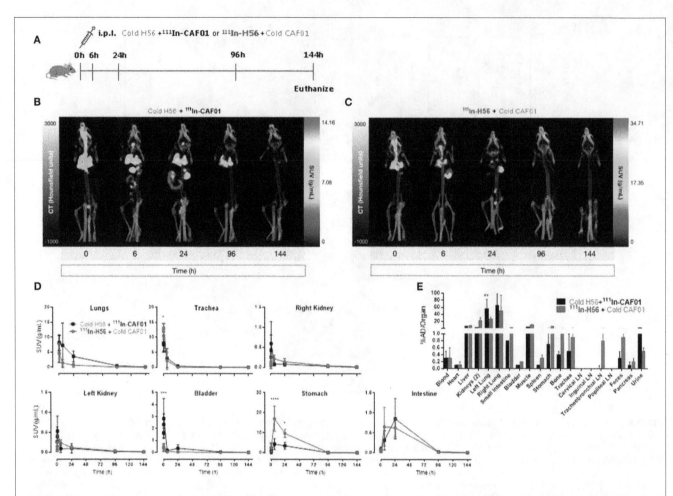

**FIGURE 2 |** The H56/CAF01 vaccine remains in the lungs following i.pulmon. administration, whereas H56 drains to the local lymph nodes. **(A)** Experimental scheme: Mice were exposed i.pulmon. to 10 μg cold H56 adjuvanted with [111]In-CAF01 (125/25 μg DDA/TDB) and 10 μg [111]In-H56 adjuvanted with cold CAF01 (125/25 μg DDA/TDB), respectively. Animals were imaged by dynamic whole-body SPECT/CT scan for the initial 40 min (10 min/frame) and after that static 40 min scans at 6 and 24 h, 60 min scan at 96 h and 90 min scan at 144 h were conducted. Animals were euthanized on day 6 after immunization for *ex vivo* quantification of the biodistribution using a gamma counter. Representative SPECT/CT images of a mouse dosed i.pulmon. with cold H56 + [111]In-CAF01 **(B)** or [111]In-H56 + cold CAF01 **(C)** and imaged over 144 h post-immunization. **(D)** Organ SUVs in g/mL of the cold H56 + [111]In-CAF01 or [111]In-H56 + cold CAF01 over 144 h post-immunization; calculated from dynamic and static SPECT/CT images. Statistical analysis: two-way ANOVA and Sidak's post-test. Data represent mean values ± s.d., $n = 3$. $^{*}p < 0.05$, $^{***}p < 0.001$, and $^{****}p < 0.0001$. **(E)** *Ex vivo* organ biodistribution [% administered dose (AD)/organ] of the cold H56 + [111]In-CAF01 or [111]In-H56 + cold CAF01 on day 6 (144 h) post-immunization. Statistical analysis: two-way ANOVA and Sidak's post-test. Bars represent mean values ± s.d., $n = 3$. $^{**}p < 0.01$.

SPECT/CT imaging at the designated time-points up to 144 h post-immunization (**Figure 3A**). Mice were euthanized 144 h post-injection for *ex vivo* quantification of the biodistribution. The SPECT/CT images clearly showed [111]In-CAF01 and [111]In-H56, respectively, in the animals at the site of injection (**Figures 3B,C**). CAF01 and H56 displayed a highly comparable biodistribution after s.c. administration, and the major part of the dose remained at the injection site for the entire duration of the experiment, suggesting the formation of a vaccine depot at the site of injection, as previously published (48). However, the activity of [111]In declined during the experiment to a minimal level 144 h post-injection. A high activity was observed at the injection site for both CAF01 and H56 (**Figure 3D**), which declined until 144 h (**Figure 3D**, upper left). However, a significantly lower activity was detected for H56, as compared

to CAF01, up to 30 min post-injection. Due to their relatively large size and cationic charge, CAF01 liposomes stayed at the injection site as previously published (48), and almost no activity of [111]In-CAF01 was observed in the kidneys and the bladder post-injection. In contrast, H56 was cleared faster from the injection site and was subsequently excreted through the kidneys, which was evident from the 6, 24, and 96 h post-injection images (**Figure 3D**, upper right and lower left) and a correspondingly higher activity for H56 in the bladder than CAF01 (**Figure 2D**, upper middle). The initial sharp increase in [111]In activity within 30 min post-injection was due to free [111]In (**Figure 2D**, upper middle) in the radiopharmaceutical. Almost no activity was observed in the stomach and the intestines following s.c. immunization (**Figure 3D**, lower middle and right). As expected, most of the radioactivity was detected at the site of injection (**Figure 3E**). For CAF01, a relatively low dose fraction of radioactivity was found in the liver, kidneys, and muscle, which was collected from the right thigh close to the site of injection. In contrast, radioactivity for H56 was observed in several other organs besides the liver, kidney and muscle. Comparing the two, the radioactivity in the kidneys was statistically significantly higher for H56 than for CAF01, which correlates well with the SPECT/CT image analyses. Hence, the SPECT/CT and the *ex vivo* biodistribution data collectively confirm that the major dose fraction of CAF01 stays at the site of injection following s.c. injection, while a small dose fraction of H56 is cleared slowly from the injection site into the blood stream and is subsequently excreted through the kidneys.

## Combined Parenteral (i.m.) Prime and Airway (i.pulmon.) Boost Immunizations Increase H56-Specific IgA Titers in the Airways

With the objective to establish an immunization protocol that generates strong local IgA responses in the airways, we compared vaccine-induced lung IgA responses using two different vaccination strategies; i.m. prime/i.m. boost and i.m. prime/i.pulmon. boost immunization. Mice were immunized twice with CAF01-adjuvanted H56 *via* the i.m./i.m. or i.m./i.pulmon. administration routes, respectively, using different doses of CAF01 to determine the optimal adjuvant dose. Subsequently, we measured H56-specific IgA, IgG1, IgG2a, IgG2b, IgG2c, and IgM antibodies in the lung homogenate supernatants, as well as the IFN-$\gamma$ and IL-17 production by H56-restimulated lung cells 2 weeks after the last booster immunization. For the antibody responses, the mid-point titers were calculated from O.D. values measured by ELISA. Significantly higher levels of H56-specific IgA responses in the lungs (**Figure 4A**) and the serum (**Figure 4B**) were measured for the three groups immunized i.m./i.pulmon, as compared to the levels measured for mice immunized three times i.m. Similarly, the lung (**Figure 4C**) and serum IgG1 responses (**Figure 4D**) were significantly higher following i.m./i.pulmon. immunization using the lowest (125/50 μg DDA/TDB) and the highest CAF01 dose (500/100 μg DDA/TDB) than 250/50 3*i.m. immunization. For the other IgG isotype responses in the lungs (**Figures 4E,G,I**), no difference was observed between i.m./i.m. vs. i.m./i.pulmon. immunization schedules, except for the IgG2b responses (**Figure 4G**), which were higher for the animals immunized using the i.m./i.pulmon. than for the animals immunized using i.m./i.m. schedule. However, the lung IgG2a responses were lower for 500/100 i.m./2*i.pulmon. as compared to 250/50 3*i.m. immunization (**Figure 4E**). In general, the serum H56-specific IgG isotype production was higher for all three groups immunized i.m./ i.pulmon., as compared to the titers for the group immunized three times i.m. (**Figures 4D,F,H,J**). However, the H56-specific IgG2b responses were lower in the 125/25 i.m./2*sngsjehdlejhdx, ki.pulmon. group (**Figure 4H**). As expected, IgM was only detected at low levels in serum and lung homogenates (**Supplementary Figure S1**).

Correlating with these findings, i.m./i.pulmon. immunization induced high IFN-$\gamma$ levels in the lungs (**Figure 4K**), and the IFN-$\gamma$ levels were significantly higher for mice vaccinated once i.m. followed by 500/100 i.m./2*i.pulmon. as compared to three i.m. immunizations (250/50). On the other hand, the IL-17 responses in the lungs were significantly lower for both 250/50 i.m./2*i.pulmon. and 500/100 i.m./2*i.pulmon. than 250/50 3*i.m. immunization (**Figure 4L**). However, the 125/25 i.m./2*i.pulmon. immunization-induced IL-17 responses were not significantly different from the responses for mice immunized three times i.m.. In contrast to the local lung responses, the systemic IFN-$\gamma$ and IL-17 responses measured in serum were significantly higher for the mice immunized three times i.m. (250/50) as compared to all three i.m./i.pulmon. immunizations (**Figures 4M,N**). Overall, i.m./i.pulmon. immunization induced higher local and systemic antibody and dose-dependent equivalent cytokine responses than 250/50 3*i.m. immunization.

## Parenteral (i.m.) Prime and Airway (i.pulmon.) Boost Immunization Cause Localization of H56-Specific Th1 and Th17 Cells in the Lung Parenchyma

Subsequently, we measured in further detail the T-cell recruitment, which takes place in i.m.-primed animals during airway mucosal boost (i.pulmon.) immunization, as compared to animals receiving an i.m. boost (**Figure 5A**). First, we examined, if H56-specific T cells were localized in the lung parenchyma or in the lung vasculature by subjecting immunized mice to *in vivo* intravascular staining. A FITC-labeled anti-CD45 mAb was injected i.v. 3 min before euthanizing the animals, which resulted in FITC staining of all intravascular, but not parenchymal lymphocytes, as previously described (49). Subsequently, we identified the i.v. CD45$^-$ and CD45$^+$ populations of H56-specific CD4$^+$CD44$^+$ T cells producing IFN-$\gamma$, TNF-$\alpha$ and IL-17, respectively, 2 weeks after the last immunization by intracellular cytokine staining. The i.m./i.pulmon. immunization strategy caused markedly elevated infiltration of CD4$^+$CD44$^+$ T cells in the lungs, as compared to i.m./i.m. immunization (**Figures 5B,C**). Most of these cells were localized in the lung parenchyma, and the percentage of IFN-$\gamma$, TNF-$\alpha$, or IL-17 cytokine-producing i.v.CD45$^-$ cells was significantly higher for 125/25 i.m./2*i.pulmon. and 250/50 i.m./2*i.pulmon. than 250/50 3*i.m. group (**Figure 5B**). A similar trend was observed when we examined the frequencies of each of the single cytokine-producing i.v. CD45$^-$CD4$^+$CD44$^+$ T cells among the different immunization groups (**Supplementary Figure S2A**). The functionality of the antigen-specific CD4$^+$CD44$^+$ T cells was determined with respect to their expression of IFN-$\gamma$, TNF-$\alpha$ and IL-17, respectively, or their combinations, for both immunization strategies by combinatorial Boolean gating analysis (**Figure 5C**). The polyfunctionality of the CD4$^+$CD44$^+$ T cells is represented pictorially by pie charts after deduction of control group responses from all immunization groups. The i.m./i.pulmon. immunization induced primarily polyfunctional T-cell populations consisting of double (IFN-$\gamma^+$TNF-$\alpha^+$ and TNF-$\alpha^+$IL-17$^+$) and triple (IFN-$\gamma^+$TNF-$\alpha^+$IL-17$^+$) positive cytokine-producing memory CD4$^+$CD44$^+$ T cells and a lower

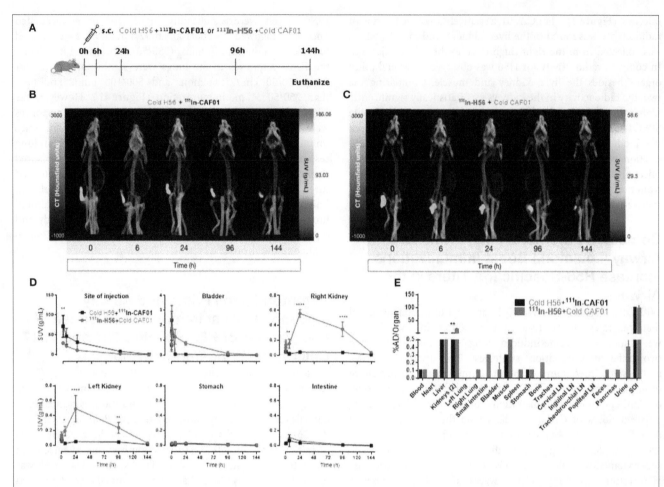

**FIGURE 3 |** The H56/CAF01 vaccine forms a depot at the site of injection following s.c. administration. **(A)** Experimental scheme: S.C. immunization was carried out with 10 μg cold H56 adjuvanted with [111]In-CAF01 (125/25 μg DDA/TDB) or 10 μg [111]In-H56 adjuvanted with cold CAF01 (125/25 μg DDA/TDB). Dynamic whole-body SPECT/CT scans were carried out for 40 min (10 min/frame) and thereafter static 40 min scans at 6 and 24 h, 60 min scan at 96 h and 90 min scan at 144 h were performed. Animals were euthanized on day 6 after immunization for *ex vivo* quantification of the biodistribution using a gamma counter. Representative SPECT/CT images of a mouse injected s.c. with cold H56 + [111]In-CAF01 **(B)** and [111]In-H56 + cold CAF01 **(C)**, imaged over 144 h post-administration. **(D)** Organ SUVs in g/mL of the cold H56 + [111]In-CAF01 or [111]In-H56 + cold CAF01 over 144 h post-immunization; calculated from dynamic and static SPECT/CT images. Statistical analysis: two-way ANOVA and Sidak's post-test. Data represent mean values ± s.d., $n = 3$. $*p < 0.05$, $**p < 0.01$, and $****p < 0.0001$. **(E)** *Ex vivo* organ biodistribution (% administered dose (AD)/organ] of the cold H56 + [111]In-CAF01 or [111]In-H56 + cold CAF01 on day 6 (144 h) post-immunization. Statistical analysis: two-way ANOVA and Sidak's post-test. Bars represent mean values ± s.d., $n = 3$. $**p < 0.01$.

frequency of single (IFN-$\gamma^+$, TNF-$\alpha^+$, or IL-17$^+$) cytokine-positive effector CD4$^+$CD44$^+$ T cells (**Figure 5C**, pies). This shows that there is a CAF01 dose-dependent increase in the frequency of terminally differentiated effector CD4$^+$CD44$^+$ T cells producing IFN-$\gamma^+$ alone (**Figure 5C**, blue pies), whereas immunization with a lower dose of CAF01 led to more IL-17 producing memory-line T cells also expressing TNF-$\alpha$ with or without expression of IFN-$\gamma$ (**Figure 5C**, red and light blue pies). However, there was a dose-dependent increase in the IFN-$\gamma^+$TNF-$\alpha^+$ producing CD4$^+$CD44$^+$ T cells (**Figure 5C**, orange pies). In agreement with the stronger antibody and cytokine responses measured above, there was a higher frequency of H56-specific, cytokine-producing memory CD4$^+$CD44$^+$ T cells in the lungs following i.m./i.pulmon. immunization, as compared to the 250/50 3*i.m. immunization, which induced very low levels of these cells (**Figure 5C**, bars). Among the

three groups immunized using i.m./i.pulmon. vaccination, immunization at the lowest CAF01 dose (125/25 μg DDA/TDB) induced consistently higher frequencies of cytokine-producing single, double, and triple cytokine-producing CD4$^+$CD44$^+$ T cells, except IFN-$\gamma^+$TNF-$\alpha^+$ subgroup, where immunization with 250/50 μg DDA/TDB induced the highest frequency of IFN-$\gamma^+$TNF-$\alpha^+$ producing CD4$^+$CD44$^+$ T cells.

T cells were also measured in the lymph nodes draining the lungs (TLNs + MLNs) in immunized mice (**Figures 5D,E**). I.m./2*i.pulmon. immunization with 125/25 and 500/100 μg DDA/TDB led to a markedly higher frequency of IFN-$\gamma$, TNF-$\alpha$, and IL-17 cytokine-producing CD4$^+$CD44$^+$ T cells as compared with 250/50 3*i.m. immunization (**Figure 5D**). At the individual cytokine level, i.m./i.pulmon. immunization with the highest CAF01 dose (500/100 μg DDA/TDB) induced the highest CD4$^+$CD44$^+$ T-cell levels (**Supplementary Figure S2B**).

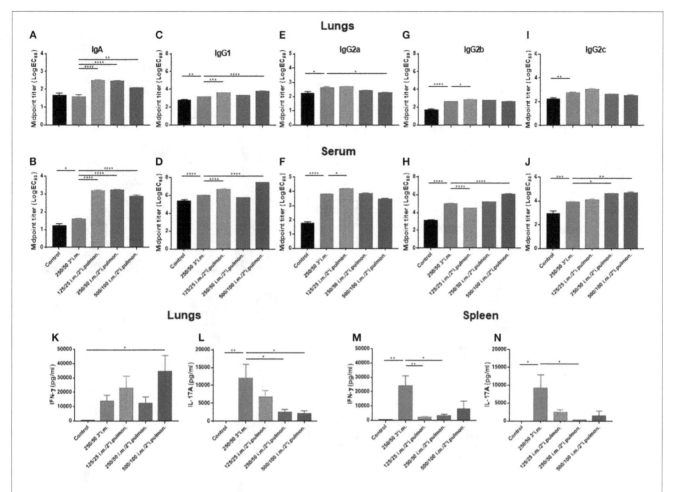

**FIGURE 4 |** Strong antibody and cytokine responses in the lungs and serum after parenteral (i.m.) prime and airway (intrapulmonary, i.pulmon.) mucosal boost immunization with H56/CAF01. Mice were primed i.m. and boosted twice i.m. (5/250/50 μg H56/DDA/TDB) or primed i.m. (5/250/50 μg H56/DDA/TDB) and boosted twice i.pulmon. (10/125/25 or 10/250/50 or 10/500/100 μg H56/DDA/TDB) at 2 weeks interval with H56 adjuvanted with different doses of CAF01 (DDA/TDB). IgA **(A,B)**, IgG1 **(C,D)**, IgG2a **(E,F)**, IgG2b **(G,H)**, and IgG2c **(I,J)** mid-point titers (log $EC_{50}$ values) were determined in homogenized lung supernatants and serum at 2 weeks after the last boost immunization. Lung cells **(K,L)** and splenocytes **(M,N)** were isolated 2 weeks after the last boost immunization and *in vitro* stimulated with H56 for 72 h and IFN-γ and IL-17 levels were determined by ELISA. Statistical analysis: one-way ANOVA and Tukey's post-test. Bars represent mean values ± s.e.m., $n = 6$. *$p < 0.05$, **$p < 0.01$, ***$p < 0.001$, and ****$p < 0.0001$.

The i.m./i.pulmon. immunization induced a polyfunctional T-cell population consisting of single (IFN-γ⁺ and TNF-α⁺, respectively) cytokine-positive effector CD4⁺CD44⁺ T cells, double (IFN-γ⁺TNF-α⁺ and TNF-α⁺IL-17⁺) positive, cytokine-producing memory CD4⁺CD44⁺ T cells and triple (IFN-γ⁺TNF-α⁺IL-17⁺) cytokine-positive CD4⁺CD44⁺ T cells (**Figure 5E**, pies). For the groups immunized i.m./i.pulmon., there was a dose-dependent decrease in the relative frequency of double-positive (TNF-α⁺IL-17⁺) and triple-positive CD4⁺CD44⁺ T cells (**Figure 5E**, red pies). In contrast to observations in the lungs, the IFN-γ⁺TNF-α⁺ producing CD4⁺CD44⁺ T cells in the draining lymph nodes did not show a dose-dependent increase after i.m./i.pulmon. immunization, and the highest fraction of cells was observed after i.m./i.pulmon. immunization with 250/50 μg DDA/TDB (**Figure 5E**, orange pies). As in the lungs, noticeably higher frequencies of memory CD4⁺CD44⁺ T cells were observed in the TLNs and MLNs

following i.m./i.pulmon. immunization, as compared to the frequencies after i.m. immunization (**Figure 5E**, bars), and immunization with 125/25 μg DDA/TDB induced higher frequencies of all subsets of cytokine-producing CD4⁺CD44⁺ T cells, except for the IFN-γ⁺TNF-α⁺ producing subset.

## H56-Specific Th1 and Th17 Cells Are Induced in the Spleen Upon Parenteral (i.m.) Prime and Airway (i.pulmon.) Boost Immunization

Systemic induction of H56-specific Th1 and Th17 cells in the spleen was also investigated (**Figure 6A**). In general, the i.m./i.pulmon. vaccination strategy resulted in induction of lower relative frequencies of CD4⁺CD44⁺ T cells in the spleen, as compared to i.m./i.m. immunization (**Figures 6B,C**). Interestingly, immunization with 125/25 μg DDA/TDB

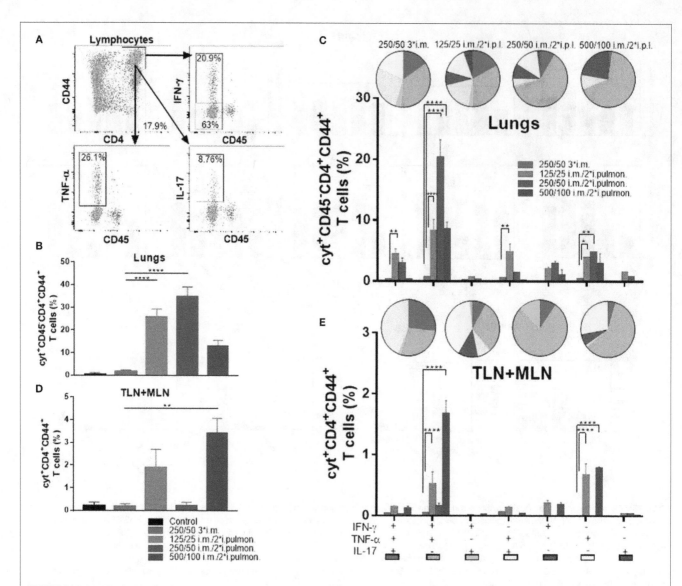

**FIGURE 5 |** Robust T-cell responses in the lungs and the lung-draining tracheobronchial and mediastinal lymph nodes (TLN + MLN) by parenteral (i.m.) priming and airway (intrapulmonary, i.pulmon.) mucosal H56/CAF01 immunization. Mice were primed i.m. and boosted twice i.m. (5/250/50 μg H56/DDA/TDB) or primed i.m. (5/250/50 μg H56/DDA/TDB) and boosted twice i.pulmon. (10/125/25 or 10/250/50 or 10/500/100 μg H56/DDA/TDB) at 2 weeks interval with H56 adjuvanted with different concentrations of CAF01 (DDA/TDB). Lung cells and the lung draining LNs (TLN + MLN) were examined for CD4+CD44+ T cells and IFN-γ, TNF-α, and IL-17 cytokines by intracellular flow cytometry analysis after stimulation with H56, 2 weeks after the last booster immunization. **(A)** Gating strategy for quantification and localization of lung-associated CD44+ T cells in immunized mice (exemplified by lung cells from an immunized mouse from the vaccine group 125/25 i.m./2*i.pulmon.). Lung cells were examined for labeling with i.v. injected FITC-conjugated anti-CD45.2 mAb 2 weeks after the last booster immunization by intracellular flow cytometry analysis after stimulation with H56. Dot plot shows IFN-γ, TNF-α, or IL-17 expression in i.v.CD45+ (intravascular) and i.v.CD45− (parenchymal) cells. **(B)** Number of cyt+CD4+CD44+ T cells (any cytokine IFN-γ, TNF-α, and IL-17), which are located in lung parenchyma (CD45−). Statistical analysis: one-way ANOVA and Tukey's post-test. Bars represent mean values ± s.e.m., n = 6. ****p < 0.0001. **(C)** After Boolean gating analysis, the frequencies of the seven possible CD4+CD44+ T cell subpopulations expressing any combination of the IFN-γ, TNF-α, and IL-17 cytokines are shown for all immunization groups. The background from the control group was subtracted. Pie charts represent the fraction of CD4+CD44+ T cells expressing different cytokine combinations. Pie chart color-coding and the subpopulation association for each color is shown below the bar graph **(E)**. Statistical analysis: two-way ANOVA and Tukey's post-test. Bars represent mean values ± s.e.m., n = 6. *p < 0.05, **p < 0.01, and ****p < 0.0001. **(D)** Number of cyt+CD4+CD44+ T cells (any cytokine IFN-γ, TNF-α, and IL-17) in the lung draining LNs (TLN+MLN). Statistical analysis: one-way ANOVA and Tukey's post-test. Bars represent mean values ± s.e.m., n = 6. **p < 0.01. **(E)** Boolean gating analysis and pie charts of CD4+CD44+ T cells expressing different cytokine combinations in the lung-draining LNs (TLN+MLN), 2 weeks after the last booster immunization. Statistical analysis: two-way ANOVA and Tukey's post-test. Bars represent mean values ± s.e.m., n = 6. ****p < 0.0001.

generated equivalent frequencies of cytokine-producing T cells as the 250/50 3*i.m. immunization (**Figure 6B**). When comparing the frequencies of CD4+CD44+ T cells

producing IFN-γ, TNF-α, and IL-17, respectively, we observed that i.m./i.pulmon. immunization with 125/25 and 250/50 μg DDA/TDB stimulated equivalent frequencies of T cells as the i.m. immunization with 250/50 μg DDA/TDB (**Supplementary Figure S2C**). Examination of the functionality of the H56-specific $CD4^+CD44^+$ T in the spleen revealed that i.m./i.pulmon. immunization with the lowest CAF01 dose (125/25 μg DDA/TDB) induced primarily a polyfunctional T cell population consisting of double ($IFN-\gamma^+TNF-\alpha^+$ and $TNF-\alpha^+IL-17^+$) and triple ($IFN-\gamma^+TNF-\alpha^+IL-17^+$) positive, cytokine-producing memory $CD4^+CD44^+$ T cells and $TNF-\alpha^+$ memory $CD4^+CD44^+$ T cells (**Figure 6C**, pies). Three i.m. immunizations promoted a comparable functionality profile. On the other hand, higher doses of CAF01 administered i.m./i.pulmon. (250/50 and 500/100 μg DDA/TDB, respectively) led to a dominant $IFN-\gamma^+TNF-\alpha^+$ producing $CD4^+CD44^+$ T cell population (**Figure 6C**, orange pies). Unlike for the lungs, i.m./i.pulmon. immunization induced comparable frequencies of H56-specific, cytokine-producing memory $CD4^+CD44^+$ T cells in the spleen as the i.m./i.m. immunization (**Figure 6C**, bars). i.m. and i.m./2*i.pulmon. immunization with 125/25 μg DDA/TDB also promoted similar frequencies of $IFN-\gamma^+$ or $TNF-\alpha^+$ producing effector $CD4^+CD44^+$ T cells.

Vaccine-induced T cells were also evaluated in the ILNs and PLNs draining the site of i.m. injection (**Figure 6A**), and we compared i.m./i.pulmon. vs. i.m./i.m. immunization, respectively. The i.m./i.m. immunization with 250/50 μg DDA/TDB induced higher but statistically indifferent cytokine-producing frequencies of $CD4^+CD44^+$ T cells in the draining LNs, as compared with i.m./i.pulmon. immunization (**Figure 6D**). There was significant differences in the frequencies of $CD4^+CD44^+$ T cells producing IFN-γ, TNF-α, or IL-17 between the groups vaccinated by i.m./i.pulmon., as compared to i.m./i.m. immunization with 250/50 μg DDA/TDB (**Supplementary Figure S2D**). However, there was a considerable difference in the functionality of the $CD4^+CD44^+$ T cells between the two immunization strategies (**Figure 6E**, pies). Whereas i.m./i.pulmon. immunization predominantly induced single cytokine-producing $CD4^+CD44^+$ T cells, i.m. immunization with 250/50 μg DDA/TDB resulted in a polyfunctional T-cell population consisting of double ($IFN-\gamma^+TNF-\alpha^+$ and $TNF-\alpha^+IL-17^+$) and triple ($IFN-\gamma^+TNF-\alpha^+IL-17^+$) positive, cytokine-producing memory $CD4^+CD44^+$ T cells and $IFN-\gamma^+$ or $TNF-\alpha^+$ effector $CD4^+CD44^+$ T cells. I.m./i.pulmon. immunization did mainly induce very low frequencies of memory $CD4^+CD44^+$ T cells and promoted single cytokine-producing effector $CD4^+CD44^+$ T cells (**Figure 6E**, bars). The frequencies of memory and effector $CD4^+CD44^+$ T cells were significantly higher after i.m. immunization with 250/50 μg DDA/TDB, as compared to the frequencies detected after i.m./i.pulmon. immunization.

## The Biodistribution of Parenteral (s.c.) Prime and Airway (i.pulmon.) Boost Administered Vaccine Mimics the Biodistribution of i.pulmon. Administered Vaccine

We used SPECT/CT to investigate the biodistribution of the H56/CAF01 vaccine following parenteral prime-airway

mucosal boost immunization and compared with our previous biodistribution results. We performed this study as we wanted to know whether there would be a faster clearance of H56 or CAF01 on i.pulmon. immunization with previously primed animals. Mice were primed s.c. with cold H56 or cold H56/CAF01, respectively, and boosted i.pulmon. 2 weeks later with $^{67}$Ga-H56 or $^{67}$Ga-H56/$^{111}$In-CAF01, respectively. Mice were imaged by SPECT/CT imaging at the designated time-points up to 144 h post-injection, and the vaccine biodistribution was visualized and quantified (**Figure 7A** and **Supplementary Figure S3A**), followed by terminal ex vivo quantification of the biodistribution on day 6 of the study. Dual-isotope labeling of H56 and CAF01 with $^{111}$In and $^{67}$Ga, respectively, followed by SPECT-CT imaging, allowed for anatomical visualization of vaccine uptake in the lungs, as well as biodistribution and pharmacokinetics (**Figures 7B,C**). The images demonstrate pronounced differences in the biodistribution of H56 and CAF01 following s.c. prime and i.pulmon. boost immunization, where H56 was cleared within 24 h post-injection. The i.pulmon. administration of unadjuvanted H56 resulted in a very fast clearance of H56 within 6 h (**Supplementary Figure S3B**). The vaccine remained in the lungs for up to 6 h, followed by a slow redistribution to the stomach and intestines up to 24 h of the study. The signal from H56 was clearly visible until 24 h (**Figure 7C**) as compared to CAF01, which could be weakly visualized up to 96 h post-injection (**Figure 7B**). The in vivo quantification of radioactivity in images through SUV values verify these findings (**Figure 7D**). In contrast to a single i.pulmon. administration of the H56/CAF01 vaccine, s.c. prime-i.pulmon. boost immunization resulted in comparable activity of H56 and CAF01 in the lungs at the designated time points (**Figure 7D**, upper left). A relatively higher activity for both H56 and CAF01 was observed in the trachea, kidneys and bladder within 30 min post-injection, which declined at later time-points. As observed previously, a high activity of both H56 and CAF01 was observed in the stomach and the intestines at 6 and 24 h post-injection. The SUVs for unadjuvanted H56 showed a very low activity in the lungs and other organs, and most of the activity was observed in the kidneys within 6 h, which reflects that immunization with unadjuvanted H56 leads to lower retention in the lungs and faster metabolism and elimination of the protein (**Supplementary Figure S3C**). Whole-body activity was measured 144 h post-i.pulmon.-boost immunization. The results are in line with the imaging-based in vivo biodistribution, and the major fraction of the radioactivity was observed in the lungs (**Figure 7E**). The biodistribution profile of unadjuvanted H56 showed relatively low H56 activity in the lungs and liver (**Supplementary Figure S3D**). For H56/CAF01 s.c. prime-i.pulmon. boost immunization, there were differences in the remaining activity ex vivo between H56 and CAF01 in the lungs with comparatively higher radioactivity for H56 than for CAF01. For all other organs than the lungs, a relatively low dose fraction of CAF01-associated radioactivity was found in the liver, kidneys and intestine, as observed previously following either a single s.c. or i.pulmon. administration (**Figure 7E**). In contrast, H56 radioactivity was detectable in relatively higher dose fractions in the liver and kidneys, which supports our prior observations of a

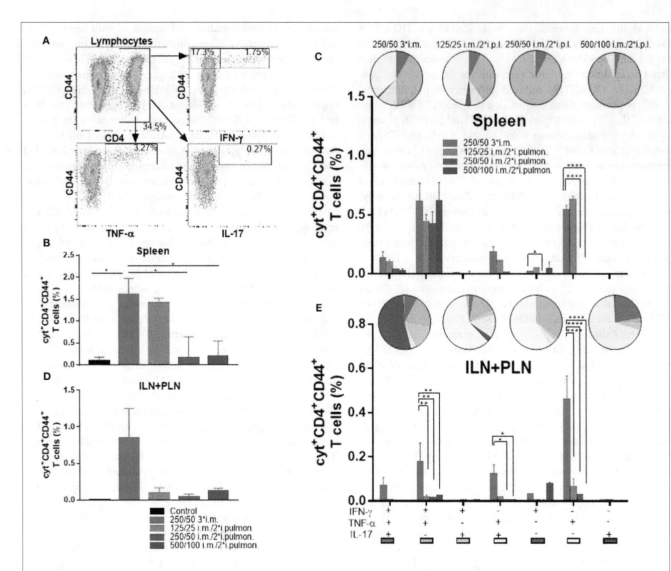

**FIGURE 6** | Parenteral (i.m.) prime and airway (i.pulmon.) mucosal boost immunization with H56/CAF01 induce equivalent T-cell responses in the spleen as parenteral (i.m.) prime-boost immunization. Mice were primed i.m. and boosted twice i.m. (5/250/50 μg H56/DDA/TDB) or primed i.m. (5/250/50 μg H56/DDA/TDB) and boosted twice i.pulmon. (10/125/25 or 10/250/50 or 10/500/100 μg H56/DDA/TDB) at 2 weeks interval with H56 adjuvanted with different concentrations of CAF01 (DDA/TDB). Spleen cells and the inguinal and popliteal lymph nodes (ILN+PLN) draining the site of i.m. injection were harvested 2 weeks after the last booster immunization, surface-stained for the CD4 and CD44 receptors and intracellular localized IFN-γ, TNF-α, and IL-17 cytokines by intracellular flow cytometry analysis after stimulation with H56. **(A)** Gating strategy for the evaluation of antigen-specific, cytokine-producing CD44+ T cells in spleen and lymph nodes of immunized mice (exemplified by TLN + MLN cells from an immunized mouse from the vaccine group 125/25 i.m./2*i.pulmon.). Dot plot shows IFN-γ, TNF-α, or IL-17 expression in CD44+ T cells. **(B)** Number of cyt+CD4+CD44+ T cells (any cytokine IFN-γ, TNF-α, and IL-17) in the spleen. Statistical analysis: one-way ANOVA and Tukey's post-test. Bars represent mean values ± s.e.m., $n = 6$. *$p < 0.05$. **(C)** After a Boolean gating analysis, the frequencies of the seven possible CD4+CD44+ T cell subpopulations expressing any combination of the IFN-γ, TNF-α, and IL-17 cytokines are shown for all immunization groups. Background from the control group was subtracted. Pie charts represent the fraction of CD4+CD44+ T cells expressing different cytokine combinations. Pie chart color-coding and the subpopulation association for each color is shown below the bar graph **(E)**. Statistical analysis: two-way ANOVA and Tukey's post-test. Bars represent mean values ± s.e.m., $n = 6$. *$p < 0.05$ and ****$p < 0.0001$. **(D)** Number of cyt+CD4+CD44+ T cells (any cytokine IFN-γ, TNF-α and IL-17) in LNs draining the site of injection (ILN + PLN). Bars represent mean values ± s.e.m., $n = 6$. **(E)** Boolean gating analysis and pie charts of CD4+CD44+ T cells expressing different cytokine combinations in the LNs draining the site of injection (ILN+PLN) 2 weeks after the last booster immunization. Statistical analysis: two-way ANOVA and Tukey's post-test. Bars represent mean values ± s.e.m., $n = 6$. *$p < 0.05$, **$p < 0.01$ and ****$p < 0.0001$.

faster clearance of H56 than CAF01 (**Figure 7E**). Proportionately higher amounts of H56 activity was also observed in organs other than the liver and the kidneys. However, no remaining activity was detected in the lung-draining LNs, as observed earlier. We also compared the activity of [67]Ga-H56 alone with

[67]Ga-H56 adsorbed to [111]In-CAF01 and observed significant differences in the pulmonary uptake and biodistribution of unadjuvanted protein, as compared to liposome-adsorbed protein (**Supplementary Figure S4**). Unadjuvanted H56 was cleared much faster than the CAF01-bound H56.

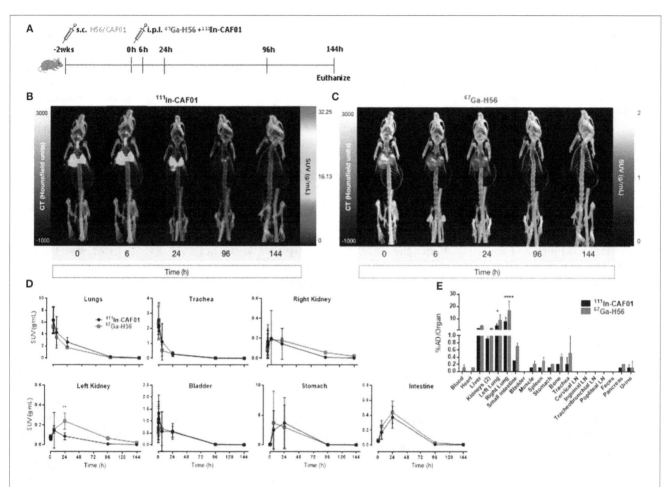

**FIGURE 7 |** H56/CAF01 vaccine biodistribution upon parenteral (s.c.) priming and airway (i.pulmon.) mucosal boosting follow a similar trend as the biodistribution following airway (i.pulmon.) mucosal prime immunization. **(A)** Experimental scheme: Mice were prime-immunized s.c. with 5 µg cold H56 adjuvanted with cold CAF01 (250/50 µg DDA/TDB). At week 2, animals were boost-immunized via intrapulmonary (i.pulmon.) route with 10 µg $^{67}$Ga-H56 adjuvanted with $^{111}$In-CAF01 (125/25 µg DDA/TDB). Animals were imaged by dynamic whole-body SPECT/CT scan for the initial 40 min (10 min/frame) and after that static 40 min scans at 6 and 24 h, 60 min scan at 96 h and 90 min scan at 144 h were conducted. Animals were euthanized on day 6 after immunization for ex vivo biodistribution using a gamma counter. Representative SPECT/CT images showing biodistribution of $^{111}$In-CAF01 **(B)** and $^{67}$Ga-H56 **(C)** of a mouse prime-immunized s.c. with H56/CAF01 and boost-immunized i.pulmon. with $^{67}$Ga-H56 + $^{111}$In-CAF01. **(D)** Organ SUVs (g/mL) were calculated from dynamic and static SPECT/CT images of the cold s.c. prime-immunized and hot ($^{67}$Ga-H56 + $^{111}$In-CAF01) i.pulmon. boost-immunized animals over 144 h post-immunization. Statistical analysis: two-way ANOVA and Sidak's post-test. Data represent mean values ± s.d., n = 3. **p < 0.01. **(E)** Ex vivo organ biodistribution [% administered dose (AD)/organ] of the cold s.c. prime-immunized and hot ($^{67}$Ga-H56 + $^{111}$In-CAF01) i.pulmon. boost-immunized animals on day 6 (144 h) post-immunization. Statistical analysis: two-way ANOVA and Sidak's post-test. Bars represent mean values ± s.d., n = 3. *p < 0.05 and ****p < 0.0001.

# DISCUSSION

Although a more efficacious vaccine is urgently needed for TB, vaccine design and development has been very challenging due to the specific requirement for induction of cell-mediated and mucosal immunity (2). It is now widely accepted that it is beneficial to stimulate Th1 and Th17 CD4$^+$ T-cell responses in the lungs for vaccine-induced protection in general (50, 51) and against Mtb infection in particular (52, 53). Mtb evades host immunity by delaying the extravasation of primed circulating antigen-specific T cells into the lung mucosa (2, 54). Antigen-specific T cells induced by parenteral vaccination remain confined to tissue compartments outside of the lung parenchyma and the airways, and are thus not capable of

mediating complete protection against Mtb (15, 55). Therefore, a vaccination strategy, which induces and maintains tissue-resident memory T cells and/or circulating T cells capable of rapid influx into the lungs upon pathogen re-exposure, may provide robust protection against Mtb infection. Parenteral administration of the TB subunit vaccine H56/CAF01 has been shown to induce promising protective efficacy in mice (29) and non-human primates (30). However, the H56/CAF01 vaccine has never been evaluated following airway (i.pulmon.) mucosal immunization. Here, we document the immunogenicity of the H56/CAF01 vaccine following parenteral (i.m.) priming and airway (i.pulmon.) boost immunization, which induces local lung and systemic memory CD4$^+$ T cells and IgA responses. We further describe, for the first time, the SPECT-CT imaging-based *in vivo* biodistribution and pharmacokinetics of the H56/CAF01 vaccine following parenteral (s.c.) or airway (i.pulmon.) priming or parenteral prime-airway mucosal boost (s.c.- i.pulmon.) immunization strategy. We observe pronounced differences in the deposition, biodistribution and clearance of H56 protein and CAF01 adjuvant. Our study provides new information on H56/CAF01 mucosal boost immunization-inducible memory CD4$^+$ T cells in the lungs and SPECT/CT imaging-based *in vivo* biodistribution of the individual vaccine components, which may assist the development of effective mucosal immunization strategies against pulmonary TB. These results also support our ongoing efforts to develop a thermostable, dry powder-based H56/CAF01 vaccine for i.pulmon. administration (43), and we envisage the potential application of such an inhalable dry powder dosage form in combination with a suitable device for mass vaccination programs against TB. Hence, the safety of airway mucosal vaccination has to be evaluated thoroughly in future studies.

It is well-known that T cells play a crucial role in the pulmonary host defense against many bacterial, viral, and fungal pathogens, and inadequate T-cell immunity may increase the likelihood of pathogen dissemination from the lungs (9). It is also well-known that MHC class II-restricted CD4$^+$ T cells producing IFN-$\gamma$ and TNF-$\alpha$ play important roles in protection against TB in experimental animal models and in humans (56, 57). In many preclinical TB challenge studies, increased CD4$^+$ central memory T cells have been associated with enhanced protection (14, 57, 58). Localization of antigen-specific CD4$^+$ T cells at the site of infection in the lung parenchyma is of ultimate importance for disease protection after vaccination (52, 56). However, *Mtb* infection greatly interferes with migration of circulating vaccine-induced antigen-specific T cells to the lungs (19), which is correlated with lack of protection (15, 59). Therefore, novel immunization strategies are needed to induce T cells that effectively home back to the lung parenchyma in the airways. In the present study, we introduce an effective immunization protocol for the H56/CAF01 vaccine, which results in induction of strong Th1, Th17, and IgA responses in the airways. We show that Th1 and Th17 cells are induced systemically after airway mucosal boost immunization of parenterally primed H56 antigen in a CAF01 dose-dependent manner, and that local lung mucosal and systemic IgA and IgG responses accompany this. We also show that mucosal immunization induces polyfunctional (IFN-$\gamma^+$TNF-$\alpha^+$IL-17$^+$) and double positive (IFN-$\gamma^+$TNF-$\alpha^+$ and TNF-$\alpha^+$IL-17$^+$) and TNF-$\alpha$ single-positive CD4$^+$ T cells in the lungs and the lung draining LNs (TLNs + MLNs) as well as the spleen. The H56/CAF01 vaccine has previously been shown to preferentially induce accumulation of TNF-$\alpha$ single-positive, double positive (IFN-$\gamma^+$TNF-$\alpha^+$ and TNF-$\alpha^+$IL-2$^+$) and triple-positive (IFN-$\gamma^+$TNF-$\alpha^+$IL-17$^+$) CD4$^+$ T cells in the lungs, which provide protection against an *Mtb* challenge (29). Our results also support previous observations that less differentiated H56-specific T-cells have increased ability to migrate into the lung parenchyma (39, 60). However, we also observe CD4$^+$ T cells with an intermediate state of differentiation (IFN-$\gamma^+$TNF-$\alpha^+$), as usually seen post-*Mtb* infection (39, 60, 61). The induction of this population following prime-boost

immunization could suggest that innate immune factors in the lung microenvironment play an important role for the extent of cell differentiation (62). However, the maintenance of an IFN-$\gamma^+$TNF-$\alpha^+$ double positive T-cell population has been associated with enhanced control of mycobacterial growth (56, 57). Similarly, parenteral prime and mucosal boost immunization were shown to induce strong mucosal and systemic immunity (16, 63, 64), accompanied by improved protection in a number of preclinical infectious disease models (65–67). Intranasal boosting of parenterally primed immune responses was associated with improved protection against *Mtb* infection, which correlated with IFN-$\gamma^+$ CD4$^+$ and CD8$^+$ T cells residing in the airway lumen of the lungs (68). Similarly, respiratory mucosal boosting of parenteral immunization resulted in improved protection against *Mtb* infection, and it was accompanied by antigen-specific T cell responses in the lungs (13, 69). Together with our data, these findings suggest that parenteral prime and mucosal boost immunization is a potentially effective strategy for inducing lung-resident CD4$^+$ T cells, which can subsequently provide an improved protection against an *Mtb* challenge. We are currently testing this strategy in an *Mtb* challenge model.

Almost all licensed vaccines against infectious diseases induce antibodies, which are correlated with disease protection (70). Antibody-mediated protective immunity is mediated by mucosal IgA, which prevents pathogen uptake across the epithelial barrier, and by serum IgG, which prevents further pathogen transmission *via* the blood (71). However, the role of B cells and their production of antibodies in the immune response to *Mtb* infection remains elusive (72–74). Recently, there is growing evidence that *Mtb*-specific antibodies may contribute to prevention of TB (75, 76), and one study reported that antibodies recovered from healthcare workers provided moderate protection against *Mtb* in mice (76). Furthermore, a number of experimental studies have shown a protective effect of antibodies against *Mtb* surface glycolipids (77, 78) and recombinant antigens (79, 80). The induction of antigen-specific IgA and IgG responses following prime-boost immunization in our study strengthens these findings. Ideally, vaccine-induced mucosal IgA antibodies present at the natural portal of entry in the lungs, which are capable of fast neutralization of *Mtb* following exposure, would be the optimal preventive strategy against TB. In line with this, passive protection by mucosally administered human IgA antibodies against *Mtb* infection in the lungs of mice has been reported (81, 82). Recently, vaccine-induced pulmonary secretory IgA has been associated with immunological protection against TB in mice (17, 83). Given the fact that antibodies are protective against many intracellular infections, further studies are required to verify the functional differences in antibodies to *Mtb* and the precise role of mucosal antibodies in the immunological protection against TB (84).

In this study, we successfully radiolabeled CAF01 liposomes with a lipophilic chelator, and developed an $^{111}$In-DTPA-CAF01 complex with high radiolabeling efficiency and purity. We also describe the successful design of $^{111}$In-DTPA-H56 and $^{67}$Ga-NOTA-H56 complexes, respectively, with high radiopurity and radiolabeling efficiency. Radiolabeling of both H56 and CAF01 was not only easy and reproducible, but did also result in preserved size and integrity of both protein and liposomes. The $^{111}$In and $^{67}$Ga radionuclides were selected due to their relatively long half-life ($^{111}$I $n$ = 2.81 and $^{67}$Ga = 3.26 days), their high photon energy, their ready and daily availability as cyclotron-produced radionuclides, and the possibility for clinical translation. Using SPECT-CT imaging, we confirmed our previous studies showing that CAF01 forms a depot at the site of injection (48). First, we show that $^{111}$In-CAF01 with surface-adsorbed cold H56 and $^{111}$In-H56 adsorbed onto cold CAF01 remain at the site of injection for up to 6 days post-s.c. injection, and we confirmed the observation through *ex vivo* biodistribution. Using the tracer molecule $^3$H-DPPC with DDA and TDB and $^{125}$I-labeled Ag85B-ESAT6 protein (so-called H1), it was shown previously that CAF01 forms a depot when injected i.m. or s.c. and promotes antigen retention at the site of injection (48). Moreover, this depot effect was correlated with the synchronization of DC uptake of antigen and activation by CAF01, which is an important element for the Th1/Th17 adjuvanticity of CAF01 (85, 86). However, in our study, there was a clear difference in the biodistribution of H56 and CAF01 following s.c. injection; H56 was cleared faster than CAF01 and was detected in the kidneys and the bladder already 6 h post-administration. Following pulmonary administration of radiolabeled H56 and CAF01, respectively, we generally observed rapid accumulation of radioactivity in the lungs and the bladder within the first hour post-administration. The observed activity in the trachea is caused by deposition of very small amounts of activity from the tip of the MicroSprayer® needle during i.pulmon. administration. At later time-points, the amount of radioactive H56 in the lungs, although lower, was detectable until 24 h, as compared to radioactive CAF01, which was observed until 96 h. For both H56 and CAF01, radioactivity was observed in the stomach and the intestines from 6 to 24 h post-injection, which could be due to cough reflux during the withdrawal of the MicroSprayer® needle from the trachea, or clearance of the dispersion from the trachea and subsequent swallowing, as previously reported (47). Nevertheless, the applied i.pulmon. administration method enables a rather uniform distribution of the aerosolized vaccine into both lung lobes as observed by SPECT imaging. This is further supported by the fact that extrapulmonary distribution following aerosolization did not influence the overall vaccine immunogenicity, and it was not associated with any apparent side effects or systemic toxicity during the study period (up to a maximum of 6 weeks).

Induction of cell-mediated immunity by vaccination is challenging. It is believed that repeated administration of the same vaccine (homologous boosting) is effective for increasing humoral but not cellular immune responses, while heterologous prime-boost immunization induces strong humoral and cellular immune responses (87, 88). However, the use of the homologous parenteral prime-mucosal boost immunization schedule has been shown to induce simultaneous robust local mucosal and systemic protective cellular and humoral immunity against mucosal pathogens, e.g., *Mtb* and HIV (13, 63, 69). Our data show that homologous parenteral priming followed by airway boosting with H56/CAF01 elicits strong antigen-specific CD4$^+$ T cell responses, both in the spleen and the lungs, and IgA responses in both serum and lungs, as compared to parenteral homologous prime-boost immunizations. Recently, it was reported that the administration route used for priming and boosting of the H56/CAF01 vaccine is important for improving and directing the vaccine-induced immune responses using either the homologous or heterologous prime-boost combinations (22). Largely, the enhanced immunity following prime-boost homologous or heterologous immunization to the target antigen is reflected predominantly by cellular events, e.g., an increased number of antigen-specific T cells, enrichment of high-avidity T cells, and subsequent increased protective efficacy against a pathogen challenge (89). Having demonstrated significantly higher CD4$^+$ T-cell- and antibody responses for homologous prime-boost immunization, we evaluated the biodistribution and pharmacokinetics of the H56/CAF01 vaccine by SPECT/CT imaging to compare pulmonary uptake and distribution between airway (i.pulmon.) prime vs. parenteral (s.c.) prime—airway (i.pulmon.) mucosal boost immunization strategies. However, the vaccine biodistribution in airway-boosted animals that were primed s.c. with the homologous vaccine was not significantly different from the biodistribution in s.c.- primed only animals. Since most of the immunological events are taking place at the cellular level initially in the lung mucosa and draining lymph nodes followed by systemic circulation, whole-body SPECT/CT imaging cannot be used to differentiate the cellular events during prime vs. prime-boost immunization. Nevertheless, the comparable vaccine biodistribution profiles upon homologous prime and prime-boost immunization underlines the reproducibility of our radiolabeling results and emphasizes the usability of the SPECT/CT imaging-based approach for quantification of the biodistribution of subunit vaccines. Our novel data represent dual-isotope radiolabeling and preclinical non-invasive and longitudinal SPECT/CT imaging of the H56/CAF01 vaccine as a readily translatable strategy, which can be integrated into a clinical workflow. In addition, this novel radiolabeling platform can be used to identify image-derived biomarkers, which could be used to image vaccine-induced immune response, where imaging of sites such as lungs, LNs and spleen can provide additional information about vaccine-induced immune response as well as safety and efficacy. Interestingly, a recent study reported a PET imaging-derived biomarker that can be used to image activated T cells to predict tumor responses to *in situ* vaccination (90). Future studies should include devising novel immuno-SPECT/CT strategies for the identification of H56/CAF01 vaccine-induced activated T cells for differentiating prime vs. prime-boost immunizations and corresponding vaccine efficacy.

From our data we can conclude that strong IgA antibody and polyfunctional Th1 and Th17 cell responses are induced in the lung mucosa and the systemic circulation upon parenteral (i.m.) priming combined with airway (i.pulmon.) mucosal boost immunization with the TB subunit vaccine H56/CAF01, as compared to parenteral (i.m.) priming combined with parenteral (i.m.) boost immunization. These data demonstrate that parenteral priming followed by airway mucosal boosting with the H56/CAF01 vaccine is a novel immunization strategy for improving vaccine immunogenicity and directing the trafficking of antigen-specific CD4$^+$ T cells to the lungs. These results warrants further preclinical and clinical development of H56/CAF01 as an inhalable and self-administrable aerosol vaccine. We conclude that there are very pronounced differences in the pharmacokinetics of H56 and CAF01 based on dual isotope ($^{111}$In/$^{67}$Ga)-based SPECT/CT imaging of the vaccine biodistribution. Our results also suggest a comparable biodistribution profile of the H56/CAF01 vaccine following airway (i.pulmon.) prime and parenteral prime (s.c.)—airway (i.pulmon.) mucosal boost immunization, respectively. We believe that immuno-SPECT/CT strategies can be developed, based on this novel radiolabeling platform, for imaging of H56/CAF01 vaccine-induced activated T cells at specific effector sites, e.g., the lungs. Overall, our findings may hold considerable implications for the rational design of effective mucosal immunization strategies against TB.

## AUTHOR CONTRIBUTIONS

AT, DC, UH, and CF designed the study. AT, CR-R, KS, FR, TE, and ZN performed the laboratory work and analyzed the data. AT, DC, UH, and CF interpreted the data. AT, CR-R, UH, and CF drafted the manuscript. AT, CR-R, KS, PA, DC, UH, and CF provided scientific input throughout the study period and draft of the manuscript.

## FUNDING

This study was supported by The Danish Council for Independent Research, Technology and Production Sciences (grant number DFF-4184-00422), the Canada Foundation for Innovation (Grant No. 25413), and the Lundbeck Foundation, Denmark (The UBC-SUND Lundbeck Foundation professorship to UH).

## ACKNOWLEDGMENTS

We thank Mette Lynggaard Rådbjerg and Mathilde Caldara from the animal facility at Department of Drug Design and Pharmacology, University of Copenhagen, for their technical assistance. We are grateful to Liselotte Norup from the Core Facility for Flow Cytometry at the University of Copenhagen for technical assistance. The authors would also like to thank the skillful team of laboratory animal technicians and veterinarians at the University of British Columbia Centre for Comparative Medicine, in particular Dr. Shelly McErlane and Dr. Jana Hodasova, for their assistance and fruitful discussions.

## REFERENCES

1. WHO. *Global Tuberculosis Report 2017*. Geneva: World Health Organization (2017).
2. Cooper AM. Cell-mediated immune responses in tuberculosis. *Annu Rev Immunol*. (2009) 27:393–422. doi: 10.1146/annurev.immunol.021908.132703
3. Kaufmann SH. Tuberculosis vaccine development: strength lies in tenacity. *Trends Immunol*. (2012) 33:373–9. doi: 10.1016/j.it.2012.03.004
4. McShane H, Jacobs WR, Fine PE, Reed SG, McMurray DN, Behr M, et al. BCG: myths, realities, and the need for alternative vaccine strategies. *Tuberculosis* (2012) 92:283–8. doi: 10.1016/j.tube.2011.12.003
5. Behr MA. BCG–different strains, different vaccines? *Lancet Infect Dis.* (2002) 2:86–92. doi: 10.1016/S1473-3099(02)00182-2
6. Jeyanathan M, Yao Y, Afkhami S, Smaill F, Xing Z. New tuberculosis vaccine strategies: taking aim at un-natural immunity. *Trends Immunol*. (2018) 39:419–33. doi: 10.1016/j.it.2018.01.006
7. Andersen P, Urdahl KB. TB vaccines; promoting rapid and durable protection in the lung. *Curr Opin Immunol*. (2015) 35:55–62. doi: 10.1016/j.coi.2015.06.001
8. Urdahl KB, Shafiani S, Ernst JD. Initiation and regulation of T-cell responses in tuberculosis. *Mucosal Immunol*. (2011) 4:288–93. doi: 10.1038/mi.2011.10
9. Chen K, Kolls JK. T cell-mediated host immune defenses in the lung. *Annu Rev Immunol*. (2013) 31:605–33. doi: 10.1146/annurev-immunol-032712-100019
10. Gengenbacher M, Nieuwenhuizen NE, Kaufmann S. BCG - old workhorse, new skills. *Curr Opin Immunol*. (2017) 47:8–16. doi: 10.1016/j.coi.2017.06.007
11. Andersen P, Woodworth JS. Tuberculosis vaccines–rethinking the current paradigm. *Trends Immunol*. (2014) 35:387–95. doi: 10.1016/j.it.2014.04.006
12. Nieuwenhuizen NE, Kaufmann SHE. Next-generation vaccines based on bacille calmette-guerin. *Front Immunol*. (2018) 9:121. doi: 10.3389/fimmu.2018.00121

13. Jeyanathan M, Shao Z, Yu X, Harkness R, Jiang R, Li J, et al. AdHu5Ag85A respiratory mucosal boost immunization enhances protection against pulmonary tuberculosis in BCG-primed non-human primates. *PLoS ONE* (2015) 10:e0135009. doi: 10.1371/journal.pone.0135009
14. Kaushal D, Foreman TW, Gautam US, Alvarez X, Adekambi T, Rangel-Moreno J, et al. Mucosal vaccination with attenuated *Mycobacterium tuberculosis* induces strong central memory responses and protects against tuberculosis. *Nat Commun*. (2015) 6:8533. doi: 10.1038/ncomms9533
15. Horvath CN, Shaler CR, Jeyanathan M, Zganiacz A, Xing Z. Mechanisms of delayed anti-tuberculosis protection in the lung of parenteral BCG-vaccinated hosts: a critical role of airway luminal T cells. *Mucosal Immunol*. (2012) 5:420–31. doi: 10.1038/mi.2012.19
16. Christensen D, Mortensen R, Rosenkrands I, Dietrich J, Andersen P. Vaccine-induced Th17 cells are established as resident memory cells in the lung and promote local IgA responses. *Mucosal Immunol*. (2017) 10:260–70. doi: 10.1038/mi.2016.28
17. Wu M, Zhao H, Li M, Yue Y, Xiong S, Xu W. Intranasal vaccination with mannosylated chitosan formulated DNA vaccine enables robust IgA and cellular response induction in the lungs of mice and improves protection against pulmonary mycobacterial challenge. *Front Cell Infect Microbiol*. (2017) 7:445. doi: 10.3389/fcimb.2017.00445
18. Beverley PC, Sridhar S, Lalvani A, Tchilian EZ. Harnessing local and systemic immunity for vaccines against tuberculosis. *Mucosal Immunol*. (2014) 7:20–6. doi: 10.1038/mi.2013.99
19. Griffiths KL, Ahmed M, Das S, Gopal R, Horne W, Connell TD, et al. Targeting dendritic cells to accelerate T-cell activation overcomes a bottleneck in tuberculosis vaccine efficacy. *Nat Commun*. (2016) 7:13894. doi: 10.1038/ncomms13894
20. Voss G, Casimiro D, Neyrolles O, Williams A, Kaufmann SHE, McShane H, et al. Progress and challenges in TB vaccine development. *F1000Res* (2018) 7:199. doi: 10.12688/f1000research.13588.1

21. Song K, Bolton DL, Wei CJ, Wilson RL, Camp JV, Bao S, et al. Genetic immunization in the lung induces potent local and systemic immune responses. *Proc Natl Acad Sci USA*. (2010) 107:22213–8. doi: 10.1073/pnas.1015536108

22. Ciabattini A, Prota G, Christensen D, Andersen P, Pozzi G, Medaglini D. Characterization of the Antigen-Specific CD4(+) T Cell Response Induced by Prime-Boost Strategies with CAF01 and CpG adjuvants administered by the intranasal and subcutaneous routes. *Front Immunol*. (2015) 6:430. doi: 10.3389/fimmu.2015.00430

23. Blazevic A, Eickhoff CS, Stanley J, Buller MR, Schriewer J, Kettelson EM, et al. Investigations of TB vaccine-induced mucosal protection in mice. *Microbes Infect*. (2014) 16:73–9. doi: 10.1016/j.micinf.2013. 09.006

24. Lewis DJ, Huo Z, Barnett S, Kromann I, Giemza R, Galiza E, et al. Transient facial nerve paralysis (Bell's palsy) following intranasal delivery of a genetically detoxified mutant of Escherichia coli heat labile toxin. *PLoS ONE* (2009) 4:e6999. doi: 10.1371/journal.pone.00 06999

25. Kallenius G, Pawlowski A, Brandtzaeg P, Svenson S. Should a new tuberculosis vaccine be administered intranasally? *Tuberculosis* (2007) 87:257–66. doi: 10.1016/j.tube.2006. 12.006

26. Willmann JK, van Bruggen N, Dinkelborg LM, Gambhir SS. Molecular imaging in drug development. *Nat Rev Drug Discov*. (2008) 7:591–607. doi: 10.1038/nrd2290

27. van der Geest T, Laverman P, Metselaar JM, Storm G, Boerman OC. Radionuclide imaging of liposomal drug delivery. *Expert Opin Drug Deliv*. (2016) 13:1231–42. doi: 10.1080/17425247.2016.12 05584

28. Srivatsan A, Chen X. Recent advances in nanoparticle-based nuclear imaging of cancers. *Adv Cancer Res*. (2014) 124:83–129. doi: 10.1016/B978-0-12-411638-2.00003-3

29. Aagaard C, Hoang T, Dietrich J, Cardona PJ, Izzo A, Dolganov G, et al. A multistage tuberculosis vaccine that confers efficient protection before and after exposure. *Nat Med*. (2011) 17:189–94. doi: 10.1038/nm.2285

30. Lin PL, Dietrich J, Tan E, Abalos RM, Burgos J, Bigbee C, et al. The multistage vaccine H56 boosts the effects of BCG to protect cynomolgus macaques against active tuberculosis and reactivation of latent Mycobacterium tuberculosis infection. *J Clin Invest*. (2012) 122:303–14. doi: 10.1172/JCI 46252

31. Luabeya AK, Kagina BM, Tameris MD, Geldenhuys H, Hoff ST, Shi Z, et al. First-in-human trial of the post-exposure tuberculosis vaccine H56:IC31 in Mycobacterium tuberculosis infected and non-infected healthy adults. *Vaccine* (2015) 33:4130–40. doi: 10.1016/j.vaccine.2015.06.051

32. Desel C, Werninghaus K, Ritter M, Jozefowski K, Wenzel J, Russkamp N, et al. The Mincle-activating adjuvant TDB induces MyD88-dependent Th1 and Th17 responses through IL-1R signaling. *PLoS ONE* (2013) 8:e53531. doi: 10.1371/journal.pone.0053531

33. Davidsen J, Rosenkrands I, Christensen D, Vangala A, Kirby D, Perrie Y, et al. Characterization of cationic liposomes based on dimethyldioctadecylammonium and synthetic cord factor from M. tuberculosis (trehalose 6,6'-dibehenate)-a novel adjuvant inducing both strong CMI and antibody responses. *Biochim Biophys Acta* (2005) 1718:22–31. doi: 10.1016/j.bbamem.2005.10.011

34. Lindenstrom T, Woodworth J, Dietrich J, Aagaard C, Andersen P, Agger EM. Vaccine-induced th17 cells are maintained long-term postvaccination as a distinct and phenotypically stable memory subset. *Infect Immun*. (2012) 80:3533–44. doi: 10.1128/IAI.00550-12

35. Knudsen NP, Olsen A, Buonsanti C, Follmann F, Zhang Y, Coler RN, et al. Different human vaccine adjuvants promote distinct antigen-independent immunological signatures tailored to different pathogens. *Sci Rep* (2016) 6:19570. doi: 10.1038/srep19570

36. Hamborg M, Kramer R, Schante CE, Agger EM, Christensen D, Jorgensen L, et al. The physical stability of the recombinant tuberculosis fusion antigens h1 and h56. *J Pharm Sci*. (2013) 102:3567–78. doi: 10.1002/jps. 23669

37. Bivas-Benita M, Zwier R, Junginger HE, Borchard G. Non-invasive pulmonary aerosol delivery in mice by the endotracheal route.

*Eur J Pharm Biopharm*. (2005) 61:214–8. doi: 10.1016/j.ejpb.2005. 04.009

38. Branderhorst W, Vastenhouw B, Beekman FJ. Pixel-based subsets for rapid multi-pinhole SPECT reconstruction. *Phys Med Biol*. (2010) 55:2023–34. doi: 10.1088/0031-9155/55/7/015

39. Woodworth JS, Cohen SB, Moguche AO, Plumlee CR, Agger EM, Urdahl KB, et al. Subunit vaccine H56/CAF01 induces a population of circulating CD4 T cells that traffic into the *Mycobacterium tuberculosis*-infected lung. *Mucosal Immunol*. (2017) 10:555–64. doi: 10.1038/mi.2016.70

40. Wern JE, Sorensen MR, Olsen AW, Andersen P, Follmann F. Simultaneous Subcutaneous and Intranasal Administration of a CAF01-adjuvanted chlamydia vaccine elicits elevated IgA and Protective Th1/Th17 responses in the genital tract. *Front Immunol*. (2017) 8:569. doi: 10.3389/fimmu.2017.00569

41. Agger EM, Rosenkrands I, Hansen J, Brahimi K, Vandahl BS, Aagaard C, et al. Cationic liposomes formulated with synthetic mycobacterial cordfactor (CAF01): a versatile adjuvant for vaccines with different immunological requirements. *PLoS ONE* (2008) 3:e3116. doi: 10.1371/journal.pone.00 03116

42. Billeskov R, Tan EV, Cang M, Abalos RM, Burgos J, Pedersen BV, et al. Testing the H56 Vaccine delivered in 4 different adjuvants as a BCG-booster in a non-human primate model of tuberculosis. *PLoS ONE* (2016) 11:e0161217. doi: 10.1371/journal.pone.0161217

43. Thakur A, Ingvarsson PT, Schmidt ST, Rose F, Andersen P, Christensen D, et al. Immunological and physical evaluation of the multistage tuberculosis subunit vaccine candidate H56/CAF01 formulated as a spray-dried powder. *Vaccine* (2018) 36:3331–9. doi: 10.1016/j.vaccine.2018. 04.055

44. Hamborg M, Jorgensen L, Bojsen AR, Christensen D, Foged C. Protein antigen adsorption to the DDA/TDB liposomal adjuvant: effect on protein structure, stability, and liposome physicochemical characteristics. *Pharm Res*. (2013) 30:140–55. doi: 10.1007/s11095-012-0856-8

45. Kallerup RS, Madsen CM, Schiot ML, Franzyk H, Rose F, Christensen D, et al. Influence of trehalose 6,6'-diester (TDX) chain length on the physicochemical and immunopotentiating properties of DDA/TDX liposomes. *Eur J Pharm Biopharm*. (2015) 90:80–9. doi: 10.1016/j.ejpb.2014. 10.015

46. Kallerup RS, Franzyk H, Schiot ML, Justesen S, Martin-Bertelsen B, Rose F, et al. Adjuvants based on synthetic mycobacterial cord factor analogues: biophysical properties of neat glycolipids and nanoself-assemblies with DDA. *Mol Pharm*. (2017) 14:2294–306. doi: 10.1021/acs.molpharmaceut.7b 00170

47. Hasegawa-Baba Y, Kubota H, Takata A, Miyagawa M. Intratracheal instillation methods and the distribution of administered material in the lung of the rat. *J Toxicol Pathol*. (2014) 27:197–204. doi: 10.1293/tox.2014-0022

48. Henriksen-Lacey M, Bramwell VW, Christensen D, Agger EM, Andersen P, Perrie Y. Liposomes based on dimethyldioctadecylammonium promote a depot effect and enhance immunogenicity of soluble antigen. *J Control Release* (2010) 142:180–6. doi: 10.1016/j.jconrel.2009. 10.022

49. Anderson KG, Mayer-Barber K, Sung H, Beura L, James BR, Taylor JJ, et al. Intravascular staining for discrimination of vascular and tissue leukocytes. *Nat Protoc*. (2014) 9:209–22. doi: 10.1038/nprot.2014.005

50. Schenkel JM, Masopust D. Tissue-resident memory T cells. *Immunity* (2014) 41:886–97. doi: 10.1016/j.immuni.2014.12.007

51. Iijima N, Iwasaki A. Tissue instruction for migration and retention of TRM cells. *Trends Immunol*. (2015) 36:556–64. doi: 10.1016/j.it.2015. 07.002

52. Sakai S, Kauffman KD, Schenkel JM, McBerry CC, Mayer-Barber KD, Masopust D, et al. Cutting edge: control of Mycobacterium tuberculosis infection by a subset of lung parenchyma-homing CD4 T cells. *J Immunol*. (2014) 192:2965–9. doi: 10.4049/jimmunol.1400019

53. Khader SA, Bell GK, Pearl JE, Fountain JJ, Rangel-Moreno J, Cilley GE, et al. IL-23 and IL-17 in the establishment of protective pulmonary CD4+ T cell responses after vaccination and during *Mycobacterium tuberculosis* challenge. *Nat Immunol*. (2007) 8:369–77. doi: 10.1038/ni1449

54. Jeyanathan M, McCormick S, Lai R, Afkhami S, Shaler CR, Horvath CN, et al. Pulmonary *M. tuberculosis* infection delays Th1 immunity via

immunoadaptor DAP12-regulated IRAK-M and IL-10 expression in antigen-presenting cells. *Mucosal Immunol.* (2014) 7:670–83. doi: 10.1038/mi.2013.86

55. Takamura S, Yagi H, Hakata Y, Motozono C, McMaster SR, Masumoto T, et al. Specific niches for lung-resident memory CD8+ T cells at the site of tissue regeneration enable CD69-independent maintenance. *J Exp Med.* (2016) 213:3057–73. doi: 10.1084/jem.20160938

56. Sharpe S, White A, Sarfas C, Sibley L, Gleeson F, McIntyre A, et al. Alternative BCG delivery strategies improve protection against Mycobacterium tuberculosis in non-human primates: protection associated with mycobacterial antigen-specific CD4 effector memory T-cell populations. *Tuberculosis* (2016) 101:174–90. doi: 10.1016/j.tube.2016.09.004

57. Lindenstrom T, Knudsen NP, Agger EM, Andersen P. Control of chronic mycobacterium tuberculosis infection by CD4 KLRG1- IL-2-secreting central memory cells. *J Immunol.* (2013) 190:6311–9. doi: 10.4049/jimmunol.13 00248

58. Perdomo C, Zedler U, Kuhl AA, Lozza L, Saikali P, Sander LE, et al. Mucosal BCG vaccination induces protective lung-resident memory T cell populations against tuberculosis. *MBio* (2016) 7:e01686-16. doi: 10.1128/mBio.01 686-16

59. Santosuosso M, McCormick S, Roediger E, Zhang X, Zganiacz A, Lichty BD, et al. Mucosal luminal manipulation of T cell geography switches on protective efficacy by otherwise ineffective parenteral genetic immunization. *J Immunol.* (2007) 178:2387–95. doi: 10.4049/jimmunol.178. 4.2387

60. Lindenstrom T, Moguche A, Damborg M, Agger EM, Urdahl K, Andersen P. T Cells Primed by live mycobacteria versus a tuberculosis subunit vaccine exhibit distinct functional properties. *EBioMedicine* (2018) 27:27–39. doi: 10.1016/j.ebiom.2017.12.004

61. Billeskov R, Lindenstrom T, Woodworth J, Vilaplana C, Cardona PJ, Cassidy JP, et al. High antigen dose is detrimental to post-exposure vaccine protection against tuberculosis. *Front Immunol.* (2017) 8:1973. doi: 10.3389/fimmu.2017.01973

62. Seder RA, Darrah PA, Roederer M. T-cell quality in memory and protection: implications for vaccine design. *Nat Rev Immunol.* (2008) 8:247–58. doi: 10.1038/nri2274

63. Cristillo AD, Ferrari MG, Hudacik L, Lewis B, Galmin L, Bowen B, et al. Induction of mucosal and systemic antibody and T-cell responses following prime-boost immunization with novel adjuvanted human immunodeficiency virus-1-vaccine formulations. *J Gen Virol.* (2011) 92(Pt 1):128–40. doi: 10.1099/vir.0.023242-0

64. Kuczkowska K, Myrbraten I, Overland L, Eijsink VGH, Follmann F, Mathiesen G, et al. Lactobacillus plantarum producing a Chlamydia trachomatis antigen induces a specific IgA response after mucosal booster immunization. *PLoS ONE* (2017) 12:e0176401. doi: 10.1371/journal.pone.0176401

65. Makitalo B, Lundholm P, Hinkula J, Nilsson C, Karlen K, Morner A, et al. Enhanced cellular immunity and systemic control of SHIV infection by combined parenteral and mucosal administration of a DNA prime MVA boost vaccine regimen. *J Gen Virol.* (2004) 85(Pt 8):2407–19. doi: 10.1099/vir.0.79869-0

66. Khalifa ME, El-Deeb AH, Zeidan SM, Hussein HA, Abu-El-Naga HI. Enhanced protection against FMDV in cattle after prime- boost vaccination based on mucosal and inactivated FMD vaccine. *Vet Microbiol.* (2017) 210:1–7. doi: 10.1016/j.vetmic.2017.08.014

67. Lorenzen E, Follmann F, Boje S, Erneholm K, Olsen AW, Agerholm JS, et al. Intramuscular priming and intranasal boosting induce strong genital immunity through secretory IgA in minipigs infected with chlamydia trachomatis. *Front Immunol.* (2015) 6:628. doi: 10.3389/fimmu.2015. 00628

68. Santosuosso M, McCormick S, Zhang X, Zganiacz A, Xing Z. Intranasal boosting with an adenovirus-vectored vaccine markedly enhances protection by parenteral *Mycobacterium bovis* BCG immunization against pulmonary tuberculosis. *Infect Immun.* (2006) 74:4634–43. doi: 10.1128/IAI.00 517-06

69. Jeyanathan M, Damjanovic D, Shaler CR, Lai R, Wortzman M, Yin C, et al. Differentially imprinted innate immunity by mucosal boost vaccination determines antituberculosis immune protective outcomes, independent of T-cell immunity. *Mucosal Immunol.* (2013) 6:612–25. doi: 10.1038/mi.2012.103

70. Thakur A, Pedersen LE, Jungersen G. Immune markers and correlates of protection for vaccine induced immune responses. *Vaccine* (2012) 30:4907–20. doi: 10.1016/j.vaccine.2012.05.049

71. Holmgren J, Svennerholm AM. Vaccines against mucosal infections. *Curr Opin Immunol.* (2012) 24:343–53. doi: 10.1016/j.coi.2012. 03.014

72. Maglione PJ, Chan J. How B cells shape the immune response against Mycobacterium tuberculosis. *Eur J Immunol.* (2009) 39:676–86. doi: 10.1002/eji.200839148

73. Achkar JM, Casadevall A. Antibody-mediated immunity against tuberculosis: implications for vaccine development. *Cell Host Microbe* (2013) 13:250–62. doi: 10.1016/j.chom.2013.02.009

74. Lu LL, Chung AW, Rosebrock TR, Ghebremichael M, Yu WH, Grace PS, et al. A functional role for antibodies in tuberculosis. *Cell* (2016) 167:433–43 e14. doi: 10.1016/j.cell.2016.08.072

75. Phuah J, Wong EA, Gideon HP, Maiello P, Coleman MT, Hendricks MR, et al. Effects of B cell depletion on early mycobacterium tuberculosis infection in cynomolgus macaques. *Infect Immun.* (2016) 84:1301–11. doi: 10.1128/IAI.00083-16

76. Li H, Wang XX, Wang B, Fu L, Liu G, Lu Y, et al. Latently and uninfected healthcare workers exposed to TB make protective antibodies against Mycobacterium tuberculosis. *Proc Natl Acad Sci USA.* (2017) 114:5023–8. doi: 10.1073/pnas.1611776114

77. Prados-Rosales R, Carreno L, Cheng T, Blanc C, Weinrick B, Malek A, et al. Enhanced control of Mycobacterium tuberculosis extrapulmonary dissemination in mice by an arabinomannan-protein conjugate vaccine. *PLoS Pathog.* (2017) 13:e1006250. doi: 10.1371/journal.ppat.10 06250

78. Prados-Rosales R, Carreno LJ, Batista-Gonzalez A, Baena A, Venkataswamy MM, Xu J, et al. Mycobacterial membrane vesicles administered systemically in mice induce a protective immune response to surface compartments of Mycobacterium tuberculosis. *MBio* (2014) 5:e01921–14. doi: 10.1128/mBio.01921-14

79. Giri PK, Verma I, Khuller GK. Enhanced immunoprotective potential of Mycobacterium tuberculosis Ag85 complex protein based vaccine against airway Mycobacterium tuberculosis challenge following intranasal administration. *FEMS Immunol Med Microbiol.* (2006) 47:233–41. doi: 10.1111/j.1574-695X.2006.00087.x

80. Kohama H, Umemura M, Okamoto Y, Yahagi A, Goga H, Harakuni T, et al. Mucosal immunization with recombinant heparin-binding haemagglutinin adhesin suppresses extrapulmonary dissemination of *Mycobacterium bovis* bacillus Calmette-Guerin (BCG) in infected mice. *Vaccine* (2008) 26:924–32. doi: 10.1016/j.vaccine.2007.12.005

81. Balu S, Reljic R, Lewis MJ, Pleass RJ, McIntosh R, van Kooten C, et al. A novel human IgA monoclonal antibody protects against tuberculosis. *J Immunol.* (2011) 186:3113–9. doi: 10.4049/jimmunol.10 03189

82. Williams A, Reljic R, Naylor I, Clark SO, Falero-Diaz G, Singh M, et al. Passive protection with immunoglobulin A antibodies against tuberculous early infection of the lungs. *Immunology* (2004) 111:328–33. doi: 10.1111/j.1365-2567.2004.01809.x

83. Ai W, Yue Y, Xiong S, Xu W. Enhanced protection against pulmonary mycobacterial challenge by chitosan-formulated polyepitope gene vaccine is associated with increased pulmonary secretory IgA and gamma-interferon(+) T cell responses. *Microbiol Immunol.* (2013) 57:224–35. doi: 10.1111/1348-0421.12027

84. Casadevall A. Antibodies to Mycobacterium tuberculosis. *N Engl J Med.* (2017) 376:283–5. doi: 10.1056/NEJMcibr1613268

85. Christensen D, Henriksen-Lacey M, Kamath AT, Lindenstrom T, Korsholm KS, Christensen JP, et al. A cationic vaccine adjuvant based on a saturated quaternary ammonium lipid have different *in vivo* distribution kinetics and display a distinct CD4 T cell-inducing capacity compared to its unsaturated analog. *J Control Release* (2012) 160:468–76. doi: 10.1016/j.jconrel.2012.03.016

86. Kamath AT, Mastelic B, Christensen D, Rochat AF, Agger EM, Pinschewer DD, et al. Synchronization of dendritic cell activation and antigen exposure is required for the induction of Th1/Th17 responses. *J Immunol.* (2012) 188:4828–37. doi: 10.4049/jimmunol.1103183

87. McShane H, Hill A. Prime-boost immunisation strategies for tuberculosis. *Microbes Infect.* (2005) 7:962–7. doi: 10.1016/j.micinf.2005.03.009

88. De Rosa SC, Thomas EP, Bui J, Huang Y, deCamp A, Morgan C, et al. HIV-DNA priming alters T cell responses to HIV-adenovirus vaccine even when responses to DNA are undetectable. *J Immunol.* (2011) 187:3391–401. doi: 10.4049/jimmunol.1101421

89. Ranasinghe C, Turner SJ, McArthur C, Sutherland DB, Kim JH, Doherty PC, et al. Mucosal HIV-1 pox virus prime-boost immunization induces high-avidity CD8+ T cells with regime-dependent cytokine/granzyme B profiles. *J Immunol.* (2007) 178:2370–9. doi: 10.4049/jimmunol.178.4.2370

90. Alam IS, Mayer AT, Sagiv-Barfi I, Wang K, Vermesh O, Czerwinski DK, et al. Imaging activated T cells predicts response to cancer vaccines. *J Clin Invest.* (2018) 128:2569–80. doi: 10.1172/JCI 98509

6

# The Profile of T Cell Responses in Bacille Calmette–Guérin-Primed Mice Boosted by a Novel Sendai Virus Vectored Anti-Tuberculosis Vaccine

Zhidong Hu[1], Ling Gu[1], Chun-Ling Li[2], Tsugumine Shu[3], Douglas B. Lowrie[1,2] and Xiao-Yong Fan[2,1]*

[1] Shanghai Public Health Clinical Center, Key Laboratory of Medical Molecular Virology of MOE/MOH, Fudan University, Shanghai, China, [2] School of Laboratory Medicine and Life Science, Wenzhou Medical University, Wenzhou, China, [3] ID Pharma, Ibaraki, Japan

*Correspondence:
Xiao-Yong Fan
xyfan008@fudan.edu.cn

The kinds of vaccine-induced T cell responses that are beneficial for protection against *Mycobacterium tuberculosis* (*Mtb*) infection are not adequately defined. We had shown that a novel Sendai virus vectored vaccine, SeV85AB, was able to enhance immune protection induced by bacille Calmette–Guérin (BCG) in a prime-boost model. However, the profile of T cell responses boosted by SeV85AB was not determined. Herein, we show that the antigen-specific CD4+ and CD8+ T cell responses were both enhanced by the SeV85AB boost after BCG. Different profiles of antigen-specific po T cell subsets were induced in the local (lung) and systemic (spleen) sites. In the spleen, the CD4+ T cell responses that were enhanced by the SeV85AB boost were predominately IL-2 responses, whereas in the lung the greater increases were in IFN-γ- and TNF-α-producing CD4+ T cells; in CD8+ T cells, although IFN-γ was enhanced in both the spleen and lung, only IL-2+TNF-α+CD8+ T subset was boosted in the latter. After a challenge *Mtb* infection, there were significantly higher levels of recall IL-2 responses in T cells. In contrast, IFN-γ-producing cells were barely boosted by SeV85AB. After *Mtb* challenge a central memory phenotype of responding CD4+ T cells was a prominent feature in SeV85AB-boosted mice. Thus, our data strongly suggest that the enhanced immune protection induced by SeV85AB boosting was associated with establishment of an increased capacity to recall antigen-specific IL-2-mediated T cell responses and confirms this Sendai virus vector system as a promising candidate to be used in a heterologous prime-boost immunization regimen against TB.

Keywords: tuberculosis, Sendai virus, vaccine, T cell responses, prime-boost, IL-2

## INTRODUCTION

Tuberculosis (TB) remains among the most deadly health challenge to humankind. Bacille Calmette–Guérin (BCG), the attenuated form of *Mycobacterium bovis*, has been used for over 80 years to protect children against severe forms of TB (1). However, its protective efficacy against pulmonary TB was found to vary from 0 to 80% in adults (2), hence a more effective vaccine is needed.

T cell responses are regarded as a critical factor in containment of *Mycobacterium tuberculosis* (*Mtb*) infection. After phagocytosis, *Mtb* preferentially resides in phagosomes, where its antigens are processed and assembled onto MHC-II molecules for presentation to CD4+ T cells (3). During the course of *Mtb*-driven differentiation, the T cells can gain the capacity to simultaneously produce two or more key cytokines and are called poly-functional T cells, which are considered to be superior effectors of protective immunity as compared to cells that produce only one cytokine (4). Specially, IFN-γ, IL-2, and TNF-α secreting CD4+ T cells, which are known as Th1 cells, are regarded as crucial for activation of effector functions to control intracellular *Mtb* and are correlated with protection (5, 6).

Although the role of CD8+ T cell-mediated immune responses against TB infection is less well defined than that of Th1 CD4+ T cells, these cells are also considered to play a crucial role in optimal immunity and protection. It was shown that CD8+ T cells were essential against *Mtb* infection in the models of mice (7, 8),

cattle (9), and macaques (10). Furthermore, vaccine-induced antigen-specific CD8+ T cell responses were found to contribute to strong or modest immune protection in several studies (11–14). Recently, we reported that a novel Sendai virus vectored vaccine, SeV85AB, induced robust T cell responses and substantial protection against *Mtb* infection, which was mainly mediated by CD8+ T cells (15).

Insufficient induction of T cell responses by BCG immunization might underlie the vaccine's inadequacies and boosting these responses by novel vaccines might be an appropriate vaccine strategy (16, 17). However, which kind of T cell responses are beneficial for the anti-TB immune protection remains controversial (18, 19); notably, the classical marker, IFN-γ, was found to play a minor role in, or even be detrimental to, the anti-TB immunity (20–22). Although we had shown that intra-nasal delivery of the SeV85AB vaccine was able to enhance immune protection induced by BCG in a prime-boost model (15), the profile of T cell responses boosted by SeV85AB was not determined. Herein, we show that SeV85AB boosting

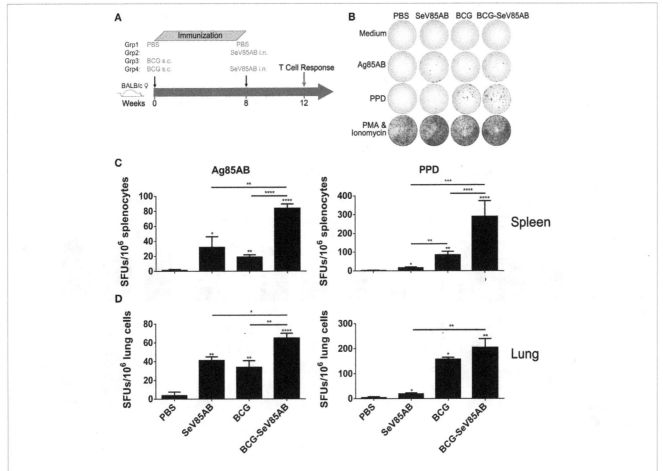

**FIGURE 1 |** Boosting with SeV85AB increased the IFN-γ responses primed by bacille Calmette–Guérin (BCG) vaccination. **(A)** Immunization and detection schedule. Mice primed by BCG were i.n. boosted with SeV85AB or not, and 4 weeks later, they were sacrificed for assays of cellular immune responses. Controls received PBS, SeV85AB, or BCG only, at the indicated time points. **(B–D)** The IFN-γ responses determined by enzyme linked immunospot assay. Representative dot plots are shown in **(B)**. Cells from spleen **(C)** and lung **(D)** were stimulated for 20 h with Ag85AB peptide pool (5 µg/ml) or PPD (10 µg/ml) in 96-well plates and then the IFN-γ-secreting cells were detected and counted. PMA plus Ionomycin stimulation was used as positive control. Data are representative of two independent experiments with at least four mice per group. *$P < 0.05$, **$P < 0.01$, ***$P < 0.001$, and ****$P < 0.0001$.

established substantial T cell responses in the lung that differed from systemic immunity; there were different profiles of antigen-specific poly-functional T cell subsets in the lung compared with the spleen. After challenge by *Mtb* infection, SeV85AB-boosted mice had significantly higher levels of recall CD4+ and CD8+ T cell responses, which were mainly mediated by IL-2. In contrast, the IFN-γ-producing cells were barely boosted by SeV85AB. The proportion of cells with central memory phenotype of peptides-responding CD4+ T cells was elevated in SeV85AB-boosted mice after *Mtb* challenge. Our study, therefore, lends strong support to the adoption of Sendai virus as a promising vector system to be used in a heterologous prime-boost immunization regimen against TB.

## MATERIALS AND METHODS

### Animals and Immunization

This study was approved by the Institutional Animal Care and Use Committee and was performed according to the guidelines of the Laboratory Animal Ethical Board of Shanghai Public Health Clinical Center. Specific pathogen-free female BALB/c mice aged 6–8 weeks were immunized with BCG subcutaneously [s.c., $5 \times 10^6$ CFU (colony forming units), in 100 μl PBS] in each hind leg and boosted intra-nasally (i.n.) with SeV85AB [$1 \times 10^7$ cell infectious units (CIU), in 20 μl PBS]. BCG, SeV85AB single immunizations, and PBS were used as controls. For the evaluation of primary cellular immune responses, 4 weeks after vaccination,

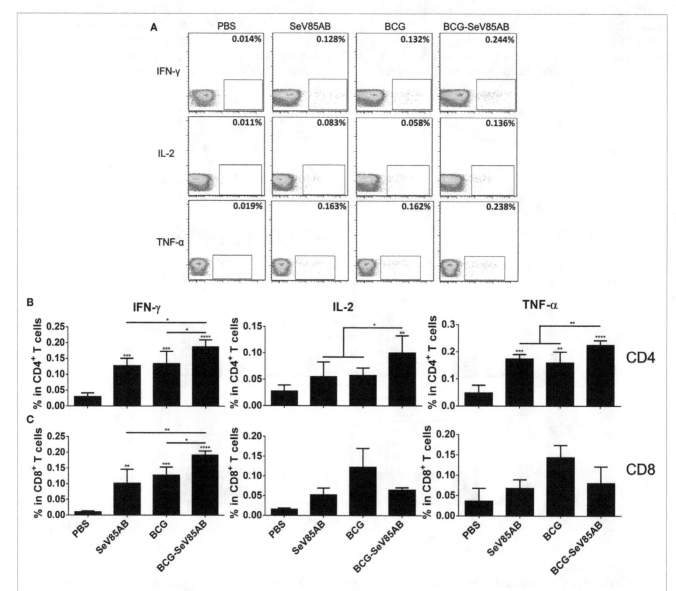

FIGURE 2 | Flow cytometric analysis of ICS in the splenocytes of vaccinated mice. Splenocytes were collected 4 weeks after the last inoculation, incubated with Ag85AB peptides (5 μg/ml) in the presence of monensin and brefeldin A, and analyzed for cytokine production by ICS assay. CD3+CD4+ cells (CD4+ T cells) and CD3+CD4− cells (CD8+ T cells) producing IFN-γ, IL-2, and TNF-α were analyzed. Representative flow cytometric plots of intracellular staining in CD4+ T cells are shown in **(A)**, and summary data of single cytokine producing CD4+ T cells **(B)** and CD8+ T cells **(C)** are shown with significant differences indicated. Data are representative of two independent experiments with at least four mice per group. *P < 0.05, **P < 0.01, ***P < 0.001, and ****P < 0.0001.

animals were sacrificed, then, the lungs and spleens were aseptically removed for antigen-specific T cell immune response assessments. For the evaluation of recall immune responses after infection, the mice were challenged through a respiratory route by the *Mtb* virulent strain H37Rv 4 weeks after immunization and maintained in a level 3 bio-containment animal facility. Five weeks later, the mice were sacrificed and lungs sampled to assess recall responses by intracellular staining (ICS) as described below.

## Harvest of Splenocytes and Lung Cells

Spleen was mechanically disrupted and single splenocytes were filtered, and then subjected to red blood cell lysis. Lung was gently minced by scissors and then incubated with DNase I (10 U, Thermo) and collagenase IV (1 mg/ml, Invitrogen) in 10 ml R10 medium (RPMI-1640 medium containing 10% fetal bovine serum and 1% Penicillin and Streptomycin) for 30 min at 37°C. The collagenase-digested tissue pieces were filtered through a 70 µm cell strainer (Fisher Scientific) by gently squashing with the plunger of a syringe. The cell suspension was centrifuged and red blood cells were lysed. The single splenocytes and lung lymphocytes were washed and re-suspended in R10 medium.

## IFN-γ Enzyme Linked Immunospot (ELISPOT) Assay

Enzyme-linked immunospot assays were performed according to IFN-γ ELISPOT kit protocols (BD Biosciences). Briefly, 96-well plates were coated with anti-mouse IFN-γ antibody at 4°C overnight. Then, they were washed and blocked with R10 medium at room temperature for 2 h. Isolated lung cells or splenocytes were added at $2 \times 10^5$ cells per well with peptide pools (5 µg/ml) or PPD (10 µg/ml). PMA (50 ng/ml, Sigma) and ionomycin (1 µg/ml, Sigma) stimulation were used as positive controls. The cells were stimulated at 37°C for 20 h. The cell suspension was aspirated and washed with PBST (PBS containing 0.5% Tween-20), and then incubated with anti-mouse IFN-γ biotinylated detection antibodies for 2 h. The cell suspension was aspirated and washed with PBST and then incubated with streptavidin-horseradish superoxidase conjugated anti-biotin antibodies for an additional 1 h. After washing with PBST and PBS, AEC substrate solution was added and incubated for 30 min before rinsing away with water. The plates were air-dried and analyzed with Immunospot Reader (Champspot III, Beijing Sage Creation Science).

## Peptides

The peptides were synthesized by GL Biochem (Shanghai, China) with 95% purity. MPVGGQSSF, 70-78aa; TFLTSELPGW-LQANRHVKPT, 99-118aa; GLSMAASSALTL, 124-125aa and YAGAMSGL, 145-152aa were used as an Ag85A peptide pool. IYAGSLSAL, 144-152aa; ALLDPSQGMGPSLIG, 151-165aa; GPSSDPAWERNDPTQQIP, 181-198aa and HSWEYWGAQLNA-MKGDLQ, 262-279aa were used as an Ag85B peptide pool.

## Intracellular Staining (ICS) and Flow Cytometry Analysis

The splenocytes or lung cells were stimulated with Ag85AB peptide pool (5 µg/ml) or PPD (10 µg/ml) in 96-well plates

at 37°C for 1 or 14 h, respectively. Then, cells were incubated for an additional 5 h after the addition of 1 µl/ml Monensin and Brefeldin A (BD Biosciences), PMA (50 ng/ml), and inonomycin (1 µg/ml) stimulation were used as positive controls. After stimulation, cells were washed with wash PBS containing 2% fetal bovine serum and then incubated on ice with the mixture of antibodies for 30 min, then washed and subjected to fixation and permeation with fix/perm buffer (BD Bioscience). After washing, the cells were incubated with antibodies against intracellular cytokines on ice for another 30 min. Then, the cells were re-suspended for flow cytometry analysis (LSRFortessa, BD Biosciences). At least 50,000 T cells were harvested.

## Antibodies

The following antibodies were used in this study: CD3-Pacific Blue (clone 17A2) from BioLegend, and CD44-FITC (clone IM7), CD62L-Percp-Cyanine 5.5 (clone MEL-14), TNF-α-PE-Cyanine 7 (clone MP6-XT22) from eBioscience, and CD4-Alexa Fluor 647 (clone RM4-5), IFN-γ-APC-Cyanine 7 (clone XMG1.2), IL-2-PE (clone JES6-5H4) from BD Biosciences.

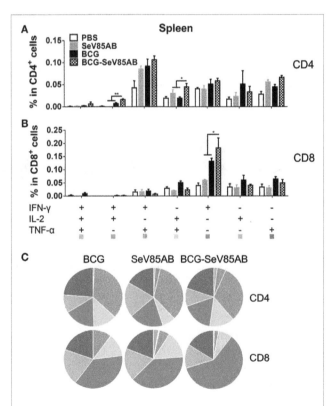

**FIGURE 3 |** Characterization of poly-functional Ag85AB-specific T cell responses in the spleen. T cells producing IFN-γ, IL-2, and TNF-α were distinguished by ICS assay as seven subpopulations based on the production of these three cytokines in any combination. The percentage of subpopulations as components of the total CD4+ **(A)** or CD8+ **(B)** T cell population and the pie chart analysis **(C)** are shown. Significant differences in frequency of poly-functional T cell subsets are indicated. Data are representative of two independent experiments with at least four mice per group. *$P < 0.05$ and **$P < 0.01$.

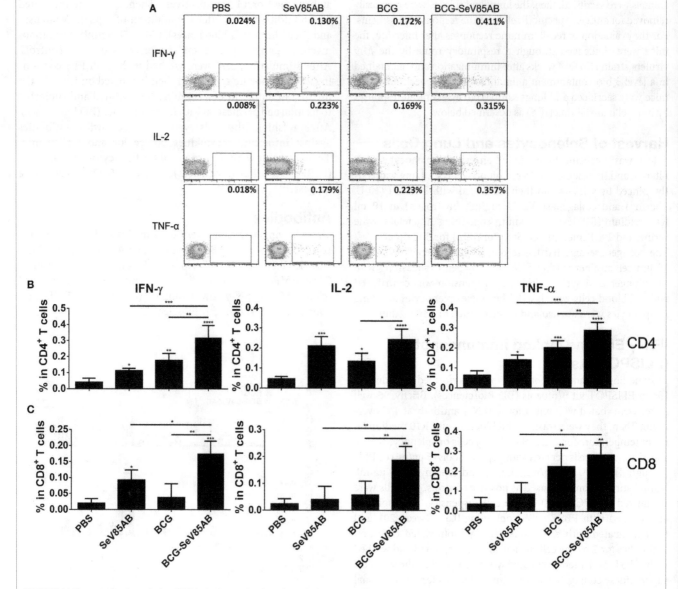

**FIGURE 4** | Flow cytometric analysis of ICS in the lung cells of vaccinated mice. Lung cells were collected, stimulated, and analyzed for cytokine production by ICS assay as described for splenocytes in **Figure 2**. Representative flow cytometric data plots from CD4+ T cells **(A)** and summarized data of single cytokine producing CD4+ T cells **(B)** and CD8+ T cells **(C)** are shown. The percentages of responding cells were compared as indicated. Data are representative of two independent experiments with at least four mice per group. *$P < 0.05$, **$P < 0.01$, ***$P < 0.001$, and ****$P < 0.0001$.

## Statistical Analysis

The statistical analysis was performed using GraphPad Prism 6 software. One-way ANOVA was used to determine the statistical significance for comparison of multiple groups, and two-way ANOVA was used for the grouped analysis.

## RESULTS

### Boosting With SeV85AB Increased the IFN-γ Responses Primed by BCG Vaccination

The experiment protocol is shown diagrammatically in **Figure 1A**. Typical IFN-γ ELISPOT results are shown in **Figure 1B**. As

expected, SeV85AB vaccination induced Ag85AB-specific immune responses, and this effect was significantly greater in BCG-primed mice, both in the spleen (**Figure 1C**) and in the lung (**Figure 1D**). Although PPD-specific cell responses were only slightly induced by SeV85AB, mice receiving SeV85AB boost secreted higher levels of IFN-γ compared with SeV85AB or BCG single immunization (**Figures 1C,D**).

### SeV85AB Boost Increased Systemic Poly-Functional T Cell Responses Primed by BCG Vaccination

At 4 weeks after vaccination, splenocytes were obtained from the different vaccination groups and stimulated with the

Ag85AB peptide pool or incubated with medium as control (The gating strategy is shown in Figure S1 in Supplementary Material, CD4+ T cells were gated as CD3+CD4+ cells and CD8+ T cells were defined as CD3+CD4− cells) and the results of flow cytometric ICS detection of IFN-γ, IL-2, and TNF-α positive T cells were compared between groups (representative mono-positive dot plots are shown in **Figure 2A** and dual-positive plots are shown in Figure S2 in Supplementary Material). Consistent with the ELISPOT assay, the production of all three cytokines in CD4+ T cells was significantly enhanced by SeV85AB boost (**Figure 2B**), whereas only IFN-γ was increased in CD8+ T cells (**Figure 2C**). The SeV85AB boost induced higher levels of antigen-specific poly-functional CD4+ T cell responses, in which the increased percentage of dual-positive IFN-γ+IL-2+ and IL-2+TNF-α+ cells were statistically significant (**Figures 3A,C**). Additionally, the mono-positive IFN-γ+CD8+ subset was significantly increased (**Figures 3B,C**).

## SeV85AB Boost Increased Poly-Functional T Cell Responses in the Lung Primed by BCG Vaccination

The representative staining results of flow cytometric ICS detection of IFN-γ, IL-2, and TNF-α mono-producing lung T cells after Ag85AB stimulation are shown in **Figure 4A** and dual-positive plots are shown in Figure S3 in Supplementary Material. The secretion of all three cytokines was significantly boosted, both in CD4+ T and CD8+ T cells (**Figures 4B,C**). The poly-functional T cell subset analysis further showed that in CD4+ T cells the dual-positive IFN-γ+TNF-α+ and mono-positive IFN-γ+ subsets were significantly boosted (**Figures 5A,C**), whereas in the CD8+ T cells, the IFN-γ+ and IL-2+TNF-α+ subsets were boosted (**Figures 5B,C**). In the spleen, SeV85AB boost dominantly increased IL-2 responses in CD4+ T cells (**Figure 3A**), whereas in the lung, the greater increases were in IFN-γ positive CD4+ T cells (**Figure 5B**). In the spleen, the CD8+ T cell responses had been only modestly enhanced (**Figure 3B**), whereas in the lung, IL-2+TNF-α+ and IFN-γ+ cells had been significantly increased by SeV85AB (**Figure 5B**). In addition, PPD-specific CD4+ T cell responses in the spleen and CD8+ T cell responses in the lung were also boosted by SeV85AB (Figure S4 in Supplementary Material). These divergences confirmed that the mucosal immunization with SeV85AB had a different capacity to establish immune memory in the systemic immune system compared with local site in the lung, confirming our previous observation (15). Taken together, these data demonstrated that SeV85AB boost induced higher levels of poly-functional antigen-specific CD4+ and CD8+ T cell responses primed by BCG vaccine.

## SeV85AB-Boosted BCG-Induced Immune Protection Was Associated With Recall of Antigen-Specific IL-2-Mediated Responses

We had shown that mucosal boosting of SeV85AB improved the protection of BCG vaccination against *Mtb* challenge in a prime-boost model (15). In this study, the protective efficacy afforded by

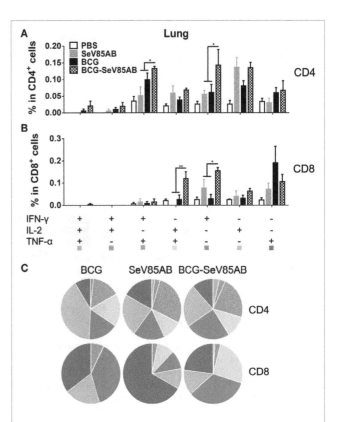

**FIGURE 5** | Characterizations of poly-functional Ag85AB-specific T cell responses in the lung. T cells secreting IFN-γ, IL-2, and TNF-α were distinguished as seven distinct subpopulations as described in **Figure 3**. The percentage of subpopulation as components of the total CD4+ **(A)** and CD8+ **(B)** T cell populations and the pie chart analysis **(C)** are shown. Significant differences in frequency of poly-functional T cell subsets are indicated. Data are representative of two independent experiments with at least four mice per group. *P < 0.05 and **P < 0.01.

SeV85AB boost was confirmed (data not shown), and the recall T cell responses that occurred upon the *Mtb* infection were especially assayed (**Figure 6A**). IFN-γ ELISPOT results showed that, at 5 weeks postinfection, mice that had received SeV85AB boosting before the infection had developed only slight, if any, overall increase of Ag85AB- (**Figure 6B**) and PPD- (**Figure 6C**) specific responses in the lung compared with the response to infection after SeV85AB or BCG single vaccination. However, SeV85AB boosting resulted in a response to infection that contained a higher percentage of Ag85AB-specific poly-functional lung T cells, notably CD4+ T cells with the phenotypes IL-2+TNF-α+/IL-2+, and CD8+ T cells of phenotypes IFN-γ+IL-2+TNF-α+/IL-2+ (**Figure 7**).

## SeV85AB Induced Elevated Central Memory Phenotype of CD4+ T Cells

The memory phenotypes of antigen-responding CD4+ T cells that secreted at least one of the cytokines IFN-γ, IL-2, or TNF-α were further determined (The gating strategy is shown in Figure S5 in Supplementary Material). As a result, SeV85AB boost led to significantly higher levels CD4+ T cells with CD44+CD62+ central

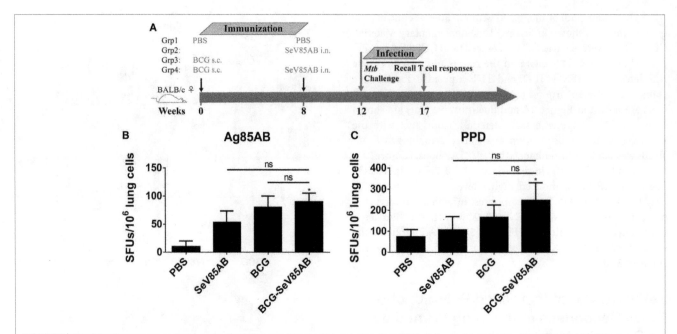

**FIGURE 6** | Recall T cell responses against specific stimulation post *Mycobacterium tuberculosis* (*Mtb*) challenge determined by IFN-γ Enzyme Linked Immunospot (ELISPOT) assay. **(A)** Immunization and infection schedule. Vaccinated mice were aerosol challenged 4 weeks later with virulent *Mtb* H37Rv. Five weeks postinfection, recall lung T cell responses were determined. **(B,C)** The IFN-γ responses by ELISPOT assay. Cells from the infected lung were stimulated for 20 h with Ag85AB peptide pool **(B)** or PPD **(C)** in 96-well plates, respectively. Significant differences in frequency between T cell subsets are indicated. Data are representative of two independent experiments with three mice per group. ns, no significant difference.

memory phenotype compared with other vaccination groups (**Figure 8**). This was paralleled by decrease in CD44⁺CD62⁻ (effector memory) among those responding CD4⁺ T cells (**Figure 8**). Thus, our data strongly suggest that the enhanced immune protection induced by SeV85AB boosting was associated with establishment of an increased capacity to recall central memory CD4⁺ T cell responses.

## DISCUSSION

Up to now, most successful vaccines against microbial pathogens have depended on humoral immunity to achieve protection or even sterile eradication. However, as is the case for many intracellular bacteria, *Mtb* is able to resist most antibody-mediated antibacterial effects by growing inside macrophages (23). Thus, T cell-mediated immune responses are crucial for the development of anti-TB vaccines.

The only available anti-TB vaccine remains the almost 100-year-old BCG. The routine administration of BCG to infants provides significant protection against miliary and meningeal TB. However, the protective efficacy is inconsistent in adults. One explanation of BCG's inadequate protection is a lack of an effective stimulation of an optimal blend of T cell populations (24). Considering that both CD4⁺ and CD8⁺ T cells play important roles in protective immunity against *Mtb* (3, 25, 26), the development of efficient memory CD4⁺ and CD8⁺ T cell responses is one of the main goals of the novel vaccine strategies against *Mtb*.

Although BCG is a strong inducer of Th1 CD4⁺ T cell immune responses, the incidence of active TB disease increases with time after BCG immunization (27), suggesting that a decline of

immunological memory after BCG vaccination is one of the causes of the vaccine's low protective efficacy. However, the waning of BCG protection was not prevented by a BCG revaccination strategy (28). Since the majority of human beings are BCG inoculated, and this seems unlikely to change, a prime-boost regimen is an attractive strategy to counter the waning immune memory post BCG. Heterologous prime-boost vaccination strategy is known to be highly effective for enhancing anti-TB T cell-mediated immunity (17, 29). For example, a vaccinia virus-vectored vaccine (MVA85A) and two adenovirus-based vaccines (AdAg85A and Crucell Ad35) are candidate booster vaccines that are under clinical evaluation. Although MVA85A was shown to be effective in boosting BCG-primed immune protection in a variety of *Mtb* animal infection models, a phase IIb clinical trial indicated that MVA85A may not be effective in humans (30). This failure suggested that novel anti-TB vaccine platforms or optimized delivery systems are urgently needed (31). Improvement would benefit from knowing which cellular responses constitute optimum protective immunity. Our analysis of the cells engaged in the enhanced protective response in the lungs of *Mtb*-challenged mice after BCG/SeV85AB prime/boost is illuminating.

In *Mtb* natural infection, T cells are initially primed in the draining lymph nodes of the infected lung, phagocytosis leads to the presentation and cross-presentation of *Mtb* peptide-loaded MHC-I and -II complexes, which provides the priming "first signal" at the DC surface (32). The "second signal," a costimulatory signal, tunes the T cell responses by decreasing the activation thresholds of T cells, and pathogen-specific inflammation provides the "third signal" that shapes the maturation of T cells (33–36). A deficiency in any of these signals might lead to the

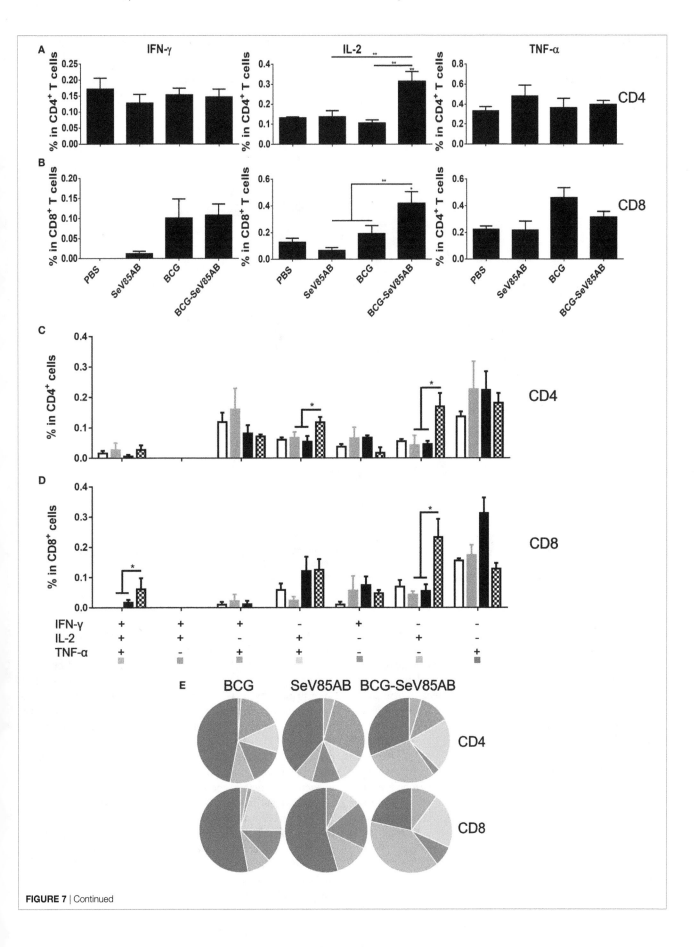

**FIGURE 7** | Continued

**FIGURE 7** | Recall T cell responses against specific stimulation post *Mycobacterium tuberculosis* challenge determined by ICS assay. The immunization and infection schedule were described in **Figure 6A**. Lung cells were stimulated *ex vivo* with Ag85AB peptides in the presence of monensin and brefeldin A and analyzed for cytokine production by ICS assay. T cells producing IFN-γ, IL-2, and TNF-α were analyzed and their percentage in CD4+ T cells **(A)** and CD8+ T cells **(B)** are shown. The percentage of seven subpopulations based on the production of three cytokines in any combination in the total CD4+ **(C)** and CD8+ **(D)** T cells and the pie chart analysis **(E)** are shown. Significant differences in frequency of T cell subsets are indicated. Data are representative of two independent experiments with three mice per group. *P < 0.05 and **P < 0.01.

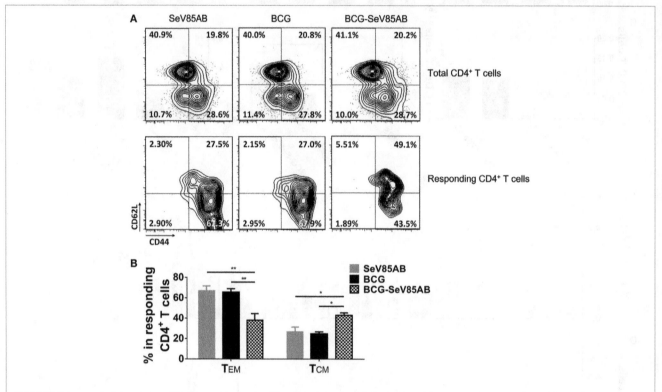

**FIGURE 8** | Memory phenotypes of recall T cell responses against *Mycobacterium tuberculosis* challenge. The memory phenotypes in total CD4+ T cells and Ag85AB-responding CD4+ T cells were assessed. The responding cells were defined as the cells that secreted at least one of the cytokines IFN-γ, IL-2, and TNF-α after Ag85AB peptide stimulation. Central memory T cells (T$_{CM}$) and effector memory T cells (T$_{EM}$) were defined as CD44+CD62L+ and CD44+CD62L−, respectively. Representative flow cytometric plots **(A)** and summarized data **(B)** are shown. Data are representative of two independent experiments with three mice per group. *P < 0.05 and **P < 0.01.

inadequate activation of anti-TB T cell immune memory (37). Sendai virus was chosen here to serve as vector of a booster anti-TB vaccine primarily because it was known that Sendai virus treatment matured dendritic cells and led to complete elimination of tumors cells *in vivo* (38). In addition, Sendai virus tests had demonstrated a potent induction of type I interferon (39) and a Sendai virus-derived RNA agonist of RIG-I had been used as an adjuvant to enhance vaccine-induced immune responses by providing an inflammatory microenvironment (40), thereby optimizing antigen-specific CD4+ and CD8+ T cell responses (41). Based on this, we initiated this program of investigation and found that the novel Sendai virus vectored vaccine, SeV85AB, did indeed induce robust T cell responses and substantial protection against *Mtb* challenge (15).

Bacille Calmette–Guérin is a strong inducer of systematic CD4+ T cell immunity but fails to induce efficient CD8+ T cells. In contrast, a single immunization of SeV85AB was able to establish antigen-specific T cells responses and CD8+ T cells

mediated immune protection (15). Here, we found that the strong antigen-specific CD4+ and modest CD8+ T cells primed by BCG vaccination were both enhanced by SeV85AB in the spleen. Most notably, the weak antigen-specific CD8+ T cell responses that were primed by BCG in the lung were significantly enhanced by the SeV85AB boosting. Heterologous prime-boost and recombinant protein anti-TB vaccine models have shown that the vaccine-induced IL-2-secreting CD4+ T cell subsets could maintain the IL-2-producing ability for at least 26 weeks post challenge infection and were associated with enhanced control of bacterial growth in mouse models (42, 43). Increased TNF-α/IFN-γ/IL-2 and decreased TNF-α/IFN-γ responses induced by BCG have been associated with protection against bovine TB (44). In this study, although the IL-2 response was not dominated in the vaccine-induced primary responses in the spleen, IL-2-producing poly-functional T cells were significantly boosted by SeV85AB, supporting the protective role of IL-2 in anti-TB vaccine-induced protection.

Moreover, it was shown that the antigen-specific IL-2$^+$CD4$^+$ T cell subsets were negative for KLRG1, which is a surface marker of terminally differentiated T cells, during *Mtb* challenge infection (42). We showed previously that the inadequacy of T cell immunity during chronic human TB infection is associated with the less-protective terminally differentiated T cell state marked by KLRG1 expression. Furthermore, the blockade of KLRG1 signaling increased CD4$^+$ T cell function through enhancement of Akt pathway in human TB infection (45, 46), supporting the protective role of IL-2 in TB infection. In this study, IL-2-producing T cells were significantly enhanced post *Mtb* infection in the BCG prime-SeV85AB boost regimen group, again showing the recall of IL-2 responses was associated with protective immunity. IL-2 enhances competitiveness for survival in CD4$^+$ T cells, thereby facilitating the development of a memory population (47). The CD4$^+$ T cells that produce IL-2 could be sustained over a prolonged period and developed into effector cells following antigen stimulation as a result of quick recall response (48). In human TB infection, active TB patients had decreased IL-2-producing CD4$^+$ T cells compared with latent TB infection, and 6 months of anti-TB treatment increased specific IL-2-producing T cells (49). In contrast, although also essential for host resistance against *Mtb*, IFN-γ responses do not always correlate with immune protection (26). Recently, Barber et al. also found that IFN-γ accounts for only ~30% of the cumulative CD4$^+$ T cell-mediated reduction in lung bacterial loads, but increasing the per capita production of IFN-γ led to the early death of the host in murine TB infection (20). Thus, although it can be regarded as a positive marker of vaccine-induced primary T cell responses, the degree of infection-induced IFN-γ production might not always be the factor limiting immune protection against TB. Instead, our data support a key positive role of IL-2 in anti-TB immune protection. Thus, perhaps recall IL-2-mediated, instead of IFN-γ-mediated

T cell responses is the critical factor normally limiting protection against TB infection.

Cumulatively, our data suggest that boosting BCG with SeV85AB might compensate for the weak induction by BCG of IL-2-dependent recall T cell immune responses in the lung. Since we showed here that an SeV85AB boost significantly enhanced the T cell immune memory induced by BCG vaccination in mice, further studies of SeV85AB in other animal models are warranted before a clinical trial of safety in humans.

## AUTHOR CONTRIBUTIONS

X-YF and TS conceive the project. X-YF and ZH designed the study, analyzed the data, and wrote the manuscript. ZH, LG, and C-LL performed the experiments. DL provided editorial input and improved the writing.

## FUNDING

This work was supported by Grants from Chinese National Mega Science and Technology Program on Infectious Diseases (2018ZX10731301, 2018ZX10302301), National Science Foundation of China (31771004, 81501365), and Shanghai Science and Technology Commission (17ZR1423900), and Shanghai Municipal Commission of Health and Family Planning (20144Y0072).

## REFERENCES

1. Rodrigues LC, Diwan VK, Wheeler JG. Protective effect of BCG against tuberculous meningitis and miliary tuberculosis: a meta-analysis. *Int J Epidemiol* (1993) 22:1154–8. doi:10.1093/ije/22.6.1154
2. Bloom BR, Fine PEM. The BCG experience: implications for future vaccines against tuberculosis. In: Bloom BR, editor. *Tuberculosis: Pathogenesis, Protection, and Control.* Washington, DC: ASM Press (1994). p. 531–57.
3. Prezzemolo T, Guggino G, La Manna MP, Di Liberto D, Dieli F, Caccamo N. Functional signatures of human CD4 and CD8 T cell responses to *Mycobacterium tuberculosis*. *Front Immunol* (2014) 5:180. doi:10.3389/fimmu.2014.00180
4. Jasenosky LD, Scriba TJ, Hanekom WA, Goldfeld AE. T cells and adaptive immunity to *Mycobacterium tuberculosis* in humans. *Immunol Rev* (2015) 264:74–87. doi:10.1111/imr.12274
5. Kaufmann SH. Tuberculosis vaccines: time to think about the next generation. *Semin Immunol* (2013) 25:172–81. doi:10.1016/j.smim.2013.04.006
6. Urdahl KB. Understanding and overcoming the barriers to T cell-mediated immunity against tuberculosis. *Semin Immunol* (2014) 26:578–87. doi:10.1016/j.smim.2014.10.003
7. van Pinxteren LA, Cassidy JP, Smedegaard BH, Agger EM, Andersen P. Control of latent *Mycobacterium tuberculosis* infection is dependent on CD8

T cells. *Eur J Immunol* (2000) 30:3689–98. doi:10.1002/1521-4141(200012)30:12<3689::AID-IMMU3689>3.0.CO;2-4
8. Sousa AO, Mazzaccaro RJ, Russell RG, Lee FK, Turner OC, Hong S, et al. Relative contributions of distinct MHC class I-dependent cell populations in protection to tuberculosis infection in mice. *Proc Natl Acad Sci U S A* (2000) 97:4204–8. doi:10.1073/pnas.97.8.4204
9. Villarreal-Ramos B, McAulay M, Chance V, Martin M, Morgan J, Howard CJ. Investigation of the role of CD8+ T cells in bovine tuberculosis in vivo. *Infect Immun* (2003) 71:4297–303. doi:10.1128/IAI.71.8.4297-4303.2003
10. Chen CY, Huang D, Wang RC, Shen L, Zeng G, Yao S, et al. A critical role for CD8 T cells in a nonhuman primate model of tuberculosis. *PLoS Pathog* (2009) 5:e1000392. doi:10.1371/journal.ppat.1000392
11. Wu Y, Woodworth JS, Shin DS, Morris S, Behar SM. Vaccine-elicited 10-kilodalton culture filtrate protein-specific CD8+ T cells are sufficient to mediate protection against *Mycobacterium tuberculosis* infection. *Infect Immun* (2008) 76:2249–55. doi:10.1128/IAI.00024-08
12. Grode L, Seiler P, Baumann S, Hess J, Brinkmann V, Nasser EA, et al. Increased vaccine efficacy against tuberculosis of recombinant *Mycobacterium bovis* bacille Calmette-Guerin mutants that secrete listeriolysin. *J Clin Invest* (2005) 115:2472–9. doi:10.1172/JCI24617
13. Wang J, Santosuosso M, Ngai P, Zganiacz A, Xing Z. Activation of CD8 T cells by mycobacterial vaccination protects against pulmonary tuberculosis

in the absence of CD4 T cells. *J Immunol* (2004) 173:4590–7. doi:10.4049/jimmunol.173.7.4590

14. Moliva JI, Hossfeld AP, Canan CH, Dwivedi V, Wewers MD, Beamer G, et al. Exposure to human alveolar lining fluid enhances *Mycobacterium bovis* BCG vaccine efficacy against *Mycobacterium tuberculosis* infection in a CD8(+) T-cell-dependent manner. *Mucosal Immunol* (2017) 11:968–78. doi:10.1038/mi.2017.80

15. Hu Z, Wong KW, Zhao HM, Wen HL, Ji P, Ma H, et al. Sendai virus mucosal vaccination establishes lung-resident memory CD8 T cell immunity and boosts BCG-primed protection against TB in mice. *Mol Ther* (2017) 25:1222–33. doi:10.1016/j.ymthe.2017.02.018

16. Nieuwenhuizen NE, Kaufmann S. Next-generation vaccines based on bacille Calmette-Guerin. *Front Immunol* (2018) 9:121. doi:10.3389/fimmu.2018.00121

17. Dalmia N, Ramsay AJ. Prime-boost approaches to tuberculosis vaccine development. *Expert Rev Vaccines* (2012) 11:1221–33. doi:10.1586/erv.12.94

18. Lewinsohn DA, Lewinsohn DM, Scriba TJ. Polyfunctional CD4(+) T cells as targets for tuberculosis vaccination. *Front Immunol* (2017) 8:1262. doi:10.3389/fimmu.2017.01262

19. Zeng G, Zhang G, Chen X. Th1 cytokines, true functional signatures for protective immunity against TB? *Cell Mol Immunol* (2018) 15:206–15. doi:10.1038/cmi.2017.113

20. Sakai S, Kauffman KD, Sallin MA, Sharpe AH, Young HA, Ganusov VV, et al. CD4 T cell-derived IFN-gamma plays a minimal role in control of pulmonary *Mycobacterium tuberculosis* infection and must be actively repressed by PD-1 to prevent lethal disease. *PLoS Pathog* (2016) 12:e1005667. doi:10.1371/journal.ppat.1005667

21. Kumar P. IFNgamma-producing CD4(+) T lymphocytes: the double-edged swords in tuberculosis. *Clin Transl Med* (2017) 6:21. doi:10.1186/s40169-017-0151-8

22. Mourik BC, Lubberts E, de Steenwinkel J, Ottenhoff T, Leenen P. Interactions between type 1 interferons and the Th17 response in tuberculosis: lessons learned from autoimmune diseases. *Front Immunol* (2017) 8:294. doi:10.3389/fimmu.2017.00294

23. Nunes-Alves C, Booty MG, Carpenter SM, Jayaraman P, Rothchild AC, Behar SM. In search of a new paradigm for protective immunity to TB. *Nat Rev Microbiol* (2014) 12(4):289–99. doi:10.1038/nrmicro3230

24. Agger EM, Andersen P. A novel TB vaccine; towards a strategy based on our understanding of BCG failure. *Vaccine* (2002) 21:7–14. doi:10.1016/S0264-410X(02)00447-4

25. Zuniga J, Torres-Garcia D, Santos-Mendoza T, Rodriguez-Reyna TS, Granados J, Yunis EJ. Cellular and humoral mechanisms involved in the control of tuberculosis. *Clin Dev Immunol* (2012) 2012:193923. doi:10.1155/2012/193923

26. Sakai S, Mayer-Barber KD, Barber DL. Defining features of protective CD4 T cell responses to *Mycobacterium tuberculosis*. *Curr Opin Immunol* (2014) 29:137–42. doi:10.1016/j.coi.2014.06.003

27. Sterne JA, Rodrigues LC, Guedes IN. Does the efficacy of BCG decline with time since vaccination? *Int J Tuberc Lung Dis* (1998) 2:200–7.

28. Karonga Prevention Trial Group. Randomised controlled trial of single BCG, repeated BCG, or combined BCG and killed *Mycobacterium leprae* vaccine for prevention of leprosy and tuberculosis in Malawi. *Lancet* (1996) 348:17–24. doi:10.1016/S0140-6736(96)02166-6

29. Brennan MJ, Clagett B, Fitzgerald H, Chen V, Williams A, Izzo AA, et al. Preclinical evidence for implementing a prime-boost vaccine strategy for tuberculosis. *Vaccine* (2012) 30:2811–23. doi:10.1016/j.vaccine.2012.02.036

30. Tameris MD, Hatherill M, Landry BS, Scriba TJ, Snowden MA, Lockhart S, et al. Safety and efficacy of MVA85A, a new tuberculosis vaccine, in infants previously vaccinated with BCG: a randomised, placebo-controlled phase 2b trial. *Lancet* (2013) 381:1021–8. doi:10.1016/S0140-6736(13)60177-4

31. Meyer J, McShane H. The next 10 years for tuberculosis vaccines: do we have the right plans in place? *Expert Rev Vaccines* (2013) 12:443–51. doi:10.1586/erv.13.19

32. Ottenhoff TH, Kaufmann SH. Vaccines against tuberculosis: where are we and where do we need to go? *PLoS Pathog* (2012) 8:e1002607. doi:10.1371/journal.ppat.1002607

33. Hu Z, Wang J, Wan Y, Zhu L, Ren X, Qiu S, et al. Boosting functional avidity of CD8+ T cells by vaccinia virus vaccination depends on intrinsic T-cell

MyD88 expression but not the inflammatory milieu. *J Virol* (2014) 88:5356–68. doi:10.1128/JVI.03664-13

34. Khan N, Gowthaman U, Pahari S, Agrewala JN. Manipulation of costimulatory molecules by intracellular pathogens: veni, vidi, vici!! *PLoS Pathog* (2012) 8:e1002676. doi:10.1371/journal.ppat.1002676

35. Etna MP, Giacomini E, Severa M, Coccia EM. Pro- and anti-inflammatory cytokines in tuberculosis: a two-edged sword in TB pathogenesis. *Semin Immunol* (2014) 26:543–51. doi:10.1016/j.smim.2014.09.011

36. Hu Z, Zhu L, Wang J, Wan Y, Yuan S, Chen J, et al. Immune signature of enhanced functional avidity CD8(+) T cells in vivo induced by vaccinia vectored vaccine. *Sci Rep* (2017) 7:41558. doi:10.1038/srep41558

37. Egen JG, Rothfuchs AG, Feng CG, Horwitz MA, Sher A, Germain RN. Intravital imaging reveals limited antigen presentation and T cell effector function in mycobacterial granulomas. *Immunity* (2011) 34:807–19. doi:10.1016/j.immuni.2011.03.022

38. Shibata S, Okano S, Yonemitsu Y, Onimaru M, Sata S, Nagata-Takeshita H, et al. Induction of efficient antitumor immunity using dendritic cells activated by recombinant Sendai virus and its modulation by exogenous IFN-beta gene. *J Immunol* (2006) 177:3564–76. doi:10.4049/jimmunol.177.6.3564

39. Buggele WA, Horvath CM. MicroRNA profiling of Sendai virus-infected A549 cells identifies miR-203 as an interferon-inducible regulator of IFIT1/ISG56. *J Virol* (2013) 87:9260–70. doi:10.1128/JVI.01064-13

40. Martinez-Gil L, Goff PH, Hai R, Garcia-Sastre A, Shaw ML, Palese P. A Sendai virus-derived RNA agonist of RIG-I as a virus vaccine adjuvant. *J Virol* (2013) 87:1290–300. doi:10.1128/JVI.02338-12

41. Seki S, Matano T. Development of a Sendai virus vector-based AIDS vaccine inducing T cell responses. *Expert Rev Vaccines* (2016) 15:119–27. doi:10.1586/14760584.2016.1105747

42. Lindenstrom T, Knudsen NP, Agger EM, Andersen P. Control of chronic *Mycobacterium tuberculosis* infection by CD4 KLRG1- IL-2-secreting central memory cells. *J Immunol* (2013) 190:6311–9. doi:10.4049/jimmunol.1300248

43. Woodworth JS, Aagaard CS, Hansen PR, Cassidy JP, Agger EM, Andersen P. Protective CD4 T cells targeting cryptic epitopes of *Mycobacterium tuberculosis* resist infection-driven terminal differentiation. *J Immunol* (2014) 192:3247–58. doi:10.4049/jimmunol.1300283

44. Maggioli MF, Palmer MV, Thacker TC, Vordermeier HM, McGill JL, Whelan AO, et al. Increased TNF-alpha/IFN-gamma/IL-2 and decreased TNF-alpha/IFN-gamma production by central memory T cells are associated with protective responses against bovine tuberculosis following BCG vaccination. *Front Immunol* (2016) 7:421. doi:10.3389/fimmu.2016.00421

45. Hu Z, Zhao HM, Li CL, Liu XH, Barkan D, Lowrie DB, et al. The role of KLRG1 in human CD4+ T-cell immunity against tuberculosis. *J Infect Dis* (2018) 217:1491–503. doi:10.1093/infdis/jiy046

46. Hu Z, Lowrie DB, Fan XY. Reply to Mahla. *J Infect Dis* (2018). doi:10.1093/infdis/jiy314

47. Dooms H, Kahn E, Knoechel B, Abbas AK. IL-2 induces a competitive survival advantage in T lymphocytes. *J Immunol* (2004) 172:5973–9. doi:10.4049/jimmunol.172.10.5973

48. Seder RA, Darrah PA, Roederer M. T-cell quality in memory and protection: implications for vaccine design. *Nat Rev Immunol* (2008) 8:247–58. doi:10.1038/nri2355

49. Day CL, Abrahams DA, Lerumo L, Janse VRE, Stone L, O'Rie T, et al. Functional capacity of *Mycobacterium tuberculosis*-specific T cell responses in humans is associated with mycobacterial load. *J Immunol* (2011) 187:2222–32. doi:10.4049/jimmunol.1101122

# 7

# Nanoparticle-Based Vaccines Against Respiratory Viruses

*Soultan Al-Halifa [1,2], Laurie Gauthier [1,2,3,4], Dominic Arpin [1,2,3,4], Steve Bourgault [1,2,4]\* and Denis Archambault [3,4]\**

[1] Département de Chimie, Université du Québec à Montréal, Montreal, QC, Canada, [2] Quebec Network for Research on Protein Function, Engineering and Applications, PROTEO, Quebec, QC, Canada, [3] Département des Sciences Biologiques, Université du Québec à Montréal, Montreal, QC, Canada, [4] Faculté de Médecine Vétérinaire, Centre de Recherche en Infectiologie Porcine et Avicole (CRIPA), Université de Montréal, St-Hyacinthe, QC, Canada

*Correspondence:*
*Steve Bourgault*
*bourgault.steve@uqam.ca*
*Denis Archambault*
*archambault.denis@uqam.ca*

The respiratory mucosa is the primary portal of entry for numerous viruses such as the respiratory syncytial virus, the influenza virus and the parainfluenza virus. These pathogens initially infect the upper respiratory tract and then reach the lower respiratory tract, leading to diseases. Vaccination is an affordable way to control the pathogenicity of viruses and constitutes the strategy of choice to fight against infections, including those leading to pulmonary diseases. Conventional vaccines based on live-attenuated pathogens present a risk of reversion to pathogenic virulence while inactivated pathogen vaccines often lead to a weak immune response. Subunit vaccines were developed to overcome these issues. However, these vaccines may suffer from a limited immunogenicity and, in most cases, the protection induced is only partial. A new generation of vaccines based on nanoparticles has shown great potential to address most of the limitations of conventional and subunit vaccines. This is due to recent advances in chemical and biological engineering, which allow the design of nanoparticles with a precise control over the size, shape, functionality and surface properties, leading to enhanced antigen presentation and strong immunogenicity. This short review provides an overview of the advantages associated with the use of nanoparticles as vaccine delivery platforms to immunize against respiratory viruses and highlights relevant examples demonstrating their potential as safe, effective and affordable vaccines.

Keywords: respiratory viruses, nanocarriers, nanovaccine, mucosal sites, immune response

## INTRODUCTION

Lower respiratory tract infections (LRTIs) constitute a major public health burden worldwide. LRTIs represent a leading cause of human mortality and morbidity, causing annually over 3 million deaths worldwide (1). Among these infections, about 80% of LRTI cases are caused by viruses (2). In most cases, these pathogens enter the host via airborne transmissions (e.g., droplets or aerosols), replicate efficiently in the respiratory tract and cause clinical manifestations, ranging from fever to bronchiolitis and pneumonia (3). In addition, LRTIs associated with viruses represent an important source of economic loss for livestock and poultry industry as these infections predispose animals to secondary bacterial infections (4–6).

Viruses infecting the human lower respiratory tract include the influenza virus, the respiratory syncytial virus (RSV), the parainfluenza virus and the adenovirus (7, 8). Seasonal influenza virus epidemics result in a significant burden of disease in children and elderlies and account for 3–5 million cases of severe illness and for nearly 290,000–650,000 deaths worldwide each year (9). RSV and parainfluenza virus infections are the leading cause of hospitalization for acute respiratory infections in young children, causing 45 and 40% of pediatric hospitalizations, respectively (10, 11). Adenovirus infections account for 3–5% of LRTIs cases in children and can be fatal for immunocompromised patients (12). In general, respiratory viruses represent a major health problem in infants, young children, immunocompromised patients and the elderly population. According to Global Burden of Diseases (GBD), 74% of deaths associated with LRTIs represent these vulnerable patient groups (13).

Vaccination remains the most cost-effective strategy to fight against infectious diseases. Conventionally, vaccine formulations consist of attenuated viruses, killed pathogens (inactivated) or subunit protein antigens, which elicit a specific immune response. These vaccine formulations have allowed the prevention, or the control, of several important diseases including rubella, yellow fever, polio and measles, and, in the case of smallpox, even eradication (14, 15). Considerable efforts have been devoted for the development of efficient vaccines against LRTIs, including inactivated/fragmented trivalent or quadrivalent seasonal vaccines against influenza type A and type B viruses such as Influvac® (16), Vaxigrip® (17), and Fluzone®(18) as well as live attenuated vaccines such as Nasovac® and Flumist® for nasal administration in young children (19, 20). Nevertheless, live-attenuated vaccines against influenza virus suffer from safety concerns due to their nature and represent a risk for elderly and immunosuppressed humans (21). Besides, killed pathogen vaccines and virus-derived subunit vaccines induce weaker immune responses and often require the use of an adjuvant to boost efficiency (22).

Several promising vaccines are currently evaluated in the clinics for different respiratory viruses (23). These new vaccine formulations aim to be safer and more efficient compared to traditional vaccines based on attenuated viruses, killed pathogens and subunits. Nevertheless, the high level of antigenic drift (genetic mutations) of some viruses, such as the influenza virus, reduces the efficacy of vaccines and needs to be addressed (24). Therefore, while improving safety and efficiency, vaccines should also be less sensitive to antigenic drift. The concept of "universal vaccine" is critical for viruses like the influenza virus, and new formulations to induce broad-spectrum immunity are being investigated. In the next sections, we discuss the advantages of using nanoparticle formulations against respiratory viruses and we highlight relevant examples of the use of nanoparticles as safe, effective, and affordable vaccines.

## NANOPARTICLES, AN ALTERNATIVE APPROACH TO CONVENTIONAL VACCINES

The use of particles as nanoplatforms displaying relevant antigenic moieties is appealing as an alternative approach to conventional vaccines. These nano-sized materials can be obtained from biological sources and/or can be synthetic.

Currently, there is a large variety of particles evaluated as antigen carriers, including inorganic and polymeric nanoparticles, virus-like particles (VLPs), liposomes and self-assembled protein nanoparticles (**Figure 1A**). The advantages of these materials reside primarily in their size (at least one dimension should be at the nanometer level), since many biological systems such as viruses and proteins are nano-sized (25). Nanoparticles can be administered via sub-cutaneous and intramuscular injections, or can be delivered through the mucosal sites (oral and intranasal), and penetrate capillaries as well as mucosal surfaces (26, 27). Recent progresses have allowed the preparation of nanoparticles with unique physicochemical properties. For instance, size, shape, solubility, surface chemistry, and hydrophilicity can be tuned and controlled, which allows the preparation of nanoparticles with tailored biological properties (28). Moreover, nanoparticles can be designed to allow the incorporation of a wide range of molecules including antigens which makes them highly interesting in vaccinology (29, 30).

Incorporation of antigens in nanoparticles can be achieved by encapsulation (physical entrapment) or by conjugation (covalent functionalization) (21). Studies have demonstrated that nanoparticles could protect the native structure of antigens from proteolytic degradation and/or improve antigen delivery to antigen-presenting cells (APCs) (31). In addition, nanoparticles incorporating antigens can exert a local depot effect, ensuring prolonged antigen presentation to immune cells (32). Interestingly, nanoparticles have also shown intrinsic immunomodulatory activity (33). For instance, nanoparticles such as carbon nanotubes (CNTs), carbon black nanoparticles, poly(lactic-co-glycolic acid) (PLGA) and polystyrene nanoparticles, titanium dioxide ($TiO_2$) nanoparticles, silicon dioxide ($SiO_2$) nanoparticles, and aluminum oxyhydroxide nanoparticles have been reported to induce NLRP3-associated inflammasome activation (34). In fact, once internalized by APCs, these nanoparticles provide signals that trigger lysosomal destabilization and the production of reactive oxygen species (ROS), leading to the release of lysosomal contents, including the cysteine protease cathepsin B. This protease is sensed by NLRP3, which subsequently activates the formation of the inflammasome complex (35–39). Subsequently, interleukins are produced as downstream signaling events, leading to the recruitment and/or activation of immune cells (35, 40–45). Taken together, these properties advocate that nanoparticles are promising antigen carriers and immune cell activators for vaccination.

## NANOPARTICLES AND THE RESPIRATORY TRACT IMMUNE SYSTEM

The respiratory mucosa represents the primary site for invasion and infection by a virus whose replication occurs in the ciliated cells of the upper respiratory tract (URT). Subsequently, infection spreads to the low respiratory tract (LRT) by virus-rich secretions and by infected cell debris from the URT (46). Nasal-associated lymphoid tissue (NALT), the first site for inhaled antigen recognition located in the URT, is an important line of defense

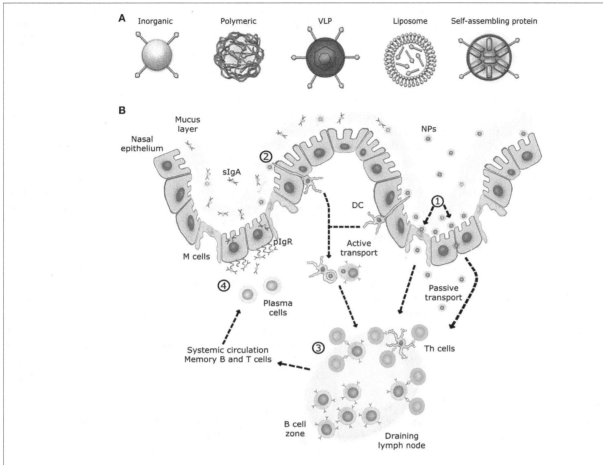

**FIGURE 1 |** Overview of the immune response in the upper respiratory tract. **(A)** Schematic view of different nanoparticles used for intranasal vaccination. **(B)** Mechanisms of NALTs immune responses in the upper respiratory tract. (1) Nanoparticles are transcytosed from the mucus layer into the nasal epithelial tissues by micro-fold cells (M cells) or passively diffuse through epithelial cell junctions. (2) Other nanoparticles are captured and internalized by DCs (dendritic cells) from their extension through epithelial junctions and by other APCs, such as B cells. (3) Cells that have encountered nanoparticles migrate to the nearest lymph node in order to activate naive T helper cells. Once activated, T helper cells activate B cells that have encountered the same antigen presented by nanoparticles. Activated B cells proliferate in the lymph node (B cell zone) and, once mature, enter systemic circulation in order to reach the inflammation site. IgA+ B cells locally differentiate into antibody-secreting plasma cells to produce IgA dimers. (4) IgA dimers are secreted via polymeric Ig receptor (pIgR) at the mucosal surface. NALT immune response induces long-lasting memory B and T cells able to trigger a rapid recall response.

against respiratory viruses. NALT is present in rodents, birds and primates (47). This structure is characterized by aggregates of lymphoid cells located in the nasopharyngeal cavity (48). In human, the Waldever's ring, made of adenoid and tonsil, is considered as the equivalent of NALT structure, which contains various narrow epithelial channels. NALT comprises aggregates of lymphoid follicles (B-cell areas), interfollicular areas (T-cell areas), macrophages and dendritic cells (DCs) (**Figure 1B**), which, when activated, support the clearance of infectious agents (46, 48, 49). Accordingly, NALT is considered as an inductive site for humoral and cellular immune responses and represents a promising target for vaccines against respiratory viruses. Ideally, nanovaccines would follow a path similar to respiratory viruses in order to efficiently deliver antigens to NALT and trigger a specific mucosal immune response. Therefore, formulation, size and antigen exposition are critical aspects when designing nanovaccines targeting NALT. Most respiratory viruses have an average diameter size ranging between 20 and 200 nm (50–53).

Thus, in addition of being safe and immunogenic on its own, a nanovaccine should have a size similar to viruses while incorporating relevant antigens (54).

Over the last decade, a number of nanoparticles have been designed to mimic respiratory viruses in terms of size, shape and surface property in order to target NALT as well as to raise humoral and cellular immune responses (21, 55, 56). First, beside a nanoparticle size of 20–200 nm in diameter to match the size of most respiratory viruses, nanoparticles should be preferably positively charged. In fact, positively charged polymeric, phospholipidic, metallic, inorganic, and protein-based nanoparticles have shown stronger immune responses compared to their negatively charged counterparts (21, 57). Second, the incorporation of antigens/epitopes within or on the surface of the nanoparticles can be challenging and requires advanced approaches in chemical and/or biological engineering (21). The most common strategy is to encapsulate or entrap antigens/epitopes within the nanoparticles. In this case, nanoparticles are used to protect the antigen/epitopes and deliver them to NALT (58–60). Nanoencapsulation can be achieved by using different procedures, including nanoprecipitation and oil in water (o/w) emulsion (61). Alternatively, antigens can be attached and exposed on the nanoparticle surface. This strategy aims at mimicking viruses. Conjugation of antigenic epitope can be performed directly on the nanoparticles using different chemical reactions like the disulfide bond and the thiolate-gold bond formation (62–64). Otherwise, it can be achieved by first preparing an epitope-functionalized self-assembling unit, which upon self-assembly form nanoparticles decorated with the antigen (65–67). Third, the formulation and administration strategies are also critical aspects to consider. Vaccines administered via subcutaneous or intramuscular injection induce systemic immunity and usually, a weak mucosal response is observed. On the other hand, mucosal vaccination, either oral or intranasal delivery, induces humoral, and cellular immune responses at the systemic level and the mucosal surfaces, which is more effective in the protection against respiratory viruses (68, 69). Studies have demonstrated that vaccination via the intranasal route provides a better protection when compared to subcutaneous immunization in the context of respiratory pathogens and mucosal immunity. Intranasal vaccination led to higher antigen-specific lymphocyte proliferation, cytokine production (interferon-γ, interleukins) and induction of antigen-specific IgA antibody (70–74). A promising formulation strategy is the intranasal spray, which delivers conveniently and safely the nanovaccines directly to the respiratory mucosa (75–77). However, the number of clinical trials using nanovaccine formulations for intranasal delivery, including spray dried nanovaccines, is limited. This is mostly associated with the difficulty of keeping the nanovaccine integrity during the entire formulation process (76). Moreover, the immune response is particularly sensitive to the nature, size, shape, and surface properties of the nanoparticles as well as to the density and the potency of the antigens. Thus, it is very challenging to predict the effect of a given nanovaccine on the immune system. In addition, nanoparticles have some limitations associated with their synthesis, or preparation, and their properties. These include limited antigen loading, low synthesis yield, poor targeting capability to immune cells, limited manufacturability, and, in some cases, toxicity (78–80). These drawbacks can lead to side effects and/or poor immunogenicity, which precludes their clinical usage. Besides, little is known about the interactions between nanoparticles and immune cells. In fact, their adjuvant effect and their ability to activate the immune system still remain unclear and need to be better understood at the molecular level (81). Nonetheless, nanoparticle formulations have recently revealed promising results against respiratory virus infections (**Table 1**) and relevant examples will now be discussed.

## POLYMERIC NANOPARTICLES

A polymer consists of a large molecule constructed from monomeric units. Depending on the construction, polymers can be linear, slightly branched or hyperbranched (3D network)

(104). Polymeric nanoparticles can be either obtained from the polymerization of monomeric units or from preformed polymers. These nanoparticles are attractive in the medical field due to their adjustable properties (size, composition, and surface properties), which allow controlled release, ability to combine both therapy and imaging (theranostics), and protection of drug molecules (105–107). For example, poly(lactic-co-glycolic acid) (PLGA) is a biodegradable and biocompatible polymer approved by the Food and Drug Administration (FDA) and European Medicines Agency (EMA) for use in humans. This is due to its ability to undergo hydrolysis *in vivo*, resulting in lactic acid and glycolic acid metabolites, which are efficiently processed by the body (108). PLGA can be engineered to form nanoparticles capable of encapsulating different types of biomolecules and release them sustainably over time (108–111). These nanoparticles can encapsulate antigens and prevent their degradation over 4 weeks under physiological conditions, which is critical for mucosal vaccination (112). Moreover, PLGA-NPs promote antigen internalization by APCs and facilitate antigen processing and presentation to naïve lymphocytes (113, 114). For instance, spherical PLGA-NPs (200–300 nm of diameter) were used to encapsulate an inactivated Swine influenza virus (SwIV) H1N2 antigens (KAg) via water/oil/water double emulsion solvent evaporation (83). It was observed that pigs vaccinated twice with this preparation and challenged with a virulent heterologous influenza virus strain, have a significantly milder disease in comparison to non-vaccinated animals. This observation correlated closely with the reduced lung pathology and the substantial clearance of the virus from the animal lungs. Other polymeric nanoparticles, such as chitosan, a natural polymer composed of randomly distributed β-(1–4)-linked d-glucosamine and N-acetyl-d-glucosamine, and N-(2-hydroxypropyl)methacrylamide/N-isopropylacrylamide (HPMA/NIPAM), were also investigated as intranasal vaccines against respiratory viruses (85–90, 115–121). Overall, polymeric nanoparticles have many advantages, including biocompatibility (122), antigen encapsulation and stabilization (123, 124), controlled release of antigens and intracellular persistence in APCs (125, 126), pathogen-like characteristics, and suitability for intranasal administration (126, 127). Nevertheless, the effect of the polymer properties (core chemistry, size, shape, surface properties) on the transport within the URT remains unknown. More studies are needed to better understand the effect of changing nanoparticle properties on their biological activities and to, ultimately, predict the fate of these nanocarriers upon their intranasal administration.

## SELF-ASSEMBLING PROTEIN NANOPARTICLES AND VLPs

Self-assembling protein nanoparticles (SAPNs) are structures obtained from the oligomerization of monomeric proteins. The protein building blocks are mostly obtained through recombinant technologies and are considered safe for biomedical applications (128). SAPNs can be engineered to have a diameter ranging from 20 to 100 nm, similar to the sizes of many

**TABLE 1 |** Nanoparticle-based vaccines against respiratory viruses delivered via the intranasal route.

| Material | Size (nm) | Virus | Antigen/Epitope | Adjuvant | References |
|---|---|---|---|---|---|
| **POLYMERIC NANOPARTICLES** | | | | | |
| PLGA | 225.4 | Bovine parainfluenza 3 virus (BPI3V) | BPI3V proteins | – | (82) |
| | 200–300 | Swine influenza virus (H1N2) | Inactivated virus H1N2 antigen | – | (83) |
| γ-PGA[a] | 100–200 | Influenza (H1N1) | Hemagglutinin | – | (84) |
| Chitosan | 140 | Influenza (H1N1) | H1N1 antigen | – | (85) |
| | 300–350 | Influenza (H1N1) | HA-Split | – | (86) |
| | 571.7 | Swine influenza virus (H1N2) | Killed swine influenza antigen | – | (87) |
| | 200–250 | Influenza (H1N1) | M2e | Heat shock protein 70c | (88) |
| HPMA/NIPAM | 12–25 | RSV | F protein | TLR-7/8 agonist | (89, 90) |
| Polyanhydride | 200–800 | RSV | F and G glycoproteins | – | (91, 92) |
| **SELF-ASSEMBLING PROTEINS AND PEPTIDE-BASED NANOPARTICLES** | | | | | |
| N nucleocapside protein of RSV | 15 | RSV | RSV phosphoprotein | R192G | (93) |
| | 15 | RSV | FsII | Montanide™ Gel 01 | (94) |
| | 15 | Influenza (H1N1) | M2e | Montanide™ Gel 01 | (95) |
| Ferritin | 12.5 | Influenza (H1N1) | M2e | – | (96) |
| Q11 | – | Influenza (H1N1) | Acid polymerase | – | (97) |
| **INORGANIC NANOPARTICLES** | | | | | |
| Gold | 12 | Influenza | M2e | CpG | (64) |
| **OTHERS** | | | | | |
| VLP | 80–120 | Influenza (H1N1) | Hemagglutinin | – | (98) |
| | 80–120 | Influenza (H1N1, H3N2, H5N1) | M2e | – | (99) |
| | 80–120 | RSV | F protein et G glycoprotein of RSV and M1 protein of Influenza | – | (100) |
| ISCOM[b] | 40 | Influenza (H1N1) | Hemagglutinin | ISCOMATRIX | (101, 102) |
| DLPC liposomes[c] | 30–100 | Influenza (H1N1) | M2, HA, NP | MPL and trehalose 6,6′ dimycolate | (103) |

[a]Poly-γ-glutamic acid.
[b]Quillaia saponin, cholesterol, phospholipid, and associated antigen.
[c]Dilauroylphosphatidylcholine.

viruses and therefore, are considered as nanovaccine candidates against viruses, including respiratory viruses (128, 129). For example, SANPs, designed to elicit an immune response against RSV, have been explored using the nucleoprotein (N) from the virus nucleocapsid. The N protein is a major target of antigen-specific cytotoxic T-cell response. The self-assembly of N protein protomers led to the formation of supramolecular nanorings of 15 nm diameter (93). This platform was modified by fusing the FsII epitope targeted by monoclonal neutralizing antibody (palivizumab) to the N-protein, in order to form chimeric nanorings with enhanced immune response and virus protection against RSV. The results showed reduced virus load in the lungs of challenged mice (94). Similarly, chimeric nanorings displaying 3 repeats of the highly conserved ectodomain of the influenza virus A matrix protein 2 (M2e), were prepared by recombinant technologies (95). When administrated via the intranasal route, these M2e-functionalized nanorings induced local production of mucosal antibodies and led to mice protection (95). These N-nanorings are interesting for intranasal delivery of antigen due to their similarities with respiratory viruses in term of size and structure (sub-nucleocapsid-like superstructures). Other examples of

SAPNs as potential nanovaccines against respiratory viruses include the capsid protein of the papaya mosaic virus (PapMV), the purified coronavirus spike protein and ferritin, which are self-assembling proteins that form rod-shaped and nearly spherical nanostructures, respectively (96, 130–140). Recently, assemblies composed of four tandem copies of M2e and headless HA proteins were prepared and stabilized by sulfosuccinimidyl propionate crosslinking, showing the possibility of generating protein nanoparticles almost entirely composed of the antigens of interest (141).

VLPs are spherical supramolecular assemblies of 20–200 nm diameter, which result from the self-assembly of viral capsid proteins. These particles are free from genetic materials and have the advantage of mimicking perfectly the structure and the antigenic epitopes of their corresponding native viruses. Therefore, this repetitive antigen display promotes efficient phagocytosis by APCs and subsequent activation (142–146). Recently, Lee and colleagues demonstrated that intranasal delivery of influenza-derived VLPs expressed in insect cells and exposing 5 repeats of the M2e epitopes, confers cross protection against different serotypes of influenza viruses by inducing humoral and cellular immune responses (99).

SAPNs and VLPs are thus attractive but their formulation into stable and spray dried vaccines for intranasal injection can be challenging and may require the use of surfactants and saccharides (147). In the last decades, self-assembling peptides (SAPs) have also been investigated as intranasal nanovaccines against respiratory viruses due to their straightforward chemical synthesis and their storage stability upon lyophilization (97).

## INORGANIC NANOPARTICLES

There are many inorganic nanoparticles suitable for biomedical applications, including superparamagnetic nanoparticles (iron oxide nanoparticles), quantum dots and plasmonic nanoparticles (gold and silver nanoparticles). Inorganic materials are mostly used as tools with improved therapeutic efficacy, biodistribution and pharmacokinetics. However, inherently, plain inorganic core nanoparticles would not be suitable in biological fluids due to particle aggregation. Therefore, in the medical field, these nanoparticles are often coated with organic molecules via adsorption or chemical reactions. In fact, these biocompatible nanoparticles can be described as complex hybrids materials with an inorganic core and an organic outer shell (148, 149). Among inorganic nanoparticles, the most commonly used for vaccination are gold nanoparticles (AuNPs). AuNPs are readily internalized by macrophages and dendritic cells, and induce their activation (150, 151). Large scale production is possible with strict control on particle size and ease of functionalization using the strong affinity between thiol groups and gold. Thiol groups can be attached to AuNP surface by forming thiolate–Au bonds (152–155). Furthermore, no immune response is elicited toward inert carriers like AuNPs (156). Thus, these nanoparticles are an appealing platform for nanovaccine engineering *via* antigen functionalization.

A wide range of molecules, including adjuvants and antigens can be conjugated on AuNPs at high density, resulting in improved immunogenicity and antigen presentation (157, 158). AuNPs can be formulated for intranasal administration and can diffuse into the lymph nodes, triggering robust antigen-specific cytotoxic T-cell immune responses (159, 160). Tao and coworkers have demonstrated that the peptide consensus M2e of influenza A viruses with a non-native cysteine residue at the C-terminal end could be attached on the AuNPs via thiolate–Au chemistry. The resulting M2e-AuNPs was administered by the intranasal route to mice with CpG (cytosine-guanine rich oligonucleotide) adjuvant, triggering a fully protective immune response against the influenza virus PR8 strain (161). More recently, it was demonstrated that this formulation could induce lung B cell activation and robust serum anti-M2e IgG response, with stimulation of both IgG1 and IgG2a

subclasses (161). Additionally, this vaccination strategy led to protection against infection by the pandemic influenza virus strain, A/California/04/2009 (H1N1pdm) pandemic strain, influenza virus A/Victoria/3/75 (H3N2) strain and the highly pathogenic avian influenza virus A/Vietnam/1203/2004 (H5N1) (64). Although gold nanoparticles constitute an attractive platform for antigen conjugation, they can accumulate in organs such as liver and spleen for a long period, which could be ultimately associated with toxicity (162). Coating with biocompatible materials reduces their toxicity, although it can lead to alterations of the physicochemical and biological properties. Therefore, safety issues of AuNPs still need to be addressed.

## CONCLUSION AND PERSPECTIVES

Engineered nanoparticles have demonstrated their potential as vaccine delivery platforms. They can be envisaged as both antigen nanocarriers and adjuvants. In all cases, intranasal administration of nanovaccines allows a convenient and safe delivery of the antigen to NALT, inducing mucosal and systemic immunity. Nonetheless, additional studies are still needed before their clinical translation. While intranasal vaccination of nanoparticles generates specific IgA antibody in the URT and leads to high survival rates in animal models, there are still limited studies on non-human primates, thus making nanoparticle's fate difficult to predict in a human URT. In addition, nanoparticle vaccines are generally functionalized with specific antigen(s), which result in an immune response targeted against these antigenic determinants. Considering antigenic drifts, the growing human population that needs to be vaccinated and the different type of viruses, the cost to address all these aspects would be too prohibitive to produce affordable vaccines. Consequently, the development of broad spectrum vaccines constitutes a critical need and we consider that nanovaccine engineering will contribute to achieve this objective.

## AUTHOR CONTRIBUTIONS

SA-H, LG, DoA, SB, and DeA have participated in writing and preparation of the manuscript, and approved it for publication.

## FUNDING

This work was supported by grants from the Natural Sciences and Engineering Research Council of Canada (NSERC; RGPIN-2016-06532 and RGPIN-2018-06209) and the International Development Research Center (IDRC; 108517) to DeA and SB.

## REFERENCES

1. World Health Organization. *Top 10 Global Causes of Deaths*. Geneva: World Health Organization (2016).
2. Seo YB, Song JY, Choi MJ, Kim IS, Yang TU, Hong KW, et al. Etiology and clinical outcomes of acute respiratory virus infection in

hospitalized adults. *Infect Chemother*. (2014) 46:67–76. doi: 10.3947/ic.2014.46.2.67
3. Kutter JS, Spronken MI, Fraaij PL, Fouchier RA, Herfst S. Transmission routes of respiratory viruses among humans. *Curr Opin Virol*. (2018) 28:142–51. doi: 10.1016/j.coviro.2018.01.001

4.  Griffin D. Economic impact associated with respiratory disease in beef cattle. *Vet Clin North Am Food Anim Pract.* (1997) 13:367–77. doi: 10.1016/S0749-0720(15)30302-9

5.  Taylor JD, Fulton RW, Lehenbauer TW, Step DL, Confer AW. The epidemiology of bovine respiratory disease: what is the evidence for predisposing factors? *Can Veterinary J.* (2010) 51:1095–102.

6.  Johnson KK, Pendell DL. Market impacts of reducing the prevalence of bovine respiratory disease in united states beef cattle feedlots. *Front Vet Sci.* (2017) 4:189. doi: 10.3389/fvets.2017.00189

7.  Walker TA, Khurana S, Tilden SJ. Viral respiratory infections. *Pediatr Clin North Am.* (1994) 41:1365–81. doi: 10.1016/S0031-3955(16)38876-9

8.  Pavia AT. Viral infections of the lower respiratory tract: old viruses, new viruses, and the role of diagnosis. *Clin Infect Dis.* (2011) 52 (Suppl. 4):S284–9. doi: 10.1093/cid/cir043

9.  World Health Organization. *Influenza (Seasonal).* World Health Organization (2018).

10. Branche AR, Falsey AR. Parainfluenza virus infection. *Semin Respir Crit Care Med.* (2016) 37:538–54. doi: 10.1055/s-0036-1584798

11. Mazur NI, Higgins D, Nunes MC, Melero JA, Langedijk AC, Horsley N, et al. The respiratory syncytial virus vaccine landscape: lessons from the graveyard and promising candidates. *Lancet Infect Dis.* (2018) 18:e295–e311. doi: 10.1016/S1473-3099(18)30292-5

12. Lu MP, Ma LY, Zheng Q, Dong LL, Chen ZM. Clinical characteristics of adenovirus associated lower respiratory tract infection in children. *World J Pediatr.* (2013) 9:346–9. doi: 10.1007/s12519-013-0431-3

13. Collaborators GL. Estimates of the global, regional, and national morbidity, mortality, and aetiologies of lower respiratory tract infections in 195 countries: a systematic analysis for the Global burden of disease study 2015. *Lancet Infect Dis.* (2017) 17:1133–61. doi: 10.1016/S1473-3099(17)30396-1

14. Fenner F, Henderson DA, Arita I, Jezek Z, Ladnyi ID. *Smallpox and its Eradication.* Geneva: World Health Organization (1988).

15. Hajj Hussein I, Chams N, Chams S, El Sayegh S, Badran R, Raad M, et al. Vaccines through centuries: major cornerstones of global health. *Front Public Health* (2015) 3:269. doi: 10.3389/fpubh.2015.00269

16. Daubeney P, Taylor CJ, Mcgaw J, Brown EM, Ghosal S, Keeton BR, et al. Immunogenicity and tolerability of a trivalent influenza subunit vaccine (Influvac) in high-risk children aged 6 months to 4 years. *Br J Clin Pract.* (1997) 51:87–90.

17. Delore V, Salamand C, Marsh G, Arnoux S, Pepin S, Saliou P. Long-term clinical trial safety experience with the inactivated split influenza vaccine, Vaxigrip. *Vaccine* (2006) 24:1586–92. doi: 10.1016/j.vaccine.2005.10.008

18. Grohskopf LA, Sokolow LZ, Olsen SJ, Bresee JS, Broder KR, Karron RA. Prevention and control of influenza with vaccines: recommendations of the advisory committee on immunization practices, United States, 2015-16 influenza season. *Morb Mortal Wkly Rep.* (2015) 64:818–25. doi: 10.15585/mmwr.mm6430a3

19. Carter NJ, Curran MP. Live attenuated influenza vaccine (FluMist(R); Fluenz): a review of its use in the prevention of seasonal influenza in children and adults. *Drugs* (2011) 71:1591–622. doi: 10.2165/11206860-000000000-00000

20. Dhere R, Yeolekar L, Kulkarni P, Menon R, Vaidya V, Ganguly M, et al. A pandemic influenza vaccine in India: from strain to sale within 12 months. *Vaccine* (2011) 29 (Suppl. 1):A16–21. doi: 10.1016/j.vaccine.2011.04.119

21. Chattopadhyay S, Chen JY, Chen HW, Hu CJ. Nanoparticle vaccines adopting virus-like features for enhanced immune potentiation. *Nanotheranostics* (2017) 1:244–60. doi: 10.7150/ntno.19796

22. Vartak A, Sucheck SJ. Recent advances in subunit vaccine carriers. *Vaccines* (2016) 4:12. doi: 10.3390/vaccines4020012

23. Papadopoulos NG, Megremis S, Kitsioulis NA, Vangelatou O, West P, Xepapadaki P. Promising approaches for the treatment and prevention of viral respiratory illnesses. *J Allergy Clin Immunol.* (2017) 140:921–32. doi: 10.1016/j.jaci.2017.07.001

24. Boni MF. Vaccination and antigenic drift in influenza. *Vaccine* (2008) 26 (Suppl. 3):C8–14. doi: 10.1016/j.vaccine.2008.04.011

25. Laval JM, Mazeran PE, Thomas D. Nanobiotechnology and its role in the development of new analytical devices. *Analyst* (2000) 125:29–33. doi: 10.1039/a907827d

26. Parveen K, Banse V, Ledwani L. Green synthesis of nanoparticles: their advantages and disadvantages. In: *5th National Conference on Thermophysical Properties: (Nctp-09).* Rajasthan (2016). p. 1249.

27. Schneider CS, Xu Q, Boylan NJ, Chisholm J, Tang BC, Schuster BS, et al. Nanoparticles that do not adhere to mucus provide uniform and long-lasting drug delivery to airways following inhalation. *Sci Adv.* (2017) 3:e1601556. doi: 10.1126/sciadv.1601556

28. Angioletti-Uberti S. Theory, simulations and the design of functionalized nanoparticles for biomedical applications: a soft matter perspective. *NPJ Comput Mater.* (2017) 3:48. doi: 10.1038/s41524-017-0050-y

29. Irvine DJ, Hanson MC, Rakhra K, Tokatlian T. Synthetic nanoparticles for vaccines and immunotherapy. *Chem Rev.* (2015) 115:11109–46. doi: 10.1021/acs.chemrev.5b00109

30. Szeto GL, Lavik EB. Materials design at the interface of nanoparticles and innate immunity. *J Mater Chem B* (2016) 4:1610–8. doi: 10.1039/C5TB01825K

31. Pachioni-Vasconcelos Jde A, Lopes AM, Apolinario AC, Valenzuela-Oses JK, Costa JS, Nascimento Lde O, et al. Nanostructures for protein drug delivery. *Biomater Sci.* (2016) 4:205–18. doi: 10.1039/C5BM00360A

32. Fredriksen BN, Grip J. PLGA/PLA micro- and nanoparticle formulations serve as antigen depots and induce elevated humoral responses after immunization of Atlantic salmon (*Salmo salar* L.). *Vaccine* (2012) 30:656–67. doi: 10.1016/j.vaccine.2011.10.105

33. Mamo T, Poland GA. Nanovaccinology: the next generation of vaccines meets 21st century materials science and engineering. *Vaccine* (2012) 30:6609–11. doi: 10.1016/j.vaccine.2012.08.023

34. Zhu M, Wang R, Nie G. Applications of nanomaterials as vaccine adjuvants. *Hum Vaccin Immunother.* (2014) 10:2761–74. doi: 10.4161/hv.29589

35. Ghiringhelli F, Apetoh L, Tesniere A, Aymeric L, Ma Y, Ortiz C, et al. Activation of the NLRP3 inflammasome in dendritic cells induces IL-1β-dependent adaptive immunity against tumors. *Nat Med.* (2009) 15:1170. doi: 10.1038/nm.2028

36. Tschopp J, Schroder K. NLRP3 inflammasome activation: the convergence of multiple signalling pathways on ROS production? *Nat Rev Immunol.* (2010) 10:210. doi: 10.1038/nri2725

37. Bruchard M, Mignot G, Derangère V, Chalmin F, Chevriaux A, Végran F, et al. Chemotherapy-triggered cathepsin B release in myeloid-derived suppressor cells activates the Nlrp3 inflammasome and promotes tumor growth. *Nat Med.* (2012) 19:57. doi: 10.1038/nm.2999

38. Abderrazak A, Syrovets T, Couchie D, El Hadri K, Friguet B, Simmet T, et al. NLRP3 inflammasome: from a danger signal sensor to a regulatory node of oxidative stress and inflammatory diseases. *Redox Biol.* (2015) 4:296–307. doi: 10.1016/j.redox.2015.01.008

39. He Y, Hara H, Núñez G. Mechanism and regulation of NLRP3 inflammasome activation. *Trends Biochem Sci.* (2016) 41:1012–21. doi: 10.1016/j.tibs.2016.09.002

40. Cassel SL, Eisenbarth SC, Iyer SS, Sadler JJ, Colegio OR, Tephly LA, et al. The Nalp3 inflammasome is essential for the development of silicosis. *Proc Natl Acad Sci USA* (2008) 105:9035. doi: 10.1073/pnas.0803933105

41. Halle A, Hornung V, Petzold GC, Stewart CR, Monks BG, Reinheckel T, et al. The NALP3 inflammasome is involved in the innate immune response to amyloid-β. *Nat Immunol.* (2008) 9:857. doi: 10.1038/ni.1636

42. Sharp FA, Ruane D, Claass B, Creagh E, Harris J, Malyala P, et al. Uptake of particulate vaccine adjuvants by dendritic cells activates the NALP3 inflammasome. *Proc Natl Acad Sci USA.* (2009) 106:870–5. doi: 10.1073/pnas.0804897106

43. Masters SL, Dunne A, Subramanian SL, Hull RL, Tannahill GM, Sharp FA, et al. Activation of the NLRP3 inflammasome by islet amyloid polypeptide provides a mechanism for enhanced IL-1β in type 2 diabetes. *Nat Immunol.* (2010) 11:897. doi: 10.1038/ni.1935

44. Niemi K, Teirila L, Lappalainen J, Rajamaki K, Baumann MH, Oorni K, et al. Serum amyloid A activates the NLRP3 inflammasome via P2X7 receptor and a cathepsin B-sensitive pathway. *J Immunol.* (2011) 186:6119–28. doi: 10.4049/jimmunol.1002843

45. Scharf B, Clement CC, Wu XX, Morozova K, Zanolini D, Follenzi A, et al. Annexin A2 binds to endosomes following organelle destabilization by particulate wear debris. *Nat Commun.* (2012) 3:755. doi: 10.1038/ncomms1754

46. Adair BM. Nanoparticle vaccines against respiratory viruses. *Wiley Interdiscip Rev Nanomed Nanobiotechnol.* (2009) 1:405–14. doi: 10.1002/wnan.45

47. Kang H, Yan M, Yu Q, Yang Q. Characteristics of nasal-associated lymphoid tissue (NALT) and nasal absorption capacity in chicken. *PLoS ONE* (2014) 8:e84097. doi: 10.1371/journal.pone.0084097

48. Marasini N, Skwarczynski M, Toth I. Intranasal delivery of nanoparticle-based vaccines. *Ther Deliv.* (2017) 8:151–67. doi: 10.4155/tde-2016-0068

49. Zuercher AW, Coffin SE, Thurnheer MC, Fundova P, Cebra JJ. Nasal-associated lymphoid tissue is a mucosal inductive site for virus-specific humoral and cellular immune responses. *J Immunol.* (2002) 168:1796. doi: 10.4049/jimmunol.168.4.1796

50. Lamb RA, Choppin PW. The gene structure and replication of influenza virus. *Annu Rev Biochem.* (1983) 52:467–506. doi: 10.1146/annurev.bi.52.070183.002343

51. Henrickson KJ. Parainfluenza viruses. *Clin Microbiol Rev.* (2003) 16:242–64. doi: 10.1128/CMR.16.2.242-264.2003

52. Utley TJ, Ducharme NA, Varthakavi V, Shepherd BE, Santangelo PJ, Lindquist ME, et al. Respiratory syncytial virus uses a Vps4-independent budding mechanism controlled by Rab11-FIP2. *Proc Natl Acad Sci USA.* (2008) 105:10209–14. doi: 10.1073/pnas.0712144105

53. Hall K, Blair Zajdel ME, Blair GE. Unity and diversity in the human adenoviruses: exploiting alternative entry pathways for gene therapy. *Biochem J.* (2010) 431:321–36. doi: 10.1042/BJ20100766

54. Gomes AC, Mohsen M, Bachmann MF. Harnessing nanoparticles for immunomodulation and vaccines. *Vaccines* (2017) 5:E6. doi: 10.3390/vaccines5010006

55. Niu Y, Yu M, Hartono SB, Yang J, Xu H, Zhang H, et al. Nanoparticles mimicking viral surface topography for enhanced cellular delivery. *Adv Mater.* (2013) 25:6233–7. doi: 10.1002/adma.201302737

56. Fogarty JA, Swartz JR. The exciting potential of modular nanoparticles for rapid development of highly effective vaccines. *Curr Opin Chem Eng.* (2018) 19:1–8. doi: 10.1016/j.coche.2017.11.001

57. Fromen CA, Robbins GR, Shen TW, Kai MP, Ting JP, Desimone JM. Controlled analysis of nanoparticle charge on mucosal and systemic antibody responses following pulmonary immunization. *Proc Natl Acad Sci USA.* (2015) 112:488–93. doi: 10.1073/pnas.1422923112

58. Rahimian S, Kleinovink JW, Fransen MF, Mezzanotte L, Gold H, Wisse P, et al. Near-infrared labeled, ovalbumin loaded polymeric nanoparticles based on a hydrophilic polyester as model vaccine: *In vivo* tracking and evaluation of antigen-specific CD8(+) T cell immune response. *Biomaterials* (2015) 37:469–77. doi: 10.1016/j.biomaterials.2014.10.043

59. Kasturi SP, Kozlowski PA, Nakaya HI, Burger MC, Russo P, Pham M, et al. Adjuvanting a simian immunodeficiency virus vaccine with toll-like receptor ligands encapsulated in nanoparticles induces persistent antibody responses and enhanced protection in TRIM5alpha restrictive macaques. *J Virol.* (2017) 91:e01844–16. doi: 10.1128/JVI.01844-16

60. Kishimoto TK, Maldonado RA. Nanoparticles for the Induction of Antigen-Specific Immunological Tolerance. *Front Immunol.* (2018) 9:230. doi: 10.3389/fimmu.2018.00230

61. Kumari A, Singla R, Guliani A, Yadav SK. Nanoencapsulation for drug delivery. *EXCLI J.* (2014) 13:265–86.

62. Hirosue S, Kourtis IC, Van Der Vlies AJ, Hubbell JA, Swartz MA. Antigen delivery to dendritic cells by poly(propylene sulfide) nanoparticles with disulfide conjugated peptides: Cross-presentation and T cell activation. *Vaccine* (2010) 28:7897–906. doi: 10.1016/j.vaccine.2010.09.077

63. Ding P, Zhang T, Li Y, Teng M, Sun Y, Liu X, et al. Nanoparticle orientationally displayed antigen epitopes improve neutralizing antibody level in a model of porcine circovirus type 2. *Int J Nanomed.* (2017) 12:5239–54. doi: 10.2147/IJN.S140789

64. Tao W, Hurst BL, Shakya AK, Uddin MJ, Ingrole RS, Hernandez-Sanabria M, et al. Consensus M2e peptide conjugated to gold nanoparticles confers protection against H1N1, H3N2 and H5N1 influenza A viruses. *Antiviral Res.* (2017) 141:62–72. doi: 10.1016/j.antiviral.2017.01.021

65. Mora-Solano C, Wen Y, Han H, Chen J, Chong AS, Miller ML, et al. Active immunotherapy for TNF-mediated inflammation using self-assembled peptide nanofibers. *Biomaterials* (2017) 149:1–11. doi: 10.1016/j.biomaterials.2017.09.031

66. Negahdaripour M, Golkar N, Hajighahramani N, Kianpour S, Nezafat N, Ghasemi Y. Harnessing self-assembled peptide nanoparticles in epitope vaccine design. *Biotechnol Adv.* (2017) 35:575–96. doi: 10.1016/j.biotechadv.2017.05.002

67. Babych M, Bertheau-Mailhot G, Zottig X, Dion J, Gauthier L, Archambault D, et al. Engineering and evaluation of amyloid assemblies as a nanovaccine against the Chikungunya virus. *Nanoscale* (2018) 10:19547–56. doi: 10.1039/C8NR05948A

68. Ichinohe T, Ainai A, Tashiro M, Sata T, Hasegawa H. PolyI:polyC12U adjuvant-combined intranasal vaccine protects mice against highly pathogenic H5N1 influenza virus variants. *Vaccine* (2009) 27:6276–9. doi: 10.1016/j.vaccine.2009.04.074

69. Lycke N. Recent progress in mucosal vaccine development: potential and limitations. *Nat Rev Immunol.* (2012) 12:592–605. doi: 10.1038/nri3251

70. Chen L, Wang J, Zganiacz A, Xing Z. Single intranasal mucosal Mycobacterium bovis BCG vaccination confers improved protection compared to subcutaneous vaccination against pulmonary tuberculosis. *Infect Immun.* (2004) 72:238–46. doi: 10.1128/IAI.72.1.238-246.2004

71. Giri PK, Sable SB, Verma I, Khuller GK. Comparative evaluation of intranasal and subcutaneous route of immunization for development of mucosal vaccine against experimental tuberculosis. *FEMS Immunol Med Microbiol.* (2005) 45:87–93. doi: 10.1016/j.femsim.2005.02.009

72. Mapletoft JW, Latimer L, Babiuk LA, Van Drunen Littel-Van Den Hurk S. Intranasal immunization of mice with a bovine respiratory syncytial virus vaccine induces superior immunity and protection compared to those by subcutaneous delivery or combinations of intranasal and subcutaneous prime-boost strategies. *Clin Vaccine Immunol.* (2010) 17:23. doi: 10.1128/CVI.00250-09

73. Kharb S, Charan S. Mucosal immunization provides better protection than subcutaneous immunization against Pasteurella multocida (B:2) in mice preimmunized with the outer membrane proteins. *Vet Res Commun.* (2011) 35:457–61. doi: 10.1007/s11259-011-9484-8

74. Mccormick AA, Shakeel A, Yi C, Kaur H, Mansour AM, Bakshi CS. Intranasal administration of a two-dose adjuvanted multi-antigen TMV-subunit conjugate vaccine fully protects mice against Francisella tularensis LVS challenge. *PLoS ONE* (2018) 13:e0194614. doi: 10.1371/journal.pone.0194614

75. Birkhoff M, Leitz M, Marx D. Advantages of intranasal vaccination and considerations on device selection. *Indian J Pharmaceut Sci.* (2009) 71:729–31.

76. Kanojia G, Have RT, Soema PC, Frijlink H, Amorij JP, Kersten G. Developments in the formulation and delivery of spray dried vaccines. *Hum Vaccin Immunother.* (2017) 13:2364–78. doi: 10.1080/21645515.2017.1356952

77. Kim SH, Jang YS. The development of mucosal vaccines for both mucosal and systemic immune induction and the roles played by adjuvants. *Clin Exp Vaccine Res.* (2017) 6:15–21. doi: 10.7774/cevr.2017.6.1.15

78. Shao K, Singha S, Clemente-Casares X, Tsai S, Yang Y, Santamaria P. Nanoparticle-based immunotherapy for cancer. *ACS Nano.* (2015) 9:16–30. doi: 10.1021/nn5062029

79. Zilker C, Kozlova D, Sokolova V, Yan H, Epple M, Überla K, et al. Nanoparticle-based B-cell targeting vaccines: tailoring of humoral immune responses by functionalization with different TLR-ligands. *Nanomedicine* (2017) 13:173–82. doi: 10.1016/j.nano.2016.08.028

80. Pan J, Wang Y, Zhang C, Wang X, Wang H, Wang J, et al. Antigen-directed fabrication of a multifunctional nanovaccine with ultrahigh antigen loading efficiency for tumor photothermal-immunotherapy. *Adv Mater.* (2018) 30:1704408. doi: 10.1002/adma.2017 04408

81. Sahdev P, Ochyl LJ, Moon JJ. Biomaterials for nanoparticle vaccine delivery systems. *Pharmaceut Res.* (2014) 31:2563–82. doi: 10.1007/s11095-014-1419-y

82. Mansoor F, Earley B, Cassidy JP, Markey B, Doherty S, Welsh MD. Comparing the immune response to a novel intranasal nanoparticle PLGA vaccine and a commercial BPI3V vaccine in dairy calves. *BMC Vet Res.* (2015) 11:220. doi: 10.1186/s12917-015-0481-y

83. Dhakal S, Hiremath J, Bondra K, Lakshmanappa YS, Shyu DL, Ouyang K, et al. Biodegradable nanoparticle delivery of inactivated swine influenza

virus vaccine provides heterologous cell-mediated immune response in pigs. *J Control Release* (2017) 247:194–205. doi: 10.1016/j.jconrel.2016.12.039

84. Okamoto S, Matsuura M, Akagi T, Akashi M, Tanimoto T, Ishikawa T, et al. Poly(gamma-glutamic acid) nano-particles combined with mucosal influenza virus hemagglutinin vaccine protects against influenza virus infection in mice. *Vaccine* (2009) 27:5896–905. doi: 10.1016/j.vaccine.2009.07.037

85. Liu Q, Zheng X, Zhang C, Shao X, Zhang X, Zhang Q, et al. Conjugating influenza a (H1N1) antigen to n-trimethylaminoethylmethacrylate chitosan nanoparticles improves the immunogenicity of the antigen after nasal administration. *J Med Virol.* (2015) 87:1807–15. doi: 10.1002/jmv.24253

86. Sawaengsak C, Mori Y, Yamanishi K, Mitrevej A, Sinchaipanid N. Chitosan nanoparticle encapsulated hemagglutinin-split influenza virus mucosal vaccine. *AAPS PharmSciTech.* (2014) 15:317–25. doi: 10.1208/s12249-013-0058-7

87. Dhakal S, Renu S, Ghimire S, Shaan Lakshmanappa Y, Hogshead BT, Feliciano-Ruiz N, et al. Mucosal immunity and protective efficacy of intranasal inactivated influenza vaccine is improved by chitosan nanoparticle delivery in pigs. *Front Immunol.* (2018) 9:934. doi: 10.3389/fimmu.2018.00934

88. Dabaghian M, Latifi AM, Tebianian M, Najminejad H, Ebrahimi SM. Nasal vaccination with r4M2e.HSP70c antigen encapsulated into N-trimethyl chitosan (TMC) nanoparticulate systems: preparation and immunogenicity in a mouse model. *Vaccine* (2018) 36:2886–95. doi: 10.1016/j.vaccine.2018.02.072

89. Lynn GM, Laga R, Darrah PA, Ishizuka AS, Balaci AJ, Dulcey AE, et al. *In vivo* characterization of the physicochemical properties of polymer-linked TLR agonists that enhance vaccine immunogenicity. *Nat Biotechnol.* (2015) 33:1201. doi: 10.1038/nbt.3371

90. Francica JR, Lynn GM, Laga R, Joyce MG, Ruckwardt TJ, Morabito KM, et al. Thermoresponsive polymer nanoparticles Co-deliver RSV F Trimers with a TLR-7/8 Adjuvant. *Bioconjug Chem.* (2016) 27:2372–85. doi: 10.1021/acs.bioconjchem.6b00370

91. Ulery BD, Phanse Y, Sinha A, Wannemuehler MJ, Narasimhan B, Bellaire BH. Polymer chemistry influences monocytic uptake of polyanhydride nanospheres. *Pharm Res.* (2009) 26:683–90. doi: 10.1007/s11095-008-9760-7

92. Mcgill JL, Kelly SM, Kumar P, Speckhart S, Haughney SL, Henningson J, et al. Efficacy of mucosal polyanhydride nanovaccine against respiratory syncytial virus infection in the neonatal calf. *Sci Rep.* (2018) 8:3021. doi: 10.1038/s41598-018-21292-2

93. Roux X, Dubuquoy C, Durand G, Tran-Tolla TL, Castagne N, Bernard J, et al. Sub-nucleocapsid nanoparticles: a nasal vaccine against respiratory syncytial virus. *PLoS ONE* (2008) 3:e1766. doi: 10.1371/journal.pone.0001766

94. Herve PL, Deloizy C, Descamps D, Rameix-Welti MA, Fix J, Mclellan JS, et al. RSV N-nanorings fused to palivizumab-targeted neutralizing epitope as a nanoparticle RSV vaccine. *Nanomedicine* (2017) 13:411–20. doi: 10.1016/j.nano.2016.08.006

95. Herve PL, Raliou M, Bourdieu C, Dubuquoy C, Petit-Camurdan A, Bertho N, et al. A novel subnucleocapsid nanoplatform for mucosal vaccination against influenza virus that targets the ectodomain of matrix protein 2. *J Virol.* (2014) 88:325–38. doi: 10.1128/JVI.01141-13

96. Qi M, Zhang XE, Sun X, Zhang X, Yao Y, Liu S, et al. Intranasal nanovaccine confers homo- and hetero-subtypic influenza protection. *Small* (2018) 14:e1703207. doi: 10.1002/smll.201703207

97. Si Y, Wen Y, Kelly SH, Chong AS, Collier JH. Intranasal delivery of adjuvant-free peptide nanofibers elicits resident CD8(+) T cell responses. *J Control Release* (2018) 282:120–30. doi: 10.1016/j.jconrel.2018.04.031

98. Quan FS, Huang C, Compans RW, Kang SM. Virus-like particle vaccine induces protective immunity against homologous and heterologous strains of influenza virus. *J Virol.* (2007) 81:3514–24. doi: 10.1128/JVI.02052-06

99. Lee YT, Ko EJ, Lee Y, Kim KH, Kim MC, Lee YN, et al. Intranasal vaccination with M2e5x virus-like particles induces humoral and cellular immune responses conferring cross-protection against heterosubtypic influenza viruses. *PLoS ONE* (2018) 13:e0190868. doi: 10.1371/journal.pone.0190868

100. Cai M, Wang C, Li Y, Gu H, Sun S, Duan Y, et al. Virus-like particle vaccine by intranasal vaccination elicits protective immunity against respiratory

101. syncytial viral infection in mice. *Acta Biochim Biophys Sin.* (2017) 49:74–82. doi: 10.1093/abbs/gmw118

101. Wee JL, Scheerlinck JP, Snibson KJ, Edwards S, Pearse M, Quinn C, et al. Pulmonary delivery of ISCOMATRIX influenza vaccine induces both systemic and mucosal immunity with antigen dose sparing. *Mucosal Immunol.* (2008) 1:489–96. doi: 10.1038/mi.2008.59

102. Coulter A, Harris R, Davis R, Drane D, Cox J, Ryan D, et al. Intranasal vaccination with ISCOMATRIX® adjuvanted influenza vaccine. *Vaccine* (2003) 21:946–9. doi: 10.1016/S0264-410X(02)00545-5

103. Tai W, Roberts L, Seryshev A, Gubatan JM, Bland CS, Zabriskie R, et al. Multistrain influenza protection induced by a nanoparticulate mucosal immunotherapeutic. *Mucosal Immunol.* (2011) 4:197–207. doi: 10.1038/mi.2010.50

104. Piluso S, Soultan AH, Patterson J. Molecularly engineered polymer-based systems in drug delivery and regenerative medicine. *Curr Pharm Des.* (2017) 23:281–94.

105. Kamaly N, Xiao Z, Valencia PM, Radovic-Moreno AF, Farokhzad OC. Targeted polymeric therapeutic nanoparticles: design, development and clinical translation. *Chem Soc Rev.* (2012) 41:2971–3010. doi: 10.1039/c2cs15344k

106. Krasia-Christoforou T, Georgiou TK. Polymeric theranostics: using polymer-based systems for simultaneous imaging and therapy. *J Mater Chem B* (2013) 1:3002. doi: 10.1039/c3tb20191k

107. Tang Z, He C, Tian H, Ding J, Hsiao BS, Chu B, et al. Polymeric nanostructured materials for biomedical applications. *Progress Polymer Sci.* (2016) 60:86–128. doi: 10.1016/j.progpolymsci.2016.05.005

108. Acharya S, Sahoo SK. PLGA nanoparticles containing various anticancer agents and tumour delivery by EPR effect. *Adv Drug Deliv Rev.* (2011) 63:170–83. doi: 10.1016/j.addr.2010.10.008

109. Mahapatro A, Singh DK. Biodegradable nanoparticles are excellent vehicle for site directed *in-vivo* delivery of drugs and vaccines. *J Nanobiotechnol.* (2011) 9:55. doi: 10.1186/1477-3155-9-55

110. Danhier F, Ansorena E, Silva JM, Coco R, Le Breton A, Preat V. PLGA-based nanoparticles: an overview of biomedical applications. *J Control Release* (2012) 161:505–22. doi: 10.1016/j.jconrel.2012.01.043

111. Silva AL, Soema PC, Slutter B, Ossendorp F, Jiskoot W. PLGA particulate delivery systems for subunit vaccines: linking particle properties to immunogenicity. *Hum Vaccin Immunother.* (2016) 12:1056–69. doi: 10.1080/21645515.2015.1117714

112. Getts DR, Shea LD, Miller SD, King NJ. Harnessing nanoparticles for immune modulation. *Trends Immunol.* (2015) 36:419–27. doi: 10.1016/j.it.2015.05.007

113. Woodrow KA, Bennett KM, Lo DD. Mucosal vaccine design and delivery. *Annu Rev Biomed Eng.* (2012) 14:17–46. doi: 10.1146/annurev-bioeng-071811-150054

114. Santos DM, Carneiro MW, De Moura TR, Soto M, Luz NF, Prates DB, et al. PLGA nanoparticles loaded with KMP-11 stimulate innate immunity and induce the killing of Leishmania. *Nanomedicine* (2013) 9:985–95. doi: 10.1016/j.nano.2013.04.003

115. Csaba N, Garcia-Fuentes M, Alonso MJ. Nanoparticles for nasal vaccination. *Adv Drug Deliv Rev.* (2009) 61:140–57. doi: 10.1016/j.addr.2008.09.005

116. Li P, Tan H, Xu D, Yin F, Cheng Y, Zhang X, et al. Effect and mechanisms of curdlan sulfate on inhibiting HBV infection and acting as an HB vaccine adjuvant. *Carbohydr Polym.* (2014) 110:446–55. doi: 10.1016/j.carbpol.2014.04.025

117. Li P, Zhang X, Cheng Y, Li J, Xiao Y, Zhang Q, et al. Preparation and *in vitro* immunomodulatory effect of curdlan sulfate. *Carbohydr Polym.* (2014) 102:852–61. doi: 10.1016/j.carbpol.2013.10.078

118. Islam S, Bhuiyan MAR, Islam MN. Chitin and chitosan: structure, properties and applications in biomedical engineering. *J Polym Environ.* (2016) 25:854–66. doi: 10.1007/s10924-016-0865-5

119. Marasini N, Giddam AK, Khalil ZG, Hussein WM, Capon RJ, Batzloff MR, et al. Double adjuvanting strategy for peptide-based vaccines: trimethyl chitosan nanoparticles for lipopeptide delivery. *Nanomedicine* (2016) 11:3223–35. doi: 10.2217/nnm-2016-0291

120. Wu M, Zhao H, Li M, Yue Y, Xiong S, Xu W. Intranasal vaccination with mannosylated chitosan formulated DNA vaccine enables robust IgA and

cellular response induction in the lungs of mice and improves protection against pulmonary mycobacterial challenge. *Front Cell Infect Microbiol.* (2017) 7:445. doi: 10.3389/fcimb.2017.00445

121. Zhang S, Huang S, Lu L, Song X, Li P, Wang F. Curdlan sulfate-O-linked quaternized chitosan nanoparticles: potential adjuvants to improve the immunogenicity of exogenous antigens via intranasal vaccination. *Int J Nanomed.* (2018) 13:2377–94. doi: 10.2147/IJN.S158536

122. Vela-Ramirez JE, Goodman JT, Boggiatto PM, Roychoudhury R, Pohl NL, Hostetter JM, et al. Safety and biocompatibility of carbohydrate-functionalized polyanhydride nanoparticles. *AAPS J.* (2015) 17:256–67. doi: 10.1208/s12248-014-9699-z

123. Carrillo-Conde B, Schiltz E, Yu J, Chris Minion F, Phillips GJ, Wannemuehler MJ, et al. Encapsulation into amphiphilic polyanhydride microparticles stabilizes Yersinia pestis antigens. *Acta Biomater.* (2010) 6:3110–9. doi: 10.1016/j.actbio.2010.01.040

124. Petersen LK, Phanse Y, Ramer-Tait AE, Wannemuehler MJ, Narasimhan B. Amphiphilic polyanhydride nanoparticles stabilize Bacillus anthracis protective antigen. *Mol Pharm.* (2012) 9:874–82. doi: 10.1021/mp2004059

125. Ulery BD, Kumar D, Ramer-Tait AE, Metzger DW, Wannemuehler MJ, Narasimhan B. Design of a protective single-dose intranasal nanoparticle-based vaccine platform for respiratory infectious diseases. *PLoS ONE* (2011) 6:e17642. doi: 10.1371/journal.pone.0017642

126. Ulery BD, Petersen LK, Phanse Y, Kong CS, Broderick SR, Kumar D, et al. Rational design of pathogen-mimicking amphiphilic materials as nanoadjuvants. *Sci Rep.* (2011) 1:198. doi: 10.1038/srep00198

127. Ross KA, Haughney SL, Petersen LK, Boggiatto P, Wannemuehler MJ, Narasimhan B. Lung deposition and cellular uptake behavior of pathogen-mimicking nanovaccines in the first 48 hours. *Adv Healthc Mater.* (2014) 3:1071–7. doi: 10.1002/adhm.201300525

128. Scheerlinck JP, Greenwood DL. Virus-sized vaccine delivery systems. *Drug Discov Today* (2008) 13:882–7. doi: 10.1016/j.drudis.2008.06.016

129. Schneider-Ohrum K, Ross TM. Virus-like particles for antigen delivery at mucosal surfaces. In: Kozlowski PA, editor. *Mucosal Vaccines: Modern Concepts, Strategies, and Challenges.* (Berlin;Heidelberg: Springer) (2012). pp. 53–73.

130. Lawson DM, Artymiuk PJ, Yewdall SJ, Smith JM, Livingstone JC, Treffry A, et al. Solving the structure of human H ferritin by genetically engineering intermolecular crystal contacts. *Nature* (1991) 349:541–4. doi: 10.1038/349541a0

131. Lee LA, Wang Q. Adaptations of nanoscale viruses and other protein cages for medical applications. *Nanomedicine* (2006) 2:137–49. doi: 10.1016/j.nano.2006.07.009

132. Li CQ, Soistman E, Carter DC. Ferritin nanoparticle technology. A new platform for antigen presentation and vaccine development. *Ind Biotechnol.* (2006) 2:143–7. doi: 10.1089/ind.2006.2.143

133. Yamashita I, Iwahori K, Kumagai S. Ferritin in the field of nanodevices. *Biochim Biophys Acta* (2010) 1800:846–57. doi: 10.1016/j.bbagen.2010.03.005

134. Yang S, Wang T, Bohon J, Gagne ME, Bolduc M, Leclerc D, et al. Crystal structure of the coat protein of the flexible filamentous papaya mosaic virus. *J Mol Biol.* (2012) 422:263–73. doi: 10.1016/j.jmb.2012.05.032

135. Babin C, Majeau N, Leclerc D. Engineering of papaya mosaic virus (PapMV) nanoparticles with a CTL epitope derived from influenza NP. *J Nanobiotechnol.* (2013) 11:10. doi: 10.1186/1477-3155-11-10

136. Kanekiyo M, Wei CJ, Yassine HM, Mctamney PM, Boyington JC, Whittle JR, et al. Self-assembling influenza nanoparticle vaccines elicit broadly neutralizing H1N1 antibodies. *Nature* (2013) 499:102–6. doi: 10.1038/nature12202

137. Coleman CM, Liu YV, Mu H, Taylor JK, Massare M, Flyer DC, et al. Purified coronavirus spike protein nanoparticles induce coronavirus neutralizing antibodies in mice. *Vaccine* (2014) 32:3169–74. doi: 10.1016/j.vaccine.2014.04.016

138. Lopez-Sagaseta J, Malito E, Rappuoli R, Bottomley MJ. Self-assembling protein nanoparticles in the design of vaccines. *Comput Struct Biotechnol J.* (2016) 14:58–68. doi: 10.1016/j.csbj.2015.11.001

139. Park H-J, Lee E-Y, Jung S, Ko HL, Lee S-M, Nam J-H. Spike nanoparticle and recombinant adenovirus 5 vaccines induce specific antibodies against the Middle East respiratory syndrome coronavirus (MERS-CoV). *J Immunol.* (2017) 198:225.

140. Therien A, Bedard M, Carignan D, Rioux G, Gauthier-Landry L, Laliberte-Gagne ME, et al. A versatile papaya mosaic virus (PapMV) vaccine platform based on sortase-mediated antigen coupling. *J Nanobiotechnol.* (2017) 15:54. doi: 10.1186/s12951-017-0289-y

141. Deng L, Mohan T, Chang TZ, Gonzalez GX, Wang Y, Kwon YM, et al. Double-layered protein nanoparticles induce broad protection against divergent influenza A viruses. *Nat Commun.* (2018) 9:359. doi: 10.1038/s41467-017-02725-4

142. Kushnir N, Streatfield SJ, Yusibov V. Virus-like particles as a highly efficient vaccine platform: diversity of targets and production systems and advances in clinical development. *Vaccine* (2012) 31:58–83. doi: 10.1016/j.vaccine.2012.10.083

143. Mathieu C, Rioux G, Dumas MC, Leclerc D. Induction of innate immunity in lungs with virus-like nanoparticles leads to protection against influenza and Streptococcus pneumoniae challenge. *Nanomedicine* (2013) 9:839–48. doi: 10.1016/j.nano.2013.02.009

144. Zeltins A. Construction and characterization of virus-like particles: a review. *Mol Biotechnol.* (2013) 53:92–107. doi: 10.1007/s12033-012-9598-4

145. Zhao Q, Li S, Yu H, Xia N, Modis Y. Virus-like particle-based human vaccines: quality assessment based on structural and functional properties. *Trends Biotechnol.* (2013) 31:654–63. doi: 10.1016/j.tibtech.2013.09.002

146. Mohsen MO, Zha L, Cabral-Miranda G, Bachmann MF. Major findings and recent advances in virus-like particle (VLP)-based vaccines. *Semin Immunol.* (2017) 34:123–32. doi: 10.1016/j.smim.2017.08.014

147. Lang R, Winter G, Vogt L, Zurcher A, Dorigo B, Schimmele B. Rational design of a stable, freeze-dried virus-like particle-based vaccine formulation. *Drug Dev Ind Pharm.* (2009) 35:83–97. doi: 10.1080/03639040802192806

148. Feliu N, Docter D, Heine M, Del Pino P, Ashraf S, Kolosnjaj-Tabi J, et al. *In vivo* degeneration and the fate of inorganic nanoparticles. *Chem Soc Rev.* (2016) 45:2440–57. doi: 10.1039/C5CS00699F

149. Giner-Casares JJ, Henriksen-Lacey M, Coronado-Puchau M, Liz-Marzán LM. Inorganic nanoparticles for biomedicine: where materials scientists meet medical research. *Mater Today* (2016) 19:19–28.

150. Bastus NG, Sanchez-Tillo E, Pujals S, Farrera C, Kogan MJ, Giralt E, et al. Peptides conjugated to gold nanoparticles induce macrophage activation. *Mol Immunol.* (2009) 46:743–8. doi: 10.1016/j.molimm.2008.08.277

151. Kang S, Ahn S, Lee J, Kim JY, Choi M, Gujrati V, et al. Effects of gold nanoparticle-based vaccine size on lymph node delivery and cytotoxic T-lymphocyte responses. *J Control Release* (2017) 256:56–67. doi: 10.1016/j.jconrel.2017.04.024

152. Hiramatsu H, Osterloh FE. A simple large-scale synthesis of nearly monodisperse gold and silver nanoparticles with adjustable sizes and with exchangeable surfactants. *Chem Mater.* (2004) 16:2509–11. doi: 10.1021/cm049532v

153. Pensa E, Cortes E, Corthey G, Carro P, Vericat C, Fonticelli MH, et al. The chemistry of the sulfur-gold interface: in search of a unified model. *Acc Chem Res.* (2012) 45:1183–92. doi: 10.1021/ar200260p

154. Spampinato V, Parracino MA, La Spina R, Rossi F, Ceccone G. Surface analysis of gold nanoparticles functionalized with thiol-modified glucose SAMs for biosensor applications. *Front Chem.* (2016) 4:8. doi: 10.3389/fchem.2016.00008

155. Belmouaddine H, Shi M, Sanche L, Houde D. Tuning the size of gold nanoparticles produced by multiple filamentation of femtosecond laser pulses in aqueous solutions. *Phys Chem Chem Phys.* (2018) 20:23403–13. doi: 10.1039/C8CP02054J

156. Wang C, Zhu W, Luo Y, Wang BZ. Gold nanoparticles conjugating recombinant influenza hemagglutinin trimers and flagellin enhanced mucosal cellular immunity. *Nanomedicine* (2018) 14:1349–60. doi: 10.1016/j.nano.2018.03.007

157. Cao-Milan R, Liz-Marzan LM. Gold nanoparticle conjugates: recent advances toward clinical applications. *Expert Opin Drug Deliv.* (2014) 11:741–52. doi: 10.1517/17425247.2014.891582

158. Jazayeri MH, Amani H, Pourfatollah AA, Pazoki-Toroudi H, Sedighimoghaddam B. Various methods of gold nanoparticles (GNPs) conjugation to antibodies. *Sens Bio Sensing Res.* (2016) 9:17–22. doi: 10.1016/j.sbsr.2016.04.002

159. Salazar-Gonzalez JA, Gonzalez-Ortega O, Rosales-Mendoza S. Gold nanoparticles and vaccine development. *Exp Rev Vaccines* (2015) 14:1197–211. doi: 10.1586/14760584.2015.1064772

160. Marques Neto LM, Kipnis A, Junqueira-Kipnis AP. Role of metallic nanoparticles in vaccinology: implications for infectious disease vaccine development. *Front Immunol.* (2017) 8:239. doi: 10.3389/fimmu.2017.00239

161. Tao W, Ziemer KS, Gill HS. Gold nanoparticle-M2e conjugate coformulated with CpG induces protective immunity against influenza a virus. *Nanomedicine* (2014) 9:237–51. doi: 10.2217/nnm.13.58

162. Boisselier E, Astruc D. Gold nanoparticles in nanomedicine: preparations, imaging, diagnostics, therapies and toxicity. *Chem Soc Rev.* (2009) 38:1759–82. doi: 10.1039/b806051g

# 8

# Neutrophils and Close Relatives in the Hypoxic Environment of the Tuberculous Granuloma: New Avenues for Host-Directed Therapies?

*Aude Remot, Emilie Doz and Nathalie Winter\**

INRA, Universite de Tours, UMR Infectiologie et Sante Publique, Nouzilly, France

*Correspondence:*
*Nathalie Winter*
*nathalie.winter@inra.fr*

Tuberculosis (TB), caused by *Mycobacterium tuberculosis* (Mtb) is one of the most prevalent lung infections of humans and kills ~1.7 million people each year. TB pathophysiology is complex with a central role played by granuloma where a delicate balance takes place to both constrain bacilli and prevent excessive inflammation that may destroy lung functions. Neutrophils reach the lung in waves following first encounter with bacilli and contribute both to early Mtb elimination and late deleterious inflammation. The hypoxic milieu where cells and bacilli cohabit inside the granuloma favors metabolism changes and the impact on TB infection needs to be more thoroughly understood. At the cellular level while the key role of the alveolar macrophage has long been established, behavior of neutrophils in the hypoxic granuloma remains poorly explored. This review will bring to the front new questions that are now emerging regarding neutrophils activity in TB. Are different neutrophil subsets involved in Mtb infection and how? How do neutrophils and close relatives contribute to shaping the granuloma immune environment? What is the role of hypoxia and hypoxia induced factors inside granuloma on neutrophil fate and functions and TB pathophysiology? Addressing these questions is key to the development of innovative host-directed therapies to fight TB.

Keywords: neutrophils, *Mycobacterium tuberculosis*, granuloma, lung, HIF, hypoxia, host-directed therapies

## INTRODUCTION

Tuberculosis caused by *Mycobacterium tuberculosis* (Mtb) is present worldwide. With estimated 10.4 million new cases and 1.7 million deaths in 2016[1], TB remains one of the most devastating respiratory disease of human kind. The key cell in Mtb lung infection is the lung alveolar macrophage (AM) that engulfs the bacilli and orchestrates the adaptive host immune response if bacilli are not eliminated (1). This is the starting point for the granuloma, set as an immune defense mechanism that eventually becomes the pathologic signature of Mtb infection. AM plays major roles in the battle between Mtb and the host and a large body of the literature is devoted to this key cell. However, mature neutrophils circulate in high numbers in blood and are also sequestered in the lung (2). As

---

[1] http://www.who.int/gho/tb/en/

they are present in the early phase of Mtb infection, before the onset of adaptive immunity, they could play important beneficial protective roles [see extensive review in (3)]. In the zebra-fish (ZF) embryo infected with *M. marinum* (Mm) as a surrogate of Mtb infection in mammals, neutrophils come in response to signals sent by Mm-infected dying macrophages (MPs). Neutrophils dispose off Mm-infected MPs by efferocytosis in the nascent granuloma and kill bacilli through NADPH oxidase-dependent mechanisms (4). We and others have shown in resistant mouse models that neutrophils come in two different waves after Mtb infection before and after the onset of adaptive immunity (5, 6). While the first wave was found to phagocytose BCG–the vaccine strain used against Mtb–*in situ* in the lung, the second T-cell dependent wave was seldom associated with bacilli. In response to virulent Mtb, T-cell dependent neutrophils did not control Mtb growth but rather established close contacts with T-cells in the granuloma (6) suggesting their role in regulation of the adaptive immune response. This is in line with their established role in the formation of the structured mature granuloma in mice (7). However, during active TB, it is now consensus that neutrophils are largely responsible for lung destruction (8). They are the most represented cell subset in sputum (9) and drive an interferon-inducible transcriptional signature in blood cells during active TB (10). Several excellent reviews recently covered neutrophils as "good and bad guys" during TB (3, 8, 11, 12). Such opposite roles may depend on several factors including timing and magnitude of neutrophil recruitment or different neutrophils subsets which respective roles in TB remain elusive. Despite the fact that neutrophils are established as key players in the TB granuloma, the impact of hypoxia on their behavior and functions is still poorly explored and we advocate in this review that this should be reconsidered. Moreover, in the granuloma, the influence of the hypoxic milieu on contribution of neutrophils to production of soluble mediators involved in TB pathophysiology needs to be reconsidered. The world is on high demand of host-directed therapies (HDTs) as adjunct to antibiotics to fight against TB and we hope that our mini review will help to design effective strategies by taking into account the impact of hypoxia on neutrophils.

## THE Mtb GRANULOMA IS A PATHOLOGICAL IMMUNOGICAL NICHE WHERE NEUTROPHILS PLAY MAJOR ROLE

For a long time, the granuloma has been considered as an uniquely host-driven response, set to constrain Mtb and prevent bacilli dissemination. This view was challenged when, in ZF embryo, virulent Mm was shown to disseminate and establish infection by manipulation of the nascent granuloma and adjacent stromal cells (13). Today, the host-pathogen mutual benefit of the granuloma is still a matter of debate (14, 15), as is the role of neutrophils in this structure. Some confounding interpretations may come from animal models, especially the mouse, most extensively used in TB research. In humans, primary TB leads to caseating granulomas that necrotize over time.

Cavities, allowing Mtb transmission, represent the most severe signature of the disease (16). Human TB granulomas are hypoxic as demonstrated by Positron Emission Tomography-Computed Tomography (PET-CT) scans using hypoxia-specific tracers in patients with active TB (17). In TB susceptible animals such as the rabbit, the guinea pig, and the non-human primate, hypoxic granulomatous lesions develop in the lung (18). By contrast, the resistant mouse lines C57BL/6 and BALB/c that have been extensively used, do not develop necrotizing hypoxic granulomas which brought the quite general belief that mice are not an adequate model for TB pathophysiology studies (19). However, extremely susceptible mice such as C3HeB/FeJ do develop central caseous necrosis in the lung (20) and these lesions are hypoxic (21). A common feature to all TB susceptible animals that develop hypoxic necrotizing granulomas is the abundance of neutrophils (22, 23). Mtb induces necrosis of human neutrophils, which depends on its main virulence factor, the small protein ESAT-6 secreted by Type VII secretion system. Necrosis is driven by neutrophil-derived Reactive Oxygen Species (ROS) and is required for Mtb growth after uptake of infected neutrophils by human macrophages (24). In C3HeB/FeJ mice, neutrophils dying by necrosis or NETosis rather than apoptosis seem to drive the caseous necrosis and liquefaction process (25). The crucial role of neutrophils and the S100A9 inflammatory protein for granuloma formation is demonstrated (26). Therefore, what "adequate" animal models and available pathology studies in humans teach us is that neutrophils and hypoxia are crucial to the development of lung lesions during TB disease.

However, some clarification is needed regarding the definition of neutrophils. These cells have long been considered as an homogenous population based on their polylobed nucleus and a minimal set of markers: in mice, they are defined by flow cytometry as Gr1, CD11b double positive cells or more recently as CD11b, Ly-6C, Ly-6G triple positive cells. In humans, they are still minimally identified as CD11b$^+$ CD14$^-$CD15$^+$ cells. The picture has become more complex with the description of Myeloid Derived Supressor Cell (MDSCs), which largely share markers with neutrophils. MDSCs are an immature and heterogeneous population present at homeostasis and accumulating in pathological situations. Originally described in cancers, MDSCs are increasingly characterized in inflammatory diseases (27, 28). MDSCs suppress T cell responses, via different mechanisms, including production of ROS, nitric oxide (NO), or arginase 1 (29). MDSCs are present as two main subsets: monocytic MDSCs and granulocytic MDSCs (Gr-MDSCs). The later display the same morphology and phenotype as *bona fide* neutrophils. They share the Ly-6G or Gr1 markers. Therefore, MDSCs can robustly be distinguished from *bona fide* neutrophils only based on their suppressive function (30). Expansion of granulocytic and monocytic MDSCs is observed in blood of active TB patients and healthy recently exposed contacts (31, 32). This correlates with enhanced L-arginine catabolism and NO production in plasma from active TB patients (33). In resistant (C57BL/6) or susceptible (129S2) strains MDSCs–defined as Gr1$^+$ cells–are identified in the lung parenchyma during the course of Mtb infection where they suppress T cells (34). They also vigorously ingest Mtb. Interestingly, in susceptible mice, Gr1$^+$ MDSCs cells accumulate in higher numbers and phagocytoze more bacilli as compared to resistant mice. Therefore, MDSCs could represent a niche for Mtb replication, helping the pathogen to escape the immune system (34). MDSCs are also associated with TB progression and lethality (35). These findings emphasize the potential of MDSCs as targets for immunotherapy. However, most studies using depletion antibodies that target the Gr1 or the Ly-6G surface marker, do not allow today a clear distinction of the role of *bona fide* neutrophils vs. MDSCs in TB pathophysiology. To add to the complexity, the low density neutrophils (LDNs) have recently been described as a new population of neutrophils. LDNs, displaying heterogeneous morphology and containing mature and immature cells, are immunosuppressive via secretion of IL-10 and expression of arginase-1 (36). Interestingly, mature high density neutrophils (HDNs) can switch to LDNs in a TGF-β dependent way, and acquire immunosuppressive functions similar to granulocytic MDSCs (37). First described in cancer (37) and pulmonary pathologies (38), LDNs have also been identified in TB and associated to the severity of the disease. Moreover, Mtb is able to convert HDNs to LDNs *in vitro*, suggesting manipulation by Mtb (39). Even though LDNs are not yet considered as granulocytic MDSCs, the largely shared purification procedure, analysis methods and markers between these two cell populations suggest possible overlaps (30). Mtb infection in mice recruits an altered "neutrophil" population defined as "Gr-1$^{int}$/Ly-6G$^{int}$" cells with lower levels of Gr1/Ly-6G as compared to classical neutrophils. These immature cells highly express the CD115 and CD135 markers and inhibit T cell proliferation (35). Whether these cells are distinct from granulocytic MDSCs remains to be clarified.

Outside from the TB research field, recent studies identified neutrophils as potential players in inflammatory angiogenesis. Neutrophils store Vascular Endothelial Growth Factor (VEGF), a key player in the process of angiogenesis, that they may release upon stimulation. By recruiting neutrophils, MIP-1α and MIP-2 act in an autocrine loop to promote this process. A new CXCR4$^{high}$ and CD49d$^{high}$ neutrophil subset, displays angiogenic properties via secretion of high concentrations of MMP-9 promoting neovascularization (40). In a model of skin hypersensitization, Tan et al. demonstrated that neutrophil MMP9 and heparanase, targeting distinct domains of the extracellular matrix, cooperate to release diverse VEGF isoforms and influence their bioavailability and bioactivity during inflammatory angiogenesis (41). In mice and humans, CD49d$^{+}$ CXCR4$^{high}$ VEGFR1$^{high}$ neutrophils are recruited specifically in hypoxic ischemic tissues in a VEGFR1 and VEGFR2 dependent way (42). Whether such neutrophils could contribute to formation of the hypoxic TB granuloma remains on open question.

## HYPOXIA-INDUCED-FACTORS ARE MASTER REGULATORS IN Mtb GRANULOMA

The tremendously exciting field of immunometabolism, which links cellular bioenergetics pathways to immune cell functions, brings new views on the fate of the TB granuloma. In response to inflammatory environment, MPs switch from oxidative phosphorylation–the mitochondrial respiration system that quiescent cells use to generate energy–to aerobic glycolysis. This shift, called the Warburg effect, was discovered in proliferating cancer cells that highly incorporate glucose, that they convert to lactate while producing ATP and cell-building blocks (43). Master regulators of this switch are Hypoxia-Induced–Factors (HIFs), a family of transcription factors that govern cell reprogrammation (44). Under normoxia, the enzymes Prolyl Hydroxylase Domains (PHD) and Factor Inhibiting HIF (FIH) repress HIFs via targeted degradation and transcriptional mechanisms. Under low $O_2$ tension, these enzymes become inactive, HIFs are stabilized and derepressed and activate a transcriptional program to adapt the cell to hypoxia. Other than $O_2$, HIFs respond to a variety of environmental factors. HIF1α$^{-/-}$ mice display enhanced Mtb burden and reduced survival (45). This could be linked to HIFs regulating the bactericidal functions of MPs and neutrophils (46). NF–kb, the master regulator of the inflammatory response, regulates transcription of the *hif1a* gene encoding one of the HIF subunits (47). In MPs, LPS binding to TLR4 activates HIF-1α that upregulates IL-1β production. The signaling occurs through succinate, one intermediate of the tricarboxylic acid cycle (48) that accumulates upon reprogrammation of the MP toward aerobic glycolysis. However, this effect cannot be generalized to all TLR- signaling pathways (49). Imaging with glucose tracers illustrates high glucose uptake after infection with Mtb in the lungs of C3HeB/FeJ mice (50) non-human primates (51) and humans (52). Aerobic glycolysis is confirmed by NMR-analysis of metabolites in mice (53) and guinea pigs (54), or global transcriptomics of genes encoding glycolytic enzymes in the lungs of mice, rabbits, and humans (55). Reprogramming of the host metabolism translates in coordinated up and down regulation of genes encoding key glycolytic enzymes and glucose transporters, reminiscent of the Warburg effect as well as regulation of HIF-1α (55). While the granuloma becomes necrotic, MPs packed with lipid droplets transform into foamy cells (56) which is driven by reprogrammation of host lipid metabolism in response to Mtb compounds (57). Interestingly, lipid droplets formation in Mtb infected MPs is driven by IFN-γ and requires HIF-1α and its target gene *hig2* (58).

Several immunopathology studies demonstrate extensive vascularization of TB granulomas in humans (59) and mice (59, 60) provided that they are not necrotic (61). The link between hypoxia, vascularization, and development of the granuloma was recently established in the ZF infected with Mm (62). In this model, HIF-1α is activated, PHD-3 expression is increased and induces production of the angiogenic factor VGEF-A, which is intimately linked to nascent granuloma formation. In human MPs infected with Mtb, a similar angiogienic signature is observed (63). Moreover, the level of VEGF-A is increased in sputum and peripheral blood of active TB patients and is proposed as a differentiating biomarker for patients progressing to active TB (64–66). Circulating angiogenic factors are markers of disease severity and are associated to the bacterial burden (67). In ZF embryos infected by Mm, CXCR4 signaling is important to initiate angiogenesis for granuloma expansion (68). Surprisingly, despite the established over-representation of neutrophils in

TB lesions, little information is available on how these cells behave in face of Mtb in the highly hypoxic and angiogenic granuloma milieu.

Neutrophils are generally seen as short-lived cells. However, the life span of neutrophils is highly increased in hypoxic milieu (69). By high consumption of oxygen during oxidative burst, neutrophils themselves contribute to generate the hypoxic milieu, which may well be the case during active TB when they invade the lung. Prolonged survival is linked to sustained expression of PHD3, in vitro and in vivo, in response to hypoxia and inflammatory stimuli (70). Interestingly, PHD3 is strongly induced in lungs of Mtb infected mice (55). HIF-2α is the most expressed in neutrophils, in contrast to MPs where HIF-1α is the most active. HIF-2α deficiency increases neutrophil apoptosis (71). MIP-1 is also identified as a novel hypoxia stimulated granulocyte survival factor (72).

In the ZF model infected with Mm, neutrophil-specific HIF-1α stabilization decreases bacterial burden via a NO-dependent mechanism. On the contrary, despite also being upregulated, HIF-2α has a negative impact on bacterial burden emphasizing opposite roles of different HIF factors (73). Therefore, it is possible that the hypoxic environment of the TB granuloma that favors extended life-span for neutrophils allows them to actively shape granuloma evolution. On one hand, this may help bacilli control as well as resolution of inflammation, since neutrophils actively participate to MP efferocytosis and the release of lipids such as LXA4. On the other hand, hypoxia increases neutrophil degranulation and confers extended activity to damage lung tissues in a PI3K dependent pathway (74). Hypoxia-induced decrease of neutrophil apoptosis

induces a delay in resolution of inflammation by maintaining active neutrophils in the inflamed tissue (75). Moreover, hypoxia impairs the ability of neutrophils to kill certain bacteria (76).

HIF-1α is a major player in an another chronic infection caused by the intracellular parasite Leishmania. HIF-1α crucially enhances immunosuppressive functions of MDSCs and decreases leishmanicidal capacity of myeloid cells (77). Even though to our knowledge no study has tackled the link between HIF-1α and MDSCs in TB, a similar important role could be discovered. Also, since hypoxia and angiogenesis are intimately linked to the granuloma development, another interesting perspective is the possible role of angiogenic neutrophils (40, 42) in the process.

## POSSIBLE INFLUENCE OF THE HYPOXIC Mtb GRANULOMA ON KEY NEUTROPHIL-RELEASED MEDIATORS

Neutrophils contribute both pro- and anti-inflammatory factors in TB (78, 79). Information on how HIF-1α stabilization in hypoxic environment influences the secretion of critical immune mediators by neutrophils is limited to granule proteases, antimicrobial peptides and TNF (46). Literature on the impact of HIF-1α stabilization on MP-released mediators is more extensive and we consider it as a source of inspiration illustrating the potential role of hypoxia on neutrophil-released mediators (**Figure 1**). In the following paragraph, we focus on how hypoxia may regulate release by neutrophils of the key mediators

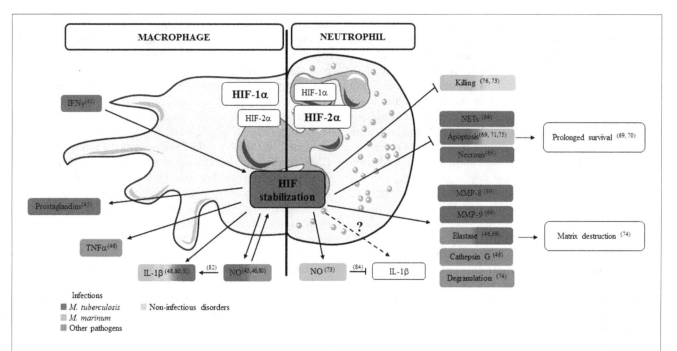

**FIGURE 1 |** Impact of HIFs on control of key mediators released by neutrophils and macrophages. Key mediators and essential cellular processes controlled by HIF stabilization in macrophage (left) or neutrophil (right) after infections with *M. tuberculosis*, *M. marinum*, or other bacteria or during non-infectious disorders are depicted (numbers refer to publications listed in the review).

**TABLE 1** | Impact of neutrophils and close relatives in cancer and TB.

| | Tumor formation and evolution | Early Mtb infection and granuloma |
|---|---|---|
| Prognosis/Pathophysiology | • Clinical evidence (neutrophil to lymphocyte ratio) mostly links neutrophils to cancer progression. Poor prognosis.<br>• Different granulocytic populations described with various functions. Anti-tumor activity of High Density Neutrophils (early stage tumor). Accumulation of immature neutrophils associated to cancer progression (Gr MDSCs or Low Density Neutrophils). Promote angiogenesis, tumor progression, and metastases (95)<br>• In many cancers, different granulocyte subpopulations are described (96). Better definition is needed | • Early phase of infection: neutrophils contribute to innate resistance (11, 97) and granuloma formation (7, 98, 99)<br>• Late phase of infection, active TB: established role of neutrophils to severe forms in preclinical models (8) and in humans (9)<br>• Gr-MDSCs accumulate during early phase Mtb infection and active TB, in blood and lung in humans (31)<br>• MDSCs may represent permissive reservoir for Mtb (34) and their accumulation associates with severe TB in mice (35) |
| Hypoxia and angiogenesis | • HIF-2α, selectively modulates neutrophil recruitment (100)<br>• Neutrophil recruitment to early-stage tumors is linked to hypoxia (101)<br>• Induction of angiogenic neutrophils in hypoxic conditions | • Hypoxia augments neutrophil degranulation and confers enhanced potential for damage to respiratory airway epithelial cells (69)<br>• Hif-1α increases NO production by neutrophils in early stage of Mm infection and is involved in control of bacterial growth (73)<br>• Granuloma formation in the ZF model coincides with angiogenesis and local hypoxia (62) |
| Modulation of T cell response | • MDSCs are major players in tumor-mediated immunosuppression<br>• Neutrophils in solid tumors are potent producers of Arg-1 and could contribute to local immune suppression (102, 103) | • MDSCs are present in lungs (3) but their role in development and evolution of granuloma remains unclear<br>• Arg-1 is associated to severe TB in mouse models (104, 105) and is detected in necrotizing granulomas in humans (106). Pathway documented in MPs, however, deciphering neutrophil contribution to Arg-1 production would be of interest. |
| Tissue Remodeling | • MMP-9 delivered by tumor-recruited neutrophils is associated to tumor angiogenesis and dissemination (107)<br>• Angiogenic neutrophils contribute to tumor growth and metastasis (108)<br>• Neutrophils through COX-2-mediated PGE2 synthesis and elastase promote tumor cell proliferation (109) | • MMPs are involved in early granuloma formation and participate to tissue destruction during late phase (110, 111)<br>• Pathogenic mycobacteria (Mm or Mtb) exploit the formation of new blood vessels to disseminate via MPs (62, 63). Neutrophils are migrating cells (112), their contribution to Mtb dissemination is not documented yet. |

in Mtb virulence: ROS, NO, IL-1β, and type I IFN. Some of these mediators may play different roles in humans and animal models and data should sometimes be interpreted with caution. In Mtb infected MPs, HIF-1α is stabilized by IFN-γ and regulates the production of prostaglandins and NO (45). In mice, NO not only acts as an antimicrobial agent and inflammatory mediator but further amplifies myeloid cell bactericidal activity via HIF-1α stabilization. NO modulates the MP response to Mtb through activation of HIF-1α and repression of NF-kB (80). HIF-1α and NO are intrinsically linked: they positively regulate each other, but display distinct roles in the regulation of inflammation. Among the mediators regulated in opposite directions, neutrophil-attracting chemokines, IL-1α and IL-1β, are all down regulated in HIF-1α$^{-/-}$ and upregulated in Nos2$^{-/-}$ Mtb infected and IFN-γ activated BMDMs (80). In the hypoxic granuloma, NO produced by IFNγ-activated MPs restricts neutrophil recruitment to avoid destructive inflammation (80). In Mm infected ZF, HIF-1α stabilization induced IL-1β production by MPs and increased neutrophil NO production that is protective against infection (81). In Mm infected NADPH oxidase 2-deficient mice (Ncf1$^{-/-}$) mice, ROS-deficiency decreases IL-1β production by MPs but induces early and extensive neutrophilic inflammation, with high elastase activity and IL-1β production (82). This also reveals a novel role for ROS in the early neutrophilic granulomatous inflammation

and the importance of neutrophil-driven IL-1β production during mycobacterial infection. In addition to MPs, neutrophils also produce ROS and NOS. Neutrophils are able to discriminate pathogens by differential production and localization of ROS, and tune their own recruitment and distribution to exquisitely tailor the anti-microbial response (83). HIF-1α stabilization in neutrophils induces NO production after infection by Mm (73). NOS and ROS production also influences the secretion of cytokines. NO inhibits NLRP3-dependent IL-1 responses (84). IL-1β signaling is also important for ROS production as Mtb-infected newly recruited neutrophils lacking IL-1R fail to produce ROS, resulting in compromised pathogen control (85). HIF-1α stabilization clearly influences ROS/NOS and IL-1β production by MPs and neutrophils, both factors are important during mycobacterial infection, but their regulation seems different in the two cell types (73, 80–82, 84, 85) (**Figure 1**). In human neutrophils stimulated with Mtb, hypoxia up-regulates secretion of MMP-8, MMP-9 and neutrophil elastase that are involved in matrix destruction. Hypoxia inhibits NETs formation and both neutrophil apoptosis and necrosis after direct stimulation by Mtb (69).

Type I IFN is a major cytokine in TB pathophysiology. Overproduction of type I IFN (IFN-I) is linked to exacerbated TB in both mouse models and humans. IFN-I triggers immunopathology by increasing the recruitment of inflammatory monocytes and neutrophils to the lung (86). Secretion of IFN-I by MPs and its effect on neutrophils is well-documented (87–89). In MPs, Mtb triggers IFN-I secretion through bacterial DNA release in the cytosol. However, strains display variable ability to activate the IFN-I pathway depending on their effective triggering of mitochondrial stress (87). Host-protective cytokines such as TNF, IL-12, and IL-1β are inhibited by exogenous IFN-I, via production of immunosuppressive IL-10 (88). By contrast, IL-1β suppresses IFN-I through eicosanoid prostaglandin E2 (90). In the inflammatory environment in mouse tumor models, IFN-I shifts neutrophils to antimetastatic phenotype (89). Therefore, IFN-I has multiple and crucial effects on neutrophils, but so far studies on IFN signaling in neutrophils in hypoxic environment are still scarce. As hypoxia leads to accumulation of cytosolic DNA via mitochondrial or nuclear DNA damage, it could favor activation of the cGAS/STING/IRF3 pathway (91). The convergence between hypoxia and IFN-I signaling is suggested by Karuppagounder et al. who identified the effect of Tilorone, a small molecule inducing IFN-I which also triggered hypoxic response in brain cells (91). Another study claims that IFN-I promotes tumorigenic properties through up-regulation of HIF functions in different cancer cell lines (92). Direct IFN-I secretion by neutrophils is proposed, where Sox2 could act as a sequence-specific DNA sensor in neutrophils during microbial infection (93). However, it is unclear if neutrophils can sense DNA via the cGAS/STING pathway (94).

Thus, even though the impact of hypoxic environment encountered in the TB granuloma on the IFN-I pathway is not documented yet, this issue could be of great interest to better understand TB pathophysiology and propose new therapies.

## NEUTROPHILS IN TB: MANY OPEN QUESTIONS

Although it is now consensus that during active TB, neutrophils are the main villains responsible for lung destruction, we–and others (3, 11)–advocate that this narrow vision is revisited. "Neutrophils" encompass different subsets with various functions that remain poorly defined. They come to infectious foci in waves of different magnitude. A better definition of neutrophil subsets, their coordinated dynamics of recruitment to the lung and their associated functions is needed. Neutrophils crosstalk with other cells and secrete a vast number of mediators thus taking full part to the regulation of the immune response against Mtb. They respond to signals sent by their environment, including hypoxia in inflamed tissues. In the hypoxic TB granuloma, light has been recently shed on the fate and behavior of MPs, under the control of the master regulator HIF-1α. However, there is currently scarce information on the fate and behavior of neutrophils in a similar context. How do neutrophils respond to hypoxia in the TB context? How do neutrophils contribute to the shaping of the granuloma? In the future, models allowing development of the hypoxic TB granuloma should be favored. A better definition

of mediators released by neutrophils in the hypoxic context of the granuloma is expected. As neutrophils are key players in the game, we believe that these questions need to be solved in order to propose new interventions to fight against TB.

## PERSPECTIVES FOR INNOVATIVE THERAPEUTICS AGAINST TB

In the era of increasing multidrug resistance of Mtb strains, HDTs sometimes represent the last hope for patients. As the hallmark of destructive inflammation, neutrophils are often considered as potential targets. Inhibiting necrotic neutrophil death could restore Mtb growth control (24). Removing neutrophils by drugs or immunotherapeutic interventions could also alleviate lung tissue destruction.

Recent studies in the TB field shed some light on parallels that could be drawn between the TB granuloma and solid tumors (**Table 1**), especially regarding the role of neutrophils. Since HDTs are more advanced in the field of cancer than they are in TB, we propose that some tracks well-developed in cancer therapy are explored to advance the field of HDTs for TB patients. Among promising avenues, we propose that metabolic changes occurring in TB granuloma are being considered (113). Modulation of the HIF pathways (114) deserves attention as it could dampen excessive protease secretion (69). PHD3 and HIF-2α that operate in neutrophils under inflammatory or hypoxic conditions (70, 71) represent more attractive targets than largely distributed HIF-1α. In cancer, another active field in the clinics is blocking angiogenesis since this pathway is key to tumor development. Angiogenesis appeared more recently as key to the development of the TB granuloma and it would be interesting to determine whether modulating angiogenesis could bring some benefit to TB patients. Along this line, we believe that recently described angiogenic neutrophils should also be investigated in TB.

TB still kills 1.7 million people each year and active TB patients continuously spread bacilli that represent threat to human kind. Development of adjunct HDTs is a promising avenue to boost current drug regimen directed against Mtb (115). We believe that addressing the questions that we raised in this review about neutrophils in TB could greatly help in the quest for innovative HDTs.

## AUTHOR CONTRIBUTIONS

All authors listed have made a substantial, direct and intellectual contribution to the work, and approved it for publication.

## FUNDING

AR is supported by a grant from Agence Nationale de la Recherche under the Carnot Program France Futur Elevage.

# REFERENCES

1. Pieters J. *Mycobacterium tuberculosis* and the macrophage: maintaining a balance. *Cell Host Microbe.* (2008) 3:399–407. doi: 10.1016/j.chom.2008.05.006

2. Kolaczkowska E, Kubes P. Neutrophil recruitment and function in health and inflammation. *Nat Rev Immunol.* (2013) 13:159–75. doi: 10.1038/nri3399

3. Lyadova IV. Neutrophils in tuberculosis: heterogeneity shapes the way? *Mediators Inflamm.* (2017) 2017:8619307. doi: 10.1155/2017/8619307

4. Yang CT, Cambier CJ, Davis JM, Hall CJ, Crosier PS, Ramakrishnan L. Neutrophils exert protection in the early tuberculous granuloma by oxidative killing of mycobacteria phagocytosed from infected macrophages. *Cell Host Microbe.* (2012) 12:301–12. doi: 10.1016/j.chom.2012.07.009

5. Appelberg R, Silva M. T cell-dependent chronic neutrophilia during mycobacterial infections. *Clin Exp Immunol.* (1989) 78:478–83.

6. Lombard R, Doz E, Carreras F, Epardaud M, Le Vern Y, Buzoni-Gatel D, et al. IL-17RA in non-hematopoietic cells controls CXCL-1 and 5 critical to recruit neutrophils to the lung of mycobacteria-infected mice during the adaptive immune response. *PLoS ONE.* (2016) 11:e0149455. doi: 10.1371/journal.pone.0149455

7. Seiler P, Aichele P, Bandermann S, Hauser A, Lu B, Gerard N, et al. Early granuloma formation after aerosol *Mycobacterium tuberculosis* infection is regulated by neutrophils via CXCR3-signaling chemokines. *Eur J Immunol.* (2003) 33:2676–86. doi: 10.1002/eji.200323956

8. Dallenga T, Schaible UE. Neutrophils in tuberculosis–first line of defence or booster of disease and targets for host-directed therapy? *Pathog Dis.* (2016) 74:ftw012. doi: 10.1093/femspd/ftw012

9. Eum SY, Kong JH, Hong MS, Lee YJ, Kim JH, Hwang SH, et al. Neutrophils are the predominant infected phagocytic cells in the airways of patients with active pulmonary TB. *Chest.* (2010) 137:122–8. doi: 10.1378/chest.09-0903

10. Berry MP, Graham CM, McNab FW, Xu Z, Bloch SA, Oni T, et al. An interferon-inducible neutrophil-driven blood transcriptional signature in human tuberculosis. *Nature.* (2010) 466:973–7. doi: 10.1038/nature09247

11. Kroon E, Coussens A, Kinnear C, Orlova M, Möller M, Seeger A, et al. Neutrophils: innate effectors of TB resistance? *Front Immunol.* (2018) 9:2637. doi: 10.3389/fimmu.2018.02637

12. Warren E, Teskey G, Venketaraman V. Effector mechanisms of neutrophils within the innate immune system in response to *Mycobacterium tuberculosis* infection. *J Clin Med.* 6:E15. doi: 10.3390/jcm6020015

13. Ramakrishnan L. Revisiting the role of the granuloma in tuberculosis. *Nat Rev Immunol.* (2012) 12:352–66. doi: 10.1038/nri3211

14. Ehlers S, Schaible UE. The granuloma in tuberculosis: dynamics of a host-pathogen collusion. *Front Immunol.* (2012) 3:411. doi: 10.3389/fimmu.2012.00411

15. Pagan AJ, Ramakrishnan L. Immunity and immunopathology in the tuberculous granuloma. *Cold Spring Harb Perspect Med.* 5:a018499. doi: 10.1101/cshperspect.a018499

16. Hunter RL. Pathology of post primary tuberculosis of the lung: an illustrated critical review. *Tuberculosis.* (2011) 91:497–509. doi: 10.1016/j.tube.2011.03.007

17. Belton M, Brilha S, Manavaki R, Mauri F, Nijran K, Hong YT, et al. Hypoxia and tissue destruction in pulmonary TB. *Thorax.* (2016) 71:1145–53. doi: 10.1136/thoraxjnl-2015-207402

18. Via LE, Lin PL, Ray SM, Carrillo J, Allen SS, Eum SY, et al. Tuberculous granulomas are hypoxic in guinea pigs, rabbits, and nonhuman primates. *Infect Immun.* (2008) 76:2333–40. doi: 10.1128/IAI.01515-07

19. Orme IM, Basaraba RJ. The formation of the granuloma in tuberculosis infection. *Semin Immunol.* (2014) 26:601–9. doi: 10.1016/j.smim.2014.09.009

20. Pan H, Yan B-S, Shebzukhov YV, Zhou H, Kobzik L. Ipr1 gene mediates innate immunity to tuberculosis. *Nature.* (2005) 434:767–72. doi: 10.1038/nature03419

21. Harper J, Skerry C, Davis SL, Tasneen R, Weir M, Kramnik I, et al. Mouse model of necrotic tuberculosis granulomas develops hypoxic lesions. *J Infect Dis.* (2012) 205:595–602. doi: 10.1093/infdis/jir786

22. Mattila JT, Maiello P, Sun T, Via LE, Flynn JL. Granzyme B-expressing neutrophils correlate with bacterial load in granulomas from *Mycobacterium tuberculosis*-infected cynomolgus macaques. *Cell Microbiol.* (2015) 17:1085–97. doi: 10.1111/cmi.12428

23. Turner OC, Basaraba RJ, Orme IM. Immunopathogenesis of pulmonary granulomas in the guinea pig after infection with *Mycobacterium tuberculosis. Infect Immun.* (2003) 71:864–71. doi: 10.1128/IAI.71.2.864-871.2003

24. Dallenga T, Repnik U, Corleis B, Eich J, Reimer R, Griffiths GW, et al. *M. tuberculosis*-tnduced necrosis of infected neutrophils promotes bacterial growth following phagocytosis by macrophages. *Cell Host Microbe.* (2017) 22:519–30.e513. doi: 10.1016/j.chom.2017.09.003

25. Marzo E, Vilaplana C, Tapia G, Diaz J, Garcia V, Cardona PJ. Damaging role of neutrophilic infiltration in a mouse model of progressive tuberculosis. *Tuberculosis.* (2014) 94:55–64. doi: 10.1016/j.tube.2013.09.004

26. Yoshioka Y, Mizutani T, Mizuta S, Miyamoto A, Murata S, Ano T, et al. Neutrophils and the S100A9 protein critically regulate granuloma formation. *Blood Adv.* (2016) 1:184–92. doi: 10.1182/bloodadvances.2016000497

27. Youn JI, Nagaraj S, Collazo M, Gabrilovich DI. Subsets of myeloid-derived suppressor cells in tumor-bearing mice. *J Immunol.* (2008) 181:5791–802. doi: 10.4049/jimmunol.181.8.5791

28. Zhang C, Lei GS, Shao S, Jung HW, Durant PJ, Lee CH. Accumulation of myeloid-derived suppressor cells in the lungs during Pneumocystis pneumonia. *Infect Immun.* (2012) 80:3634–41. doi: 10.1128/IAI.00668-12

29. Gabrilovich DI, Nagaraj S. Myeloid-derived suppressor cells as regulators of the immune system. *Nat Rev Immunol.* (2009) 9:162–74. doi: 10.1038/nri2506

30. Bronte V, Brandau S, Chen SH, Colombo MP, Frey AB, Greten TF, et al. Recommendations for myeloid-derived suppressor cell nomenclature and characterization standards. *Nat Commun.* (2016) 7:12150. doi: 10.1038/ncomms12150

31. du Plessis N, Loebenberg L, Kriel M, von Groote-Bidlingmaier F, Ribechini E, Loxton AG, et al. Increased frequency of myeloid-derived suppressor cells during active tuberculosis and after recent *Mycobacterium tuberculosis* infection suppresses T-cell function. *Am J Respir Crit Care Med.* (2013) 188:724–32. doi: 10.1164/rccm.201302-0249OC

32. Yang B, Wang X, Jiang J, Zhai F, Cheng X. Identification of CD244-expressing myeloid-derived suppressor cells in patients with active tuberculosis. *Immunol Lett.* (2014) 158:66–72. doi: 10.1016/j.imlet.2013.12.003

33. El Daker S, Sacchi A, Tempestilli M, Carducci C, Goletti D, Vanini V, et al. Granulocytic myeloid derived suppressor cells expansion during active pulmonary tuberculosis is associated with high nitric oxide plasma level. *PLoS ONE.* (2015) 10:e0123772. doi: 10.1371/journal.pone.0123772

34. Knaul JK, Jorg S, Oberbeck-Mueller D, Heinemann E, Scheuermann L, Brinkmann V, et al. Lung-residing myeloid-derived suppressors display dual functionality in murine pulmonary tuberculosis. *Am J Respir Crit Care Med.* (2014) 190:1053–66. doi: 10.1164/rccm.201405-0828OC

35. Tsiganov EN, Verbina EM, Radaeva TV, Sosunov VV, Kosmiadi GA, Nikitina IY, et al. Gr-1dimCD11b+ immature myeloid-derived suppressor cells but not neutrophils are markers of lethal tuberculosis infection in mice. *J Immunol.* (2014) 192:4718–27. doi: 10.4049/jimmunol.1301365

36. Cloke T, Munder M, Taylor G, Muller I, Kropf P. Characterization of a novel population of low-density granulocytes associated with disease severity in HIV-1 infection. *PLoS ONE.* (2012) 7:e48939. doi: 10.1371/journal.pone.0048939

37. Sagiv JY, Michaeli J, Assi S, Mishalian I, Kisos H, Levy L, et al. Phenotypic diversity and plasticity in circulating neutrophil subpopulations in cancer. *Cell Rep.* (2015) 10:562–73. doi: 10.1016/j.celrep.2014.12.039

38. Fu J, Tobin MC, Thomas LL. Neutrophil-like low-density granulocytes are elevated in patients with moderate to severe persistent asthma. *Ann Allergy Asthma Immunol.* (2014) 113:635–40.e632. doi: 10.1016/j.anai.2014.08.024

39. Deng Y, Ye J, Luo Q, Huang Z, Peng Y, Xiong G, et al. Low-density granulocytes are elevated in mycobacterial infection and associated with the severity of tuberculosis. *PLoS ONE.* (2016) 11:e0153567. doi: 10.1371/journal.pone.0153567

40. Christoffersson G, Vagesjo E, Vandooren J, Liden M, Massena S, Reinert RB, et al. VEGF-A recruits a proangiogenic MMP-9-delivering neutrophil subset that induces angiogenesis in transplanted hypoxic tissue. *Blood.* (2012) 120:4653–62. doi: 10.1182/blood-2012-04-421040

41. Tan KW, Chong SZ, Wong FH, Evrard M, Tan SM, Keeble J, et al. Neutrophils contribute to inflammatory lymphangiogenesis by increasing

VEGF-A bioavailability and secreting VEGF-D. *Blood*. (2013) 122:3666–77. doi: 10.1182/blood-2012-11-466532

42. Massena S, Christoffersson G, Vagesjo E, Seignez C, Gustafsson K, Binet F, et al. Identification and characterization of VEGF-A-responsive neutrophils expressing CD49d, VEGFR1, and CXCR4 in mice and humans. *Blood*. (2015) 126:2016–26. doi: 10.1182/blood-2015-03-631572

43. O'Neill LA, Kishton RJ, Rathmell J. A guide to immunometabolism for immunologists. *Nat Rev Immunol*. (2016) 16:553–65. doi: 10.1038/nri.2016.70

44. Taylor CT, Colgan SP. Regulation of immunity and inflammation by hypoxia in immunological niches. *Nat Rev Immunol*. (2017) 17:774–85. doi: 10.1038/nri.2017.103

45. Braverman J, Sogi KM, Benjamin D, Nomura DK, Stanley SA. HIF-1α is an essential mediator of IFN-γ-dependent immunity to *Mycobacterium tuberculosis*. *J Immunol*. (2016) 197:1287–97. doi: 10.4049/jimmunol.1600266

46. Peyssonnaux C, Datta V, Cramer T, Doedens A, Theodorakis EA, Gallo RL, et al. HIF-1α expression regulates the bactericidal capacity of phagocytes. *J Clin Invest*. (2005) 115:1806–15. doi: 10.1172/JCI23865

47. Rius J, Guma M, Schachtrup C, Akassoglou K, Zinkernagel AS, Nizet V, et al. NF-kappaB links innate immunity to the hypoxic response through transcriptional regulation of HIF-1α. *Nature*. (2008) 453:807–11. doi: 10.1038/nature06905

48. Tannahill GM, Curtis AM, Adamik J, Palsson-McDermott EM, McGettrick AF, Goel G, et al. Succinate is an inflammatory signal that induces IL-1β through HIF-1α. *Nature*. (2013) 496:238–42. doi: 10.1038/nature11986

49. Lachmandas E, Boutens L, Ratter JM, Hijmans A, Hooiveld GJ, Joosten LA, et al. Microbial stimulation of different Toll-like receptor signalling pathways induces diverse metabolic programmes in human monocytes. *Nat Microbiol*. (2016) 2:16246. doi: 10.1038/nmicrobiol.2016.246

50. Davis SL, Nuermberger EL, Um PK, Vidal C, Jedynak B, Pomper MG, et al. Noninvasive pulmonary [18F]-2-fluoro-deoxy-D-glucose positron emission tomography correlates with bactericidal activity of tuberculosis drug treatment. *Antimicrob Agents Chemother*. (2009) 53:4879–84. doi: 10.1128/AAC.00789-09

51. Coleman M, Maiello P, Tomko J, Frye L, Fillmore D, Janssen C, et al. Early Changes by (18)Fluorodeoxyglucose positron emission tomography coregistered with computed tomography predict outcome after *Mycobacterium tuberculosis* infection in cynomolgus macaques. *Infect Immun*. (2014) 82:2400–4. doi: 10.1128/IAI.01599-13

52. Kim IJ, Lee JS, Kim SJ, Kim YK, Jeong YJ, Jun S, et al. Double-phase 18F-FDG PET-CT for determination of pulmonary tuberculoma activity. *Eur J Nucl Med Mol Imaging*. (2008) 35:808–14. doi: 10.1007/s00259-007-0585-0

53. Shin JH, Yang JY, Jeon BY, Yoon YJ, Cho SN, Kang YH, et al. (1)H NMR-based metabolomic profiling in mice infected with *Mycobacterium tuberculosis*. *J Proteome Res*. (2011) 10:2238–47. doi: 10.1021/pr101054m

54. Somashekar BS, Amin AG, Rithner CD, Troudt J, Basaraba R, Izzo A, et al. Metabolic profiling of lung granuloma in *Mycobacterium tuberculosis* infected guinea pigs: *ex vivo* 1H magic angle spinning NMR studies. *J Proteome Res*. (2011) 10:4186–95. doi: 10.1021/pr2003352

55. Shi L, Eugenin EA, Subbian S. Immunometabolism in tuberculosis. *Front Immunol*. (2016) 7:150. doi: 10.3389/fimmu.2016.00150

56. Russell DG, Cardona PJ, Kim MJ, Allain S, Altare F. Foamy macrophages and the progression of the human tuberculosis granuloma. *Nat Immunol*. (2009) 10:943–8. doi: 10.1038/ni.1781

57. Kim MJ, Wainwright HC, Locketz M, Bekker LG, Walther GB, Dittrich C, et al. Caseation of human tuberculosis granulomas correlates with elevated host lipid metabolism. *EMBO Mol Med*. (2010) 2:258–74. doi: 10.1002/emmm.201000079

58. Knight M, Braverman J, Asfaha K, Gronert K, Stanley S. Lipid droplet formation in *Mycobacterium tuberculosis* infected macrophages requires IFN-γ/HIF-1α signaling and supports host defense. *PLoS Pathog*. (2018) 14:e1006874. doi: 10.1371/journal.ppat.1006874

59. Tsai MC, Chakravarty S, Zhu G, Xu J, Tanaka K, Koch C, et al. Characterization of the tuberculous granuloma in murine and human lungs: cellular composition and relative tissue oxygen tension. *Cell Microbiol*. (2006) 8:218–32. doi: 10.1111/j.1462-5822.2005.00612.x

60. Aly S, Laskay T, Mages J, Malzan A, Lang R, Ehlers S. Interferon-γ-dependent mechanisms of mycobacteria-induced pulmonary immunopathology: the role of angiostasis and CXCR3-targeted chemokines for granuloma necrosis. *J Pathol*. (2007) 212:295–305. doi: 10.1002/path.2185

61. Ulrichs T, Kosmiadi G, Jörg S, Pradl L, Titukhina M, Mishenko V, et al. Differential organization of the local immune response in patients with active cavitary tuberculosis or with non-progressive tuberculoma. *J Infect Dis*. (2005) 192:89–97. doi: 10.1086/430621

62. Oehlers SH, Cronan MR, Scott NR, Thomas MI, Okuda KS, Walton EM, et al. Interception of host angiogenic signalling limits mycobacterial growth. *Nature*. (2015) 517:612–5. doi: 10.1038/nature13967

63. Polena H, Boudou F, Tilleul S, Dubois-Colas N, Lecointe C, Rakotosamimanana N, et al. *Mycobacterium tuberculosis* exploits the formation of new blood vessels for its dissemination. *Sci Rep*. (2016) 6:33162. doi: 10.1038/srep33162

64. Abe Y, Nakamura M, Oshika Y, Hatanaka H, Tokunaga T, Ohkubo Y, et al. Serum levels of vascular endothelial growth factor and cavity formation in active pulmonary tuberculosis. *Respiration*. (2001) 68:496–500. doi: 10.1159/000050557

65. Alatas F, Alatas O, Metintas M, Ozarslan A, Erginel S, Yildirim H. Vascular endothelial growth factor levels in active pulmonary tuberculosis. *Chest*.(2004) 125:2156–9. doi: 10.1378/chest.125.6.2156

66. Ota M, Mendy J, Donkor S, Togun T, Daramy M, Gomez M, et al. Rapid diagnosis of tuberculosis using *ex vivo* host biomarkers in sputum. *Eur Respir J*. (2014) 44:254–7. doi: 10.1183/09031936.00209913

67. Kumar NP, Banurekha VV, Nair D, Babu S. Circulating angiogenic factors as biomarkers of disease severity and bacterial burden in pulmonary tuberculosis. *PLoS ONE*. (2016) 11:e0146318. doi: 10.1371/journal.pone.0146318

68. Torraca V, Tulotta C, Snaar-Jagalska BE, Meijer AH. The chemokine receptor CXCR4 promotes granuloma formation by sustaining a mycobacteria-induced angiogenesis programme. *Sci Rep*. (2017) 7:45061. doi: 10.1038/srep45061

69. Ong CWM, Fox K, Ettorre A, Elkington PT, Friedland JS. Hypoxia increases neutrophil-driven matrix destruction after exposure to *Mycobacterium tuberculosis*. *Sci Rep*. (2018) 8:11475. doi: 10.1038/s41598-018-29659-1

70. Walmsley SR, Chilvers ER, Thompson AA, Vaughan K, Marriott HM, Parker LC, et al. Prolyl hydroxylase 3 (PHD3) is essential for hypoxic regulation of neutrophilic inflammation in humans and mice. *J Clin Invest*. (2011) 121:1053–63. doi: 10.1172/JCI43273

71. Thompson AA, Elks PM, Marriott HM, Eamsamarng S, Higgins KR, Lewis A, et al. Hypoxia-inducible factor 2α regulates key neutrophil functions in humans, mice, and zebrafish. *Blood*. (2014) 123:366–76. doi: 10.1182/blood-2013-05-500207

72. Walmsley SR, Print C, Farahi N, Peyssonnaux C, Johnson RS, Cramer T, et al. Hypoxia-induced neutrophil survival is mediated by HIF-1α-dependent NF-kappaB activity. *J Exp Med*. (2005) 201:105–15. doi: 10.1084/jem.20040624

73. Elks PM, Brizee S, van der Vaart M, Walmsley SR, van Eeden FJ, Renshaw SA, et al. Hypoxia inducible factor signaling modulates susceptibility to mycobacterial infection via a nitric oxide dependent mechanism. *PLoS Pathog*. (2013) 9:e1003789. doi: 10.1371/journal.ppat.1003789

74. Hoenderdos K, Lodge KM, Hirst RA, Chen C, Palazzo SG, Emerenciana A, et al. Hypoxia upregulates neutrophil degranulation and potential for tissue injury. *Thorax*. (2016) 71:1030–8. doi: 10.1136/thoraxjnl-2015-207604

75. Elks PM, van Eeden FJ, Dixon G, Wang X, Reyes-Aldasoro CC, Ingham PW, et al. Activation of hypoxia-inducible factor-1α (Hif-1α) delays inflammation resolution by reducing neutrophil apoptosis and reverse migration in a zebrafish inflammation model. *Blood*. (2011) 118:712–22. doi: 10.1182/blood-2010-12-324186

76. McGovern NN, Cowburn AS, Porter L, Walmsley SR, Summers C, Thompson AAR, et al. Hypoxia selectively inhibits respiratory burst activity and killing of *Staphylococcus aureus* in human neutrophils. *J Immunol*. (2011) 186:453–63. doi: 10.4049/jimmunol.1002213

77. Hammami A, Abidin BM, Charpentier T, Fabie A, Duguay AP, Heinonen KM, et al. HIF-1α is a key regulator in potentiating suppressor activity and limiting the microbicidal capacity of MDSC-like cells during visceral leishmaniasis. *PLoS Pathog*. (2017) 13:e1006616. doi: 10.1371/journal.ppat.1006616

78. Etna MP, Giacomini E, Severa M, Coccia EM. Pro- and anti-inflammatory cytokines in tuberculosis: a two-edged sword in TB pathogenesis. *Semin Immunol.* (2014) 26:543–51. doi: 10.1016/j.smim.2014.09.011

79. Domingo-Gonzalez R, Prince O, Cooper A, Khader SA. Cytokines and chemokines in *Mycobacterium tuberculosis* infection. *Microbiol Spectr.* (2016) 4:1–37. doi: 10.1128/microbiolspec.TBTB2-0018-2016

80. Braverman J, Stanley SA. Nitric oxide modulates macrophage responses to *Mycobacterium tuberculosis* infection through activation of HIF-1α and repression of NF-kappaB. *J Immunol.* (2017) 199:1805–16. doi: 10.4049/jimmunol.1700515

81. Ogryzko NV, Lewis A, Wilson HL, Meijer AH, Renshaw SA, Elks PM. Hif-1α-induced expression of Il-1β protects against mycobacterial infection in zebrafish. *J Immunol.* (2019) 202:494–502. doi: 10.4049/jimmunol.1801139

82. Chao WC, Yen CL, Hsieh CY, Huang YF, Tseng YL, Nigrovic PA, et al. Mycobacterial infection induces higher interleukin-1β and dysregulated lung inflammation in mice with defective leukocyte NADPH oxidase. *PLoS ONE.* (2017) 12:e0189453. doi: 10.1371/journal.pone.0189453

83. Warnatsch A, Tsourouktsoglou TD, Branzk N, Wang Q, Reincke S, Herbst S, et al. Reactive oxygen species localization programs inflammation to clear microbes of different size. *Immunity.* (2017) 46:421–32. doi: 10.1016/j.immuni.2017.02.013

84. Mishra BB, Rathinam VA, Martens GW, Martinot AJ, Kornfeld H, Fitzgerald KA, et al. Nitric oxide controls the immunopathology of tuberculosis by inhibiting NLRP3 inflammasome-dependent processing of IL-1β. *Nat Immunol.* (2013) 14:52–60. doi: 10.1038/ni.2474

85. Di Paolo NC, Shafiani S, Day T, Papayannopoulou T, Russell DW, Iwakura Y, et al. Interdependence between interleukin-1 and tumor necrosis factor regulates TNF-dependent control of *Mycobacterium tuberculosis* infection. *Immunity.* (2015) 43:1125–36. doi: 10.1016/j.immuni.2015.11.016

86. Dorhoi A, Yeremeev V, Nouailles G, Weiner JIII, Jorg S, Heinemann E, et al. Type I IFN signaling triggers immunopathology in tuberculosis-susceptible mice by modulating lung phagocyte dynamics. *Eur J Immunol.* (2014) 44:2380–93. doi: 10.1002/eji.201344219

87. Wiens KE, Ernst JD. The mechanism for type I interferon induction by *Mycobacterium tuberculosis* is bacterial strain-dependent. *PLoS Pathog.* (2016) 12:e1005809. doi: 10.1371/journal.ppat.1005809

88. McNab FW, Ewbank J, Howes A, Moreira-Teixeira L, Martirosyan A, Ghilardi N, et al. Type I IFN induces IL-10 production in an IL-27-independent manner and blocks responsiveness to IFN-γ for production of IL-12 and bacterial killing in *Mycobacterium tuberculosis*-infected macrophages. *J Immunol.* (2014) 193:3600–12. doi: 10.4049/jimmunol.1401088

89. Pylaeva E, Lang S, Jablonska J. The essential role of type I interferons in differentiation and activation of tumor-associated neutrophils. *Front Immunol.* (2016) 7:629. doi: 10.3389/fimmu.2016.00629

90. Mayer-Barber KD, Andrade BB, Oland SD, Amaral EP, Barber DL, Gonzales J, et al. Host-directed therapy of tuberculosis based on interleukin-1 and type I interferon crosstalk. *Nature.* (2014) 511:99–103. doi: 10.1038/nature13489

91. Karuppagounder S, Zhai Y, Chen Y, He R, Ratan R. The interferon response as a common final pathway for many preconditioning stimuli: unexpected crosstalk between hypoxic adaptation and antiviral defense. *Condition. Med.* (2018) 1:143–50. Available online at: http://www.conditionmed.org/Data/View/1626

92. Yeh YH, Hsiao HF, Yeh YC, Chen TW, Li TK. Inflammatory interferon activates HIF-1α-mediated epithelial-to-mesenchymal transition via PI3K/AKT/mTOR pathway. *J Exp Clin Cancer Res.* (2018) 37:70. doi: 10.1186/s13046-018-0730-6

93. Xia P, Wang S, Ye B, Du Y, Huang G, Zhu P, et al. Sox2 functions as a sequence-specific DNA sensor in neutrophils to initiate innate immunity against microbial infection. *Nat Immunol.* (2015) 16:366–75. doi: 10.1038/ni.3117

94. Yu Z, Chen T, Cao X. Neutrophil sensing of cytoplasmic, pathogenic DNA in a cGAS–STING-independent manner. *Cell Mol Immunol.* (2015) 13:411–4. doi: 10.1038/cmi.2015.34

95. Zilio S, Serafini P. Neutrophils and granulocytic MDSC: the janus god of cancer immunotherapy. *Vaccines.* (2016) 4:E31. doi: 10.3390/vaccines4030031

96. Kiss M, Van Gassen S, Movahedi K, Saeys Y, Laoui D. Myeloid cell heterogeneity in cancer: not a single cell alike. *Cell Immunol.* (2018) 330:188–201. doi: 10.1016/j.cellimm.2018.02.008

97. Martineau AR, Newton SM, Wilkinson KA, Kampmann B, Hall BM, Nawroly N, et al. Neutrophil-mediated innate immune resistance to mycobacteria. *J Clin Invest.* (2007) 117:1988–94. doi: 10.1172/JCI31097

98. Okamoto Yoshida Y, Umemura M, Yahagi A, O'Brien RL, Ikuta K, Kishihara K, et al. Essential role of IL-17A in the formation of a mycobacterial infection-induced granuloma in the lung. *J Immunol.* (2010) 184:4414–22. doi: 10.4049/jimmunol.0903332

99. Umemura M, Yahagi A, Hamada S, Begum M, Watanabe H, Kawakami K, et al. IL-17-mediated regulation of innate and acquired immune response against pulmonary Mycobacterium bovis bacille Calmette-Guerin infection. *J Immunol.* (2007) 178:3786–96. doi: 10.4049/jimmunol.178.6.3786

100. Triner D, Xue X, Schwartz AJ, Jung I, Colacino JA, Shah YM. Epithelial hypoxia-inducible factor 2α facilitates the progression of colon tumors through recruiting neutrophils. *Mol Cell Biol.* 37:e00481-16. doi: 10.1128/MCB.00481-16

101. Blaisdell A, Crequer A, Columbus D, Daikoku T, Mittal K, Dey SK, et al. Neutrophils oppose uterine epithelial carcinogenesis via debridement of hypoxic tumor cells. *Cancer Cell.* (2015) 28:785–99. doi: 10.1016/j.ccell.2015.11.005

102. Rodriguez P, Quiceno D, Zabaleta J, Ortiz B, Zea A, Piazuelo M, et al. Arginase I production in the tumor microenvironment by mature myeloid cells inhibits T-cell receptor expression and antigen-specific T-cell responses. *Cancer Res.* (2004) 64:5839–49. doi: 10.1158/0008-5472.CAN-04-0465

103. Hurt B, Schulick R, Edil B, El Kasmi KC, Barnett C Jr. Cancer-promoting mechanisms of tumor-associated neutrophils. *Am J Surg.* (2017) 214:938–44. doi: 10.1016/j.amjsurg.2017.08.003

104. El Kasmi KC, Qualls JE, Pesce JT, Smith AM, Thompson RW, Henao-Tamayo M, et al. Toll-like receptor-induced arginase 1 in macrophages thwarts effective immunity against intracellular pathogens. *Nat Immunol.* (2008) 9:1399–406. doi: 10.1038/ni.1671

105. Monin L, Griffiths KL, Lam WY, Gopal R, Kang DD, Ahmed M, et al. Helminth-induced arginase-1 exacerbates lung inflammation and disease severity in tuberculosis. *J Clin Invest.* (2015) 125:4699–713. doi: 10.1172/JCI77378

106. Pessanha AP, Martins RA, Mattos-Guaraldi AL, Vianna A, Moreira LO. Arginase-1 expression in granulomas of tuberculosis patients. *FEMS Immunol Med Microbiol.* (2012) 66:265–8. doi: 10.1111/j.1574-695X.2012.01012.x

107. Bekes EM, Schweighofer B, Kupriyanova TA, Zajac E, Ardi VC, Quigley JP, et al. Tumor-recruited neutrophils and neutrophil TIMP-free MMP-9 regulate coordinately the levels of tumor angiogenesis and efficiency of malignant cell intravasation. *Am J Pathol.* (2011) 179:1455–70. doi: 10.1016/j.ajpath.2011.05.031

108. Deryugina EI, Zajac E, Juncker-Jensen A, Kupriyanova TA, Welter L, Quigley JP. Tissue-infiltrating neutrophils constitute the major *in vivo* source of angiogenesis-inducing MMP-9 in the tumor microenvironment. *Neoplasia.* (2014) 16:771–88. doi: 10.1016/j.neo.2014.08.013

109. Houghton AM, Rzymkiewicz DM, Ji H, Gregory AD, Egea EE, Metz HE, et al. Neutrophil elastase-mediated degradation of IRS-1 accelerates lung tumor growth. *Nat Med.* (2010) 16:219–23. doi: 10.1038/nm.2084

110. Ong CW, Elkington PT, Brilha S, Ugarte-Gil C, Tome-Esteban MT, Tezera LB, et al. Neutrophil-derived MMP-8 drives AMPK-dependent matrix destruction in human pulmonary tuberculosis. *PLoS Pathog.* (2015) 11:e1004917. doi: 10.1371/journal.ppat.1004917

111. Elkington PT, Ugarte-Gil CA, Friedland JS. Matrix metalloproteinases in tuberculosis. *Eur Respir J.* (2011) 38:456–64. doi: 10.1183/09031936.00015411

112. Abadie V, Badell E, Douillard P, Ensergueix D, Leenen PJ, Tanguy M, et al. Neutrophils rapidly migrate via lymphatics after *Mycobacterium bovis* BCG intradermal vaccination and shuttle live bacilli to the draining lymph nodes. *Blood.* (2005) 106:1843–50. doi: 10.1182/blood-2005-03-1281

113. Qualls JE, Murray PJ. Immunometabolism within the tuberculosis granuloma: amino acids, hypoxia, and cellular respiration. *Semin Immunopathol.* (2016) 38:139–52. doi: 10.1007/s00281-015-0534-0

114. Balamurugan K. HIF-1 at the crossroads of hypoxia, inflammation, and cancer. *Int J Cancer.* (2016) 138:1058–66. doi: 10.1002/ijc.29519

115. Ndlovu H, Marakalala MJ. Granulomas and inflammation: host-directed therapies for tuberculosis. *Front Immunol.* (2016) 7:434. doi: 10.3389/fimmu.2016.00434

# 9

# Recombinant BCG Vaccines Reduce Pneumovirus-Caused Airway Pathology by Inducing Protective Humoral Immunity

Jorge A. Soto[1†], Nicolás M. S. Gálvez[1†], Claudia A. Rivera[1], Christian E. Palavecino[1], Pablo F. Céspedes[1], Emma Rey-Jurado[1], Susan M. Bueno[1] and Alexis M. Kalergis[1,2]*

[1] Departamento de Genética Molecular Microbiología, Facultad de Ciencias Biológicas, Millennium Institute of Immunology and Immunotherapy, Pontificia Universidad Católica de Chile, Santiago, Chile, [2] Departamento de Endocrinología, Facultad de Medicina, Pontificia Universidad Católica de Chile, Santiago, Chile

*Correspondence:
Alexis M. Kalergis
akalergis@bio.puc.cl

† These authors have contributed equally in this work

The Human Respiratory Syncytial Virus (hRSV) and the Human Metapneumovirus (hMPV) are two pneumoviruses that are leading agents causing acute lower respiratory tract infections (ALRTIs) affecting young infants, the elderly, and immunocompromised patients worldwide. Since these pathogens were first discovered, many approaches for the licensing of safe and effective vaccines have been explored being unsuccessful to date. We have previously described that immunization with recombinant strains of *Mycobacterium bovis* Bacillus Calmette-Guérin (rBCG) expressing the hRSV nucleoprotein (rBCG-N) or the hMPV phosphoprotein (rBCG-P) induced immune protection against each respective virus. These vaccines efficiently promoted viral clearance without significant lung damage, mainly through the induction of a T helper 1 cellular immunity. Here we show that upon viral challenge, rBCG-immunized mice developed a protective humoral immunity, characterized by production of antibodies specific for most hRSV and hMPV proteins. Further, isotype switching from IgG1 to IgG2a was observed in mice immunized with rBCG vaccines and correlated with an increased viral clearance, as compared to unimmunized animals. Finally, sera obtained from animals immunized with rBCG vaccines and infected with their respective viruses exhibited virus neutralizing capacity and protected *naïve* mice from viral replication and pulmonary disease. These results support the notion that the use of rBCG strains could be considered as an effective vaccination approach against other respiratory viruses with similar biology as hRSV and hMPV.

Keywords: hRSV, hMPV, antibodies, humoral immune response, vaccine, respiratory virus, BCG

## INTRODUCTION

For almost a century, *Mycobacterium bovis* Bacillus Calmette-Guérin (BCG) has been widely used to prevent Tuberculosis and has also been characterized as an effective T helper type 1 (Th1) inducer (1). Further, BCG has been shown to be safe in adults, infants, and newborns. The approach of using BCG as a vector for recombinant expression of heterologous antigens has been previously tested for several pathogens, such as measles virus, rotavirus, hepatitis B virus, *Plasmodium yoelii*, *Bordetella pertussis*, and *Toxoplasma gondii*, exhibiting promising results in mouse models for those diseases (2–7).

Worldwide, human Respiratory Syncytial Virus (hRSV) is the leading cause of acute lower respiratory tract infections (ALRTIs). HRSV was first identified in 1956 and mainly afflicts infants, young children, elderly, and immunocompromised patients, causing about 34 millions of ALRTIs and ~200,000 deaths per year (8). Next to hRSV, human Metapneumovirus (hMPV) is the second cause of ALRTIs (9) and was first identified in 2001 (10). Although the overall burden in hospitalization remains poorly characterized for hMPV, as it was recently identified, it has been estimated that about a 7–19% of children hospitalization can be due solely to this virus (11, 12). Furthermore, clinical studies have shown that by the age of 5, virtually every child has been infected with both of these viruses, exhibiting classical ALRTI manifestations, which include fever, cough, wheezing, and some clinical manifestation like bronchiolitis, laryngotracheitis, acute bronchitis, and pneumonia (8, 10–14) with an increase in the mucus production, obstruction of bronchoalveolar spaces, exacerbated inflammatory response, and the generation of airway hyper-responsiveness (15–17). In addition, prospective surveillance studies have suggested that children affected by severe hMPV infections usually require longer recovery periods at intensive care units than do children infected with hRSV (11–14). Both hRSV and hMPV are RNA single-stranded, negative sense enveloped viruses, belonging to the *Pneumoviridae* family, particularly the *Orthopneumovirus* genus and the *Metapneumovirus* genus, respectively (15). Furthermore, hRSV has been recently renamed as human Orthopneumovirus (15).

Some reports have suggested that the host immune system is unable to generate an effective and protective immunological memory against either of these viruses, which after disease resolution, prompts the acquisition of repeated infections throughout life (18, 19). Accordingly, it has been described that the nucleoprotein of hRSV (N-hRSV) is able to inhibit the assembly of an effective immunological synapse, apparently by clustering with the pMHC-TCR complex (20). Also, N-hRSV blunts the interferon response by interacting with MDA5 and MAVS, pivotal elements in the main pathways associated with the viral clearance (21). On the other hand, the phosphoprotein of hMPV (P-hMPV) has been described as a crucial component for the assembly of the virus replication core (22). It has been reported that P of hMPV-B1 serotype could interfere with the RIG-I pathway, prompting the inhibition of the interferon I pathway (23). Considering this, both proteins have been previously suggested as possible candidate antigens for the induction of a strong and protective cellular immune response against either hRSV or hMPV infections when used for immunization, respectively (24, 25).

Our group has previously reported that recombinant BCG strains (rBCG) expressing either N-hRSV (rBCG-N) or P-hMPV (rBCG-P) as heterologous antigens, can protect against infection by hRSV or hMPV, respectively (24, 25). In this work, we evaluated the previously unexplored humoral immune response induced in mice immunized with either rBCG-N and rBCG-P. We observed that the post-challenge antibody response is enhanced by the established immunity elicited by both rBCG vaccines (rBCG-N or rBCG-P). This concerted response was able to significantly decrease viral replication and disease by promoting the secretion of neutralizing antibodies specific against the attachment and the fusion glycoproteins of both paramyxoviruses. These results suggest that rBCG strains are good vaccine candidates able to induce a cellular immune response capable of boosting the humoral immune response against unrelated antigens and to prevent the disease cause by both pneumoviruses.

## MATERIALS AND METHODS

### hRSV and hMPV Propagation and Titration

HEp-2 cells (American Type Culture Collection, CCL-23™) and LLC-MK2 (American Type Culture Collection, CCL-7™) were used to propagate hRSV serogroup A2, strain 13018–8 (clinical isolate obtained from the *Instituto de Salud Pública de Chile*) and hMPV serogroup A, strain CZ0107 (clinical isolate obtained from the *Laboratorio de Infectología y Virología* of the *Hospital Clínico, Pontificia Universidad Católica de Chile*) (26, 27). Briefly, cell monolayers were grown in T75 flasks with DMEM (Life Technologies Invitrogen, Carlsbad, CA) supplemented with 10% FBS (Gibco Invitrogen Corp, Carlsbad) for HEp-2 cells and Opti-MEM supplemented with 5% FBS for LLC-MK2 cells, until 80–90% confluence. Flasks containing 5 mL of infection medium [DMEM 1% FBS for hRSV and Opti-MEM 5% FBS medium, supplemented with $CaCl_2$ (100 μg/mL) for hMPV] were inoculated with $2 \times 10^5$ Plaque formation units (PFU) of the respective virus and incubated at 37°C. After viral adsorption (2 h), supernatants were replaced with fresh medium (DMEM 1% FBS and Opti-MEM) and incubated for 48 h for hRSV and 72 h for hMPV, until visible cytopathic effect was observed. For harvesting, cells were scraped, and the flask content was pooled and centrifuged first at $300 \times g$ for 10 min and then at $500 \times g$ for 10 min in order to remove cell debris. In parallel, supernatants of non-infected cells monolayers (HEp-2 and LLC-MK2) were collected as previously described and used as non-infectious control (Mock). Viral titers of supernatants were determined by immunocytochemistry in 96-well plates with HEp-2 and LLC-MK2 cells monolayers, as previously described (26–29). hRSV and hMPV inoculums were routinely evaluated for lipopolysaccharide and *Mycoplasma* contamination.

### Doses of BCG-WT, rBCG-N, and rBCG-P for Immunization

Vaccine doses of BCG-WT (Danish 1331 strain), rBCG-N, and rBCG-P (both of them obtained as previously described (24, 25) were prepared by growing the mycobacteria on 7H9 liquid medium (Sigma-Aldrich, M0178-500G), supplemented with 10% OADC (Sigma-Aldrich, M0678-1VL) and Kanamycin only for the recombinant bacteria [20 μg/mL] (Sigma-Aldrich, 60615), until reaching an OD600 equal to 0.8. Then, the mycobacteria cultures were washed three times with 1X PBS-0.05% Tween 80, resuspended with 1X PBS-glycerol 50% at a final concentration of $4 \times 10^8$ CFU per vial and frozen at −80°C until their use. For immunization, vials were centrifuged at 14,000 g and resuspended in saline solution prior to injection.

## Dot-Blot Assays

Lysates obtained from BCG-WT and rBCG strains expressing either N-hRSV or the P-hMPV, as well as purified N and P proteins as positive controls and 1X PBS as a negative control, were spotted into nitrocellulose membranes. Loaded membranes were incubated for 1 h at 4°C. Membranes were then blocked with a solution 1X PBS and 5% non-fat milk solution for 2 h at RT. Then, membranes were incubated for 1 h with an hRSV anti-N protein monoclonal antibody (1E9/D1 clone 1.48 mg/mL) and hMPV anti-P protein polyclonal antibody (6B12 clone 1.2 mg/mL) diluted in 1X PBS and 5% non-fat milk at a final dilution for both antibodies of 1:750. As a secondary antibody, an HRP-Goat anti-mouse IgG (H+L) (1.5 mg/mL) (Life Technologies, N. Meridian rd., Rockford, IL 61101, USA) was used diluted in 1X PBS, 5% non-fat milk, at a final dilution of 1:2,000, for 1 h. Membranes were washed with 1X PBS, 0.05% Tween 20, three times after every step. Finally, membranes were incubated with the HRP Chemiluminescent Substrate (Invitrogen, Carlsbad, CA 92008, USA) and proteins were visualized with the gel documenter myECL Imager (ThermoFischer Scientific).

## Mouse Immunization and Viral Infection

Six to eight-week-old BALB/cJ mice received a sub-cutaneous injection in the right dorsal flank with $1 \times 10^8$ CFU of BCG WT or rBCG strains expressing N-hRSV or P-hMPV, respectively, in a final volume of 100 μL per dose ($n = 6$ per group) (**Figures 2A,G**). After 14 days, mice were boosted with the respective BCG strain. Twenty-one days post immunization, mice were intraperitoneally anesthetized with a mixture of ketamine and xylazine (80 and 4 mg/kg, respectively), and challenged by intranasal instillation with $\sim 1 \times 10^7$ PFU of hRSV A2, strain 13018-8 or $\sim 1 \times 10^6$ PFU of hMPV A, strain CZ0107, accordingly to the vaccine injected, in a final volume of <100 μL per mouse. Blood samples were obtained from these animals before immunization, boost, challenge, and at 7 days post-infection (dpi) and 14 dpi. For hRSV infected mice, lung samples, and Bronchoalveolar Lavage (BAL) were obtained at 7 and 14 dpi. For hMPV-infected mice, blood samples, lung samples, and BAL were obtained at 28 dpi, and 21 days post re-infection with $\sim 1 \times 10^6$ PFU of hMPV (49 dpi). All animals were treated and manipulated with supervision of a veterinarian and according to the institutional guidelines of the Pontificia Universidad Católica de Chile and the "Guide for the care and use of laboratory animals".

## Quantification of IgG Isotypes

Ninety-six well ELISA plates were separately coated with the following antigens overnight at 4°C: 50 μL/well of hRSV or hMPV (previously UV-inactivated for 45 min and sonicated by 10 min to expose as many antigens as possible), 100 ng/well of N-hRSV purified protein or 100 ng/well of F-, G- and P-hRSV proteins (SinoBiological, Beijing, China). For hMPV ELISA, plates were coated with 200 ng/well of P-, M-, and M2.1- proteins purified.

Plates were blocked with 200 μL of 1X PBS, 2% Fish gelatine. After 1 h at RT, plates were washed three times with 200 μL of 1X PBS, 0.05% Tween 20 and incubated for 1 h at RT with 100

μL of the different serum samples previously diluted at 1:500 in triplicate (14 dpi for hRSV and 28 dpi for hMPV). Then, the plates were washed three times and incubated with 50 μL of 1:2,000 dilution of HRP-Goat anti-mouse IgG (H+L) (Life Technologies, N. Meridian rd., Rockford, IL 61101, USA) for 1 h at RT. Afterwards, plates were washed and revealed with 50 μL of 1 mg/mL 3-39-5-59-tetramethylbenzidine (TMB, Merck) at RT in the darkness. After 10 min, 50 μL of $H_2SO_4$ solution were added to stop the reaction. Plates were analyzed in an ELISA reader at 450 nm (Multiskan Ex, Thermo Labsystems).

Immunoglobulin isotypes were also analyzed from the same sera samples in similar conditions. 96-well ELISA plates were coated overnight at 4°C with 50 μL of hRSV or hMPV, previously UV-inactivated by 45 min and sonicated by 10 min. After blocking and washing as previously described, the plates were incubated with 50 μL of 1:500 dilution of sera sample in triplicate (14 dpi for hRSV and 49 dpi for hMPV) 1 h at RT. Biotinylated Rat anti-Mouse IgG2a (Clone RMG2a-62, Biolegend, San Diego, CA) and IgG1 (Clone RMG1-1, Biolegend, San Diego, CA) antibodies were used to assess the titers of circulating anti-hRSV IgG isotype in vaccinated and control mice. Plates were read at 450 nm and data was represented as a ratio of the IgG2a concentration/IgG1 concentration. The concentration of different IgG, IgG1, and IgG2a isotypes, was measured interpolating the absorbance values in a curve of mice purified IgG-antibody. The production of the hybridomes was made by GrupoBios, Chile.

## Determination of Linked Recognition Mechanism

Six to eight-week-old BALB/cJ mice received a sub-cutaneous injection in the right dorsal flank with $1 \times 10^8$ CFU of either BCG WT or rBCG-N strains ($n = 5$ for each group). Other mice were immunized with purified N-hRSV protein in Freund adjuvant or purified N-hRSV protein in Aluminum Hydroxide adjuvant (**Supplementary Figure 2**). After 14 days, animals were boosted with the same dose and at day 21 post-immunization, mice were euthanized. Spleens were collected and plated at a final concentration equal to $1 \times 10^6$ cells/mL in 24 well plates. Then, cells were stimulated with purified N-hRSV protein (1 μg/mL) and after 72 h T cells were purified by MACS columns following the manufacturer instructions (mouse CD4$^+$ T cell isolation kit, Miltenyl Biotec). Purified T cells were transferred to a total of 5 naïve mice per group and 1 day post-transfer, animals were either treated with mock or infected with hRSV. Animal body weight loss was monitored and at 7 dpi mice were euthanized (Data not shown). Sera samples were used to measure antibody secretion against the whole virus and the N, F, and G hRSV proteins by indirect ELISA, as described above.

## Serum Neutralization Assays

HEp-2 or LLC-MK2 cells were grown until 80–90% of confluence. Then, the sera from 14 dpi in the hRSV-infected animals or 21 days post-second infection (49 dpi) in the hMPV-infected animals were pooled and incubated at 56°C for 30 min to inactivate the complement system. Sera were then incubated with GFP-recombinant viruses (hRSV or hMPV), respectively, at 37°C for 1 h. The mixtures were added to the respective cell culture and incubated for 1 h at 37°C in 5% of $CO_2$ supplement. Then supernatants were replaced with fresh DMEM 1% FBS for the HEP-2 cells and Opti-MEM for the LLC-MK2 cells. Cells were incubated for 48 h at 37°C with a 5% of $CO_2$ supplement. GFP expression in both cells was visualized by epifluorescence microscopy and the plaque-forming units (PFU) were quantified as previously described (30). As a positive control, cells were treated with GFP-expressing virus without sera, and as negative control cells were treated with Mock.

## Passive Transfer of Immune IgG From rBCG-Vaccinated Mice to Naive Animals

Six to eight-week-old BALB/cJ mice were intravenously transferred with 100 μg of total IgG from the sera of the following animal groups: non-immunized but hRSV-infected (nt-hRSV), BCG-WT immunized hRSV-infected, rBCG-N immunized hRSV-infected, non-immunized but hMPV-infected (nt-hMPV), BCG-WT hMPV-infected, and rBCG-P immunized hMPV-infected mice ($n = 6$ for each group). Serum samples used for these experiments were collected at 14 dpi (hRSV) and 49 dpi (hMPV). One day after the transfer, animals were intraperitoneally anesthetized with a mixture of ketamine and xylazine (80 and 4 mg/kg, respectively) and challenged by intranasal instillation with $1 \times 10^7$ PFU of hRSV or $1 \times 10^6$ PFU of hMPV, respectively. In both cases, Mock treatments were used as negative control and virus infected non-transferred (nt) as an infection-control. In order to evaluate the effect of the protection, animals were immunized with 100 μg of palivizumab (intraperitoneal route) as a positive antiviral control against hRSV. Weight loss was daily measured in both experiments (Data not shown). At 7 dpi, animals were terminally anesthetized by i.p. injection of a mixture of ketamine and xylazine (20 and 1 mg/kg, respectively) and BALs and lungs were collected.

## Evaluation of hRSV- and hMPV-Associated Disease Parameters

To determine the infiltration of polymorphonuclear cells, BALs were collected as previously described (24). Briefly, lung samples were collected, clamping the non-lobed section of the lung, stored in 4% PFA and later used to histological analyzes, as previously described (24). A lower section of the lobate lung was collected and stored in TRIzol (Life Technologies), and the RNA was extracted following the manufacture conditions. The rest of the lung was collected and incubated with collagenase IV for 30 min at 37°C, then PBS-1X/1%FBS was added to stop the collagenase reaction. Lung samples were homogenized using a 70 μm cell strainer (BD Biosciences) and centrifugated at 0.3 g for 5 min at 4°C. Supernatants were discarded, and pellets were incubated for 5 min with an ACK solution at RT. The cells were washed with PBS/1%FBS and centrifuged once again. Finally, samples were resuspended in 1 mL of PBS/1%FBS and used for flow cytometry. BAL samples were collected by gently instilling 1 mL of PBS with a tuberculin syringe through the trachea of the animals and subsequently recovered (twice), while the lung was pinched. The final volume was centrifuged at 0.3 g for 5 min at 4°C.

Supernatant was stored at −80°C and pellets were resuspended in 300 μL of PBS/1%FBS. Finally, the cells from Lungs and BALs were incubated in 96 six-well plates and centrifugated at 0.3 g for 5 min at 4°C, then the samples were stained with anti–CD11b PerCP-Cy 5.5 (clone M1/70, BD Pharmingen), anti–CD11c APC (clone HL3, BD Pharmingen), and anti-Ly6G FITC (Clone 1A8, BD Pharmingen) antibodies. Data were acquired on FACSCanto II cytometer (BD Biosciences) and analyzed using FlowJo v10.0.7 software (BD Biosciences). Viral loads were detected in the lungs by qRT-PCR as previously described (24, 25). Also, lung samples were stored in 4% PFA, maintained at 4°C, embedded in paraffin, cut, and stained with H&E as previously described (24).

## Statistical Analyses

All statistical analyses were performed using GraphPad Prism version 6.0 Software. Statistical significance was assessed using One-way ANOVA with a posteriori Tukey test or Two-way ANOVA test with a posteriori Tukey test.

# RESULTS

## rBCG-N and rBCG-P Vaccines Are Able to Reduce Disease-Associated Parameters Caused by hRSV or hMPV Infection

The expression of the hRSV N protein or the hMPV P protein in rBCG-N or rBCG-P strains, respectively, was corroborated by dot blot assays. Both recombinant BCG strains expressed significant amounts of the respective proteins, as compared to negative and BCG-WT controls (**Supplementary Figure 1**).

The hRSV- and hMPV-associated disease parameters were evaluated post-immunization to evaluate the protective capacity of the rBCG strains against each respective viral infection (**Figure 1**). The immunization scheme is described at the Materials and Methods section (Mouse immunization and viral infection) and is also shown in **Figure 2A**. As shown in **Figure 1A**, infection with $1 \times 10^7$ PFU of hRSV induces body weight loss in all infected animals 1 day post-infection (dpi). Importantly, rBCG-N-immunized and hRSV-infected mice started recovering their original body weight at 2 dpi and recovered their original body weight by day 5 pi. On the contrary, the non-immunized and hRSV-infected group (hRSV) was not able to recover their initial weight by 7 dpi.

Likewise, as seen for the rBCG-N immunized and hRSV-infected mice (rBCG-N+hRSV), vaccination was able to drastically decrease viral loads in the lungs of the hRSV-infected animals as compared to the non-immunized but infected group (hRSV) (**Figure 1B**). Further, the BCG-WT immunized and hRSV-infected mice (BCG-WT+ hRSV) showed a significant decrease in the viral loads, as compared to hRSV mice, although this decrease was less pronounced than the observed for the rBCG-N+hRSV mice (**Figure 1B**). Remarkably, the number of BAL neutrophils (CD11b$^+$ Ly6G$^+$ cells) infiltrating the lungs of rBCG-N-vaccinated animals was lower than those vaccinated with BCG-WT or hRSV-infected, naïve mice (**Figure 1C**).

A similar protective response was found for the hMPV-infected animals with a similar body weight loss and recovery

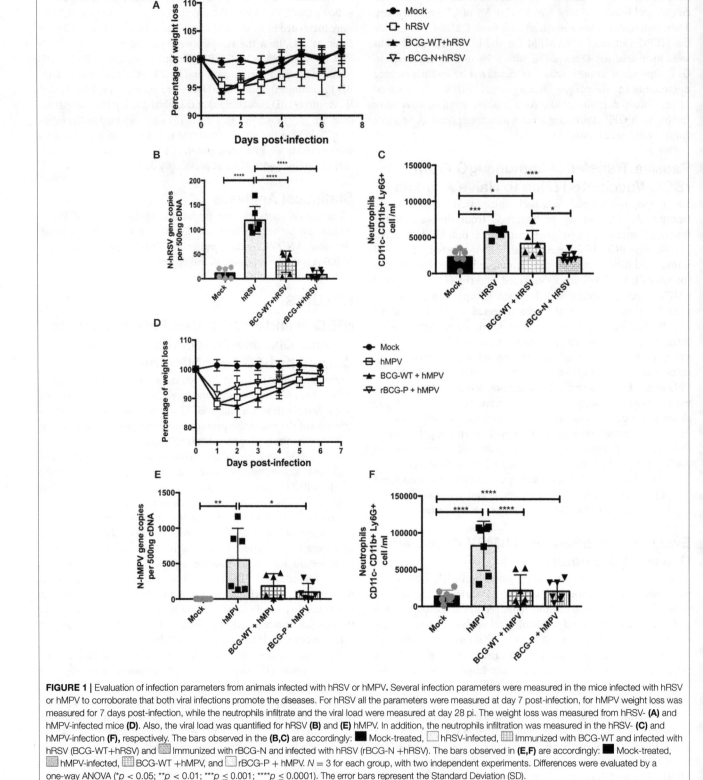

**FIGURE 1 |** Evaluation of infection parameters from animals infected with hRSV or hMPV. Several infection parameters were measured in the mice infected with hRSV or hMPV to corroborate that both viral infections promote the diseases. For hRSV all the parameters were measured at day 7 post-infection, for hMPV weight loss was measured for 7 days post-infection, while the neutrophils infiltrate and the viral load were measured at day 28 pi. The weight loss was measured from hRSV- **(A)** and hMPV-infected mice **(D)**. Also, the viral load was quantified for hRSV **(B)** and **(E)** hMPV. In addition, the neutrophils infiltration was measured in the hRSV- **(C)** and hMPV-infection **(F)**, respectively. The bars observed in the **(B,C)** are accordingly: ■ Mock-treated, ☐ hRSV-infected, ▦ Immunized with BCG-WT and infected with hRSV (BCG-WT+hRSV) and ▨ Immunized with rBCG-N and infected with hRSV (rBCG-N +hRSV). The bars observed in **(E,F)** are accordingly: ■ Mock-treated, ▦ hMPV-infected, ▦ BCG-WT +hMPV, and ☐ rBCG-P + hMPV. $N = 3$ for each group, with two independent experiments. Differences were evaluated by a one-way ANOVA (*$p < 0.05$; **$p < 0.01$; ***$p \leq 0.001$; ****$p \leq 0.0001$). The error bars represent the Standard Deviation (SD).

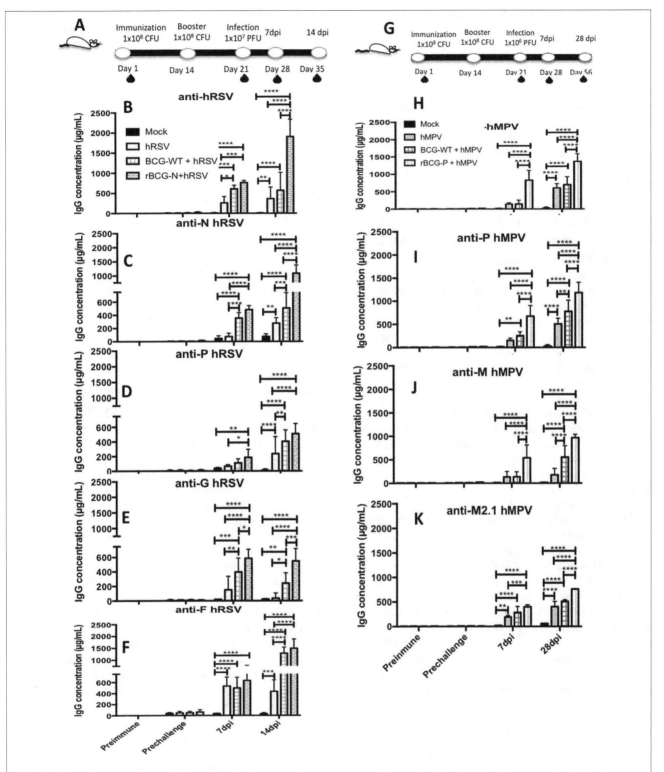

**FIGURE 2** | Evaluation of the induction of IgG specific-antibodies against viral antigens after a viral infection. IgG for different antigens were evaluated from the sera obtained at different time points: Prior to immunization (Preimmune), prior to virus infection (Prechallenge), 7 and 14 days post-infection (7 dpi and 14 dpi) for hRSV or 7 dpi and 28 dpi for hMPV, respectively **(A, G)**. Specific antibodies levels were determined by ELISA assay against hRSV **(B)**, N protein **(C)**, P protein **(D)**, G protein **(E)**, F protein **(F)**. Similarly, this same ELISA assays were done against hMPV **(H)**, P protein **(I)**, M2.1 protein **(J)**, and M protein **(K)**. The bars observed in the **(B–F)** are accordingly: ■ Mock-treated, ☐ hRSV-infected, ▦ BCG-WT +hRSV, and ▨ rBCG-N +hRSV. On the other hand, the bars observed in **(H–K)** are accordingly: ■ Mock-treated, ▨ hMPV-infected, ▦ BCG-WT +hMPV, and ☐ rBCG-P +hMPV. The measure was made at 450 nm. The sera from 6 different animals for each group was used for the ELISA assay, with each serum tested in 3 replicates. $N = 3$ for each group, with two independent experiments. Differences were evaluated by a two-way ANOVA ($*p < 0.05$; $**p < 0.01$; $***p \leq 0.001$; $****p \leq 0.0001$). The error bars represent the Standard Deviation (SD).

(**Figure 1D**). Also, the rBCG-P immunized and hMPV-infected mice (rBCG-P+hMPV) showed a significant decrease in viral loads as compared to the non-immunized and hMPV-infected mice (hMPV) (**Figure 1E**) and a decrease in the number of infiltrating neutrophils in the BALs (**Figure 1F**). Remarkably, no significant differences were detected in the BALs of BCG-WT+hMPV when compared with the hMPV-infected naive mice. Therefore, and as described previously, immunization with recombinant rBCG vaccines significantly decrease disease parameters associated to hRSV and hMPV infection, such as body weight loss, viral loads, and neutrophil infiltration in the lungs.

## Immunization With rBCG Strains Enhances Post-challenge Antibody Responses for Several Viral Proteins

To evaluate whether the immune protection induced by the rBCG vaccines involves a humoral-mediated response, the presence of anti-hRSV or -hMPV antibodies in sera from immunized mice (BCG-WT, rBCG-N, and rBCG-P groups) was measured (**Figure 2**). An increase in the total anti-hRSV antibodies was observed in the rBCG-N+hRSV sera at both 7 and 14 dpi, as compared to all the other treatments (**Figure 2B**). BCG-WT+hRSV treated mice showed a significant increase in anti-hRSV antibodies as compared to mock-treated and the hRSV-infected mice at 14 dpi (**Figure 2B**). However, this increase was not as pronounced as the one observed for the rBCG-N+hRSV treated mice. No significant differences were detected between hRSV- and the mock-treated animals at day 7 post-infection, although there is a clear tendency to an increase in the quantity of IgG.

Since the production of total antibodies against hRSV was significantly higher in infected mice previously immunized with rBCG-N, we measured the specific antibody production against various individual hRSV proteins, such as N, P, G, and F proteins (**Figures 2C–F**). We observed that at 7 and 14 dpi rBCG-N+hRSV treated mice secreted more anti-N antibody as compared with all the other groups (with the exception of the BCG-WT+hRSV group at 7 dpi). At 14 dpi BCG-WT+hRSV also showed an increase in the anti-N antibody secretion, as compared to mock-treated and the hRSV mice (**Figure 2C**). A significantly higher antibody secretion against P-, G-, and F-hRSV proteins was detected at 7 and 14 dpi for the rBCG-N+hRSV treated mice as compared to the mock controls (**Figures 2D–F**). Remarkably, this increase was statistically higher when compared to all the other treatments at 14 dpi, with the exception of BCG-WT+hRSV for the F-protein (**Figure 2F**). The IgG concentration for the F protein was as high as the one detected for the total hRSV antibodies (about 1,500–2,000 µg/mL), indicating that this protein is one of the major antigenic determinants of the virus, accordingly to what has been previously described (31).

When the humoral response induced by the rBCG-P vaccine was evaluated, high antibody titers were observed starting from 28 dpi against total hMPV, P-, M2.1-, and M-proteins for the rBCG-P+hMPV, when compared with all the other

treatments, with the exception of the BCG-WT+hMPV treated mice for the total anti-hMPV (**Figures 2H–K**). Likewise, the BCG-WT+hMPV treated mice also showed significantly higher anti-hMPV antibody titers as compared to the mock-treated mice at 28 dpi (**Figure 2H**). Remarkably, a higher secretion of anti-M antibodies was detected for the rBCG-P+hMPV treated mice as early as 7 dpi, as compared to all the other treatments (**Figure 2J**). Finally, the BCG-WT+hMPV treated mice and the hMPV infected naïve mice showed higher levels of anti-M2.1 antibodies as compared to the mock treated-mice at 28 dpi (**Figures 2I–K**). Again, post-infection IgG levels for all the proteins evaluated was significantly higher in rBCG-P-immunized mice as compared to the other groups, suggesting that the effect was induced by both vaccination and infection.

The low IgG levels detected in the sera from mock-treated mice against both G and F proteins, could be associated with the assay methodology properties, as ELISA may have shown unspecific interactions (**Figure 2**). These results suggest that immunization with rBCG vaccines, upon challenge with the pathogen, is able to promote the secretion of antibodies against several proteins of each respective virus.

## Transfer of Activated N-hRSV Protein-Specific T Cells From Immunized Mice to Challenged Mice Leads to Diversification of the Antibody Response Against Viral Proteins

As shown above, a significant increase in the secretion of antibodies specific against proteins different than those expressed by the rBCG vaccines was detected upon immunization and viral challenge (**Figure 2**). Therefore, to elucidate whether the secretion of antibodies against the different proteins was an effect of either the expressed proteins by themselves or an effect of the vaccine prototypes as a whole, we measured the secretion of antibodies by hRSV-infected mice that were previously adoptively transferred with T cells derived from rBCG-N immunized mice (**Figure 3** and **Supplementary Figure 3**). Briefly, mice were immunized with $1 \times 10^8$ CFU of either BCG-WT or rBCG-N, then at day 14 post-immunization mice were boosted with the same vaccine dose. Unimmunized or mice immunized with purified hRSV Nucleoprotein with either Freund adjuvant or Aluminum Hydroxide adjuvant, were included as controls (**Supplementary Figure 2**). At day 21 after the first immunization, animals were euthanized, spleens were collected and 72 h-long splenocyte cultures were performed stimulating with purified hRSV nucleoprotein. Next, T cells were purified and immediately transferred to *naïve* mice. Animals were then infected and euthanized at 7 dpi, sera were collected, and the secretion of specific antibodies was measured.

We detected that mice receiving T cells from the rBCG-N immunized group and then infected with hRSV (rBCG-N+hRSV) induced the higher antibody secretion against the proteins evaluated, as compared to control animals (**Figure 3**). The anti-hRSV antibody titers were higher in the rBCG-N-transferred mice, exhibiting a significant increase when compared to most of the other groups, except the one

Recombinant BCG Vaccines Reduce Pneumovirus-Caused Airway Pathology by Inducing Protective Humoral...

121

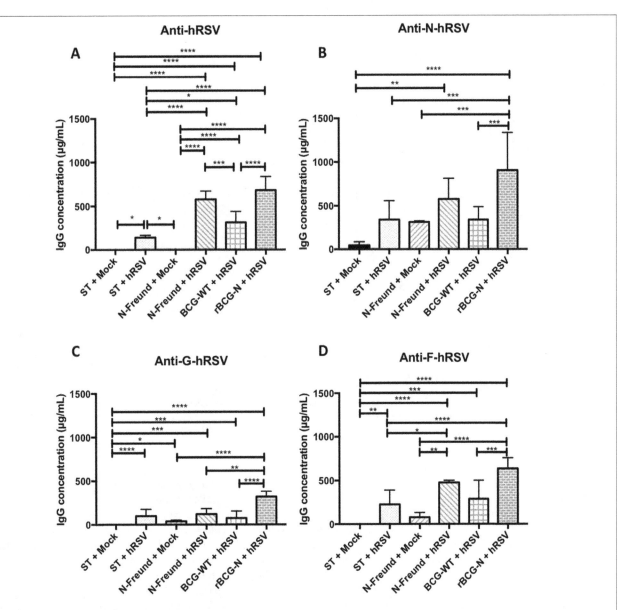

**FIGURE 3** | The rBCG-N vaccine promotes the secretion of antibodies against several antigens through the Linked Recognition mechanism. The secretion of specific antibodies against the whole virus and the N, F, and G hRSV proteins were measured by indirect ELISA from the sera collected of the T cell transferred and infected mice after 7 dpi. The anti- hRSV **(A)**, anti-N-hRSV **(B)**, anti-F-hRSV **(C)** and anti-G-hRSV **(D)** were evaluated and measured at 450 nm. The bars observed in the **(A–D)** are accordingly: ■ Non-transferred and Mock-treated (ST+Mock), □ Non-transferred, and hRSV-infected (ST+hRSV), ▨ T cells transferred from mice immunized with hRSV-N protein in Freund adjuvant, treated with mock (N-Freund+Mock), ▨ T cells transferred from mice immunized with hRSV-N protein in Freund adjuvant, infected with hRSV(N-Freund+hRSV), ▦ T cells transferred from mice immunized with BCG-WT and then infected with hRSV (BCG-WT + hRSV) and ▦ T cells transferred from mice immunized with rBCG-N and then infected with hRSV (rBCG-N +hRSV). The sera from five different animals for each group was used for the ELISA assay, with each serum tested in three replicates. Data combinate from two independent experiment for ST+mock, ST+hRSV, BGC-WT+hRSV and rBCG-N+hRSV groups ($N = 9$), and one independent experiment for N-Freund+Mock, N-Freund+hRSV groups ($N = 5$). Differences were evaluated by a one-way ANOVA (*$p < 0.05$; **$p < 0.01$; ***$p \leq 0.001$; ****$p \leq 0.0001$). The error bars represent the Standard Deviation (SD).

immunized with purified hRSV-N protein with Freund as adjuvant and then infected with hRSV (N-Freund+hRSV), were no significant differences were detected. Remarkably, mice receiving T cells from the BCG-WT immunized and then infected with hRSV (BCG-WT+hRSV) showed no significant differences as compared to the N-Freund group (**Figure 3A**).

A similar response was observed when the anti-N antibody secretion was evaluated, as only rBCG-N+hRSV transferred

mice showed a rise in antibody titers, as compared to all other experimental groups. No significant differences were observed between the mock-treated, hRSV-infected and BCG-WT+hRSV transferred groups (**Figure 3B**). Regarding the other viral proteins, we identified an increase in the anti-F and anti-G antibody secretion for the rBCG-N+hRSV transferred mice as compared to mock-treated mice, whether they were immunized or not (**Figures 3C,D**).

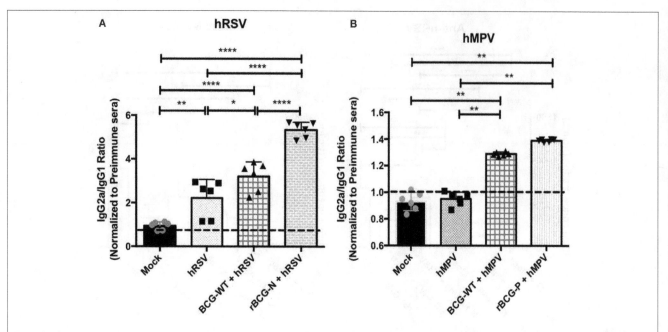

**FIGURE 4 |** The rBCG strains induce a strong IgG2a isotype switching after a viral infection. The secretion of specific antibody isotype IgG2a and IgG1 was measured in both vaccines by indirect ELISA. The assay was done using a total virus extract and expressed as the ratio between the IgG2a and IgG1 in animals infected with hRSV **(A)** and hMPV **(B)**. Secretion of this specific antibody was measured from sera at 14 dpi (hRSV) or 49 dpi (hMPV) using total extract of each virus to incubate the plate. The bars observed in the **(A)** are accordingly: ■ Mock-treated, ▢ hRSV-infected, ▦ BCG-WT +hRSV, and ▧ rBCG-N +hRSV. On the other hand, the bars observed in **(B)** are accordingly: ■ Mock-treated, ▨ hMPV-infected, ▦ BCG-WT +hMPV, and ▢ rBCG-P +hMPV. The measure was made at 450 nm. The sera from six different animals for each group was used for the ELISA assay, with each serum tested in three replicates. $N = 3$ for each group, with two independent experiment. Differences among groups were evaluated by a one-way ANOVA (*$p \leq 0.05$; **$p \leq 0.01$; ***$p \leq 0.001$; ****$p \leq 0.0001$). The error bars represent the Standard Deviation (SD).

As controls, we also included animals immunized with the nucleoprotein of hRSV, along with either the Freund Adjuvant—a Th-1 inducer—or Aluminum hydroxide Adjuvant—a Th-2 inducer (32, 33) (**Supplementary Figures 2, 3**). Remarkably, the total anti-hRSV, anti-F and anti-G antibodies secretion was statistically higher in the mice transferred with the T cells from the animals immunized with the Aluminum hydroxide adjuvant, as compared to all the other groups. This effect was not seen when the specific anti-N antibodies were measured, as the rBCG-N+hRSV transferred animals exhibited a significantly higher antibody secretion as compared to all the groups except for the Aluminum hydroxide (**Supplementary Figure 3**). These results suggest that, although animals are being immunized with a particular antigen, the vaccine elicited T helper response seems to promote the activation of B cells specific for viral antigens beyond those encoded by these recombinant proteins. As such, these data also suggest the normal presentation of nucleoprotein and phosphoprotein peptides by the B cells of hRSV and hMPV infected mice, respectively.

## rBCG Vaccines Induce an Efficient Antibody Class Switching Upon Viral Infection

Since antibody class switching also depends on the help provided by CD4+ T cells, we sought to evaluate whether this phenomenon is also promoted by the cellular immunity induced by rBCG vaccination. Sera obtained from the experimental

groups presented in **Figure 2** were analyzed by ELISA and the IgG2a/IgG1 antibody ratio was determined for virus-specific antibodies. Similar responses were observed for both rBCG vaccines as compared with their respective control groups (**Figure 4**). rBCG-N+hRSV treated mice showed the highest IgG2a/IgG1 ratio for virus-specific IgGs as compared to all of the others control mice (**Figure 4A**). Nevertheless, the BCG-WT+hRSV treated mice also showed an increased IgG2a/IgG1 ratio as compared to mock-treated and hRSV mice, although this rise was not as high as the observed for the sera derived from rBCG-N+hRSV-treated mice (**Figure 4A**). Additionally, the hRSV infected naïve mice only showed an increase in the antibody ratio when compared with the mock-treated animals (**Figure 4A**).

As stated above, a similar pattern was observed in the sera derived from rBCG-P-vaccinated mice (**Figure 4B**). The rBCG-P+hMPV treated mice also showed an increase in the IgG2a/IgG1 antibody ratio, as compared with mock-treated and hMPV infected naïve mice (**Figure 4B**). Further, a higher IgG2a/IgG1 antibody ratio was observed for the BCG-WT+hMPV treated mice as compared to hMPV-infected and mock-treated mice. Remarkably, no differences were detected in the ratio among the sera from mock-treated and hMPV infected naïve mice. These results indicate that antibodies secreted by animals immunized with rBCG vaccines undergo significant isotype switching that may contribute to their viral clearance capacity.

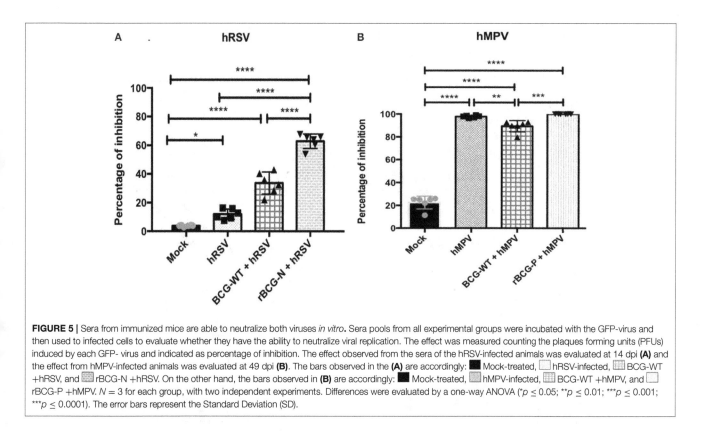

**FIGURE 5 |** Sera from immunized mice are able to neutralize both viruses *in vitro*. Sera pools from all experimental groups were incubated with the GFP-virus and then used to infected cells to evaluate whether they have the ability to neutralize viral replication. The effect was measured counting the plaques forming units (PFUs) induced by each GFP- virus and indicated as percentage of inhibition. The effect observed from the sera of the hRSV-infected animals was evaluated at 14 dpi **(A)** and the effect from hMPV-infected animals was evaluated at 49 dpi **(B)**. The bars observed in the **(A)** are accordingly: ■ Mock-treated, ☐ hRSV-infected, ▦ BCG-WT +hRSV, and ▦ rBCG-N +hRSV. On the other hand, the bars observed in **(B)** are accordingly: ■ Mock-treated, ▦ hMPV-infected, ▦ BCG-WT +hMPV, and ☐ rBCG-P +hMPV. $N = 3$ for each group, with two independent experiments. Differences were evaluated by a one-way ANOVA (*$p \leq 0.05$; **$p \leq 0.01$; ***$p \leq 0.001$; ***$p \leq 0.0001$). The error bars represent the Standard Deviation (SD).

## rBCG-Induced Antibodies Show Virus Neutralizing Capacity *ex vivo*

To evaluate whether the antibodies generated by the rBCG immunization are able to neutralize hRSV or hMPV replication *ex-vivo*, sera collected from the immunized and infected animals were incubated with hRSV or hMPV and later used to infect cells (Hep-2 for hRSV and LLC-MK2 for hMPV), then PFUs were evaluated (**Figure 5**). Sera obtained from rBCG-N+hRSV-treated, BCG-WT+hRSV-treated and hRSV-infected mice led to a decrease in the number of viral PFUs, represented as an increase in the percentage of inhibition of viral loads, as compared to mock-treated mice. Furthermore, sera from rBCG-N+hRSV-treated mice showed a higher antiviral effect when compared with sera derived from hRSV-infected and BCG-WT+hRSV-treated animals (**Figure 5A**). As for hMPV-infected animals, rBCG-P+hMPV-treated, BCG-WT+hMPV-treated, and hMPV-infected mice showed a significant increase in the percentage of inhibition, as compared to mock-treated mice. Moreover, rBCG-P+hMPV-treated and hMPV-infected mice showed significantly higher percentage of inhibition as compared to sera from BCG-WT+hMPV-treated animals. However, no differences were found among rBCG-P+hMPV and hMPV mice (**Figure 5B**). These data suggest that immunization with rBCG promotes the secretion of antibodies with enhanced capacities to neutralize virus in cell culture experiments.

Antibodies triggered by rBCG vaccination followed by virus challenge protect *naïve* mice from viral-induced lung pathology.

After evaluating the neutralizing effect of the sera obtained from the immunized mice *ex-vivo*, we sought to evaluate the capacity of these sera to protect from a viral infection *in vivo*. With this aim, sera were transferred from immunized to *naïve* mice, which in turn were challenged with the respective virus. As shown in **Figure 6A**, a significant viral load reduction was observed for mice transferred with sera from rBCG-N+hRSV-treated mice as compared to non-transferred but hRSV-infected mice (nt-hRSV). The adoptive transfer of sera from rBCG-N+hRSV-treated mice led to similar levels of protection as compared to the transfer of Palivizumab, a commercially available humanized anti-hRSV-F mAb (**Figure 6A**). Further, a significant decrease in the infiltration of neutrophils to the lungs was observed for mice that had received sera from rBCG-N+hRSV-treated animals (**Figure 6B**).

Additionally, H&E staining of histopathological lung samples showed that nt-hRSV and hRSV animals exhibited a loss of lung structure and a high cellular infiltration (**Figure 6C**). In contrast, animals transferred either with Palivizumab, sera from BCG-WT+hRSV-treated mice or sera from hRSV-infected mice and then challenged with hRSV, showed reduced pathological signs as compared to nt-hRSV mice (**Figure 6C**). When mice transferred with sera from rBCG-N+hRSV-treated mice were evaluated, signs of improvement in the lung structure and a decrease in the cellular infiltration were observed as compared to nt-hRSV, being similar to the infiltration found in the lungs from mock-treated mice (**Figure 6C**).

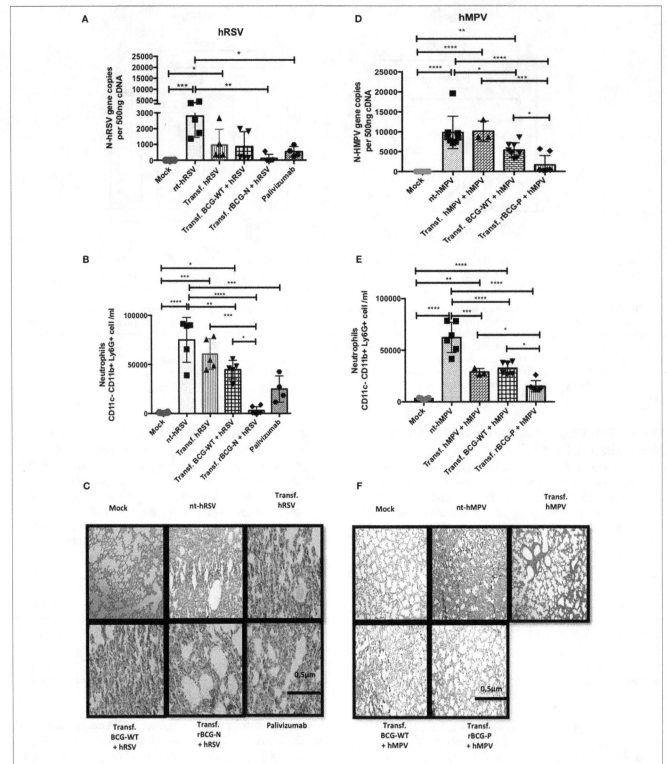

**FIGURE 6 |** Passive immunity transfer from sera of previously rBCG immunized mice protects naïve mice from hRSV- and hMPV-associated pathology. Sera from 14 dpi (hRSV) or 49 dpi (hMPV) was passively transferred to naïve mice. Then mice were then infected with hRSV or hMPV, respectively. As a control, a non-transferred group was also infected (nt-hRSV or nt-hMPV). Parameters as viral load in lung by RT-qPCR **(A** for hRSV and **D** for hMPV), neutrophils infiltrated in BALs **(B** for hRSV and **E** for hMPV) and histopathological lung H&E staining **(C** for hRSV and **F** for hMPV) were evaluated. For hRSV, Palivizumab was used as a positive control. The bars observed in the **(B,C)** are accordingly: ■ Mock-treated, ▢ nt-hRSV, ▥ Transf. hRSV, ▦ Transf. BCG-WT +hRSV, and ▩ Transf. rBCG-N +hRSV and ▨ Palivizumab. On the other hand, the bars observed in **(E,F)** are accordingly: ■ Mock-treated, ▨ nt-hMPV, ▥ Transf. hMPV ▦ Transf. BCG-WT +hMPV, and ▢ Transf. rBCG-P +hMPV. Differences were evaluated by a one-way ANOVA (*$p \leq 0.05$; **$p \leq 0.01$; ***$p \leq 0.001$; ****$p \leq 0.0001$). These results are from two independent experiments with 3 animals by group. The error bars represent the Standard Deviation (SD).

Equivalent parameters were evaluated for animals transferred with sera from rBCG-P+hMPV-treated mice. As seen in mock-treated mice, we observed almost no hMPV replication and significantly lower viral loads in mice that received sera from rBCG-P+hMPV-treated mice, as compared to non-transferred but hMPV-infected (nt-hMPV), mice transferred with sera from hMPV-infected mice, and from BCG-WT+hMPV-treated mice (**Figure 6D**). Further, animals transferred with BCG-WT+hMPV-treated mice also showed a decrease in viral loads relative to nt-hMPV, although this was not seen against hMPV-transferred + hMPV mice. Neutrophil infiltration into the lungs was also evaluated for the rBCG-P vaccine. Importantly, sera transfer from rBCG-P+hMPV-treated mice led to a reduced infiltration of neutrophils into lungs, similar to the values seen in mock-treated mice. Further, nt-hMPV mice, mice transferred with sera from hMPV-treated and BCG-WT+hMPV-treated mice showed higher values of neutrophil infiltration, as compared to mice receiving sera from rBCG-P+hMPV-treated mice (**Figure 6E**). Although animals transferred with sera from BCG-WT+hMPV-treated mice also showed a slight reduction in neutrophil infiltration as compared with the sera from nt-hMPV mice, the value of neutrophils was significantly higher than in those transferred with sera from rBCG-P+hMPV transferred mice (**Figure 6E**). No significant differences were detected between the hMPV-transferred group and nt-hMPV mice. These data were consistent with the observation that mice receiving sera from rBCG-P+hMPV mice showed a healthier lung structure, similar to the control mock-treated mice, with signs of significantly lower inflammatory cell infiltration, as seen in the histopathological lung samples (**Figure 6F**). In contrast, mice from groups nt-hMPV, hMPV-transferred, and BCG-WT+hMPV transferred showed a significant loss of lung structure and an increase of inflammatory cell infiltration (**Figure 6F**). These data suggest that passive transfer of humoral immunity from rBCG-vaccinated mice into *naïve* animals is able to significantly reduce virus-associated pathology symptoms, characterized by viral loads, neutrophil infiltration, and lung structure damage.

## DISCUSSION

Both hRSV and hMPV are respiratory viruses identified as the leading cause of most pathologies affecting the upper and lower respiratory tract of infants, children, elderly and immunocompromised people (10). Both hRSV and hMPV cause bronchiolitis, bronchitis, pneumonia, and high rates of hospitalizations, with hMPV as an emergent pathogen (8, 10–15). Nowadays, no vaccines against these viral pathogens are available. Thus, we developed two vaccines prototype using recombinant BCG strains (rBCG) that incorporate the genes codifying either the N protein (rBCG-N) of hRSV or the P protein (rBCG-P) of hMPV, respectively (24, 25). In this present work, we sought to evaluate whether the previously found cell-mediated immune response protection against hRSV and hMPV was also accompanied by a virus-specific neutralizing antibodies production after viral infection.

Both rBCG-N and rBCG-P have been previously reported as protectors from lung damage, neutrophils infiltration to the lungs and viral replication. Further, these rBCG vaccines were shown to elicit a Th-1 response and induce the proliferation of specific CD4$^+$ and CD8$^+$ IFN$\gamma^+$ producers T cells (24, 25, 34). Also, rBCG-N has been found to induce a Th-17 response and a long-lasting immunity in mice (34). In the present work, we observed that rBCG-N and rBCG-P were able to induce high antibody titers specific for hRSV and hMPV, respectively, as well as for several of the viral proteins. Interestingly, antibodies against hRSV were found before viral challenge in sera from rBCG-N immunized mice, but no antibodies against hMPV were found in sera from rBCG-P immunized mice before the viral challenge. Further, titers of anti-hMPV, anti-P, anti-M2, and anti-M antibodies were found at 28 dpi in the sera of rBCG-P immunized and hMPV-infected mice. Consistently, it has been previously reported that hMPV displays a biphasic replication cycle and infection peaks fluctuating from 7 to 14 dpi and it is possible to find neutralizing antibodies throughout 28 dpi and until 60 dpi (30). The different behaviors seen between hRSV and hMPV could be associated with the capacity of the N protein of hRSV to migrate to the surface of the host cells, a characteristic that could also enhance its capacity to be presented as an antigen by immune cells (20), when compared with the P protein of hMPV (35). Another reason that could explain the antibody secretion differences found could be associated with the capacity of the BCG to achieve a proper folding of these proteins.

Mature B cells are activated upon B cell receptor (BCR) binding to antigen, which is processed and presented to effector helper T cells (36). Activated B cells will produce antibodies against this antigen. Significantly, even when the concentration and affinity of the antigen is very low, it has been reported that insoluble antigens may congregate in a region of the immunological synapse along with cytoplasmic effectors polarizing inside the B cell, which enhance antigen processing and presentation to T cells (36). We observed that both vaccines induced significant antibody secretion against viral proteins different than those expressed by the rBCGs. Remarkably, the secretion of antibodies against hRSV was significantly higher in the immunized animals (BCG-WT + hRSV and rBCG-N + hRSV), as compared to the unimmunized and infected mice. It has been reported that both hRSV and hMPV infections do not induce an effective humoral immune response, promoting a low antibody secretion with a non-protective isotype (37). On the contrary, we found that BCG-WT, rBCG-N, and rBCG-P promote an increase in antibody secretion throughout time. Such antibody secretion could be explained by the immunogenic capacity of BCG to induce a strong Th-1 profile, prompting the secretion of IFN-γ in higher levels than IL-4 (38). Such Th-1 driving, in turn, promotes the proliferation and differentiation of the B cells population into an effector plasma cell profile, which increase the secretion of antibodies (39, 40). In addition, BCG vaccination by itself has been associated to the selection and survival of B cells and their subsequent maturation toward plasma cell and memory B cell by Follicular B-helper T cell (TFH), which could explain the high antibody titers detected for the mice immunized with the BCG-WT (41). Furthermore, it has been previously described that the immunization with BCG is able to induce the secretion of IgG2a antibodies by itself, therefore explaining the isotope switching detected. Also, the antibodies increase found in rBCG-N when compared to the BCG-WT could be associated with the nature of the antigen and the capacity of the host to present this antigen (39) that could, in turn, promote the enhancement of these capacities of the rBCG, when compared to the BCG-WT strain. Also, it is possible for B cells to be activated recognizing the specific recombinant antigen in their B cell receptor (BCR), while presenting another viral antigen in their Major Histocompatibility complex II (MHC-II) to T cells, for their later activation. These activated T cells will aid naïve B cells to maturate and differentiate into plasma cells, that will secrete high levels of antibodies, as compared with the BCG-WT- which did not express the recombinant antigen- after the viral infection (36). Higher antibody concentrations in sera from hMPV- compared to hRSV-infected mice were found. Such differences could be attributed to the times of collected samples, as the hMPV sera were collected at 28 dpi and the hRSV sera were collected at 14 dpi (40).

Production of IgG specific for an antigen different than the one used for the immunization has been previously reported for other pathogens (42–44). Such phenomenon, known as "linked recognition," takes place when two or more proteins have epitopes spatially close to each other in a manner that the B cell presents on MHC-II one of those linked antigens to the T cell. As a result, the B cell that receives help from the T cell becomes activated and reacts to the secondary antigen—not the one presented to the T cell—and generates antibodies against this linked antigen. Therefore, it is likely that linked recognition takes place after rBCG-N and rBCG-P immunization, as IgGs specific for other antigens, such as P, F, and G proteins for hRSV and M and M2.1 for hMPV, were produced. These proteins are all closely expressed on the surface of infected cells, along with the N protein during early stages of the replication cycle of hRSV (20). Importantly, the anti-F antibody secretion at 14 dpi from BCG-WT+hRSV and rBCG-N+hRSV mice is significantly higher (about 1,500–2,000 µg/mL) than the one seen for all the other proteins (about 500 µg/mL). Such large antibody titers could be explained by the capacity of both BCG and F protein to activate the TLR4 signaling pathway, which eventually can induce IL-6 secretion (31, 45) and promote secretion of protein specific IgGs by B cells (46).

To corroborate that the linked recognition antibody secretion against the different viral proteins were an effect of the vaccine as a whole and not just an effect of the expressed proteins, we compared the response induced by the transfer of T cells purified from rBCG-N immunized, BCG-WT immunized, and hRSV-infected mice 7 dpi, the point when we detect an early IgG secretion. We also included other groups such as N-hRSV + Freund Adjuvant –as a Th-1 inducer adjuvant- and N-hRSV + Aluminum hydroxide (Alum) Adjuvant – as a Th-2 inducer adjuvant (**Supplementary Figure 2**). The data obtained indicates that rBCG-N vaccine promotes the highest antibodies secretion when compared with all the other groups, even against N-hRSV protein + Freund Adjuvant

–whose adjuvant formulation is based on an extract of BCG.

These results suggest that the live-attenuated vaccine as a whole is required to induce an increase in the humoral immune response. Remarkably, N-hRSV + Alum Adjuvant showed higher levels of antibodies secretion when compared to the other control groups in three of the four analyses made (**Supplementary Figure 3**). A possible reason for this could be associated with the capacity of this adjuvant to promote a Th-2 immune profile, through the IL-4 secreted by the monocytes –instead of IFN-γ- promoting and strong but not protective humoral response (47). Moreover, it has been reported that the effect of Alum is dependent of several variables, such as the adsorption capacity of the antigen and the protein content of the vaccine, among others (48). Although the IgG measurement was performed at both 7 and 14 dpi, we decided to perform the linked recognition assay at 7 dpi, as we detected that as early as this time point the CD4+ T cell population was already activated, therefore the mechanism we suggest could occur at this time (**Supplementary Figure 4**).

A signature immune response against respiratory viruses, such as hRSV and hMPV, is the antibody secretion of IgG1 and IgG3 isotypes (49, 50). Importantly, although these subclasses can opsonize and neutralize these viruses, they are not suitable for the induction of an effective antiviral response, thereby not being optimal for the control of the infection. Importantly, several studies have demonstrated that IgG2a is the adequate isotype against these infections since it increases the opsonization and exhibits enhanced neutralizing capacities when compared to the IgG1 isotype (51). Interestingly, we found that the use of rBCG strains promotes an isotype switching from IgG1 to IgG2a, which has been previously reported to be associated with an efficient immune response due to the neutralizing activity of these antibodies and the activation of the complement pathway (4). Such isotype changes –along with the Th-1 driving- have already been reported after rBCG immunization (1, 24, 25, 34, 52). Interestingly, we found that rBCG-N vaccine enhanced isotype switching, prompting to an even better humoral response. Also, rBCG-P and BCG-WT promoted the isotype switching seen in rBCG-N—for hMPV-infected mice—but in lower levels when compared with rBCG-N. Such a difference among viruses could be explained because IgG2a displays a faster viral clearance as compared to IgG1, thereby allowing rapid elimination of the pathogen (40). Further, the differences could also be associated to the fact that the IgG2a/IgG1 ratio was determined for the sera obtained at 14 dpi for hRSV and at 28 dpi for hMPV, promoting in this way the decrease of the total circulating IgG.

The use of IFN-α previous to an hRSV-infection has been associated with an increase in the IgA secretion in neonatal and adult mice, accompanied by a strong B cell activation and maturation (53). This effect has also been observed after the BCG vaccination where, using blood samples from neonatal vaccinated children, it was found that BCG promotes the secretion of type I IFN by the plasmacytoid dendritic cells. This might explain why

BCG is a good vaccine against viral and intracellular pathogens as we have found in our study (54). The neonatal immune response induced by hRSV-infection promotes an inefficient antibody secretion during the first infection, as compared with adult mice (55). Such a response is characterized with low levels of IgM and IgG in the sera, with a peak at day 28 post-infection, instead of the 7-day post-infection peak detected in adult mice (55). A possible explanation for this behavior is the associated age response dependent-limitation. Also, the antibody levels increase faster after a second infection (55). Therefore, there seem to be differences in the immune response of neonatal compared to adult mice, which could vary the response to the vaccination. For this reason, further studies in neonatal mice are needed to better understand the response of vaccines against hRSV to be intended finally to vaccinate newborns.

As we determined that both rBCG were able to induce the secretion of several types of antibodies, we then sought to evaluate their neutralizing capacities. We found that sera from rBCG-N+hRSV and BCG-WT+hRSV mice at 14 dpi were able to neutralize hRSV-GFP in Hep-2 cell culture since the hRSV PFUs in these cells significantly decreased, shown as an increase in the percentage of inhibition. Importantly, such inhibition was also found in BCG-WT+hRSV sera but its effect was not as high as the one seen in rBCG-N+hRSV sera, suggesting that the BCG could promote the isotype antibodies switching, inducing an inhibitory effect on the capacity of hRSV to infect cells *ex vivo*. Likewise, rBCG-P+hMPV and BCG-WT+hMPV displayed higher percentage of inhibition when compared with mock-treated sera. The hMPV sera also presented significantly higher capacities to neutralize hMPV-GFP in cell culture. These data suggest that a second challenge with hMPV could induce a positive effect on the neutralizing capacity of IgG2a antibodies promoting the control of the viral replication in both the infection alone and the rBCG-P vaccine. Also, although the neutralizing levels in those three groups—hMPV, BCG-WT+hMPV, and rBCG-P+hMPV—were similar, the quantity of secreted antibodies was significantly different among them, suggesting that the vaccine not only promoted the isotype switching, but also a higher secretion of these antibodies.

Given that both vaccines showed neutralizing capacity of the secreted antibodies *ex vivo*, we used these sera to perform a passive transference of immunity to *naïve* mice. In the sera transfer experiments, sera from hRSV-infected mice resulted in a mildly decrease of neutrophils infiltration to the lungs, but only sera from rBCG-N and hRSV-infected mice induce a reduction of neutrophils to mock-like levels. Remarkably, we observed that sera from previously rBCG-N and rBCG- P immunized mice were able to reduce viral load, neutrophils infiltration to lungs and protected from lung damage when compared to their respective control groups.

Currently, the most effective FDA approved treatment against hRSV is palivizumab, a monoclonal antibody that targets a region of F protein that is highly conserved between both antigenic groups of the virus. Further, such antibody is currently used as a prophylactic method, mainly for high-risk infants (51). However, a major concern about this treatment is its price/effectiveness relation, since at least five doses are required in order to achieve a passive immune response. Moreover, even after the administration of five doses, only a 50% of the cases reported a decrease in the hRSV-associated disease parameters. Accordingly, no memory immune response has been reported after administration of palivizumab (19, 51, 56). Importantly, in the sera transfer experiment we found that our rBCG-N strain is able to induce an even more pronounced humoral-mediated protection than palivizumab. Such protection could be associated with the high levels of anti-viral antibodies in the sera of immunized animals and the significant isotype switching, which in turn promote an effective antiviral response, as well as the activation of complement pathway (19).

In conclusion, the use of BCG as a vector could be considered as a promising vaccine approach against respiratory viruses, promoting an efficient humoral response characterized by high titers of neutralizing and protecting antibodies. Thus, our rBCG strains are not inducing only a cellular response, as previously described, but also a humoral response, mediated by neutralizing antibodies against several viral proteins, that promotes an effective immune response when those are transferred to *naïve* recipient mice.

## AUTHOR CONTRIBUTIONS

JS and NG are equal contributors in the experimental development and design, data organization, data analysis, writing, and revision of this manuscript. CR, CP, and PC supported in organization and experimental design, along with manuscript writing, and revision. ER-J and SB supported in experimental design along with manuscript revision. AK is the leading investigator and supported in the organization, experimental design, and full manuscript revision.

## FUNDING

This work was supported by COMISIÓN NACIONAL DE INVESTIGACIÓN CIENTÍFICA Y TECNOLÓGICA (CONICYT) N°21151028, CONICYT/FONDECYT POSTDOCTORADO No. 3160249, the Millennium Institute on Immunology and Immunotherapy (P09/016-F) and Fondecyt grant No 1150862.

## ACKNOWLEDGMENTS

We thank María Jose Altamirano for her support in the handling and caring of the animals used. We also thank Natalia Muñoz and Francisco Salazar for their help with experimental support and design.

# REFERENCES

1. Zhang G, Wang P, Qiu Z, Qin X, Lin X, Li N, et al. Distant lymph nodes serve as pools of Th1 cells induced by neonatal BCG vaccination for the prevention of asthma in mice. *Allergy Eur J Allergy Clin Immunol.* (2013) 68:330–8. doi: 10.1111/all.12099

2. Dennehy M, Bourn W, Steele D, Williamson AL. Evaluation of recombinant BCG expressing rotavirus VP6 as an anti-rotavirus vaccine. *Vaccine* (2007) 25:3646–57. doi: 10.1016/j.vaccine.2007.01.087

3. Fennelly GJ, Flynn JL, Ter Meulen V, Liebert UG, Bloom BR. Recombinant bacille calmette-guérin priming against measles. *J Infect Dis.* (1995) 172:698–705. doi: 10.1093/infdis/172.3.698

4. Matsumoto S, Yukitake H, Kanbara H, Yamada H, Kitamura A, Yamada T. *Mycobacterium bovis* bacillus calmette-guerin induces protective immunity against infection by *Plasmodium yoelii* at blood-stage depending on shifting immunity toward Th1 type and inducing protective IgG2a after the parasite infection. *Vaccine* (2000) 19:779–87. doi: 10.1016/S0264-410X(00)00257-7

5. Rezende CAF, De Moraes MTB, De Souza Matos DC, Mcintoch D, Armoa GRG. Humoral response and genetic stability of recombinant BCG expressing hepatitis B surface antigens. *J Virol Methods* (2005) 125:1–9. doi: 10.1016/j.jviromet.2004.11.026

6. Medeiros MA, Armôa GRG, Dellagostin OA, McIntosh D. Induction of humoral immunity in response to immunization with recombinant *Mycobacterium bovis* BCG expressing the S1 subunit of *Bordetella pertussis* toxin. *Can J Microbiol.* (2005) 51:1015–20. doi: 10.1139/w05-095

7. Wang H, Liu Q, Liu K, Zhong W, Gao S, Jiang L, et al. Immune response induced by recombinant *Mycobacterium bovis* BCG expressing ROP2 gene of *Toxoplasma gondii*. *Parasitol Int.* (2007) 56:263–8. doi: 10.1016/j.parint.2007.04.003

8. Nair H, Nokes DJ, Gessner BD, Dherani M, Madhi SA, Singleton RJ, et al. Global burden of acute lower respiratory infections due to respiratory syncytial virus in young children: a systematic review and meta-analysis. *Lancet* (2010) 375:1545–55. doi: 10.1016/S0140-6736(10)60206-1

9. Lefebvre A, Manoha C, Bour J-B, Abbas R, Fournel I, Tiv M, et al. Human metapneumovirus in patients hospitalized with acute respiratory infections: a meta-analysis. *J Clin Virol.* (2016) 81:68–77. doi: 10.1016/j.jcv.2016.05.015

10. Berry M, Gamieldien J, Fielding B. Identification of new respiratory viruses in the new millennium. *Viruses* (2015) 7:996–1019. doi: 10.3390/v7030996

11. Edwards KM, Zhu Y, Griffin MR, Weinberg GA, Hall CB, Szilagyi PG, et al. Burden of human metapneumovirus infection in young children. *N Engl J Med.* (2013) 368:633–43. doi: 10.1056/NEJMoa1204630

12. Williams JV, Harris PA, Tollefson SJ, Halburnt-Rush LL, Pingsterhaus JM, Edwards KM, Wright PF, Crowe JE. Human metapneumovirus and lower respiratory tract disease in otherwise healthy infants and children. *N Engl J Med.* (2004) 350:443–50. doi: 10.1056/NEJMoa025472

13. Tregoning JS, Schwarze J. Respiratory viral infections in infants: causes, clinical symptoms, virology, and immunology. *Clin Microbiol Rev.* (2010) 23:74–98. doi: 10.1128/CMR.00032-09

14. Hahn A, Wang W, Jaggi P, Dvorchik I, Ramilo O, Koranyi K, et al. Human metapneumovirus infections are associated with severe morbidity in hospitalized children of all ages. *Epidemiol Infect.* (2013) 141:2213–23. doi: 10.1017/S0950268812002920

15. Afonso CL, Amarasinghe GK, Bányai K, Bào Y, Basler CF, Bavari S, et al. Taxonomy of the order Mononegavirales: update 2016. *Arch Virol.* (2016) 161:2351–60. doi: 10.1007/s00705-016-2880-1

16. Collins PL, Melero JA. Progress in understanding and controlling respiratory syncytial virus: still crazy after all these years. *Virus Res.* (2011) 162:80–99. doi: 10.1016/j.virusres.2011.09.020

17. Mukherjee S, Lukacs NW. Innate immune responses to respiratory syncytial virus infection. *Curr Top Microbiol Immunol.* (2013) 372:139–54. doi: 10.1007/978-3-642-38919-1_7

18. Espinoza JA, Bueno SM, Riedel CA, Kalergis AM. Induction of protective effector immunity to prevent pathogenesis caused by the respiratory syncytial virus. Implications on therapy and vaccine design. *Immunology* (2014) 143:1–12. doi: 10.1111/imm.12313

19. Gomez RS, Guisle-Marsollier I, Bohmwald K, Bueno SM, Kalergis AM. Respiratory syncytial virus: pathology, therapeutic drugs and prophylaxis. *Immunol Lett.* (2014) 162:237–47. doi: 10.1016/j.imlet.2014.09.006

20. Céspedes PF, Bueno SM, Ramírez BA, Gomez RS, Riquelme SA, Palavecino CE, et al. Surface expression of the hRSV nucleoprotein impairs immunological synapse formation with T cells. *Proc Natl Acad Sci USA.* (2014) 111:E3214–23. doi: 10.1073/pnas.1400760111

21. Caly L, Ghildyal R, Jans DA. Respiratory virus modulation of host nucleocytoplasmic transport; target for therapeutic intervention? *Front Microbiol.* (2015) 6:848. doi: 10.3389/fmicb.2015.00848

22. Derdowski A, Peters TR, Glover N, Qian R, Utley TJ, Burnett A, et al. Human metapneumovirus nucleoprotein and phosphoprotein interact and provide the minimal requirements for inclusion body formation. *J Gen Virol.* (2008) 89:2698–708. doi: 10.1099/vir.0.2008/004051-0

23. Goutagny N, Jiang Z, Tian J, Parroche P, Schickli J, Monks BG, et al. Cell type-specific recognition of human metapneumoviruses (HMPVs) by retinoic acid-inducible gene I (RIG-I) and TLR7 and viral interference of RIG-I ligand recognition by HMPV-B1 phosphoprotein. *J Immunol.* (2010) 184:1168–79. doi: 10.4049/jimmunol.0902750

24. Bueno SM, González PA, Cautivo KM, Mora JE, Leiva ED, Tobar HE, et al. Protective T cell immunity against respiratory syncytial virus is efficiently induced by recombinant BCG. *Proc Natl Acad Sci USA.* (2008) 105:20822–7. doi: 10.1073/pnas.0806244105

25. Palavecino CE, Cespedes PF, Gomez RS, Kalergis AM, Bueno SM, Céspedes PF, et al. Immunization with a recombinant bacillus calmette-guerin strain confers protective Th1 immunity against the human metapneumovirus. *J Immunol.* (2014) 192:214–23. doi: 10.4049/jimmunol.1300118

26. Espinoza JA, Bohmwald K, Cespedes PF, Gomez RS, Riquelme SA, Cortes CM, et al. Impaired learning resulting from respiratory syncytial virus infection. *Proc Natl Acad Sci USA.* (2013) 110:9112–7. doi: 10.1073/pnas.1217508110

27. Reina J, Ferres F, Alcoceba E, Mena A, de Gopegui ER, Figuerola J. Comparison of different cell lines and incubation times in the isolation by the shell vial culture of human metapneumovirus from pediatric respiratory samples. *J Clin Virol.* (2007) 40:46–9. doi: 10.1016/j.jcv.2007.06.006

28. Tollefson SJ, Cox RG, Williams JV. Studies of culture conditions and environmental stability of human metapneumovirus. *Virus Res.* (2010) 151:54–9. doi: 10.1016/j.virusres.2010.03.018

29. Céspedes PF, Gonzalez PA, Kalergis AM. Human metapneumovirus keeps dendritic cells from priming antigen-specific naive T cells. *Immunology* (2013) 139:366–76. doi: 10.1111/imm.12083

30. Alvarez R, Harrod KS, Shieh WJ, Zaki S, Tripp RA. Human metapneumovirus persists in BALB/c mice despite the presence of neutralizing antibodies. *J Virol.* (2004) 78:14003–11. doi: 10.1128/JVI.78.24.14003-14011.2004

31. Marr N, Turvey SE. Role of human TLR4 in respiratory syncytial virus-induced NF-κB activation, viral entry and replication. *Innate Immun.* (2012) 18:856–65. doi: 10.1177/1753425912444479

32. Lindblad EB. Aluminium adjuvants - in retrospect and prospect. *Vaccine* (2004) 22:3658–68. doi: 10.1016/j.vaccine.2004.03.032

33. Egli A, Santer DM, Barakat K, Zand M, Levin A, Vollmer M, et al. Vaccine adjuvants - understanding molecular mechanisms to improve vaccines. *Swiss Med Wkly.* (2014) 144:w1394. doi: 10.4414/smw.2014.13940

34. Céspedes PF, Rey-Jurado E, Espinoza JA, Rivera CA, Canedo-Marroquín G, Bueno SM, et al. A single, low dose of a cGMP recombinant BCG vaccine elicits protective T cell immunity against the human respiratory syncytial virus infection and prevents lung pathology in mice. *Vaccine* (2017) 35:757–66. doi: 10.1016/j.vaccine.2016.12.048

35. Oliveira AP, Simabuco FM, Tamura RE, Guerrero MC, Ribeiro PGG, Libermann TA, et al. Human respiratory syncytial virus N, P, and M protein interactions in HEK-293T cells. *Virus Res.* (2013) 177:108–12. doi: 10.1016/j.virusres.2013.07.010

36. Batista FD, Iber D, Neuberger MS. B cells acquire antigen from target cells after synapse formation. *Nature* (2001) 411:489–94. doi: 10.1038/35078099

37. Freitas GRO, Silva DAO, Yokosawa J, Paula NT, Costa LF, Carneiro BM, et al. Antibody response and avidity of respiratory syncytial virus-specific total IgG, IgG1, and IgG3 in young children. *J Med Virol.* (2011) 83:1826–33. doi: 10.1002/jmv.22134

38. Finkelman FD, Holmes J, Katona IM, Urban JF, Beckmann MP, Park LS, et al. Lymphokine control of *in vivo* immunoglobulin isotype selection. *Annu Rev Immunol.* (1990) 8:303–33. doi: 10.1146/annurev.iy.08.040190.001511

39. Drowart A, Selleslaghs J, Yernault JC, Valcke C, De Bruyn J, Huygen K, et al. The humoral immune response after BCG vaccination: an immunoblotting

study using two purified antigens. *Tuber Lung Dis.* (1992) 73:137–40. doi: 10.1016/0962-8479(92)90146-B

40. Mattes MJ, Natale A, Goldenberg DM, Mattes MJ. Rapid blood clearance of immunoglobulin G2a and immunoglobulin G2b in nude mice. *Cancer Res* (1991) 51:3102–7.

41. Moliva JI, Turner J, Torrelles JB. Immune responses to bacillus Calmette-Guérin vaccination: why do they fail to protect against *mycobacterium tuberculosis? Front Immunol.* (2017) 8:407. doi: 10.3389/fimmu.2017.00407

42. Davies JD, Leong LY, Mellor A, Cobbold SP, Waldmann H. T cell suppression in transplantation tolerance through linked recognition. *J Immunol.* (1996) 156:3602–7.

43. Morse K, Norimine J, Palmer GH, Sutten EL, Baszler TV, Brown WC. Association and evidence for linked recognition of type IV secretion system proteins VirB9-1, VirB9-2, and VirB10 in Anaplasma marginale. *Infect Immun.* (2012) 80:215–27. doi: 10.1128/IAI.05798-11

44. Fucs R, Jesus JT, Souza Junior PH, Franco L, Vericimo M, Bellio M, et al. Frequency of natural regulatory CD4+CD25+ T lymphocytes determines the outcome of tolerance across fully mismatched MHC barrier through linked recognition of self and allogeneic stimuli. *J Immunol.* (2006) 176:2324–9. doi: 10.4049/jimmunol.176.4.2324

45. Begum NA, Ishii K, Kurita-Taniguchi M, Tanabe M, Kobayashi M, Moriwaki Y, et al. *Mycobacterium bovis* BCG cell wall-specific differentially expressed genes identified by differential display and cDNA subtraction in human macrophages. *Infect Immun.* (2004) 72:937–48. doi: 10.1128/IAI.72.2.937-948.2004

46. Suematsu S, Matsuda T, Aozasa K, Akira S, Nakano N, Ohno S, et al. IgG1 plasmacytosis in interleukin 6 transgenic mice. *Proc Natl Acad Sci USA.* (1989) 86:7547–51. doi: 10.1073/pnas.86.19.7547

47. Ulanova M, Tarkowski A, Hahn-Zoric M, Hanson LÅ. The common vaccine adjuvant aluminum hydroxide up-regulates accessory properties of human monocytes via an interleukin-4-dependent mechanism. *Infect Immun.* (2001) 69:1151–9. doi: 10.1128/IAI.69.2.1151-11 59.2001

48. al-Shakhshir R, Regnier F, White JL, Hem SL. Effect of protein adsorption on the surface charge characteristics of aluminium-containing adjuvants. *Vaccine* (1994) 12: 472–4. doi: 10.1016/0264-410X(94)90127-9

49. Knudson CJ, Hartwig SM, Meyerholz DK, Varga SM. RSV vaccine-enhanced disease is orchestrated by the combined actions of distinct CD4 T cell subsets. *PLoS Pathog.* (2015) 11:e1004757. doi: 10.1371/journal.ppat.1004757

50. Cseke G, Wright DW, Tollefson SJ, Johnson JE, Crowe JE, et al. Human metapneumovirus fusion protein vaccines that are immunogenic and protective in cotton rats. *J Virol.* (2007) 81:698–707. doi: 10.1128/JVI.00844-06

51. Huang K, Incognito L, Cheng X, Ulbrandt ND, Wu H. Respiratory syncytial virus-neutralizing monoclonal antibodies motavizumab and palivizumab inhibit fusion. *J Virol.* (2010) 84:8132–40. doi: 10.1128/JVI.02699-09

52. Cautivo KM, Bueno SM, Cortes CM, Wozniak A, Riedel CA, Kalergis AM. Efficient lung recruitment of respiratory syncytial virus-specific Th1 cells induced by recombinant bacillus calmette-guerin promotes virus clearance and protects from infection. *J Immunol.* (2010) 185:7633–45. doi: 10.4049/jimmunol.0903452

53. Hijano DR, Siefker DT, Shrestha B, Jaligama S, Vu LD, Tillman H, et al. Type I interferon potentiates IgA immunity to respiratory syncytial virus infection during infancy. *Sci Rep.* (2018) 8: 11034. doi: 10.1038/s41598-018-29456-w

54. Kativhu CL, Libraty DH. A model to explain how the bacille calmette guérin (BCG) vaccine drives interleukin-12 production in neonates. *PLoS ONE* (2016) 11:e0162148. doi: 10.1371/journal.pone.0162148

55. Tasker L, Lindsay RWB, Clarke BT, Cochrane DWR, Hou S. Infection of mice with respiratory syncytial virus during neonatal life primes for enhanced antibody and T cell responses on secondary challenge. *Clin Exp Immunol.* (2008) 153:277–88. doi: 10.1111/j.1365-2249.2008.03591.x

56. Hamelin ME, Couture C, Sackett M, Kiener P, Suzich JA, Ulbrandt N, et al. The prophylactic administration of a monoclonal antibody against human metapneumovirus attenuates viral disease and airways hyperresponsiveness in mice. *Antivir Ther.* (2008) 13:39–46.

# 10

# Porous Nanoparticles with Self-Adjuvanting M2e-Fusion Protein and Recombinant Hemagglutinin Provide Strong and Broadly Protective Immunity Against Influenza Virus Infections

Valentina Bernasconi[1], Beatrice Bernocchi[2], Liang Ye[3], Minh Quan Lê[2],
Ajibola Omokanye[1], Rodolphe Carpentier[2], Karin Schön[1], Xavier Saelens[4,5],
Peter Staeheli[3,6], Didier Betbeder[2,7] and Nils Lycke[1]*

[1] Mucosal Immunobiology and Vaccine Center, Department of Microbiology and Immunology, Institute of Biomedicine, Sahlgrenska Academy, University of Gothenburg, Gothenburg, Sweden, [2] Lille Inflammation Research International Center – U995, University of Lille, INSERM and CHU Lille, Lille, France, [3] Institute of Virology, University Medical Center Freiburg, Freiburg, Germany, [4] VIB-UGent Center for Medical Biotechnology, Ghent, Belgium, [5] Department of Biomedical Molecular Biology, Ghent University, Ghent, Belgium, [6] Faculty of Medicine, University of Freiburg, Freiburg, Germany, [7] Faculté des Sciences du Sport, University of Artois, Arras, France

*Correspondence:
Nils Lycke
nils.lycke@microbio.gu.se

Due to the high risk of an outbreak of pandemic influenza, the development of a broadly protective universal influenza vaccine is highly warranted. The design of such a vaccine has attracted attention and much focus has been given to nanoparticle-based influenza vaccines which can be administered intranasally. This is particularly interesting since, contrary to injectable vaccines, mucosal vaccines elicit local IgA and lung resident T cell immunity, which have been found to correlate with stronger protection in experimental models of influenza virus infections. Also, studies in human volunteers have indicated that pre-existing CD4[+] T cells correlate well to increased resistance against infection. We have previously developed a fusion protein with 3 copies of the ectodomain of matrix protein 2 (M2e), which is one of the most explored conserved influenza A virus antigens for a broadly protective vaccine known today. To improve the protective ability of the self-adjuvanting fusion protein, CTA1-3M2e-DD, we incorporated it into porous maltodextrin nanoparticles (NPLs). This proof-of-principle study demonstrates that the combined vaccine vector given intranasally enhanced immune protection against a live challenge infection and reduced the risk of virus transmission between immunized and unimmunized individuals. Most importantly, immune responses to NPLs that also contained recombinant hemagglutinin (HA) were strongly enhanced in a CTA1-enzyme dependent manner and we achieved broadly protective immunity against a lethal infection with heterosubtypic influenza virus. Immune protection was mediated by enhanced levels of lung resident CD4[+] T cells as well as anti-HA and -M2e serum IgG and local IgA antibodies.

Keywords: mucosal vaccination, influenza A virus, CTA1-DD, maltodextrin nanoparticles, targeted adjuvant, nasal immunization, Universal vaccine

## INTRODUCTION

The quest for a broadly protective influenza vaccine is ongoing. Whereas many different strategies have been employed to design a novel vaccine, a common denominator for these has been to identify conserved viral epitopes that could serve as effective vaccine components (1). Attention has been given to epitopes from the hemagglutinin (HA) stem region in order to raise neutralizing antibodies against conserved structures of the protein (2–6). The prevailing idea is that protective antibodies are largely neutralizing antibodies, but also antibodies acting through antibody-dependent cell-mediated cytotoxicity (ADCC) could prevent disease, as shown in experimental models (7–9). To the latter category of ADCC-acting antibodies we count antibodies against the ectodomain of the influenza A matrix protein 2 (M2e), an ion channel protein which, in fact, is one of the most explored vaccine subcomponents for a universal influenza vaccine today (10–13) M2e as part of a virus-like particle or a fusion protein has been shown to stimulate strong protection against homologous as well as heterologous influenza virus infections in different animal models (14–16). Furthermore, clinical studies have indicated that cell-mediated immune responses, more than antibodies, may be critical for a broadly protective influenza vaccine and, hence, not only M2e, but also several internal structural proteins have been considered for a universal flu vaccine (10, 13). While both memory CD4$^+$ and CD8$^+$ T cells have been found to correlate with protection against heterosubtypic influenza virus strains, experimental evidence in this regard points to a particularly critical function of lung resident memory T cells for protection (17–20). Most influenza vaccines are injectable vaccines, but these are poor inducers of lung resident memory T cells (13, 21). Therefore, many researchers have focused efforts on mucosal vaccines, which have been found superior to injectable vaccines at stimulating lung resident memory T cells, concomitant with strong secretory IgA (sIgA) and significant systemic IgG immune responses (22).

We have previously developed a universal influenza vaccine candidate by incorporating the M2e-peptide into the non-toxic CTA1-DD adjuvant molecule (16). The CTA1-DD molecule exploits the full immunomodulating ability of CTA1, which is the ADP-ribosylating enzyme from cholera toxin (CT), linked in a fusion protein (FPM2e) that employs the D-fragment from *Staphylococcus aureus* protein A as a cell targeting unit (23–25) CTA1-3M2e-DD was found to strongly protect against a challenge infection with a heterosubtypic influenza A virus strain (H1N1/PR8) (26). Our vaccine adjuvant molecule is lacking the CTB pentamer of CT and cannot bind to the GM1-ganglioside receptors present on most nucleated cells, including nerve cells (27, 28). This way, CTA1-3M2e-DD is completely safe and non-toxic even when given intranasally (i.n) contrary to CT or other GM1-binding toxin adjuvants that can cause facial nerve paralysis, also described as Bell's palsy (29). Interestingly, the CTA1-3M2e-DD not only stimulated strong M2e-specific serum IgG and mucosal IgA antibody responses, but we also identified a critical induction of lung resident M2e-specific memory CD4$^+$ T cells (16, 26). We observed that M2e-specific CD4$^+$T cells were dominated by Th17 cells, which conveyed protection

against influenza that was independent of anti-M2e-antibodies. Accordingly, we believe the CTA1-3M2e-DD, generating both lung resident memory CD4$^+$T cells and M2e-specific antibodies, is a good candidate for a broadly protective influenza vaccine.

However, to improve vaccine stability and mucosal delivery of the fusion protein, we sought to explore the combination of the FPM2e with a nanoparticle (30). We used our well established technology to incorporate CTA1-3M2e-DD into porous maltodextrin nanoparticles (NPLs) to further improve the immunogenicity and disease protective functions of the vaccine candidate (31). Apart from shielding the protein against degradation, we speculated that the combined FPM2e:NPL vaccine formulation would facilitate breaching of the mucosal membrane barrier and, in this way, augment antigen uptake in migrating dendritic cells (DC) (32, 33). The positively charged NPLs used in this work have three main components: the reticulated maltodextrin, the anionic lipid (DPPG) and the protein, which are all linked together by non-covalent interactions (Van der Waals forces and electrostatic interactions). Hence, the NPL hosts a negative hydrophobic core surrounded by a positively charged polysaccharide shell (34). We have reported previously that nasal immunizations with similar NPL preparations could stimulate significant protection against *Toxoplasma gondii* in mice (35, 36). An additional advantage of the NPL technology is that it allows for loading of multiple proteins in the same particle. This gave us the opportunity to explore whether anti-influenza protection could be improved with NPLs that carry both the CTA1-3M2e-DD and recombinant HA. Thus, the present study was undertaken to investigate whether the combined HA:FPM2e:NPL vaccine vector, hosting the CTA1-3M2e-DD and recombinant HA, stimulated enhanced protective immunity against influenza virus infections. A special focus was given to the uptake and antigen-processing of the combined vector by DCs, which are the essential primers of CD4$^+$ T cell immunity (37).

## MATERIALS AND METHODS
### Mice and Immunizations
Age- and sex-matched BALB/c, C57BL/6 or DBA/2 mice were obtained from Harlan (The Netherlands) or Janvier Laboratories (France). The Eα-specific T cell receptor transgenic B6.Cg-Tg(Tcrα,Tcrβ)3Ayr/J mice were obtained from The Jackson Laboratories (USA). Mice were maintained under specific pathogen-free conditions at the Laboratory for Experimental Biomedicine (EBM) (University of Gothenburg, Sweden) or at the Laboratory of Virology (University of Freiburg, Germany). Experiments were ethically approved by local committees regulating animal ethics at the universities of Gothenburg and Freiburg, respectively. A single or three immunizations with 10 days between immunizations were given intranasally (i.n) to 4–6 weeks old mice. As indicated, an i.n antigen dose of 1 or 5 µg of protein was given in a volume of 20 µl i.n to each mouse. Mice were sacrificed after 1–2 weeks following the final immunization or virus challenge infection and spleens, mediastinal lymph nodes (mLN), serum, and broncheoalveolar lavage (BAL) were

collected. Serum and BAL were taken at times indicated and stored at $-20°C$ until further analyzed.

## Fusion Protein Construction

CTA1(C189A)-3M2e-DD, with enzymatic activity, CTA1(R9K)-3M2e-DD, the enzymatically inactive mutant, CTA1-DD and CTA1(C189A)-3Eα-DD were produced in *E. coli* by MIVAC Development AB, Sweden, as previously described (16). The first two constructs carry three copies of the extracellular domain of the influenza virus M2 protein (SLLTEVETPIRNEWGSRSNDSSD) derived from the A/Victoria/3/75 (H3N2) virus strain. CTA1(C189A)-3Eα-DD carries 3 copies of the Eα 52-68 peptide (ASFEAQGALANIAVDKA). The fusion proteins were routinely tested for the presence of endotoxin, using the limulus amebocyte lysate assay (LAL Endochrome TM Charles River Endosafe, USA) and found to be <100 endotoxin units/mg protein (EU/mg). The enzymatic ADP-ribosyltransferase activity was determined by the NAD:agmatine assay (38). Protein analysis was performed with SDS-PAGE, and concentrations were determined using the Bio-Rad DC protein assay (Bio-Rad, USA), according to the manufacturer's instructions.

## Nanoparticle Preparation

Nanoparticles (NPLs) were produced as described by Paillard et al. (34). Briefly, maltodextrin (Roquette, France) was dissolved in 2N sodium hydroxide by magnetic stirring at room temperature. A mixture of epichlorohydrin and glycidyltrimethylammonium chloride (GTMA, a cationic ligand; both from Sigma-Aldrich, France) was added to the polysaccharide leading to the formation of a gel. After neutralization by means of acetic acid, the gel was crushed with a high pressure homogenizer (Emulsiflex C3, Avestin, Germany). The newly obtained NPLs were purified by tangential flow ultra-filtration (Centramate Minim II PALL, France) using a 300 kDa membrane (PALL, France) to remove oligosaccharides, low-molecular weight reagents and salts. Purified NPLs were freeze dried. Lyophilized NPLs were dissolved in water and a 1,2-dipalmitoyl-sn-glycero-3-phosphatidylglycerol (DPPG) lipid (Lipoid, Germany) was loaded into NPLs at a temperature above the liquid phase transition temperature of the lipid.

## CTA1-3M2e-DD and HA Loading Into Nanoparticles

The fusion proteins or trimeric HA were loaded into premade NPL at a mass ratio 1:5 (protein:NPL), by mixing the proteins with NPLs followed by incubation for 30 min at room temperature. The recombinant extracellular domain (Met 1-Gln 528) of the hemagglutinin (HA1+HA2) was derived from Influenza A Virus H1N1 (A/Puerto Rico/8/34 virus strain) fused with a C-terminal polyhistidine tag (Sino Biological Inc., China) was resuspended in 1.98% Empigen® BB (N,N- Dimethyl-N-dodecylglycine betaine, Sigma-Aldrich, France) obtaining a protein concentration of 1 mg/ml. Then HA was incubated with either NPL or CTA1-3M2e-DD:NPL at r.t. to obtain a formulation with a mass ratio 1:5 (protein:NPL).

## Size, Zeta Potential, and Long Term Stability

We determined the efficiency of protein incorporation into NPLs by native polyacrylamide gel electrophoresis (PAGE). Proteins and NPLs were dissolved in electrophoresis buffer (Tris-HCl 125Mm (pH 6.8), 10% glycerol, 0.06% bromophenol blue) and run on a 10% acrylamide-bisacrylamide gel. The gel was stained by silver nitrate to detect unbound proteins. The size and the zeta potential of the proteins and NPLs were assessed by dynamic light scattering and electrophoretic mobility with a Zetasizer nanoZS (Malvern Instruments, France). Proteins or NPLs were kept in low volume quartz batch cuvettes (ZEN2112, Malvern Instrument, France) for particle size purposes. For assessments of zeta potential samples were diluted in water to a final volume of 750 µl and loaded into a disposable folded capillary cell (DTS1070, Malvern Instrument, France). The molecular stability of CTA1-3M2e-DD (FPM2e) or the different NPLs, was assessed after 3 months, under accelerated (40°C) or standard (4°C) conditions, or after >12 months in 4°C, "sterile setting." The molecular stability was determined by change in size or zeta potential as measured by dynamic light scattering and laser doppler velocimetry. The stability of the protein incorporated into NPLs was evaluated by native PAGE analysis, as described above. Antigen degradation was assessed by SDS-PAGE, using a denaturing buffer (Tris–HCL 125 mm (pH 6.8), 20% glycerol, 10% SDS, 2.5% β-mercaptoethanol and 0.06% bromophenol blue). The gels were stained by silver nitrate.

## *In vitro* Antigen Presentation Assays

The D1 cell line, a long-term growth factor-dependent immature myeloid (CD11b+, CD8α-) DC line of splenic origin derived from a female C57BL/6 mouse, was generously provided by prof. P. Ricciardi-Castagnoli (University of Milan-Bicocca, Italy) (39). The D1 cells were cultured in 24-well plates (Nunc, A/S Roskilde, Denmark) in Iscove's medium (Biochrom KG, Germany), supplemented with 10% heat-inactivated fetal calf serum (Biochrom KG, Germany), 50 µM 2-mercaptoethanol (Sigma Aldrich, Sweden), 1 mM L-glutamine (Biochrom KG, Germany) and 50 µg/ml Gentamycin (Sigma Aldrich, Sweden) and stimulated for different times with 0. 2 µM of CTA1-3Eα-DD soluble protein or when incorporated into NPLs. To assess the processing efficiency of fusion protein we determined the cell surface expression of peptide plus MHC II complex by incubating D1 cells with anti-Eα(52-68):I-A$^b$ complex-specific Y-Ae biotin-labeled antibody (eBiosciences, USA). Flow cytometric analysis was performed after incubation with streptavidin-APC and anti-CD11c-PE, 7AAD, MHCII-FITC at 4°C for 30 min (eBiosciences, USA). We analyzed 100,000 events using a BD-FACS LSR II instrument (BD Bioscience, USA) and the data were analyzed with FlowJo (TreeStar, USA) software.

## Antigen Processing by Migratory DCs and CD4$^+$ T Cell Priming *in vivo*

Four to 6 weeks old, age, and sex-matched TCR transgenic B6.Cg-Tg(Tcrα,Tcrβ)3Ayr/J mice were immunized i.n. with 50 µg of protein using the fusion proteins alone or incorporated into

NPLs. At 24 h after a single i.n administration of fusion protein or NPLs, mice were sacrificed and the mediastinal lymph nodes (mLN) were extracted and single cell suspensions were prepared. To assess the level of Eα loaded MHCII molecules on isolated migratory DCs we incubated the cells with biotin-labeled Y-Ae anti-mouse Eα(52-68):I-A$^b$ Mab. In the second step we used streptavidin-APC, anti-Ly6c-BV605, anti-CD11c-BV421, anti-MHCII (I-Ab)-FITC, anti-CD11b-APC, anti-CD103-PE, 7AAD for 30 min. at 4°C (antibodies from eBiosciences, USA). We also performed adoptive transfer experiments with $2 \times 10^6$ TCR transgenic CD4$^+$ T cells injected i.v into recipient C57BL/6 mice after isolation using a CD4$^+$ T Cell Isolation Kit (Miltenyi Biotec, Sweden). Prior to transfer the cells were stained with $5 \mu$M CFSE and the mice were immunized i.n. with $5 \mu$g of fusion protein alone or incorporated into NPLs. On days 2,4,6 and 8 after immunizations the mLNs were isolated and single cell suspensions were prepared followed by labeling with anti-CD3-efluor 780, anti-CD4-BV711, anti-TCR Vα2-PE, anti-TCR Vβ6-APC, and 7AAD for 30 min at 4°C (all Mabs from eBiosciences, USA). Proliferating CD4$^+$TCR Vα2$^+$ Vβ6$^+$ cells were identified by reduced CFSE-staining. Flow cytometry analysis was performed on 500,000 events using a BD-FACS LSR II instrument (BD Bioscience, USA) and the FlowJo (TreeStar, USA) software program.

## Virus Transmission and Challenge Experiments

Female BALB/c mice (index animals) in groups of 10 individuals were either unimmunized or immunized i.n as described above and 8 weeks later all mice were infected i.n with $3 \times 10^4$ PFU H3N2 Udorn virus (A/Udorn/307/1972 (H3N2)). After 24 h these infected mice were co-housed with unimmunized uninfected DBA/2 mice (contact animals) and the level of virus transmission was determined. After 4 days the snouts and lungs of both index and contact animals were collected and viral loads were determined by the plaque assay. Briefly, tissue samples were homogenized in cold PBS using FastPrep® spheres (MP Biomedicals, Germany), and centrifuged for 10 min at 9,000 rpm at 4°C. Sample dilutions were done with OptiMEM (Thermo Fisher Scientific, USA) supplemented with 0.3% bovine serum albumin (BSA) and inoculated in 12 well plates with confluent MDCK cells and incubated for 1–2 h at room temperature. The number of plaques in the confluent cell layer was counted in the respective dilution to calculate the virus titer and then given as plaque-forming units (pfu) per ml.

Influenza virus challenge experiments were performed in groups of 10 mice at 2 weeks after the last immunization. We used a lethal i.n dose of $4 \times$ LD50, corresponding to $2.5 \times 10^3$ TCID$_{50}$, of PR8 A/Puerto Rico/8/34 (H1N1) virus or the mouse adapted X47 virus (a reassortant between A/Victoria/3/75 (H3N2) and A/Puerto Rico/8/34 (H1N1)). Morbidity (body weight) and mortality were monitored daily for 2 weeks. Mice were sacrificed when reaching a weight loss >25–30%.

## CD4$^+$ T Cell Immune Responses

We assessed the CD4$^+$ T cell response after immunizations by two different analyses. The first analysis used flow cytometry and

the PE-labeled M2e-tetramer, specifically designed for the study by the NIH Tetramer Core Facility (Bethesda, USA) to identify the CD4$^+$ T cells that specifically recognize and react to M2e in the context of MHC class II I-A$^b$. Briefly, 2 weeks after a challenge infection lung tissue was treated with a Lung Dissociation Kit (Miltenyi Biotec Norden AB, Sweden) and single cell suspensions were prepared. Lung cells were incubated with the specific M2e-tetramer-PE and labeled with anti-CD4-Alexa700, anti-CD19-FITC, anti-F4/80-FITC, anti-CD8-APC/Cy7 Mabs and 7AAD at 4°C for 30 min (all Mabs from eBiosciences, USA). We collected 100,000 events on the BD-FACS LSR II instrument (BD Bioscience, USA) and analyzed the data using the FlowJo (TreeStar, USA) software. The second analysis used in vitro M2e-peptide recall responses in single cell suspensions from spleen and mLN from immunized and control mice. Briefly, $2 \times 10^6$ cells/ml were cultured in plain medium or together with $1 \mu$M of M2e peptide (Pepscan, The Netherlands) in triplicates in 96-well microtiter plates (Nunc, Denmark) in Iscove's medium (Biochrom KG, Germany), supplemented with 10% heat-inactivated fetal calf serum (Biochrom KG, Germany), $50 \mu$M 2-mercaptoethanol (Sigma Aldrich, Sweden), 1 mM L-glutamine (Biochrom KG, Germany) and $50 \mu$g/ml Gentamycin (Sigma Aldrich, Sweden) for 72 h at 37°C in 5% CO$_2$. After 72 h we added [3H]-thymidine (PerkinElmer, USA) to the cultures for the last 6 h and [3H]-thymidine uptake was determined using a scintillation counter (Beckman, Sweden). Prior to the addition of [3H]-thymidine we collected supernatants that were stored at −80°C for further analysis of cytokine contents. We assessed IFNy and IL-17 concentrations by ELISA using 96-well plates (Dynatech Laboratories, Inc., USA) coated with $5 \mu$g/ml of rat anti-mouse IFN-γ or IL-17 (JES5–2A5, PharMingen, USA). After washing polyclonal rabbit anti-mouse IFN-γ or anti-IL-17 antibodies (PharMingen, Denmark) at 1 μg/ml in 0.1% BSA/PBS were added to each well and the p-nitrophenyl phosphatase (Sigma Aldrich, Sweden) reaction was visualized using a Titertek Multiscan spectrophotometer (Labsystems, Sweden) at 450 nm. The concentrations of cytokines in the supernatants were expressed in pg/ml, as calculated from plotted standard curves of serial dilutions of recombinant cytokines.

## Antibody Responses

Serum and BAL were collected from individual mice at indicated time points. M2e- and HA-specific IgG and IgA antibody determinations were performed by ELISA. Briefly, we used 96-well microtiter plates (MaxiSorp, Nunc, Denmark) coated with $5 \mu$g/ml of M2e or $1 \mu$g/ml of recombinant HA (same as described above) in 50 mM sodium bicarbonate buffer pH 9,7 and incubated overnight at 4°C. Serum or BAL were diluted 1:25 and 1:2, respectively, in 0.1% BSA/PBS and serial dilutions 1:3 in corresponding sub-wells were performed. Wells were then incubated with alkaline phosphatase-conjugated rabbit anti-mouse IgA or IgG antibodies (Southern Biotechnology, USA) at 1:1000 dilution overnight. Nitro phenyl (NPP) phosphatase substrate (1 mg/ml, Sigma Aldrich, Sweden) in ethanolamine buffer, pH 9.8, was added to each well and the reaction was read at 405 nm using a Titertek Multiscan spectrophotometer (Labsystems, Sweden). Log$_{10}$ titers were defined as the interpolated OD-reading giving rise to an absorbance 0.4 above background, which consistently gave values on the linear part of the curve.

## Statistical Analysis

Analyses of significance were done in Prism (GraphPad Software) using unpaired *t*-test. All reported *P*-values are two-sided and values of less than 0.05 were considered to indicate statistical significance. $*p < 0.05$, $**p < 0.01$, and $***p < 0.005$.

## RESULTS

### Dendritic Cells Effectively Take Up and Process the Combined Fusion Protein/Nanoparticle Vector

The fusion protein CTA1-3M2e-DD (FPM2e) has previously been demonstrated to stimulate strong protective immunity against challenge with different influenza A virus subtype strains when administered intranasally (i.n) (26). However, it appeared that formulating this very effective influenza virus vaccine candidate in a suitable nanoparticle would increase its efficiency and stability as a vaccine vector even further (40). Therefore, we combined the FPM2e with porous NPLs that previously have been found effective for i.n immunizations (30, 34). Since little is known about DC uptake and presentation of antigens delivered with these nanoparticles, we initially focused on the DCs (41). A panel of formulations with different ratios between loaded protein and the NPLs was produced and their physico-chemical properties were characterized. Of this panel, we selected NPLs with a 1:5 protein:NPL mass ratio (FPM2e:NPL) as the optimal construct to be used for the continued studies. The FPM2e:NPL vector consisted of three main components: the maltodextrin scaffold (NP+), the lipid (DPPG) and the FPM2e, which were linked together by non-covalent interactions (**Figure 1A**). The FPM2e:NPL vector had an average size of 160 nm with a zeta potential of +45.63 ± 1.65 mV, i.e., highly positively charged, while the FPM2e itself was negatively charged (-19.47 ± 0.85 mV) (**Figure 1B**, left and middle panel). We found that most of the FPM2e had been bound to the NPLs, as shown by the absence of free FPM2e in the native PAGE analysis (**Figure 1B**, right panel). The combination vector was stable at different temperatures for up to 1 year with no detectable loss of FPM2e and both size and zeta-potential were kept intact (**Supplementary Figures 1, 2**).

To analyze antigen uptake and processing, we established an *in vitro* screening system based on NPLs carrying a fusion protein with incorporated Eα-peptide, i.e., CTA1-3Eα-DD, termed FPEα. The Eα peptide can be detected when bound to MHC class II surface molecules on DCs by using a labeled Y-Ae antibody that detects the complex (42). Therefore, the FPEα:NPL vectors were used to follow uptake and presentation of the Eα-peptide on the surface of DCs. This way, we could monitor the whole process from uptake to peptide presentation kinetically and, hence, determine what the T cell receptor would recognize on the DC surface. The initial experiments were undertaken using an immature DC cell line, D1 cells (of C57BL/6 origin), to assess the ability to present peptides to CD4+ T cells (39). The mean

fluorescence intensity (MFI) of the bound Y-Ae antibody was assessed by FACS at different time points and from 1 h onwards we consistently observed a 2–3-fold higher MFI and also MHC class II-expression on DCs exposed to the combined vector as opposed to when the FPEα was used alone (**Figure 1C**, left and middle panels). Noteworthy, the CTA1-3Eα-DD given alone had a 2-fold enhancing effect on MHC class II-expression, attesting to its immunomodulating ability (**Figure 1C**, right panel). Thus, the combined FPEα:NPL vector was superior to soluble CTA1-3Eα-DD alone for MHC class II peptide presentation by DCs *in vitro*.

The next experiment evaluated the priming ability of DCs stimulated by FPEα:NPLs for Eα peptide-specific recognition by TCR transgenic CD4+ T cells (I-A$^b$) *in vivo*. We used the B6.Cg-Tg(TCRα,TCRβ)3Ayr/J mice, which host TCR transgenic CD4+ T cells that recognize the Eα peptide bound to MHC class II. First, we determined whether the combined formulation was taken up by DCs *in vivo*. Following i.n. administration of 50 μg of the vector or soluble FPEα, we isolated the mediastinal lymph node (mLN) 24 h later and assessed the presence of DCs labeled with Y-Ae antibody (**Figure 1D**, left panel). We observed strong labeling with antibody in 20% of the migratory DCs (MHC II$^{high}$, CD11c+) while resident DCs (MHC II$^{low}$, CD11c+) did not carry the Eα-peptide and, thus, had not taken up the vaccine vector that was given i.n (**Figure 1D**, middle panel). Migratory DCs were found to carry the Eα peptide also when the FPEα was given i.n alone and the surface expression of the peptide/MHC II-complex was similar to that found in mice receiving the combined FPEα:NPL vector (**Figure 1D**, right panel). In an adoptive transfer experiment where B6.Cg-Tg(TCRα,TCRβ)3Ayr/J CD4+ T cells were injected into wild type C57BL/6 mice, we followed the expansion of TCR Tg CFSE-labeled CD4+ T cells on days 2, 4, 6, 8, 10, and 12 after the i.n immunization. We found that peptide-specific CD4+ T cells in the mLN, were strongly proliferating in FPEα immunized mice at the early time points, while mice given the combined FPEα:NPL vector showed similar proliferation on day 8, which was sustained until at least day 12 after immunization, when proliferation to FPEα only was minimal (**Figure 1E**, upper panel). Hence, peak CD4+ T cell proliferation to FPEα (80%) was observed on day 8 while FPEα:NPL (80%) immunized mice peaked on day 12 (**Figure 1E**, lower panel). Thus, the FPEα:NPL vector stimulated slower but prolonged CD4+ T cell activation in the draining mLN after i.n immunizations compared to that stimulated by FPEa alone.

### Enhanced Immunogenicity and Protective Function of the Combined Fusion Protein/Nanoparticle Vector

Given that the combined vector effectively primed peptide-specific CD4+ T cells *in vivo*, we addressed whether the FPM2e:NPL vector was also effective at stimulating protective immunity against infection. We produced FPM2e:NPL vectors with CTA1-3M2e-DD and determined their immunogenicity in BALB/c mice. Following i.n immunizations with 5 or 1 μg of FPM2e or FPM2e:NPL, we assessed the protective efficacy

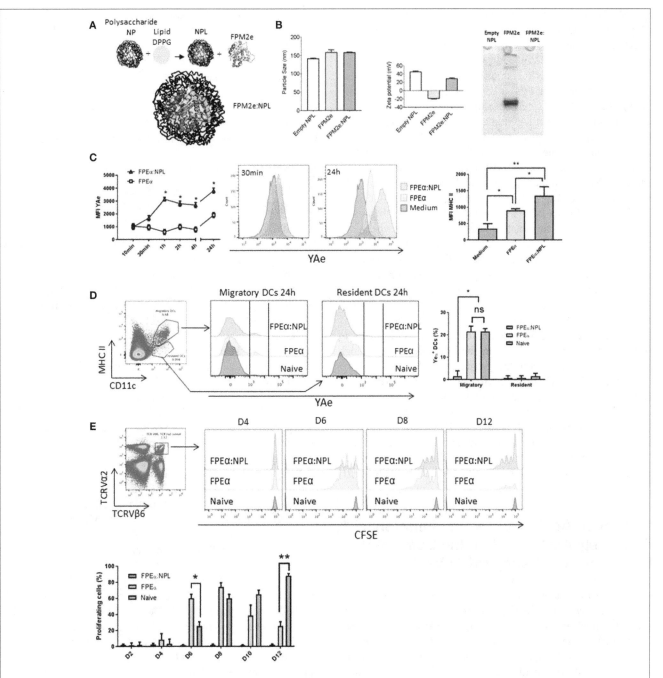

**FIGURE 1 |** Efficient uptake and presentation of the combined NPL vaccine vector by DCs. **(A)** Schematic representation of the design of the FPM2e:NPL vaccine vector. **(B)** FPM2e:NPLs were characterized with regard to particle size (left panel), zeta potential (middle panel) and native-PAGE electrophoresis analysis (right panel). **(C)** The uptake, processing and surface presentation of Eα peptide and MHC class II complexes by D1 dendritic cells (DC) at different time points after stimulation with 0. 2 μM of FPEa or FPEa:NPL. Surface expression of peptide/MHC II complexes were analyzed by flow cytometry using the mean fluorescent intensity (MFI) of labeled Y-Ae Mab plotted as means ± SD of 3 experiments (left panel). Representative histograms of Y-Ae MFI after 30 min and 24 h stimulation are shown (middle panel). MFI values of anti-MHC II Mab labeling of the D1 cell surface after stimulation with FPEa or FPEa:NPL are given as means ± SD of 3 experiments (right panel). **(D)** Gating strategy used for migratory and resident DCs in the mediastinal lymph node (mLN) (left panel). Representative FACS histograms of Y-Ae MFI in migratory (MHC II^high, CD11c+) and resident (MHC II^low, CD11c+) DCs 24 h after a single i.n immunization (middle panel). The percentage of Y-Ae+ cells in migratory and resident DC populations was calculated in 3 independent experiments and given as means ± SD (right panel). **(E)** Gating strategy used to identify proliferation in Eα-specific CFSE-labeled TCR Tg CD4+ T cells following i.n immunization (left panel). Representative FACS histograms of proliferating TCRVα2+TCRVβ6+CFSE+ T cells in the mLN at 4, 6, 8, and 12 days after a single i.n immunization with 5 μg of FPEα or FPEα:NPL in C57Bl/6 mice adoptively transferred on day 0 with 2 × 10^6 TCRVα2+TCRVβ6+CFSE+ CD4+ T cells (right panel). The percentage of proliferating TCRVα2+TCRVβ6+CFSE+ CD4+ T cells was calculated and given as means ± SD (lower panel). These data are from at least 3 independent experiments giving similar results. Statistical significance was calculated by unpaired t-test and p-values are given as *p < 0.05 and **p < 0.01.

against a challenge with $4xLD_{50}$ of the X47 virus strain, a mouse adapted reassortant A/Victoria/3/75 (H3N2) virus strain (43, 44). Infected mice were monitored for weight loss and survival for 15 days post-infection. We found that mice immunized with the 5 µg/dose of FPM2e:NPL exhibited 100% protection, whereas mice immunized with FPM2e alone were less well protected (80%) (**Figure 2A**). Protection was clearly reduced (50%) in mice immunized with 1 µg FPM2e or FPM2e:NPL (**Figure 2B**). Furthermore, immunogenicity was assessed by M2e-peptide-recall responses of splenic $CD4^+$ T cells isolated from immunized mice. Whereas a low dose of FPM2e:NPL (1µg/dose) was more effective than a comparable dose of FPM2e alone, both the 5 µg and 1 µg doses of FPM2e:NPL gave similar $CD4^+$ T cell priming (**Figure 2C**). Importantly, the augmenting effect of the FPM2e:NPL formulation was dependent on the ADP-ribosylating ability of CTA1-3M2e-DD, because the combined vector with the enzymatically inactive CTA1(R9K)-3M2e-DD preparation was significantly less immunogenic (**Figure 2C**). The protective effect of FPM2e:NPL was associated with a strong $CD4^+$ T cell priming effect for IFN-γ and IL-17 production, as assessed in culture supernatants *ex vivo* (**Figures 2D,E**, respectively). Finally, the presence of resident memory M2e-tetramer-specific $CD4^+$ T cells in the lung was similarly high in mice immunized with the combined FPM2e:NPL vector or FPM2e alone (**Figures 2F, G**). In addition, strong and comparable M2e-specific antibody responses in serum were found in both FPM2e alone and the combined FPM2e:NPL vector immunized mice (**Figure 2H**). However, by contrast, anti-M2e IgA titers in bronchoalveolar lavage (BAL) were highest in FPM2e:NPL immunized mice, also with 1 mcg doses, clearly identifying a benefit of the NPL formulation (**Figure 2I**) (45, 46).

## Protection Against Virus Transmission Is Effectively Achieved With the Combined Fusion Protein/Nanoparticle Vector

An effective vaccine against influenza infection should preferentially also stop virus transmission between individuals. To this end, we tested the ability of the combined FPM2e:NPL vector to impair virus transmission between animals. We used a recently established mouse transmission model (47) with highly susceptible DBA/2 mice (48) as contact animals. Following a challenge infection with Udorn virus (H3N2) immunized and unimmunized Balb/c mice (index mice) were co-housed with the DBA/2 contact mice for 4 days (**Figure 3A**). Virus transmission was assessed by monitoring the influenza virus titres in the snouts and lungs of both Balb/c index and DBA/2 contact mice. We found lower virus titres in the snouts of the contact mice co-housed with index mice immunized with FPM2e:NPL (**Figure 3B**). However, protection against infection in the index mice was comparable between FPM2e alone and FPM2e:NPL (**Figure 3B**). Of note, unimmunized (PBS) mice or index mice immunized with CTA1-DD without the M2e-peptide failed to influence transmission of virus to the contact mice. The results from the analysis of the virus titers in the lungs of index or contact mice were less compelling, but also in

the lung we found the least transmission from FPM2e:NPL immunized mice (**Figure 3C**). Anti-M2e serum antibody titers were comparable between index mice immunized with FPM2e or FPM2e:NPL (**Figure 3D**). Taken together the combined FPM2e:NPL vector gave the strongest protection against virus transmission, although the Balb/c index mice immunized with FPM2e:NPL or FPM2e alone exhibited comparable virus titers, suggesting that virus from FPM2e:NPL immunized mice was less infective, maybe due to local anti-M2e IgA antibodies (49).

## Co-incorporated Recombinant HA Improves the Protective Capacity of the Combined Fusion Protein/Nanoparticle Vector

The combined FPM2e:NLP vector was found to be highly immunogenic and induced strong protection against virus transmission. However, we asked whether we could improve the protective ability of the combined vector even further by incorporating recombinant hemagglutinin (HA) from Influenza A Virus H1N1 (A/Puerto Rico/8/34) into the vector (**Figure 4A**). We formulated NPLs with equal amounts of CTA1-M2e-DD and HA. The HA:FPM2e:NPL vector had a size of 130 nm and a zeta potential of +27 mV (**Figure 4B**, left and middle panels). Noteworthy, the soluble HA protein had a particle size of around 50 nm and was negatively charged (−10 mV) (**Figure 4B**, left and middle panels). We found that most of the HA was incorporated into the FPM2e:NPLs (**Figure 4B**, right panel). Mice immunized i.n with the combined HA:FPM2e:NPL vector were fully protected against a challenge infection with the highly virulent PR8 virus (A/Puerto Rico/8/34 (H1N1), whereas none of the HA:NPL, FPM2e:NPL, or FPM2e alone immunized mice were protected (**Figure 4C**). Interestingly, i.n. administration of the NPL formulated CTA1-3M2e-DD (FPM2e:NPL) together with HA:NPLs still resulted in 100% protection against PR8 challenge, showing that the adjuvant CTA1 component was effective even if not physically linked to the HA:NPL (**Figure 4C**). By contrast, a challenge infection with the H3N2 X47 virus strain resulted in partial protection in mice immunized i.n with HA:NPL, and only to achieve 100% protection the adjuvant active FPM2e was needed (**Figure 4D**). As seen previously, FPM2e:NPL and FPM2e alone gave excellent protection against X47 virus infection (**Figures 2A,B, 4D**). Noteworthy, the frequency and absolute numbers of lung resident $M2e-tetramer^+$ $CD4^+$ T cells were lower in mice immunized with HA:M2e:NPL than in FPM2e:NPL or FPM2e alone immunized mice (**Figure 4E**). Again, we observed that the FPM2e:NPLs with an enzymatically inactive fusion protein (CTA1(R9K)-3M2e-DD) were poorly immunogenic, indicating that the performance of the NPL vector was critically dependent on the ADP-ribosylating ability of the FPM2e (**Figure 4F**). In fact, it was clear that the immunogenicity of the incorporated HA greatly benefitted from the adjuvant enhancing effects of the HA:FPM2e:NPL vector as anti-HA serum IgG titers were almost 10-fold higher than in HA:NLPs without the FPM2e (**Figure 4G**). Interestingly, though, this effect was seen only when the FPM2e was in the same particle as the HA and not when the FPM2e was co-administered in

Porous Nanoparticles with Self-Adjuvanting M2e-Fusion Protein and Recombinant Hemagglutinin Provide...

137

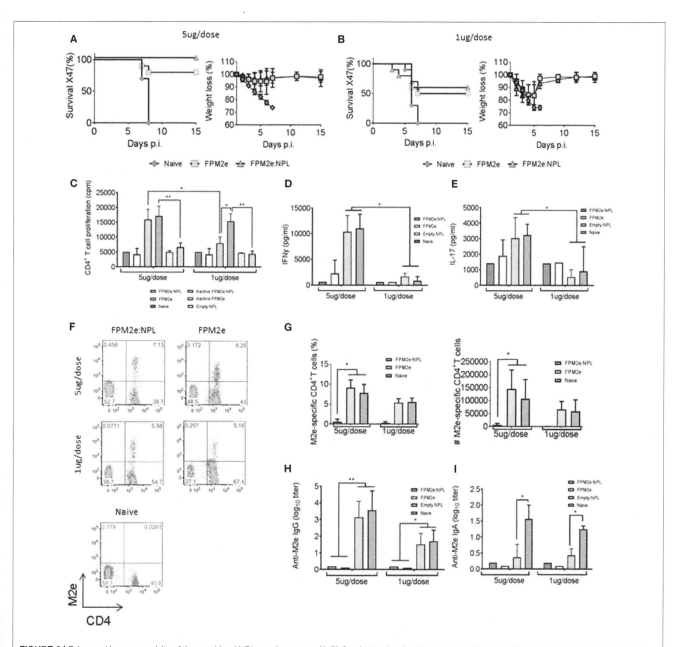

**FIGURE 2 |** Enhanced immunogenicity of the combined NPL vaccine vector. **(A,B)** Survival and weight loss were monitored in influenza virus challenged Balb/c mice following three i.n immunizations with 5 µg **(A)** or 1 µg **(B)** of FPM2e or FPM2e:NPL. The percent of surviving mice (left panel) and body weight loss (right panel) following a challenge infection with 4 × LD50 of the mouse adapted X47 virus strain are plotted. **(C)** Recall responses to M2e-peptide in primed CD4+ T cells following i.n immunizations with 5 or 1 µg of enzymatically active or inactive mutant FPM2e or FPM2e:NPL or empty NPL w/o FPM2e, as indicated. Mean proliferation in isolated splenocytes to M2e peptide is given as mean c.p.m ± S.E.M. **(D,E)** The production of IFN-γ **(D)** or IL-17A **(E)** to recall stimulation with M2e-peptide of the primed CD4+ T cells (as in **C**) is given in pg/ml ± SD. **(F,G)** Representative FACS plots of M2e-tetramer+ CD4+ T cells in the lungs of i.n immunized and challenged mice as indicated **(F)**. The percentage (left panel) and absolute number (right panel) of antigen primed M2e+ tetramer CD4+ T cells **(G)**. **(H,I)** M2e specific IgG antibodies in serum **(H)** or IgA antibodies in BAL **(I)** were measured by ELISA in Balb/c mice immunized i.n. with FPM2e, FPM2e:NPL or PBS (naïve), as indicated, and given as mean log10-titers ± SD of 3 independent experiments giving similar results. Statistical significance was calculated by unpaired t-test and p-values are given as *p < 0.05 and **p < 0.01.

a separate NPL (**Figure 4G**). The M2e-specific IgG responses in serum and IgA-responses in BAL were reduced in HA-containing NPLs as compared to FPM2e:NPLs without the HA (**Figure 4H**). Thus, the FPM2e:NPL vector can be further improved by incorporating additional proteins into the vector and the HA:FPM2e:NPLs vaccine vector was found to exhibit superior protective capacity against a virulent PR8 influenza virus infection, where neither NPLs with HA nor CTA1-3M2e-DD gave any protection. Importantly, the immunogenicity and protective capacity of the combined HA:FPM2e:NPL vector was critically dependent on the enzymatic activity of CTA1 in the FPM2e.

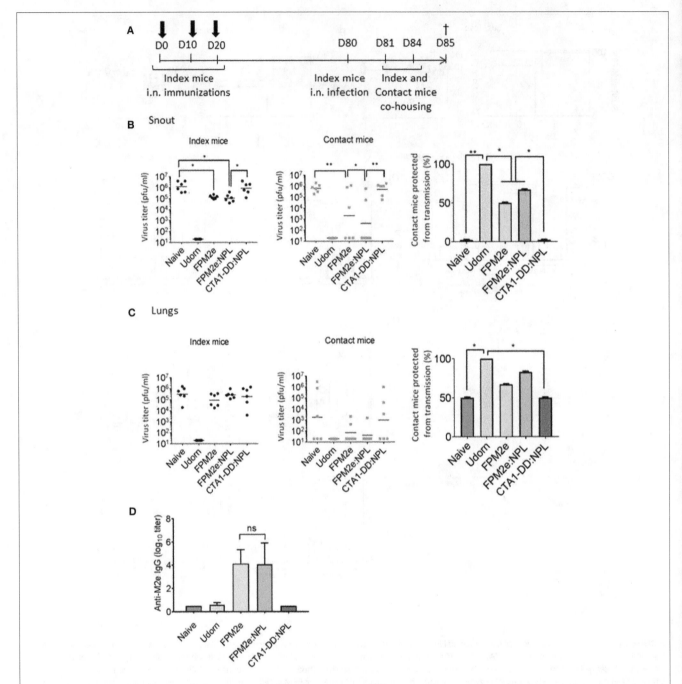

**FIGURE 3** | Reduction of viral transmission following intranasal immunizations with the combined NPL vaccine vector. **(A)** A schematic representation of the experimental protocol used for virus transmission experiments. BALB/c mice (index mice) were immunized three times with 10 days apart with split Udorn virus, 5 $\mu$g per dose of FPM2e alone, FPM2e:NPL, or FP:NPL w/o M2e. Index mice were infected 2–4 weeks after the final immunization with A/Udorn/307/1972 (H3N2) and co-housed with DBA/2 mice (contact mice). **(B,C)** The viral titers in snouts **(B)** or lungs **(C)** of index (left panel) and contact (middle panel) mice and the mean percentages of contact mice protected from virus transmissions (right panel) are shown. **(D)** M2e-specific IgG antibodies in serum were measured by ELISA in index mice and the results are given as mean $\log_{10}$ titers $\pm$ SD. These are representative results from 3 experiments giving similar results and the statistical significance was calculated using unpaired $t$-test and $p$-values are $*p < 0.05$ and $**p < 0.01$.

## DISCUSSION

The present proof-of-principle study demonstrates that an effective broadly protective anti-influenza mucosal vaccine vector can be developed when HA and the enzyme-active CTA1-3M2e-DD adjuvant are incorporated into NPLs. We found that the novel combined HA:FPM2e:NPL vector stimulated strong protective immune responses against homologous and heterologous infections with significantly better survival compared to mice immunized i.n with HA:NPL,

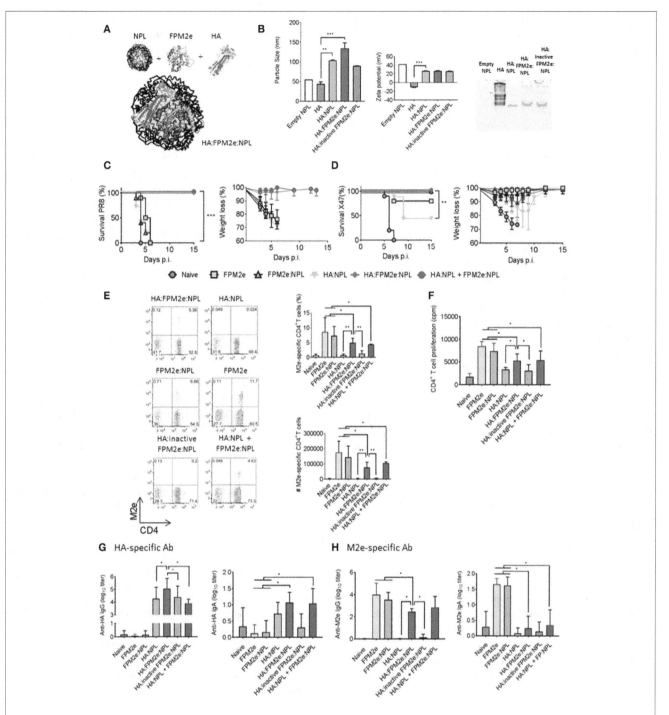

**FIGURE 4 |** Enhanced immunogenicity and protection by co-incorporation of recombinant HA and FPM2e in the combined NPL vaccine vector. **(A)** A schematic representation of the HA:FPM2e:NPL vaccine vector. **(B)** The combined HA:FPM2e:NPL vector was characterized with regard to particle size (left panel), zeta potential (middle panel) and native-PAGE electrophoresis analysis (right panel). **(C,D)** Survival and weight loss was monitored in influenza virus challenged Balb/c mice following three i.n immunizations with 5 μg of vaccine formulations as indicated. The percent of surviving mice (left panel) and body weight loss (right panel) following a challenge infection with 4×LD50 of the mouse adapted X47 **(C)** or PR8 **(D)** virus strains. **(E)** Representative FACS plots of M2e-tetramer+ CD4+ T cells in the lungs of i.n immunized and challenged mice are shown. The percentage and absolute numbers (right panels) of antigen primed M2e+ tetramer CD4+ T cells in the lung. **(F)** Recall responses of primed M2e-specific CD4+ T cells in the spleens of immunized mice are given as mean cpm± SD of 3 independent experiments. **(G,H)** HA- **(G)** or M2e-specific **(H)** IgG antibodies in serum (left panel) and IgA antibodies in BAL (right panel) were determined by ELISA in immunized mice as indicated and the mean log₁₀-titers± SD are given. These are representative results from three experiments giving similar results and the statistical significance was calculated using unpaired *t*-test and *p*-values are *$p < 0.05$, **$p < 0.01$ and ***$p < 0.005$.

FPM2e:NPL, or FPM2e alone. The vector hosted some critical features brought together in a single physical unit, namely the powerful CTA1 adjuvant, the M2e and recombinant HA for broad cross-protection and the particle formulation, facilitating mucosal delivery, stability, and uptake by DCs. These elements combined contributed to the strong protective immune response following i.n immunizations that we observed. Whereas many previous studies have reported on promising mucosal vaccine candidates against influenza, this is the first to describe the combination of an enzyme-active adjuvant system incorporated into nanoparticles (50–52). The NPL incorporation technique used did not damage the ADP-ribosylating ability of the CTA1-enzyme.

Several of the mucosal vaccine candidates against influenza that have been, or are being, tested have explored various other forms of nanoparticle formulations (53–58). Among the more successful ones are chitosan nanoparticles, that have been developed for immunizations of pigs, and which were reported to stimulate mucosal IgA as well as effector $CD4^+$ T cell immunity (49, 59). Contrary to our combined vector, these nanoparticles carried multiple killed swine H1N1 antigens while we explored only the M2e-peptide and recombinant HA. However, this and several other studies support the concept of multiple influenza antigens encapsulated into nanoparticles as a promising way forward for a broadly protective influenza vaccine (60, 61). In this context, it is noteworthy that nanoparticles with killed whole-inactivated virus antigens have consistently been found to be poor inducers of T cell mediated responses and, hence, have provided only weak protection against heterologous influenza strains (62). Our study demonstrates that strong $CD4^+$ T cell responses can be achieved with the present combined NPL. An explanation for the weak protection could be that injectable vaccines give poor lung resident T cell immunity, which is thought to be critical for a broadly protective influenza vaccine (4).

The porous NPL technology has been successfully used for several i.n vaccine formulations in the past, including a vaccine candidate against toxoplasma infection (31). It has repeatedly been found that the use of particulate antigens can be more effective than soluble proteins at stimulating strong immune responses and affording long-term protection (34, 35, 63–66). However, previous work with porous NPLs has not explored adding an independent adjuvant active vaccine component, such as the CTA1-3M2e-DD molecule. Here, we report that this greatly augmented the immunogenicity of the NPL vector. We observed that HA:FPM2e:NPLs achieved a 10-fold stronger anti-HA IgG serum titer when the HA was co-incorporated into NPLs with CTA1-3M2e-DD. This enhancing effect is what we regularly have observed with the CTA1-DD adjuvant in other systems (23, 24, 28). The augmenting effect required an active ADP-ribosylating enzyme, because the inactive CTA1(R9K)-3M2e-DD mutant failed to augment immunogenicity, which agrees well with results from our previous studies (67). The latter finding also identified that nanoparticles can achieve much improved immunogenicity if complemented with adjuvant active molecules, such as chitosan, flagellin or CTA1-DD (68–70). Interestingly, this augmenting effect on anti-HA IgG serum antibodies was not seen when the FPM2e and HA were provided

in separate NPLs, suggesting that this effect required physical contact between HA and the FPM2e. While excellent protection was achieved also in vaccine regimens with NPLs where HA and FPM2e formulations where separated and both protocols induced comparable M2e-immunity, we can speculate that anti-HA-specific cell-mediated immunity was responsible for the improved protection against influenza virus challenge infection. We did not determine HA-specific T cell immunity in the present study, but the result is in agreement with a direct effect of the CTA1-3M2e-DD on the follicular dendritic cells (FDC) in the germinal center, which could only work if expanding HA-specific B cells were recruited to CTA1-3M2e-DD exposed FDCs (71, 72). We have recently found that this effect of the CTA1-DD adjuvant on FDCs is mediated through an up-regulation of gene transcription and, in particular, the CXCL13 gene, which encodes the main chemokine to attract activated B cells to the GC (73). However, the adjuvant effect on CD4+ T cell priming is likely to be through enhancing DC functions, which is effectively achieved with the FPM2e and would not necessarily require that HA and FPM2e are physically co-formulated in the same NPL. Additional studies are required to dissect the detailed mechanisms behind the strong adjuvanticity that we observed with the combined NPL vaccine vector.

A special focus was given to DCs for the binding and uptake of the combined NPL vector. We observed in vitro that Eα-peptide in the FPEα incorporated in NPLs was more efficiently taken up and/or processed and presented by DCs than when provided as soluble FPEα. The FPEα:NPL formulation gave up-regulated MHC class II expression and Eα-peptide presentation on the surface of the DCs. In vivo, we identified that migratory DCs were the cell subset responsible for Eα peptide priming of the specific $CD4^+$ T cells in the draining mLN. With a relatively larger dose (50 μg) of FPEα:NPL than used for i.n immunizations (5 μg) we could detect Eα-presenting DC in the draining mLN. Hence, this result provides strong evidence that migratory DCs are the prime effectors of the augmented FPEα:NPL response. However, while the effect in vitro indicated a dramatic improvement of peptide expression in exposed DCs, the in vivo expression in migratory DC was comparable between FPEα alone and FPEα:NPL. The protective ability was similar between FPM2e and M2e:NPL, which was supported by comparable levels of resident M2e-specific $CD4^+$ T cells in the lung and IgG-specific M2e-antibodies in serum. To reconcile these observations, it may be postulated that NPL formulations are retained in the nasal mucosa longer than the FPM2e alone and that this leads to a slower and more prolonged priming of specific $CD4^+$ T cells in the mLN when FPEa:NPLs are given. Also earlier studies have observed a depot-effect and retention of $CD4^+$ T cell priming in draining lymph nodes when NPL formulations were used (74). Therefore, it may be possible to improve the performance of the FPM2e:NPL vector further by altering the chemical composition of the NPL or by adding chitosan or some known component with an effect on the penetration of the mucosal barrier (72, 75–77).

In vivo, we found that a higher M2e-specific $CD4^+$ T cell priming effect was achieved with the lower FPM2e:NPL dose as compared to an equivalent FPM2e dose. This was evident from recall responses to M2e-peptide in isolated splenocytes from immunized mice. Strong support for the requirement of an active ADP-ribosylating activity of the CTA1 enzyme was also found in these experiments. The enhanced response showed augmented levels of IFN-$\gamma$ and IL-17 production from the M2e-specific CD4$^+$ T cells, which are the cardinal features of strong heterosubtypic protection in the mouse model of influenza infection (78–82). We could identify the presence of lung resident M2e tetramer-specific CD4$^+$ T cells in these well protected mice, which confirms the pattern that we previously identified with the FPM2e and places emphasis on the very important role of these tissue resident M2e-specific CD4 T cells for heterosubtypic protection (26). Also, M2e-specific IgA antibody titers in BAL were higher in mice immunized with the FPM2e:NPL. However, because both FPM2e alone and FPM2e:NPL induced protection against virus transmission in immunized mice, albeit slightly better in FPM2e:NPL mice, the protective role of IgA anti-M2e antibodies is not clear. Other studies, such as that from Hervé et al, have suggested that an enhanced anti-M2e IgA antibody response after i.n immunizations could be protective (49). Noteworthy, though, is the fact that IgA antibodies are likely not mediating ADCC reactions and, hence, the role of local respiratory tract anti-M2e IgA for protection is at present poorly defined. Nonetheless, mucosal IgA anti-HA following i.n immunizations with in HA:FPM2e:NPL may well play a protective role, as suggested in several other studies (52, 83, 84). In addition, our recent study with M2e-specific lung resident memory CD4$^+$ T cells has clearly pointed to a critical protective function of these cells, which are only generated after i.n immunizations (26). Hence, the co-existence of local IgA and influenza-specific resident memory CD4$^+$ T cells makes it difficult to identify the relative contribution each of these elements for protection, but ongoing studies in our laboratory is attempting to better dissect this question (85, 86).

In the present study we have convincingly shown that co-incorporation of adjuvant active molecules and influenza specific target antigens into porous NPLs is more broadly effective against influenza virus infections than either component used alone. Hence, we would like to continue developing the NPL vector with additional components known to exert broad protection against influenza. In particular, we will test the addition of the nucleoprotein (NP), which can elicit strong cytotoxic CD8$^+$ T cells (4). In addition, instead of whole recombinant HA, we propose to include a stabilized HA stem region, as recently reported using ferritin nanoparticles, which stimulated protection against a heterosubtypic challenge infection in both mice and ferrets (5, 66). In addition, we noticed that the presence of recombinant HA in the NPL formulation significantly reduced the anti-M2e antibody and CD4$^+$ T cell responses, suggesting that we need to increase the FPM2e component in future combined NPL vectors. This way we may also achieve improved adjuvanticity for HA-immune responses. Future studies will reveal if the favorable effects observed with the combined HA:FPM2e:NPL i.n vaccine vector for broad protection against influenza can be translated into a human vaccine.

## AUTHOR CONTRIBUTIONS

VB, XS, PS, DB, and NL designed the study, analyzed data and wrote the manuscript. BB, ML, and RC prepared the formulations. VB, LY, AO, and KS performed the experiments and analysis of the data.

## FUNDING

The study received funding from the People Programme (Marie Curie Actions) of the European Union's Seventh Framework Programme FP7/2007-2013/ under REA grant agreement number 607690. It was also supported in parts by research funds from the Knut and Alice Wallenberg Foundation KAW 2013.0030, Swedish Foundation for Strategic Research SB12-0088, The Swedish Cancer Foundation, The Swedish Research Council, the EU project UNISEC, LUA/ALF ALFGBG-531021 and the Lundberg foundation.

## ACKNOWLEDGMENTS

The authors would like to thank Jan-Olof Andersson and Richard Christison for helping with expression and purification of fusion proteins. Special thanks to the NIH Tetramer Core Facility for producing the unique MHC class II restricted M2e tetramer: I-A(d) Influenza A M2 2-17 SLLTEVETPIRNEWGS varC>S. We also thank staff at the Laboratory for Experimental Biomedicine at the University of Gothenburg for valuable help with the studies.

## SUPPLEMENTARY MATERIAL

**Supplementary Figure 1** | FPM2e:NPL vaccine vectors are stable up to 12 months.**(A)** Characterization of the stability of FPM2e:NPL by native PAGE analysis after 3 months of storage at 4°C (left panel) or 40°C (middle panel) or after 12 months at 4°C (right panel). **(B)** Characterization of the stability of FPM2e:NPL by SDS-PAGE analysis after 3 months of storage at 4°C (left panel) or 40°C (middle panel) or after 12 months at 4°C (right panel). These are representative experiments out of 3 with similar results.

**Supplementary Figure 2** | Size and charge of FPM2e:NPL is stable after 3 months storage. **(A)** Characterization of the size stability of FPM2e:NPLs after 3 months of storage at 4°C (left panel) or 40°C (right panel). **(B)** Characterization of the charge stability of FPM2e:NPL after 3 months of storage at 4°C (left panel) or 40°C (right panel). These are representative experiments out of 3 with similar results.

# REFERENCES

1. Sautto GA, Kirchenbaum GA, Ross TM. Towards a universal influenza vaccine: different approaches for one goal. *Virol J.* (2018) 15:17. doi: 10.1186/s12985-017-0918-y

2. Impagliazzo A, Milder F, Kuipers H, Wagner MV, Zhu X, Hoffman RM, et al. A stable trimeric influenza hemagglutinin stem as a broadly protective immunogen. *Science* (2015) 349:1301–6. doi: 10.1126/science.aac7263

3. Nachbagauer R, Liu WC, Choi A, Wohlbold TJ, Atlas T, Rajendran M, et al. A universal influenza virus vaccine candidate confers protection against pandemic H1N1 infection in preclinical ferret studies. *NPJ Vaccines* (2017) 2:26. doi: 10.1038/s41541-017-0026-4

4. Saletti G, Gerlach T, Rimmelzwaan GF. Influenza vaccines: 'tailor-made' or 'one fits all'. *Curr Opin Immunol.* (2018) 53:102–10. doi: 10.1016/j.coi.2018.04.015

5. Yassine HM, Boyington JC, McTamney PM, Wei CJ, Kanekiyo M, Kong WP, et al. Hemagglutinin-stem nanoparticles generate heterosubtypic influenza protection. *Nat Med.* (2015) 21:1065–70. doi: 10.1038/nm.3927

6. Khanna M, Sharma S, Kumar B, Rajput R. Protective immunity based on the conserved hemagglutinin stalk domain and its prospects for universal influenza vaccine development. *Biomed Res Int.* (2014) 2014:546274. doi: 10.1155/2014/546274

7. Laursen NS, Wilson IA. Broadly neutralizing antibodies against influenza viruses. *Antiviral Res.* (2013) 98:476–83. doi: 10.1016/j.antiviral.2013.03.021

8. To KK, Zhang AJ, Hung IF, Xu T, Ip WC, Wong RT, et al. High titer and avidity of nonneutralizing antibodies against influenza vaccine antigen are associated with severe influenza. *Clin Vaccine Immunol.* (2012) 19:1012–8. doi: 10.1128/CVI.00081-12

9. Carragher DM, Kaminski DA, Moquin A, Hartson L, Randall TD. A novel role for non-neutralizing antibodies against nucleoprotein in facilitating resistance to influenza A virus. *J Immunol.* (2008) 181:4168–76. doi: 10.4049/jimmunol.181.6.4168

10. Zheng M, Luo J, Chen Z. Development of universal influenza vaccines based on influenza virus M and NP genes. *Infection* (2014) 42:251–62. doi: 10.1007/s15010-013-0546-4

11. Kolpe A, Schepens B, Fiers W, Saelens X. M2-based influenza vaccines: recent advances and clinical potential. *Exp Rev Vaccines* (2017) 16:123–36. doi: 10.1080/14760584.2017.1240041

12. Berlanda Scorza F, Tsvetnitsky V, Donnelly JJ. Universal influenza vaccines: Shifting to better vaccines. *Vaccine* (2016) 34:2926–33. doi: 10.1016/j.vaccine.2016.03.085

13. Houser K, Subbarao K. Influenza vaccines: challenges and solutions. *Cell Host Microbe.* (2015) 17:295–300. doi: 10.1016/j.chom.2015.02.012

14. Lee YT, Ko EJ, Lee Y, Kim KH, Kim MC, Lee YN, et al. Intranasal vaccination with M2e5x virus-like particles induces humoral and cellular immune responses conferring cross-protection against heterosubtypic influenza viruses. *PLoS ONE* (2018) 13:e0190868. doi: 10.1371/journal.pone.0190868

15. Kim YJ, Lee YT, Kim MC, Lee YN, Kim KH, Ko EJ, et al. Cross-protective efficacy of influenza virus M2e containing virus-like particles is superior to hemagglutinin vaccines and variable depending on the genetic backgrounds of mice. *Front Immunol.* (2017) 8:1730. doi: 10.3389/fimmu.2017.01730

16. Eliasson DG, El Bakkouri K, Schon K, Ramne A, Festjens E, Lowenadler B, et al. CTA1-M2e-DD: a novel mucosal adjuvant targeted influenza vaccine. *Vaccine* (2008) 26:1243–52. doi: 10.1016/j.vaccine.2007.12.027

17. Zens KD, Chen JK, Farber DL. Vaccine-generated lung tissue-resident memory T cells provide heterosubtypic protection to influenza infection. *JCI Insight* (2016) 1:e85832. doi: 10.1172/jci.insight.85832

18. Slutter B, Van Braeckel-Budimir N, Abboud G, Varga SM, Salek-Ardakani S, Harty JT. Dynamics of influenza-induced lung-resident memory T cells underlie waning heterosubtypic immunity. *Sci Immunol.* (2017) 2:eaag2031. doi: 10.1126/sciimmunol.aag2031

19. McMaster SR, Wilson JJ, Wang H, Kohlmeier JE. Airway-resident memory CD8 T cells provide antigen-specific protection against respiratory virus challenge through Rapid IFN-gamma production. *J Immunol.* (2015) 195:203–9. doi: 10.4049/jimmunol.1402975

20. Wu T, Hu Y, Lee YT, Bouchard KR, Benechet A, Khanna K, et al. Lung-resident memory CD8 T cells (TRM) are indispensable for optimal cross-protection against pulmonary virus infection. *J Leukoc Biol.* (2014) 95:215–24. doi: 10.1189/jlb.0313180

21. Genton B, D'Acremont V. Intranasal versus injectable influenza vaccine. *Clin Infect Dis.* (2004) 39:754:author reply:754–5. doi: 10.1086/422879

22. Lycke N. Recent progress in mucosal vaccine development: potential and limitations. *Nat Rev Immunol.* (2012) 12:592–605. doi: 10.1038/nri3251

23. Mowat AM, Donachie AM, Jagewall S, Schon K, Lowenadler B, Dalsgaard K, et al. CTA1-DD-immune stimulating complexes: a novel, rationally designed combined mucosal vaccine adjuvant effective with nanogram doses of antigen. *J Immunol.* (2001) 167:3398–405. doi: 10.4049/jimmunol.167.6.3398

24. Agren LC, Ekman L, Lowenadler B, Nedrud JG, Lycke NY. Adjuvanticity of the cholera toxin A1-based gene fusion protein, CTA1-DD, is critically dependent on the ADP-ribosyltransferase and Ig-binding activity. *J Immunol.* (1999) 162:2432–40.

25. Agren LC, Ekman L, Lowenadler B, Lycke NY. Genetically engineered nontoxic vaccine adjuvant that combines B cell targeting with immunomodulation by cholera toxin A1 subunit. *J Immunol.* (1997) 158:3936–46.

26. Eliasson DG, Omokanye A, Schon K, Wenzel UA, Bernasconi V, Bemark M, et al. M2e-tetramer-specific memory CD4 T cells are broadly protective against influenza infection. *Mucosal Immunol.* (2017) 11:273–89. doi: 10.1038/mi.2017.14

27. De Filette M, Fiers W, Martens W, Birkett A, Ramne A, Lowenadler B, et al. Improved design and intranasal delivery of an M2e-based human influenza a vaccine. *Vaccine* (2006) 24:6597–601. doi: 10.1016/j.vaccine.2006.05.082

28. Eriksson AM, Schon KM, Lycke NY. The cholera toxin-derived CTA1-DD vaccine adjuvant administered intranasally does not cause inflammation or accumulate in the nervous tissues. *J Immunol.* (2004) 173:3310–9. doi: 10.4049/jimmunol.173.5.3310

29. Connell TD. Cholera toxin, LT-I, LT-IIa and LT-IIb: the critical role of ganglioside binding in immunomodulation by type I and type II heat-labile enterotoxins. *Expert Rev Vaccines* (2007) 6:821–34. doi: 10.1586/14760584.6.5.821

30. Bernocchi B, Carpentier R, Lantier I, Ducournau C, Dimier-Poisson I, Betbeder D. Mechanisms allowing protein delivery in nasal mucosa using NPL nanoparticles. *J Control Release* (2016) 232:42–50. doi: 10.1016/j.jconrel.2016.04.014

31. Csaba N, Garcia-Fuentes M, Alonso MJ. Nanoparticles for nasal vaccination. *Adv Drug Deliv Rev.* (2009) 61:140–57. doi: 10.1016/j.addr.2008.09.005

32. Zhang T, Xu Y, Qiao L, Wang Y, Wu X, Fan D, et al. Trivalent Human Papillomavirus (HPV) VLP vaccine covering HPV type 58 can elicit high level of humoral immunity but also induce immune interference among component types. *Vaccine* (2010) 28:3479–87. doi: 10.1016/j.vaccine.2010.02.057

33. Woodrow KA, Bennett KM, Lo DD. Mucosal vaccine design and delivery. *Annu Rev Biomed Eng.* (2012) 14:17–46. doi: 10.1146/annurev-bioeng-071811-150054

34. Paillard A, Passirani C, Saulnier P, Kroubi M, Garcion E, Benoit JP, et al. Positively-charged, porous, polysaccharide nanoparticles loaded with anionic molecules behave as 'stealth' cationic nanocarriers. *Pharm Res.* (2010) 27:126–33. doi: 10.1007/s11095-009-9986-z

35. Dimier-Poisson I, Carpentier R, N'Guyen TT, Dahmani F, Ducournau C, Betbeder D. Porous nanoparticles as delivery system of complex antigens for an effective vaccine against acute and chronic *Toxoplasma gondii* infection. *Biomaterials* (2015) 50:164–75. doi: 10.1016/j.biomaterials.2015.01.056

36. Dombu C, Carpentier R, Betbeder D. Influence of surface charge and inner composition of nanoparticles on intracellular delivery of proteins in airway epithelial cells. *Biomaterials* (2012) 33:9117–26. doi: 10.1016/j.biomaterials.2012.08.064

37. Kim TS, Sun J, Braciale TJ. T cell responses during influenza infection: getting and keeping control. *Trends Immunol.* (2011) 32:225–31. doi: 10.1016/j.it.2011.02.006

38. Spangler BD. Structure and function of cholera toxin and the related Escherichia coli heat-labile enterotoxin. *Microbiol Rev.* (1992) 56:622–47.

39. Winzler C, Rovere P, Rescigno M, Granucci F, Penna G, Adorini L, et al. Maturation stages of mouse dendritic cells in growth factor-dependent long-term cultures. *J Exp Med.* (1997) 185:317–28. doi: 10.1084/jem.185.2.317

40. Bernasconi V, Norling K, Bally M, Hook F, Lycke NY. Mucosal vaccine development based on liposome technology. *J Immunol Res.* (2016) 2016:5482087. doi: 10.1155/2016/5482087

41. Bernocchi B, Carpentier R, Betbeder D. Nasal nanovaccines. *Int J Pharm.* (2017) 530:128–38. doi: 10.1016/j.ijpharm.2017.07.012

42. Murphy DB, Lo D, Rath S, Brinster RL, Flavell RA, Slanetz A, et al. A novel MHC class II epitope expressed in thymic medulla but not cortex. *Nature* (1989) 338:765–8. doi: 10.1038/338765a0

43. Vanlandschoot P, Beirnaert E, Neirynck S, Saelens X, Jou WM, Fiers W. Molecular and immunological characterization of soluble aggregated A/Victoria/3/75 (H3N2) influenza haemagglutinin expressed in insect cells. *Arch Virol.* (1996) 141:1715–26. doi: 10.1007/BF01718294

44. Thangavel RR, Bouvier NM. Animal models for influenza virus pathogenesis, transmission, and immunology. *J Immunol Methods* (2014) 410:60–79. doi: 10.1016/j.jim.2014.03.023

45. Zhang L, Yang W, Hu C, Wang Q, Wu Y. Properties and applications of nanoparticle/microparticle conveyors with adjuvant characteristics suitable for oral vaccination. *Int J Nanomed.* (2018) 13:2973–87. doi: 10.2147/IJN.S154743

46. Zhao L, Seth A, Wibowo N, Zhao CX, Mitter N, Yu C, et al. Nanoparticle vaccines. *Vaccine* (2014) 32:327–37. doi: 10.1016/j.vaccine.2013.11.069

47. Klinkhammer J, Schnepf D, Ye L, Schwaderlapp M, Gad HH, Garcin D, et al. IFN-γ prevents influenza virus spread from the upper airways to the lungs and limits virus transmission. *eLife* (2018). 7:e33354. doi: 10.7554/eLife.33354

48. Pica N, Iyer A, Ramos I, Bouvier NM, Fernandez-Sesma A, Garcia-Sastre A, et al. The DBA.2 mouse is susceptible to disease following infection with a broad, but limited, range of influenza A and B viruses. *J Virol.* (2011) 85:12825–9. doi: 10.1128/JVI.05930-11

49. Herve PL, Raliou M, Bourdieu C, Dubuquoy C, Petit-Camurdan A, Bertho N, et al. A novel subnucleocapsid nanoplatform for mucosal vaccination against influenza virus that targets the ectodomain of matrix protein 2. *J Virol.* (2014) 88:325–38. doi: 10.1128/JVI.01141-13

50. Rose MA, Zielen S, Baumann U. Mucosal immunity and nasal influenza vaccination. *Expert Rev Vaccines* (2012) 11:595–607. doi: 10.1586/erv.12.31

51. Hasegawa H, Ichinohe T, Tamura S, Kurata T. Development of a mucosal vaccine for influenza viruses: preparation for a potential influenza pandemic. *Expert Rev Vaccines* (2007) 6:193–201. doi: 10.1586/14760584.6.2.193

52. van Riet E, Ainai A, Suzuki T, Hasegawa H. Mucosal IgA responses in influenza virus infections; thoughts for vaccine design. *Vaccine* (2012) 30:5893–900. doi: 10.1016/j.vaccine.2012.04.109

53. Babai I, Barenholz Y, Zakay-Rones Z, Greenbaum E, Samira S, Hayon I, et al. A novel liposomal influenza vaccine (INFLUSOME-VAC) containing hemagglutinin-neuraminidase and IL-2 or GM-CSF induces protective anti-neuraminidase antibodies cross-reacting with a wide spectrum of influenza A viral strains. *Vaccine* (2001) 20:505–15. doi: 10.1016/S0264-410X(01)00326-7

54. Barnier-Quer C, Elsharkawy A, Romeijn S, Kros A, Jiskoot W. Adjuvant effect of cationic liposomes for subunit influenza vaccine: influence of antigen loading method, cholesterol and immune modulators. *Pharmaceutics* (2013) 5:392–410. doi: 10.3390/pharmaceutics5030392

55. Even-Or O, Joseph A, Itskovitz-Cooper N, Samira S, Rochlin E, Eliyahu H, et al. A new intranasal influenza vaccine based on a novel polycationic lipid-ceramide carbamoyl-spermine (CCS). II. Studies in mice and ferrets and mechanism of adjuvanticity. *Vaccine* (2011) 29:2474–86. doi: 10.1016/j.vaccine.2011.01.009

56. Joseph A, Itskovitz-Cooper N, Samira S, Flasterstein O, Eliyahu H, Simberg D, et al. A new intranasal influenza vaccine based on a novel polycationic lipid–ceramide carbamoyl-spermine (CCS) I. Immunogenicity and efficacy studies in mice. *Vaccine* (2006) 24:3990–4006. doi: 10.1016/j.vaccine.2005.12.017

57. Sawaengsak C, Mori Y, Yamanishi K, Mitrevej A, Sinchaipanid N. Chitosan nanoparticle encapsulated hemagglutinin-split influenza virus mucosal vaccine. *AAPS PharmSciTech.* (2014) 15:317–25. doi: 10.1208/s12249-013-0058-7

58. Waeckerle-Men Y, Allmen EU, Gander B, Scandella E, Schlosser E, Schmidtke G, et al. Encapsulation of proteins and peptides into biodegradable poly(D,L-lactide-co-glycolide) microspheres prolongs and enhances antigen presentation by human dendritic cells. *Vaccine* (2006) 24:1847–57. doi: 10.1016/j.vaccine.2005.10.032

59. Dhakal S, Renu S, Ghimire S, Shaan Lakshmanappa Y, Hogshead BT, Feliciano-Ruiz N, et al. Mucosal immunity and protective efficacy of intranasal inactivated influenza vaccine is improved by chitosan nanoparticle delivery in pigs. *Front Immunol.* (2018) 9:934. doi: 10.3389/fimmu.2018.00934

60. Patterson DP, Rynda-Apple A, Harmsen AL, Harmsen AG, Douglas T. Biomimetic antigenic nanoparticles elicit controlled protective immune response to influenza. *ACS Nano* (2013) 7:3036–44. doi: 10.1021/nn4006544

61. Hiremath J, Kang KI, Xia M, Elaish M, Binjawadagi B, Ouyang K, et al. Entrapment of H1N1 influenza virus derived conserved peptides in PLGA nanoparticles enhances T cell response and vaccine efficacy in Pigs. *PLoS ONE* (2016) 11:e0151922. doi: 10.1371/journal.pone.0151922

62. Vincent AL, Perez DR, Rajao D, Anderson TK, Abente EJ, Walia RR, et al. Influenza A virus vaccines for swine. *Vet Microbiol.* (2017) 206:35–44. doi: 10.1016/j.vetmic.2016.11.026

63. Hagenaars N, Mastrobattista E, Glansbeek H, Heldens J, van den Bosch H, Schijns V, et al. Head-to-head comparison of four nonadjuvanted inactivated cell culture-derived influenza vaccines: effect of composition, spatial organization and immunization route on the immunogenicity in a murine challenge model. *Vaccine* (2008) 26:6555–63. doi: 10.1016/j.vaccine.2008.09.057

64. Patel JM, Vartabedian VF, Kim MC, He S, Kang SM, Selvaraj P. Influenza virus-like particles engineered by protein transfer with tumor-associated antigens induces protective antitumor immunity. *Biotechnol Bioeng.* (2015) 112:1102–10. doi: 10.1002/bit.25537

65. Vanloubbeeck Y, Pichyangkul S, Bayat B, Yongvanitchit K, Bennett JW, Sattabongkot J, et al. Comparison of the immune responses induced by soluble and particulate Plasmodium vivax circumsporozoite vaccine candidates formulated in AS01 in rhesus macaques. *Vaccine* (2013) 31:6216–24. doi: 10.1016/j.vaccine.2013.10.041

66. Deng L, Mohan T, Chang TZ, Gonzalez GX, Wang Y, Kwon YM, et al. Double-layered protein nanoparticles induce broad protection against divergent influenza A viruses. *Nat Commun.* (2018) 9:359. doi: 10.1038/s41467-017-02725-4

67. Eliasson DG, Helgeby A, Schon K, Nygren C, El-Bakkouri K, Fiers W, et al. A novel non-toxic combined CTA1-DD and ISCOMS adjuvant vector for effective mucosal immunization against influenza virus. *Vaccine* (2011) 29:3951–61. doi: 10.1016/j.vaccine.2011.03.090

68. Kim JR, Holbrook BC, Hayward SL, Blevins LK, Jorgensen MJ, Kock ND, et al. Inclusion of flagellin during vaccination against influenza enhances recall responses in nonhuman primate neonates. *J Virol.* (2015) 89:7291–303. doi: 10.1128/JVI.00549-15

69. Holbrook BC, D'Agostino RB Jr, Parks GD, Alexander-Miller MA. Adjuvanting an inactivated influenza vaccine with flagellin improves the function and quantity of the long-term antibody response in a nonhuman primate neonate model. *Vaccine* (2016) 34:4712–17. doi: 10.1016/j.vaccine.2016.08.010

70. Ghendon Y, Markushin S, Vasiliev Y, Akopova I, Koptiaeva I, Krivtsov G, et al. Evaluation of properties of chitosan as an adjuvant for inactivated influenza vaccines administered parenterally. *J Med Virol.* (2009) 81:494–506. doi: 10.1002/jmv.21415

71. Allen CD, Cyster JG. Follicular dendritic cell networks of primary follicles and germinal centers: phenotype and function. *Semin Immunol.* (2008) 20:14–25. doi: 10.1016/j.smim.2007.12.001

72. Kranich J, Krautler NJ. How follicular dendritic cells shape the B-cell antigenome. *Front Immunol.* (2016) 7:225. doi: 10.3389/fimmu.2016.00225

73. Mattsson J, Yrlid U, Stensson A, Schon K, Karlsson MC, Ravetch JV, et al. Complement activation and complement receptors on follicular dendritic cells are critical for the function of a targeted adjuvant. *J Immunol.* (2011) 187:3641–52. doi: 10.4049/jimmunol.1101107

74. Henriksen-Lacey M, Bramwell VW, Christensen D, Agger EM, Andersen P, Perrie Y. Liposomes based on dimethyldioctadecylammonium promote a depot effect and enhance immunogenicity of soluble antigen. *J Control Release* (2010) 142:180–6. doi: 10.1016/j.jconrel.2009.10.022

75. Barua S, Mitragotri S. Challenges associated with penetration of nanoparticles across cell and tissue barriers: a review of current status and future prospects. *Nano Today* (2014) 9:223–43. doi: 10.1016/j.nantod.2014.04.008

76. Shan W, Zhu X, Liu M, Li L, Zhong J, Sun W, et al. Overcoming the diffusion barrier of mucus and absorption barrier of epithelium by self-assembled nanoparticles for oral delivery of insulin. *ACS Nano* (2015) 9:2345–56. doi: 10.1021/acsnano.5b00028

77. Battaglia L, Panciani PP, Muntoni E, Capucchio MT, Biasibetti E, De Bonis P, et al. Lipid nanoparticles for intranasal administration: application to nose-to-brain delivery. *Expert Opin Drug Deliv.* (2018) 15:369–378. doi: 10.1080/17425247.2018.1429401

78. Crowe CR, Chen K, Pociask DA, Alcorn JF, Krivich C, Enelow RI, et al. Critical role of IL-17RA in immunopathology of influenza infection. *J Immunol.* (2009) 183:5301–10. doi: 10.4049/jimmunol.0900995

79. Way EE, Chen K, Kolls JK. Dysregulation in lung immunity - the protective and pathologic Th17 response in infection. *Eur J Immunol.* (2013) 43:3116–24. doi: 10.1002/eji.201343713

80. Das S, Khader S. Yin and yang of interleukin-17 in host immunity to infection. *F1000Res* (2017) 6:741. doi: 10.12688/f1000research.10862.1

81. Bot A, Bot S, Bona CA. Protective role of gamma interferon during the recall response to influenza virus. *J Virol.* (1998) 72:6637–45.

82. Killip MJ, Fodor E, Randall RE. Influenza virus activation of the interferon system. *Virus Res.* (2015) 209:11–22. doi: 10.1016/j.virusres.2015.02.003

83. Gould VMW, Francis JN, Anderson KJ, Georges B, Cope AV, Tregoning JS. Nasal IgA provides protection against human influenza challenge in volunteers with low serum influenza antibody titre. *Front Microbiol.* (2017) 8:900. doi: 10.3389/fmicb.2017.00900

84. Isaka M, Zhao Y, Nobusawa E, Nakajima S, Nakajima K, Yasuda Y, et al. Protective effect of nasal immunization of influenza virus hemagglutinin with recombinant cholera toxin B subunit as a mucosal adjuvant in mice. *Microbiol Immunol.* (2008) 52:55–63. doi: 10.1111/j.1348-0421.2008.00010.x

85. Trieu MC, Zhou F, Lartey S, Jul-Larsen A, Mjaaland S, Sridhar S, et al. Long-term maintenance of the influenza-specific cross-reactive memory CD4+ T-Cell responses following repeated annual influenza vaccination. *J Infect Dis.* (2017) 215:740–49. doi: 10.1093/infdis/jiw619

86. Anderson RJ, Li J, Kedzierski L, Compton BJ, Hayman CM, Osmond TL, et al. Augmenting influenza-specific T Cell memory generation with a natural killer T Cell-dependent glycolipid-peptide vaccine. *ACS Chem Biol.* (2017) 12:2898–905. doi: 10.1021/acschembio.7b00845

# 11

# Bifunctional Small Molecules Enhance Neutrophil Activities Against *Aspergillus fumigatus in vivo* and *in vitro*

*Caroline N. Jones [1†‡], Felix Ellett [1†], Anne L. Robertson [2], Kevin M. Forrest [3], Kevin Judice [3], James M. Balkovec [3], Martin Springer [3], James F. Markmann [1,4], Jatin M. Vyas [5], H. Shaw Warren [5] and Daniel Irimia [1\*]*

[1] BioMEMS Resource Center, Department of Surgery, Massachusetts General Hospital, Harvard Medical School, Boston, MA, United States, [2] Boston Children's Hospital, Harvard Medical School, Boston, MA, United States, [3] Cidara Therapeutics, San Diego, CA, United States, [4] Division of Transplantation, Massachusetts General Hospital, Boston, MA, United States, [5] Division of Infectious Diseases, Massachusetts General Hospital, Harvard Medical School, Boston, MA, United States

*Correspondence:*
*Daniel Irimia*
*Dirimia@mgh.harvard.edu*

[†] These authors have contributed
equally to this work

[‡] Present Address:
*Caroline N. Jones,*
*Department of Biological Sciences,*
*Virginia Tech, Blacksburg, VA,*
*United States*

Aspergillosis is difficult to treat and carries a high mortality rate in immunocompromised patients. Neutrophils play a critical role in control of infection but may be diminished in number and function during immunosuppressive therapies. Here, we measure the effect of three bifunctional small molecules that target *Aspergillus fumigatus* and prime neutrophils to generate a more effective response against the pathogen. The molecules combine two moieties joined by a chemical linker: a targeting moiety (TM) that binds to the surface of the microbial target, and an effector moiety (EM) that interacts with chemoattractant receptors on human neutrophils. We report that the bifunctional compounds enhance the interactions between primary human neutrophils and *A. fumigatus in vitro*, using three microfluidic assay platforms. The bifunctional compounds significantly enhance the recruitment of neutrophils, increase hyphae killing by neutrophils in a uniform concentration of drug, and decrease hyphal tip growth velocity in the presence of neutrophils compared to the antifungal targeting moiety alone. We validated that the bifunctional compounds are also effective *in vivo*, using a zebrafish infection model with neutrophils expressing the appropriate EM receptor. We measured significantly increased phagocytosis of *A. fumigatus* conidia by neutrophils expressing the EM receptor in the presence of the compounds compared to receptor-negative cells. Finally, we demonstrate that treatment with our lead compound significantly improved the antifungal activity of neutrophils from immunosuppressed patients *ex vivo*. This type of bifunctional compounds strategy may be utilized to redirect the immune system to destroy fungal, bacterial, and viral pathogens.

Keywords: neutrophil, fungi (mycelium and spores), *Aspergillus fumigatus* (*A. fumigatus*), bifunctional molecules, cloudbreak, microfluidic, zebrafish

## INTRODUCTION

Humans are continuously exposed to airborne spores of the saprophytic fungus *Aspergillus fumigatus* (*A. fumigatus*). In healthy individuals, pulmonary host defense mechanisms efficiently eliminate this mold. However, the incidence of invasive pulmonary aspergillosis (IPA) has risen in recent decades, reflecting the increasing number of immunosuppressive medical interventions such as chemotherapy, hematopoietic stem cell and solid organ transplants (1, 2). Even with appropriate antimicrobial therapy, the mortality rate of IPA remains as high as 50% (3, 4). In a recent clinical study of patients with acute lymphoblastic leukemia (ALL), 6.7% of patients developed invasive fungal infections within a median time of 20 days after induction of chemotherapy, with a high (19.2%) 12-week mortality after diagnosis of invasive aspergillosis (IA) (5). There is an increasing demand for novel therapeutic strategies aimed at enhancing or restoring antifungal immunity (6).

Recently, exploration has begun into the promise of using immunotherapy to combat IA, with use of cytokines and granulocyte transfusions, alone or in combination with antifungal therapy. In the past, chemokines have been tested to modify effector and antigen presenting cells in the context of cancer (7). Modulation of neutrophil functions are an especially promising immunotherapeutic strategy (8). Colony stimulating factors (CSFs) and cytokines, mainly IFN-γ, have been utilized in the clinical management of fungal diseases. CSFs and granulocyte transfusions are used to augment the number and function of circulating neutrophils in neutropenic patients (9). Other *in vivo* studies report on the anti-Aspergillus activity of neutrophils, including the rapid resolution of IPA following recovery of chemotherapy-induced neutropenia (10, 11). *Ex vivo* loading of the antifungal drug posaconazole into HL60s, a neutrophil-like cell line, enhanced activity against *A. fumigatus*, and transfusion of these cells improved survival outcome in a mouse model of IPA (12).

Neutrophils are one of the key targets for fungal immunotherapy because of their critical role in preventing infections. In different immunocompromised murine models, myeloid (notably neutrophils and macrophages), but not lymphoid cells, were strongly recruited to the lungs upon infection. Other myeloid cells, particularly dendritic cells and monocytes, were only recruited to lungs of corticosteroid treated mice, which developed a strong pulmonary inflammation after infection (13). Both macrophages and neutrophils are known to kill conidia, whereas hyphae are killed mainly by neutrophils (14, 15). Some evidence suggests that killing of conidia by neutrophils *in vitro* depends whether or not the conidia are in a "resting" or "swollen" state (16). *In vivo*, early recruitment of neutrophils to the lung is important to inhibit germination of *A. fumigatus* conidia and to restrict growth of hyphae (17). Since hyphae are too large to be engulfed, neutrophils possess an array of extracellular killing mechanisms, including the creation of swarms surrounding the fungi and the formation of neutrophil extracellular traps (NETs), which consist of nuclear DNA decorated with fungicidal proteins (18, 19).

Microfluidics are emerging as an important tool for precisely quantifying neutrophil-pathogen interactions (20). We have recently reported on microfluidic devices that enabled the measurement of neutrophil-fungus interactions at single-cell resolution. We found that human neutrophils have a limited ability to migrate toward and block the growth of *A. fumigatus* conidia (21) and that the growth-blocking ability of human neutrophils is significantly enhanced by peptide chemoattractants such as N-Formyl-Met-Leu-Phe (fMLP), which act through the Formyl Peptide Receptor (FPR1) on neutrophils. This effect of chemoattractants is significantly larger in the presence of chemoattractant gradients compared to uniform concentrations (21). To study interactions between neutrophils and hypha in detail, we have developed an "infection-on-a-chip" device, which enabled the detailed analysis of neutrophil-hypha interaction at single-cell resolution over time and revealed the importance of hypha branching, neutrophil recruitment, and iron sequestration on blocking hypha growth (22).

Here, we present a novel immunotherapy strategy that aims to enhance the interactions between neutrophils and fungi and direct the natural innate immune system to achieve control over fungal infection. Using microfluidic platforms, we quantify a significant increase in recruitment of neutrophils and hyphae killing in both gradients and uniform concentrations of bifunctional compounds that bind both to fungi and neutrophils. We measure decreased hyphal tip growth velocity in the presence of bifunctional compounds compared to the antifungal targeting moiety alone. Using a zebrafish model of conidial phagocytosis, we demonstrate molecular specificity for drug action through human FPR1 *in vivo*. Finally, we demonstrate that these bifunctional compounds significantly improve the antifungal activity of neutrophils from immunosuppressed patients *ex vivo*.

## RESULTS

Bifunctional compounds are molecules with two binding sites: a targeting moiety (TM), which recognizes a target on the surface of microbes, and an effector moiety (EM), which binds to a receptor on the surface of the immune cells (7, 23, 24) (**Figure 1A**). Here, we tested bifunctional compounds that used caspofungin (CAS) and amphotericin B (AmB) as TMs with affinity to known fungal targets: (1-3)-*β*-*D*-*glucan synthase* and *ergosterol*, respectively. These compounds were linked to the EM fMLP, which is an FPR1 ligand (**Figure 1B**, **Figure S1**). The coupling of the TM to the EM results in bifunctional compounds designed to decorate fungal targets with potent activators of innate immune cells, with the goal of enhancing antifungal activity (**Figure 1C**). To visualize decoration of fungal hyphae via antifungal TMs, we utilized a boron-dipyrromethane (BODIPY) labeled caspofungin (TM-BODIPY) conjugate. Treatment of RFP-expressing fungal hyphae for 30 min with TM-BODIPY [10 mM] augmented the BODIPY fluorescent signal at the hyphal interface (**Figure 1D**ii). This effect is most likely due to the specific binding and accumulation of antifungal TM on the surface of the fungi, and was not observed for a BODIPY-labeled formyl peptide (EM-BODIPY) negative control (**Figure 1D**i).

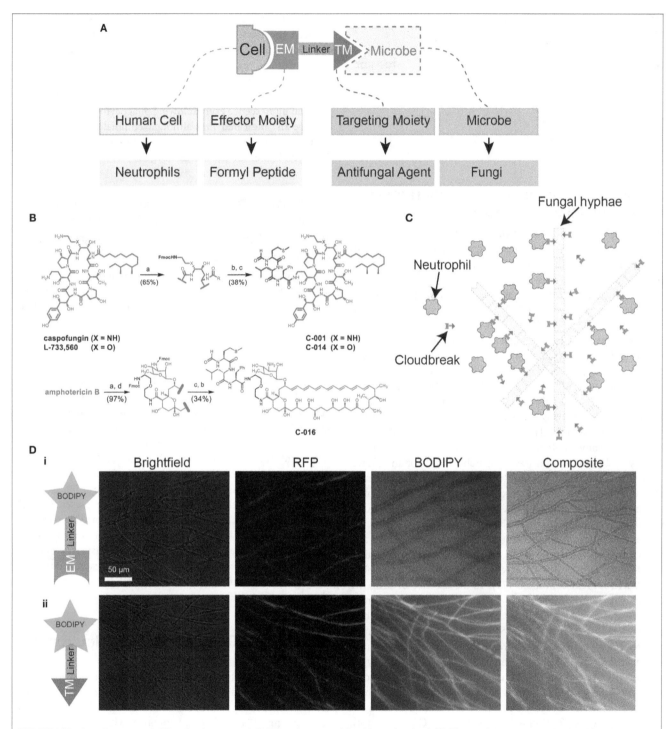

**FIGURE 1 |** Design of immunogenic bifunctional compounds for enhancing neutrophil activity against fungi. **(A)** Diagram shows conceptual basis of bifunctional compounds design to stimulate interactions between specific immune cell types and microbes. The bifunctional compounds used in this study utilize antifungal TMs and a formyl peptide EM with the aim of stimulating neutrophil activity against fungi. **(B)** Chemical structures detailing synthesis of C-001/C-014 and C-016 by fusion of an fMLP EM with caspofungin (CAS) and amphotericin B (AmB) TM, respectively. Detailed synthesis methods can be found in the **Supplementary Material**. **(C)** Hypothesized mode of action: Binding of formyl peptides enhances neutrophil activation, while molecules decorating the fungal surface further stimulate their anti-microbial activities. **(D)** Targeting of compounds to the fungal surface via the antifungal TM caspofungin. Following 30 min of treatment with caspofungin-BODIPY conjugate, RFP-expressing hyphal structures are clearly labeled with the fluorescent signal from BODIPY **(ii)**. This specific decoration of the fungal surface does not occur using a BODIPY-conjugated formyl peptide control **(i)**. Scale as shown.

**TABLE 1** | MIC/MEC values (μM) for conjugates and control compounds.

| | A. fumigatus | | |
|---|---|---|---|
| Compound | MAY-3626 | MAY-4609 | ATCC 13073 |
| CAS | >29/0.055 | >29/0.11 | >29/0.11 |
| C-014 | >20/0.16 | >20/0.076 | >20/0.16 |
| AmB | 0.54 | 0.54 | 0.54 |
| C-016 | 1.4/1.4 | 2.8/0.7 | 2.8/1.4 |

71.8 ± 10.4% and AmB: 83.4 ± 4.2%). Neutrophils alone reduced the fraction of conidia germination to 47.9 ± 7.8% ($N = 8$). Remarkably, human neutrophils further reduced the fraction of conidia germinating in the presence of C-001 (13.2 ± 3.4, $N = 10$), C-014 (16.0 ± 9.7%, $N = 4$), and C-016 (11.2 ± 6.0%, $N = 4$) (**Figure 2D**, **Movies S2, S3**). Maintained conidial fluorescence even following phagocytosis by neutrophils (**Figure 2B**) indicated that although conidial germination was suppressed, some of these spores likely remained viable within neutrophils over the timeframe imaged.

## Bifunctional Compounds Amplify Human Neutrophil Migration Toward *A. fumigatus* and Suppression of Fungal Growth

To confirm that the bifunctional compounds interact with human neutrophils via FPR1, we tested the ability of the compounds to induce neutrophil chemotaxis. First, we calculated the minimum inhibitory concentrations (MICs) and minimum effective concentration (MEC) of our compounds against *A. fumigatus* (AF293) in the absence of neutrophils (see Supplemental Materials). Compounds C-001 and C-014 (CAS-formyl peptide conjugates), as well as C-016 (a AmB-formyl peptide conjugate) demonstrated potent MIC/MEC values, which suggested excellent affinity of the TMs (**Table 1**).

Next, we validated that these concentrations also induced maximum chemotaxis of human neutrophils. Measurement of healthy-donor neutrophil recruitment showed that C-001, C-014, and C-016 retained potent chemotactic activity. The chemotactic activity of the compounds was comparable to that of an optimal concentration of fMLP (25), with [10 nM] C-001, and [100 nM] of C-016 or fMLP inducing maximum neutrophil migration in the microfluidic assay (**Figure 2C**). Importantly, CAS and AmB were not chemotactic to neutrophils (**Figure 2C**).

To investigate the interactions between neutrophils and fungi at single-cell resolution, we utilized our microfluidic infection-on-chip platforms, which provide well-controlled microenvironment conditions (21). In the absence of drug, we observed that low numbers of neutrophils migrate naturally toward *A. fumigatus* hyphae in the chemotaxis-chambers (**Figure 2B** top panel **Movie S1**). We tested that human neutrophils are activated in the presence bifunctional compounds by measuring the change in circularity and reactive oxygen species (ROS) production (**Figure S2**). We also ran a dose-response experiment to identify the optimal concentration of C-001, C-014, and C-016 to induce neutrophil chemotaxis in the presence of *A. fumigatus* (**Figures S3, S4**). C-001 [10 nM], C-014 [10 nM], and C-016 [100 nM] were able to produce a significant influx of neutrophils compared to *A. fumigatus* alone. The bifunctional compounds were less chemotactic than the fMLP [100 nM] positive control in the presence of *A. fumigatus*, likely due to the lower [10 nM] concentration used for C-001 and C-014 (**Figure 2C**).

In the chemotaxis-chamber devices, in the absence of neutrophils, 80.7 ± 4.6% of the conidia germinated within 6 h. The antifungal backbone alone had minimal effect on the germination of conidia within the same time interval (CAS:

## Uniform Concentrations of Bifunctional Compounds Significantly Enhance the Activity of Human Neutrophils Against Growing Hyphae

To measure the interactions between human neutrophils and fungi in uniform concentrations of drug, we confined these interactions within nanowells (300 μm wide × 500 μm long × 50 μm deep) (**Figure 3A**). We loaded fungi into the wells and allowed the conidia to germinate for 7 h. We added isolated human neutrophils to the wells (average concentration: 30 neutrophils/well), in the presence and absence of uniform concentrations of bifunctional compounds and control chemoattractants, and monitored the interactions between neutrophils and fungi for 18 h. The ability of neutrophils to block conidia germination was enhanced in the presence of C-016 [10 nM – 1.7% conidia germination] compared with uniform concentrations of fMLP [100 nM – 21.4 % conidia germination] (**Figure 3C**). Strikingly, we also observed a significant increase in the number of neutrophil "swarms" (clusters of more than 6 neutrophils) in the presence of C-016 (**Figures 3B,D**), which correlated with enhanced suppression of hyphal growth in that condition. This "swarming" effect might have been facilitated by the shorter distances between neutrophils and germinating conidia and faster recruitment of larger neutrophil numbers compared to the chemotaxis-chamber assay.

## Bifunctional Compounds Help Neutrophils Block Hyphal Tip Extension

We have previously described the ability of neutrophils to interact with growing hyphal tips and suppress their growth (22). Using similar microfluidic devices (22) that allow fungi to grow for 18 h before interactions with neutrophils and confine growing hyphae into channels, we tested whether bifunctional compounds enhance the interaction between neutrophils and hyphae. We found that the velocity of hypha growth was drastically reduced from ~11 to ~0.5–1.5 μm/min by the presence of human neutrophils and bifunctional compounds ($P = 0.05$, $N = 10$) (**Figures 4A,B**, **Figure S5**, **Movies S4, S5**). The velocity of hypha growth was not altered in the presence of antifungal controls and was only reduced to ~6 μm/min in the presence of neutrophils without the bifunctional compounds.

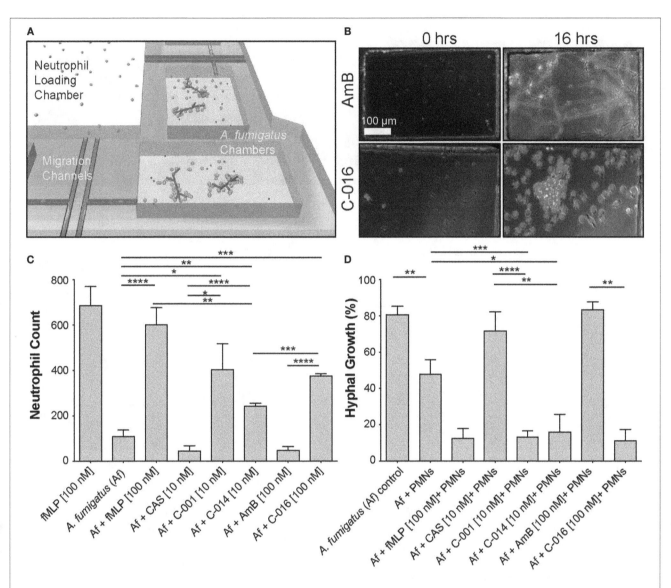

FIGURE 2 | Gradients of bifunctional compounds enhance human neutrophil recruitment and their ability to suppress A. fumigatus hyphal growth. (A) A previously published device consisting of fungal growth chambers connected via migration channels to one central neutrophil reservoir are used to test neutrophil chemotaxis in response to gradients of bifunctional compounds (21). (B) Representative images show A. fumigatus (red, RFP) hyphal growth and neutrophil (blue, Hoechst) recruitment in chambers at 0 and 16 h in the presence of C-016 (bifunctional conjugate with amphotericin B TM and formyl peptide EM, lower panels) or amphotericin B (AmB, upper panels) controls. Gradients of C-016 resulted in enhanced neutrophil recruitment and effective suppression of hyphal growth compared to amphotericin B alone. Scale as shown (C). Quantification of neutrophil recruitment at 16 h in response to bifunctional compounds compared to relevant controls. Chemotaxis of neutrophils was enhanced in the presence of the formyl peptide control (fMLP [100 nM]) and all three bifunctional formyl peptide conjugates compared to untreated and antifungal-treated controls. (D) Quantification of hyphal growth at 16 h following treatment with bifunctional compounds in the presence of neutrophils compared to relevant controls. Only partial suppression of hyphal growth was observed in the presence of neutrophils alone. This was significantly enhanced by treatment with all three bifunctional conjugates and the formyl peptide control, as previously described (20). Antifungal controls used at the relevant concentrations did not affect fungal growth. Bar graphs show mean and standard error from pooled experimental replicates. Statistics: two-tailed T-test. *p ≤ 0.05, **p ≤ 0.01, ***p ≤ 0.001, and ****p < 0.0001.

## Bifunctional Compounds Enhance Phagocytosis of Conidia by Humanized Zebrafish Neutrophils

To assess whether bifunctional compounds could enhance neutrophil responses in vivo, we utilized an established zebrafish infection model that has been used to study the activity of innate immune cells in response to A. fumigatus conidia and

hyphae (26–28). In this model, conidial phagocytosis is heavily predominated by macrophages rather than neutrophils (26, 28). Consequently, reducing macrophage numbers (via knockdown of spi1 expression using antisense oligonucleotides that block translation of spi1 mRNA) was required for isolating the effect of neutrophil activities on A. fumigatus conidia phagocytosis and clearance (26, 27).

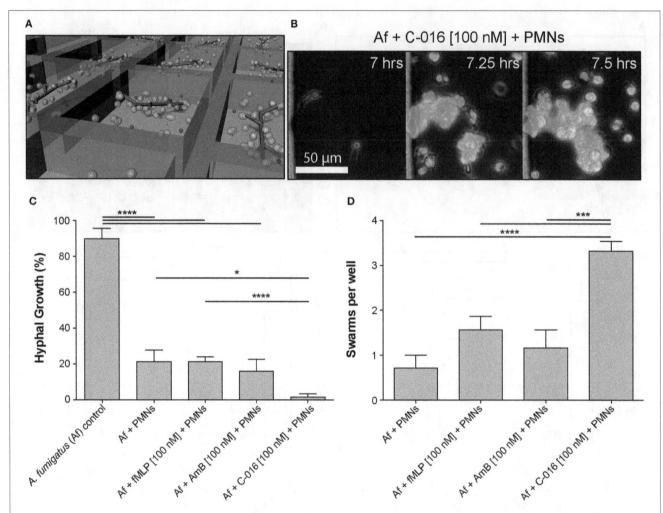

**FIGURE 3 |** Uniform concentrations of bifunctional compounds enhance the ability of human neutrophils to suppress hyphal growth and stimulate neutrophil swarming. **(A)** Diagram of previously described nanowell device designed to test drug activity at uniform concentrations (21). Fungal conidia are allowed to germinate and grow for 7 h prior to addition of neutrophils in the presence or absence of neutrophils. **(B)** Representative images show swarming of neutrophils (polymorphonucleocytes, PMNs, blue, Hoechst) around *A. fumigatus* hyphae induced by the presence of C-016. **(C)** Quantification of hyphal growth in this device demonstrates significant suppression by neutrophils, either in the presence or absence of fMLP or AmB treatment. This suppression was further enhanced in the presence of C-016. **(D)** Quantification of neutrophil swarms around growing *A. fumigatus* hyphae shows a significant increase in the presence of C-016 vs. control conditions. Bar graphs show mean and standard error from pooled experimental replicates. Statistics: two-tailed *T*-test. *$p \leq 0.05$, ***$p \leq 0.001$, and ****$p < 0.0001$.

FPR1 sensitivity has been shown to vary widely between mammalian species, with mouse and rat neutrophils exhibiting poor recruitment in response to fMLP compared to human cells (29). There is evidence that zebrafish neutrophils do respond to formylated peptides (30, 31), although experiments in this model have been complicated by inability to distinguish direct responses to chemoattractant from recruitment to injured tissue at the site of microinjection. To avoid this complication in our experiments, we delivered pre-treated conidia at one site (the duct of Cuvier) and analyzed neutrophil responses at a spatially distant site (the caudal venous plexus) (**Figure 5Ai**).

To test whether bifunctional compounds could enhance phagocytosis of *A. fumigatus* conidia, we microinjected pre-treated and control conidia along with test or control compounds into the circulation, then imaged the caudal venous plexus 2 h

post-infection (hpi) (**Figure S7A**). Despite effective suppression of the macrophage lineage by treatment with antisense oligonucleotides targeting *spi-1* mRNA transcripts (*spi1*-MO) (**Figure S7B**) and comparable numbers of neutrophils (**Figure S7B**) and conidia (**Figure S7C**) present in all groups, no significant increase in the percent of phagocytic neutrophils (**Figure S7D**) or the number of engulfed conidia (**Figure S7E**) was observed following pretreatment with bifunctional compounds.

Colony forming units (CFU) provide a poor readout of infectious burden for hyphal pathogens, because unlike single-cell organisms like bacteria or yeast, fungal filaments cannot be reliably homogenized into individual viable units. To assess whether fungal burden might be suppressed following treatment, we therefore scored larvae at 24 hpi for RFP-positive hyphae

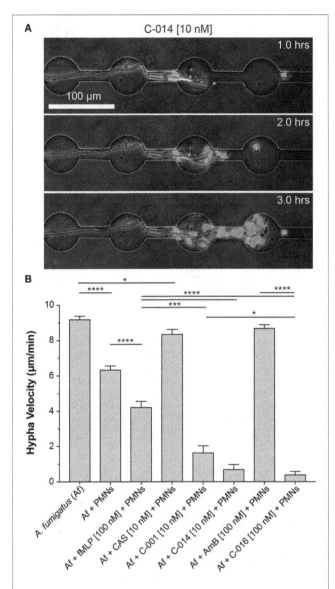

**FIGURE 4 |** Bifunctional compounds enhance the ability of human neutrophils to suppress hyphal tip extension. **(A)** Representative images show suppression of hyphal tip (red, RFP) elongation by neutrophils (blue, Hoechst) in the presence of C-014 [10 nM]. **(B)** Quantification of hyphal growth velocity demonstrates significant suppression in the presence of bifunctional compounds C-001 [10 nM], C-014 [10 nM], and especially C-016 [100 nM] compared to control conditions—including fMLP [100 nM]. Bar graphs show mean and standard error from pooled experimental replicates. Statistics: two-tailed $T$-test. $^{*}p \leq 0.05$, $^{***}p \leq 0.001$, and $^{****}p < 0.0001$.

Comparison of protein sequence identity between receptor homologs in humans, mice, rats and zebrafish revealed that while the conservation between mammalian homologs was higher than 70%, conservation between mammals and zebrafish was <40% (**Figure S6**). To test whether expression of human FPR1 in zebrafish neutrophils could enhance the neutrophil response in the presence of bifunctional compounds, we mosaically expressed human FPR1 under the control of the leukocyte-specific zebrafish *lyzC* promoter (33) using Tol2-mediated transgenesis. Expression of the protein was traced using mCherry linked to the receptor using the self-cleaving T2A peptide, allowing separation of the fluorophore and thus unimpeded receptor function. The transgene DNA construct and Tol2 transposase mRNA were co-injected with an antisense morpholino oligonucleotide targeting *irf8*, knockdown of which results in enhanced specification of neutrophils at the expense of macrophages (34). Injection into Tg(*mpx*:EGFP) embryos at the one-cell stage resulted in both on-target expression of FPR1/mCherry in GFP-labeled neutrophils (GFP/mCherry+ cells), as well as off-target expression in tissues such as the somite (**Figure 5Aii**). To test whether the FPR1-expressing dual-labeled cells would exhibit an enhanced response to bifunctional compounds, we inoculated control or pre-treated conidia into the circulation FPR1/mCherry-expressing larvae at 3 dpf, and scored phagocytosis at 2 h post-infection in the caudal venous plexus. Because mosaic larvae contained both FPR1-positive (GFP+/mCherry+) and FPR1-negative (GFP(only)+) neutrophils, this approach provided an internal control when assessing phagocytosis of pre-treated conidia.

Pre-treatment of conidia with C-016 prior to inoculation significantly enhanced phagocytosis by GFP+ neutrophils expressing human FPR1 and mCherry (**Figure S7E**). Furthermore, comparison of per-cell phagocytosis rates demonstrated that pre-treatment of conidia with either C-001 or C-016 (but not DMSO or fMLP) resulted in significantly higher rates of phagocytosis by FPR1/mCherry-expressing GFP+ leukocytes compared to GFP(only)+ cells in the same larvae (**Figure 5B**). As expected, conidial delivery, leukocyte numbers, and phagocytosis by GFP(only)+ cells (expressing the native zebrafish FPR1) were not significantly different between treatment groups (**Figures S7A–D**). These observations suggest that using fMLP as an effector moiety on immunotherapy compounds confers species-specific neutrophil responses mediated by differential formyl-peptide receptor activity.

## Bifunctional Compounds Improve Fungicidal Activity of Neutrophils From Immunosuppressed Patients

Our previous studies have shown that stimulation of neutrophils with chemoattractants presented as spatial gradients, enhanced neutrophil activity against fungal pathogens (20). We therefore assessed the efficacy of C-016, our most promising candidate, in enhancing fungicidal activity of neutrophils isolated from kidney transplant patients using our microfluidic host-pathogen platform. The patients were undergoing various regimes of immunotherapy (**Table 2**). For healthy donors without stimulation, an average of 194.2 ± 100 neutrophils migrated

using fluorescence microscopy (**Figure S8**). In *spi1*-MO treated larvae, which had neutrophils but reduced macrophages, we observed hyphae in 10–20% of surviving infected larvae, with no significant difference between drug-treated and control groups (**Figure S8B**). In *spi1-MO/csf3r-MO* treated zebrafish, which had reduced neutrophils as well as macrophages (32), we observed hyphae in 80–90% of larvae, highlighting the important role that neutrophils play in suppressing hyphae in this model. Again, no significant difference was observed between treated and control groups in this context.

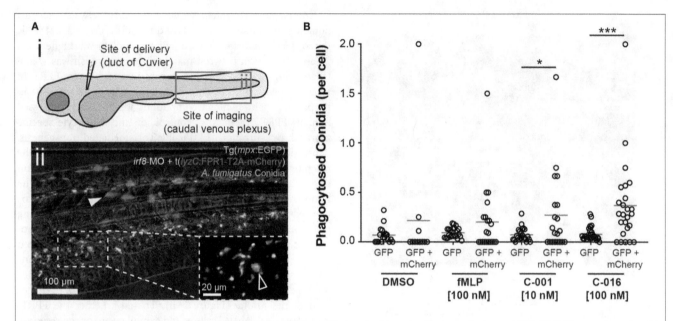

**FIGURE 5 |** Bifunctional compounds enhance phagocytosis of *A. fumigatus* conidia by zebrafish neutrophils expressing human FPR1. **(A) (i)** Diagram of experimental approach: Calcofluor-stained *A. fumigatus* conidia (blue) are co-delivered with treatments into the circulation via the Duct of Cuvier at 3 days post-fertilization. Imaging is performed at 2 h post-infection at a distal site, the caudal venous plexus, which is rich in leukocytes. **(ii)** Example image of 3 dpf *irf8*-MO treated Tg(*mpx*:EGFP) larva (GFP-labeled neutrophils) with mosaic expression of human FPR1 (traced by mCherry, red fluorescence), 2 h following delivery of calcofluor-labeled (blue fluorescent) *A. fumigatus* conidia. A GFP/mCherry co-labeled leukocyte containing phagocytosed conidia is indicated in magnified panel (open white arrowhead). Off-target expression of the transgene was also observed in tissues including the somites (full white arrowhead). **(B)** Treatment with C-001 and C-016 resulted in significantly increased phagocytosis of conidia by GFP/mCherry+ (human FPR1-expressing) neutrophils compared to GFP(only) wild-type cells. Each point represents an infected larva. *N* ≥ 40 larva scored per condition. Data collated from multiple experiments. Statistics: two-tailed *T*-test. *$p \leq 0.05$, ***$p \leq 0.001$.

to the chambers. After stimulation with C-016, an order of magnitude higher number of neutrophils migrated to the chamber (1,966 ± 158.3 cells, $p = 0.002$). For kidney transplant patients without stimulation, an average of 133.5 ± 70.35 neutrophils migrated to the chambers. After stimulation with C-016, an order of magnitude higher number of neutrophils migrated to the chamber (1,053 ± 233.5 cells, $p = 0.012$) (**Figure 6A**). The increase in migration and stimulation of healthy neutrophils by C-016 resulted in <1% conidia germination, compared with 26.1 ± 5.1% in the presence of neutrophils without compound. In kidney transplant patients, conidia germination decreased from 45.66 ± 8.8% (neutrophils alone) to 6.47 ± 4.6% (neutrophils and compound) (**Figure 6B**). One of the transplant patient's neutrophils did not respond to C-016 (Patient #4). In this patient, only 4% of the average number of neutrophils migrated to the chamber, and this was not a sufficient number to control *A. fumigatus* hyphae growth.

## DISCUSSION

We tested the efficiency of bifunctional compounds consisting of a TM that binds to the surface of *A. fumigatus* and an EM that interacts with FPR1 chemoattractant receptor on human neutrophils in an immunotherapy strategy to amplify neutrophil anti-fungal activities. We found that the bifunctional compounds enhanced the activity of neutrophils

against *A. fumigatus* both *in vitro* and *in vivo*. We also measured a significant improvement in the response of human neutrophils isolated from immunosuppressed kidney transplant patients, in *ex vivo* experiments in the presence of bifunctional compound C-016.

We also show that zebrafish models recently developed for the detailed study of leukocyte-fungi interaction during infection (28) are effective tools for evaluating bifunctional compounds *in vivo*. The direct visualization of host-pathogen interactions is facilitated by the use of Tg(*mpx*:EGFP/*mpeg1*:mCherry) compound transgenic larvae on a *nacre*$^{-/-}$ mutant background with reduced pigmentation (35) to enhance imaging. This compound transgenic line has green fluorescent neutrophils and red fluorescent macrophages (36). Rather than delivering conidia into the zebrafish brain as previously described (26, 27), we instead microinjected fungal conidia directly into the circulation and measured phagocytosis at a spatially distant site. This methodology enabled us to measure neutrophil activity in the absence of damage signals from a nearby wound. Delivery into the circulation resulted in a dominant macrophage phagocytic response, consistent with previous studies (28) and the higher efficiency of macrophages vs. neutrophils at phagocytosing pathogens from zebrafish circulation (37). To allow measurement of neutrophil responses in isolation, macrophage numbers were suppressed by morpholino-mediated knockdown of genes driving macrophage specification from the anterior lateral plate mesoderm (*spi1*) (38), or differentiation

**TABLE 2 |** Kidney transplant patient data summary.

| Patient | Time from transplant | ANC (K/uL) | Treatment (daily doses) | Neutrophil response to *A. fumigatus* | | | |
|---|---|---|---|---|---|---|---|
| | | | | No compound | | With C-016 | |
| | | | | Neutrophils recruited | %Fungus alive | Neutrophils recruited | %Fungus alive |
| #1 | 6 months | 12.24 | Prograf 4 mg, Prednisone 20 mg, MMF 1 g | 222 | 56.6% | 1,648 | 2% |
| #2 | 6 years | 1.93 | Prograf 4.5 mg, Prednisone 5 mg, MMF 1 g | 447 | 3.6% | 806 | 0.4% |
| #3 | 14 years | 4.58 | Prograf 0.5 mg, Prednisone 2.5 mg, Cell Cept 500 mg | 18 | 61.6% | 1166 | 2% |
| #4 | 1 month | 0.95 | Prograf 6 mg, Prednisone 15 mg, Cell Cept 750 mg, Cefepime, Valcyte and Bactrim | 17 | 55.7% | 52 | 29.3% |
| #5 | 7 years | 2.47 | Prograf 3 mg, Cell Cept 500 mg, Prednisone 5 mg | 71 | 43.2% | 1496 | 5.1% |
| #6 | 3 years | 9.34 | Cyclosporine 125 mg, Cell Cept 500 mg, Prednisone 5 mg | 26 | 53.3% | 1,152 | 0% |
| Average Transplant Patients | | | | 133.5 ± 70.4 | 45.67 ± 8.8 | 1,053 ± 233.5 | 6.47 ± 4.6 |
| Average Healthy Controls | | | | 194.2 ± 100 | 26.1 ± 5.1 | 1,966 ± 158.3 | 0.58 ± 0.2 |
| *Comparison between with and without C-0016* | | | | | | $p = 0.012$ | $p = 0.006$ |

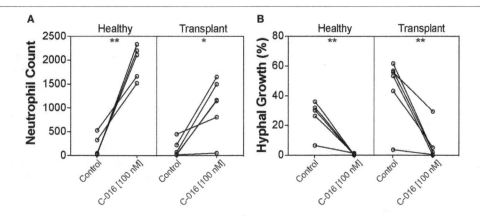

**FIGURE 6 |** C-016 enhances the anti-fungal activity of neutrophils from immunosuppressed patients. **(A)** Quantification of neutrophil recruitment demonstrated that gradients of C-016 enhanced migration of cells from both healthy donors and transplant patients to Aspergillus chambers compared to unstimulated controls. **(B)** Quantification of hyphal growth showed enhanced suppression by C-016 treated neutrophils from healthy donors and transplant patients compared to unstimulated controls. Each point represents an individual neutrophil donor. $N = 5$ healthy donors and $N = 6$ kidney transplant patient donors tested. Statistics: paired $T$-test. $^*p \leq 0.05$, $^{**}p \leq 0.01$.

from the neutrophil-macrophage common precursor (*irf8*) (34). In theory, the absence of a significant response from zebrafish neutrophils to untreated conidia provided an ideal environment to test enhancement by bifunctional compounds. However, our experiments in zebrafish demonstrate that use of fMLP as an effector moiety provides highly specific activity via the human FPR1.

The modular composition of bifunctional compounds allows for rapid exploration of combinations of TM, EM, and linker domains, potentially enabling efficient discovery of anti-infective molecules with the desired potency, specificity and physical properties. These experiments also highlight the power of utilizing both *ex vivo* and *in vivo* models to test activity, specificity, and mode of action. Together, microfluidics and zebrafish offer complementary imaging-based platforms for measuring leukocyte activity, allowing intuitive translation, and comparison of experimental findings between models.

Bifunctional small molecules represent promising immunotherapies for the treatment of aspergillosis and other fungal infections. Enhancing the host response against fungi is important in situations where the efficacy of the innate immune response is deficient and the degree of the immune suppression in the patient becomes the major host determinant (39). Further study of these agents is warranted. While our current study focusses on enhancing the activity of neutrophils, which express high levels of FPR-1, other cells, such as monocytes, macrophages, dendritic cells, and even vascular endothelial cells and keratinocytes are known to express FPR-1, albeit at lower levels (40). It is possible that activation of these other immune cell lineages *in vivo* may provide further protection against fungi. Treatment with bifunctional compounds may also be limited to topical or localized delivery, for example: to treat dermatophyte infection. Bifunctional compounds may be useful as adjunctive therapy along with standard of care regimens to augment neutrophil killing potential and improve protection against fungal infections. The same compound design principles used here may also be applied to other infectious diseases to redirect the immune system to destroy fungal, bacterial, or viral pathogens. The compendium of microfluidic devices developed to probe neutrophil-fungi interactions (21, 22) could be utilized to prescreen drug candidates and predict the effectiveness of bifunctional compound immunotherapies in individual patients. Theoretically, this type of measurement could also be used to tune the immune system by immunosuppressive therapy drug dosages high enough to avoid organ rejection and low enough to ward off fungal infections.

## MATERIALS AND METHODS

### Bifunctional Compound Synthesis

Compounds were prepared as described in detail in the (**Figure S1**). Preparation of C-001: mono-Fmoc-protected caspofungin was prepared from commercial caspofungin acetate by treating with 9-fluorenylmethyl-N-hydroxysuccinimidyl carbonate (Fmoc-OSu) in DMF. The purified product was coupled with N-formyl-L-methioninyl-L-leucyl-L-phenylalanine N-hydroxysuccinimide ester (fMLF-OSu). The Fmoc group was removed from that product by stirring with 10% piperidine to give C-001 after HPLC purification. Preparation of C-014: C-014 was prepared using a procedure analogous to that for C-001 above but replacing caspofungin with L-733,560 (41). Preparation of C-016: The diaminoethylether amide of amphotericin B was prepared by Fmoc derivatization of the mycosamine of amphotericin B followed by coupling with N-Fmoc-diaminoaminoethyl amine and removal of the Fmoc groups with piperidine. Treatment of the product with fMLF-OSu gave C-016 after reversed phase purification. fMet-Leu-Phe (fMLP) was obtained commercially.

### Fungal Strains

*Aspergillus fumigatus* strain 293 expressing cytosolic RFP or GFP was grown on Sabouraud dextrose agar plates supplemented with 100 μg/mL ampicillin at 30°C for 3–4 days. Conidia were harvested by gentle scraping, followed by washing in ice-cold phosphate-buffered saline (PBS) 3 times. Conidia were immediately used or stored at 4°C for up to 1 week before use. To enable visualization following zebrafish infection, conidia were briefly stained with Calcofluor White as previously described (28).

### Zebrafish

Zebrafish stocks were maintained and mated according to standard protocols (42) and following the rules of the Massachusetts General Hospital Subcommittee on Research Animal Care. Transgenic strains—*Tg(mpx:GFPuwm1)* (43) and *Tg(mpeg1:mCherry)* (36), were on the *nacre*$^{-/-}$ background (35), and were a kind gift from Elliott Hagedorn and Leonard Zon. Human formyl-peptide receptor (FPR1) was sub-cloned from pBGSA FPR1-EGFP (Addgene ID:62604) into a middle entry vector and combined with existing 5′ (lyzC promoter) and 3′ (T2A-mCherry) vectors using standard Gateway approaches. Mosaic expression of FPR1 was achieved by Tol2 transposase-mediated transgenesis (44). Briefly, fertilized eggs were co-injected with transgene DNA (50 ng/μl) and Tol2 transposase mRNA (25 ng/μL) into the cell at the single-cell stage. For infection, embryos were raised to 52 h post-fertilization, conidia delivered into the duct of Cuvier by microinjection as previously described (28), and imaging performed on the caudal venous plexus 2 h post-infection to assess phagocytosis. For knockdown studies, fertilized eggs were microinjected with 1 nL of morpholino at the one-cell stage. To enable better measurement of neutrophil-specific responses, primitive macrophage differentiation was restricted by blocking translation of *spi1* or *irf8* using anti-sense morpholino oligonucleotides (*spi1*-MO) as previously described (34, 38). The morphant larvae were raised to 2 days post-fertilization, and then microinjected into the vasculature with a solution of *A. fumigatus* conidia pre-stained with Calcofluor together with C-001 (10 nM), C-016 (100 nM), or DMSO, using microstructured surface arrays developed for this purpose (31, 45). Imaging was performed on a fully automated Nikon TiE microscope. For each larva, a 21-slice z-stack (100 μm at 5 μm intervals) was captured of the caudal venous plexus at 10x magnification for 4 channels: DAPI—conidia, GFP—neutrophils, TRITC—macrophages, and brightfield. Analysis was performed manually using NIS Elements and ImageJ.

### Microfluidic Device Fabrication

Microfluidic devices used to measure leukocyte migration in response to *Aspergillus fumigatus* with or without drug (C-001, C-014, C-016), anti-fungal control (Caspofungin) and/or chemoattractant (fMLP) gradients were manufactured using standard microfabrication techniques. Two layers of photoresist (SU8; Microchem), the first one 10 μm thin (corresponding to the migration channels) and the second one 70 μm thick (corresponding to the FCCs) were patterned on one silicon wafer sequentially using two photolithographic masks and processing cycles according to the instructions from the manufacturer. The wafer with patterned photoresist was used as a mold to produce polydimethylsiloxane (PDMS) (Fisher Scientific) devices, which were then bonded to the base of glass-bottom 12- or 24-well plates, using an oxygen plasma machine (Nordson-March).

## Primary Human Neutrophil Isolation

Peripheral blood samples were collected in 3 mL tubes containing a final concentration of 5 mM ethylenediaminetetraacetic acid (EDTA, Vacutainer; Becton Dickinson) and processed within 2 h of collection.

Using standard sterile techniques, we isolated neutrophils from whole blood by use of HetaSep followed by the EasySep human neutrophil enrichment kit (Stemcell Technologies) in accordance with the manufacturer's protocol. The purity of neutrophils was assessed to be >98%, using the Sysmex KX-21N Hematology Analyzer (Sysmex America). White blood cells (WBCs) were isolated using Hetasep, followed by a 5-min spin-down cycle and washing with $1 \times$ PBS. WBCs were stained with Hoechst fluorescent dye ($32.4 \mu M$; Sigma-Aldrich). The final aliquots of WBCs were re-suspended in Roswell Park Memorial Institute (RPMI) medium plus 10% fetal bovine serum (FBS; stock 50 mL of FBS/450 mL of RPMI; Sigma-Aldrich) at a concentration of 4,000 cells/2 $\mu L$ and kept at 37°C. Cells were then immediately introduced into the microfluidic device for the chemotaxis and A. fumigatus assay. All experiments were repeated at least 3 times with neutrophils or WBCs from 3 different healthy donors.

## Microfluidic Neutrophil Chemotaxis and A. fumigatus Killing Assay Preparation

Immediately after bonding to the well plate, donut-shaped devices were filled with A. fumigatus conidia (MYA-4609) expressing red fluorescent protein (RFP) at a concentration of $10^6$ cells/mL$^{+/-}$ drug [10 nM], anti-fungal control [10 nM] and/or chemoattractant solution of fMLP [100 nM] (Sigma-Aldrich, St. Louis, MO) in IMDM + 20% FBS. The device was then placed in a vacuum for 15 min. The chemoattractant filled all of the FCCs as the air was displaced. The devices were then vigorously washed five times with $1\times$ PBS to remove any residual A. fumigatus conidia, K2 Therapeutics drug or chemoattractant that was outside of the focal chemotaxis chambers (FCCs). The device was then submerged in 0.5 mL of cell media. Neutrophils or white blood cells (20,000 cells/2 $\mu L$) were then pipetted into the cell loading chamber (CLC) using a gel-loading pipette tip and could reach the fungus only after migrating through a 600 $\mu$m long channel between the cell-loading well and the drug-treated fungi chambers (**Figure 2A**). Neutrophil migration into the migration channel toward the FCC started immediately and was recorded

using time-lapse imaging for 18 h on a fully automated Nikon TiE microscope (10× magnification) with biochamber heated to 37°C with 5% carbon dioxide gas. Image analysis of cell migration counts and fungal growth was analyzed by hand using Image J software.

## Statistical Analysis of Neutrophil Chemotaxis and A. fumigatus Killing

Image analysis of cell migration counts and fungi growth was analyzed by hand using Image J software. Neutrophils in each chamber were counted every 15 min for the first 2 h of the experiment and then every hour for the remaining 16 h. Percentage of conidia to convert to hyphal growth was measured by counting conidia loaded per chamber before neutrophils or WBCs are loaded into the chamber and counting numbers of these conidia that grow hyphae by 18 h. Fungal growth velocity was calculated using Image J. For experiments with neutrophils from transplant patients, the 16 chambers in each device ($n = 3$) were analyzed for at least three different healthy donors. Data was analyzed for statistical significance using paired two-tailed $t$-tests. For zebrafish experiments, data was tested for normality using the D'Agostino & Pearson normality test. Normally distributed data was analyzed using two-tailed unpaired $t$-tests for pairwise comparisons, or ordinary one-way ANOVA with Tukey's multiple comparisons test. Non-normal data was compared using Kruskal-Wallis test for multiple comparisons. All statistical analysis was performed using Prism Version 7.0a (GraphPad).

## AUTHOR CONTRIBUTIONS

CJ and FE performed experiments. AR, KF, KJ, JB, MS, JM, JV, and HW provided reagents and oversight. DI provided direct supervision of the work.

## FUNDING

Funding support for this project was provided in part by Cidara Therapeutics and grants from the National Institute of Health: EB002503 and GM092804. The funders had no role in study design, data collection and analysis, decision to publish, or preparation of the manuscript.

# ACKNOWLEDGMENTS

We would like to thank Kerry Crisalli, R.N. for assistance collecting patient blood samples, and Nida Khan for her assistance in the culture of *A. fumigatus*. We would also like to thank Julian Tailhades, Jennifer Payne, and Max Cryle for providing BODIPY-labeled formyl peptides, Elliott Hagedorn, and Leonard Zon for providing zebrafish lines, and David Langenau for aquarium space.

# REFERENCES

1. Taccone FS, Van den Abeele AM, Bulpa P, Misset B, Meersseman W, Cardoso T, et al. Epidemiology of invasive aspergillosis in critically ill patients: clinical presentation, underlying conditions, and outcomes. *Crit Care*. (2015) 19:7. doi: 10.1186/s13054-014-0722-7

2. Garnacho-Montero J, Olaechea P, Alvarez-Lerma F, Alvarez-Rocha L, Blanquer J, Galvan B, et al. Epidemiology, diagnosis and treatment of fungal respiratory infections in the critically ill patient. *Rev Esp Quimioter*. (2013) 26:173–88.

3. Lehrnbecher T, Kalkum M, Champer J, Tramsen L, Schmidt S, Klingebiel T. Immunotherapy in invasive fungal infection–focus on invasive aspergillosis. *Curr Pharm Des*. (2013) 19:3689–712. doi: 10.2174/1381612811319200010

4. Herbrecht R, Denning DW, Patterson TF, Bennett JE, Greene RE, Oestmann JW, et al. Voriconazole versus amphotericin B for primary therapy of invasive aspergillosis. *N Engl J Med*. (2002) 347:408–15. doi: 10.1056/NEJMoa020191

5. Mariette C, Tavernier E, Hocquet D, Huynh A, Isnard F, Legrand F, et al. Epidemiology of invasive fungal infections during induction therapy in adults with acute lymphoblastic leukemia: a GRAALL-2005 study. *Leuk Lymphoma*. (2017) 58:586–93. doi: 10.1080/10428194.2016.1204652

6. van de Veerdonk FL, Joosten LA, Netea MG. The interplay between inflammasome activation and antifungal host defense. *Immunol Rev*. (2015) 265:172–80. doi: 10.1111/imr.12280

7. Coscia M, Biragyn A. Cancer immunotherapy with chemoattractant peptides. *Semin Cancer Biol*. (2004) 14:209–18. doi: 10.1016/j.semcancer.2003.10.008

8. Carvalho A, Cunha C, Bistoni F, Romani L. Immunotherapy of aspergillosis. *Clin Microbiol Infect*. (2012) 18:120–5. doi: 10.1111/j.1469-0691.2011.03681.x

9. Roilides E, Lamaignere CG, Farmaki E. Cytokines in immunodeficient patients with invasive fungal infections: an emerging therapy. *Int J Infect Dis*. (2002) 6:154–63. doi: 10.1016/S1201-9712(02)90104-9

10. Mehrad B, Strieter RM, Moore TA, Tsai WC, Lira SA, Standiford TJ. CXC chemokine receptor-2 ligands are necessary components of neutrophil-mediated host defense in invasive pulmonary aspergillosis. *J Immunol*. (1999) 163:6086–94.

11. Todeschini G, Murari C, Bonesi R, Pizzolo G, Verlato G, Tecchio C, et al. Invasive aspergillosis in neutropenic patients: rapid neutrophil recovery is a risk factor for severe pulmonary complications. *Eur J Clin Invest*. (1999) 29:453–7. doi: 10.1046/j.1365-2362.1999.00474.x

12. Baistrocchi SR, Lee MJ, Lehoux M, Ralph B, Snarr BD, Robitaille R, et al. Posaconazole-loaded leukocytes as a novel treatment strategy targeting invasive pulmonary aspergillosis. *J Infect Dis*. (2017) 215:1734–41. doi: 10.1093/infdis/jiw513

13. Kalleda N, Amich J, Arslan B, Poreddy S, Mattenheimer K, Mokhtari Z, et al. Dynamic immune cell recruitment after murine pulmonary aspergillus fumigatus infection under different immunosuppressive regimens. *Front Microbiol*. (2016) 7:1107. doi: 10.3389/fmicb.2016.01107

14. Rex JH, Bennett JE, Gallin JI, Malech HL, Melnick DA. Normal and deficient neutrophils can cooperate to damage *Aspergillus fumigatus* hyphae. *J Infect Dis*. (1990) 162:523–8. doi: 10.1093/infdis/162.2.523

15. Mircescu MM, Lipuma L, van Rooijen N, Pamer EG, Hohl TM. Essential role for neutrophils but not alveolar macrophages at early time points following *Aspergillus fumigatus* infection. *J Infect Dis*. (2009) 200:647–56. doi: 10.1086/600380

16. Levitz SM, Diamond RD. Mechanisms of resistance of *Aspergillus fumigatus* conidia to killing by neutrophils *in vitro*. *J Infect Dis*. (1985) 152:33–42. doi: 10.1093/infdis/152.1.33

17. Bonnett CR, Cornish EJ, Harmsen AG, Burritt JB. Early neutrophil recruitment and aggregation in the murine lung inhibit germination of *Aspergillus fumigatus* conidia. *Infect Immun*. (2006) 74:6528–39. doi: 10.1128/IAI.00909-06

18. Bruns S, Kniemeyer O, Hasenberg M, Aimanianda V, Nietzsche S, Thywissen A, et al. Production of extracellular traps against *Aspergillus fumigatus in vitro* and in infected lung tissue is dependent on invading neutrophils and influenced by hydrophobin RodA. *PLoS Pathog*. (2010) 6:e1000873. doi: 10.1371/journal.ppat.1000873

19. McCormick A, Heesemann L, Wagener J, Marcos V, Hartl D, Loeffler J, et al. NETs formed by human neutrophils inhibit growth of the pathogenic mold *Aspergillus fumigatus*. *Microbes Infect*. (2010) 12:928–36. doi: 10.1016/j.micinf.2010.06.009

20. Berthier E, Lim FY, Deng Q, Guo CJ, Kontoyiannis DP, Wang CC, et al. Low-volume toolbox for the discovery of immunosuppressive fungal secondary metabolites. *PLoS Pathog*. (2013) 9:e1003289. doi: 10.1371/journal.ppat.1003289

21. Jones CN, Dimisko L, Forrest K, Judice K, Poznansky MC, Markmann JF, et al. Human neutrophils are primed by chemoattractant gradients for blocking the growth of *Aspergillus fumigatus*. *J Infect Dis*. (2016) 213:465–75. doi: 10.1093/infdis/jiv419

22. Ellett F, Jorgensen J, Frydman GH, Jones CN, Irimia D. Neutrophil interactions stimulate evasive hyphal branching by *Aspergillus fumigatus*. *PLoS Pathog*. (2017) 13:e1006154. doi: 10.1371/journal.ppat.1006154

23. Kermer V, Hornig N, Harder M, Bondarieva A, Kontermann RE, Muller D. Combining antibody-directed presentation of IL-15 and 4–1BBL in a trifunctional fusion protein for cancer immunotherapy. *Mol Cancer Ther*. (2014) 13:112–21. doi: 10.1158/1535-7163.MCT-13-0282

24. Chu D, Zhao Q, Yu J, Zhang F, Zhang H, Wang Z. Nanoparticle targeting of neutrophils for improved cancer immunotherapy. *Adv Healthc Mater*. (2016) 5:1088–93. doi: 10.1002/adhm.201500998

25. Chandrasekaran A, Ellett F, Jorgensen J, Irimia D. Temporal gradients limit the accumulation of neutrophils toward sources of chemoattractant. *Microsyst Nanoeng*. (2017) 3:16067. doi: 10.1038/micronano.2016.67

26. Knox BP, Deng Q, Rood M, Eickhoff JC, Keller NP, Huttenlocher A. Distinct innate immune phagocyte responses to *Aspergillus fumigatus* conidia and hyphae in zebrafish larvae. *Eukaryot Cell*. (2014) 13:1266–77. doi: 10.1128/EC.00080-14

27. Rosowski EE, Raffa N, Knox BP, Golenberg N, Keller NP, Huttenlocher A. Macrophages inhibit *Aspergillus fumigatus* germination and neutrophil-mediated fungal killing. *PLoS Pathog*. (2018) 14:e1007229. doi: 10.1371/journal.ppat.1007229

28. Ellett F, Pazhakh V, Pase L, Benard EL, Weerasinghe H, Azabdaftari D, et al. Macrophages protect *Talaromyces marneffei* conidia from myeloperoxidase-dependent neutrophil fungicidal activity during infection establishment *in vivo*. *PLoS Pathog*. (2018) 14:e1007063. doi: 10.1371/journal.ppat.1007063

29. Jones CN, Hoang AN, Martel JM, Dimisko L, Mikkola A, Inoue Y, et al. Microfluidic assay for precise measurements of mouse, rat, and human neutrophil chemotaxis in whole-blood droplets. *J Leukoc Biol*. (2016) 100:241–7. doi: 10.1189/jlb.5TA0715-310RR

30. Yang CT, Cambier CJ, Davis JM, Hall CJ, Crosier PS, Ramakrishnan L. Neutrophils exert protection in the early tuberculous granuloma by oxidative killing of mycobacteria phagocytosed from infected macrophages. *Cell Host Microbe*. (2012) 12:301–12. doi: 10.1016/j.chom.2012.07.009

31. Ellett F, Irimia D. Microstructured devices for optimized microinjection and imaging of zebrafish larvae. *J Vis Exp.* (2017) e56498. doi: 10.3791/56498

32. Pase L, Layton JE, Wittmann C, Ellett F, Nowell CJ, Reyes-Aldasoro CC, et al. Neutrophil-delivered myeloperoxidase dampens the hydrogen peroxide burst after tissue wounding in zebrafish. *Curr Biol.* (2012) 22:1818–24. doi: 10.1016/j.cub.2012.07.060

33. Hall C, Flores MV, Storm T, Crosier K, Crosier P. The zebrafish lysozyme C promoter drives myeloid-specific expression in transgenic fish. *BMC Dev Biol.* (2007) 7:42. doi: 10.1186/1471-213X-7-42

34. Li L, Jin H, Xu J, Shi Y, Wen Z. Irf8 regulates macrophage versus neutrophil fate during zebrafish primitive myelopoiesis. *Blood.* (2011) 117:1359–69. doi: 10.1182/blood-2010-06-290700

35. Lister JA, Robertson CP, Lepage T, Johnson SL, Raible DW. Nacre encodes a zebrafish microphthalmia-related protein that regulates neural-crest-derived pigment cell fate. *Development.* (1999) 126:3757–67.

36. Ellett F, Pase L, Hayman JW, Andrianopoulos A, Lieschke GJ. mpeg1 promoter transgenes direct macrophage-lineage expression in zebrafish. *Blood.* (2011) 117:e49–56. doi: 10.1182/blood-2010-10-3 14120

37. Colucci-Guyon E, Tinevez JY, Renshaw SA, Herbomel P. Strategies of professional phagocytes *in vivo*: unlike macrophages, neutrophils engulf only surface-associated microbes. *J Cell Sci.* (2011) 124(Pt 18):3053–9. doi: 10.1242/jcs.082792

38. Rhodes J, Hagen A, Hsu K, Deng M, Liu TX, Look AT, et al. Interplay of pu.1 and gata1 determines myelo-erythroid progenitor cell fate in zebrafish. *Dev Cell.* (2005) 8:97–108. doi: 10.1016/j.devcel.2004.11.014

39. Ravikumar S, Win MS, Chai LY. Optimizing outcomes in immunocompromised hosts: understanding the role of immunotherapy in invasive fungal diseases. *Front Microbiol.* (2015) 6:1322. doi: 10.3389/fmicb.2015.01322

40. Becker EL, Forouhar FA, Grunnet ML, Boulay F, Tardif M, Bormann BJ, et al. Broad immunocytochemical localization of the formylpeptide receptor in human organs, tissues, and cells. (1998) 292:129–35. doi: 10.1007/s004410051042

41. Bouffard FA, Zambias RA, Dropinski JF, Balkovec JM, Hammond ML, Abruzzo GK, et al. Synthesis and antifungal activity of novel cationic pneumocandin B(o) derivatives. *J Med Chem.* (1994) 37:222–5. doi: 10.1021/jm00028a003

42. Westerfield M. *The Zebrafish Book: A Guide for the Laboratory Use of Zebrafish.* Available online at: http://zfin org/zf_info/zfbook/zfbk html. 2000

43. Mathias JR, Perrin BJ, Liu TX, Kanki J, Look AT, Huttenlocher A. Resolution of inflammation by retrograde chemotaxis of neutrophils in transgenic zebrafish. *J Leukoc Biol.* (2006) 80:1281–8. doi: 10.1189/jlb.0506346

44. Kwan KM, Fujimoto E, Grabher C, Mangum BD, Hardy ME, Campbell DS, et al. The Tol2kit: a multisite gateway-based construction kit for Tol2 transposon transgenesis constructs. *Dev Dyn.* (2007) 236:3088–99. doi: 10.1002/dvdy.21343

45. Ellett F, Irimia D. Microstructured surface arrays for injection of zebrafish larvae. *Zebrafish.* (2017) 14:140–5. doi: 10.1089/zeb.2016.1402

# 12

# The Role of Pre-Existing Cross-Reactive Central Memory CD4 T-Cells in Vaccination with Previously Unseen Influenza Strains

Mikalai Nienen [1,2,3*], Ulrik Stervbo [4], Felix Mölder [5], Sviatlana Kaliszczyk [4],
Leon Kuchenbecker [6], Ludmila Gayova [7], Brunhilde Schweiger [8], Karsten Jürchott [2],
Jochen Hecht [9,10], Avidan U. Neumann [11], Sven Rahmann [5], Timm Westhoff [12],
Petra Reinke [2,13], Andreas Thiel [2] and Nina Babel [2,4,13*]

[1] Institute for Medical Immunology, Charité University Medicine Berlin, Berlin, Germany, [2] Berlin-Brandenburg Center for Regenerative Therapies, Charité University Medicine Berlin, Berlin, Germany, [3] Labor Berlin-Charité Vivantes GmbH, Berlin, Germany, [4] Center for Translational Medicine, Immunology and Transplantation, Marien Hospital Herne, Ruhr University Bochum, Herne, Germany, [5] Genome Informatics, Institute of Human Genetics, University Hospital Essen, University of Duisburg-Essen, Essen, Germany, [6] Applied Bioinformatics, Tübingen University, Tübingen, Germany, [7] Bogomolets National Medical University, Kyiv, Ukraine, [8] Robert-Koch Institute, Berlin, Germany, [9] Centre for Genomic Regulation (CRG), The Barcelona Institute of Science and Technology, Barcelona, Spain, [10] Universitat Pompeu Fabra (UPF), Barcelona, Spain, [11] Institute of Environmental Medicine, German Research Center for Environmental Health, Helmholtz Zentrum München, Augsburg, Germany, [12] Department of Internal Medicine, Marien Hospital Herne, Ruhr University Bochum, Herne, Germany, [13] Department of Nephrology and Intensive Care, Charité University Medicine Berlin, Berlin, Germany

*Correspondence:
Mikalai Nienen
mikalai.nienen@charite.de
Nina Babel
nina.babel@charite.de

Influenza vaccination is a common approach to prevent seasonal and pandemic influenza. Pre-existing antibodies against close viral strains might impair antibody formation against previously unseen strains–a process called original antigenic sin. The role of this pre-existing cellular immunity in this process is, despite some hints from animal models, not clear. Here, we analyzed cellular and humoral immunity in healthy individuals before and after vaccination with seasonal influenza vaccine. Based on influenza-specific hemagglutination inhibiting (HI) titers, vaccinees were grouped into HI-negative and -positive cohorts followed by in-depth cytometric and TCR repertoire analysis. Both serological groups revealed cross-reactive T-cell memory to the vaccine strains at baseline that gave rise to the majority of vaccine-specific T-cells post vaccination. On the contrary, very limited number of vaccine-specific T-cell clones was recruited from the naive pool. Furthermore, baseline quantity of vaccine-specific central memory helper T-cells and clonotype richness of this population directly correlated with the vaccination efficacy. Our findings suggest that the deliberate recruitment of pre-existing cross-reactive cellular memory might help to improve vaccination outcome.

Keywords: influenza vaccination, vaccination efficacy, pre-existing cross-reactive T-cells, central memory T-cell, clonotype diversity

# INTRODUCTION

Influenza infection is a major cause of acute respiratory infections (1, 2). While healthy individuals manage the infection efficiently, several groups, including elder, immunosuppressed, and chronically ill individuals, have a significant risk of prolonged and complicated infection course and high mortality (2, 3).

Vaccination with trivalent inactivated vaccine (TIV) or live attenuated vaccine (LAV) is the common approach to raise protective antibody titers against influenza and is generally accepted as the most relevant protection factor (4, 5). However, it is not rare that the post vaccination antibody levels are insufficient. Even though several clinical conditions are associated with low vaccination efficacy (e.g., chronic inflammatory and metabolic disorders, immune deficiencies), the scenario of insufficient or failed vaccination also affects the healthy population (6–8).

The exact prerequisites and correlates of efficient vaccination are not completely understood so far but have been attributed to the vaccine origin, its composition and application mode (9–14). In case of a primary immune response the contact with previously unseen pathogenic antigens leads to an inflammatory process and the recruitment of T- and B-cells from naive pools. Besides generation of effector cells this leads to formation of the immune memory, both cellular and humoral. In case of a secondary immune response, pre-existing memory B- and T-cells promptly proliferate, differentiate and perform numerous effector functions, resulting in a rapid raise of antibodies titers and pathogen clearance. For influenza however, the situation is somewhat special. The previous contacts with influenza leave long-lasting and sometimes life-long cellular and humoral immunity. However, due to antigenic drift and shift new viral strains are continuously created which are no longer recognized by the pre-existing memory, what helps the virus to bypass the pre-existing immunity (15–18). The exact role of pre-existing immune memory in the development of sufficient protection against novel epitopes is not clear, yet. Numerous findings indicate that it can be detrimental and lead to impaired formation of neutralizing antibody against previously unseen influenza strains. This phenomenon known as the original antigenic sin (OAS) was initially linked to the pre-existing cross-reactive antibodies and cognate memory B-cells (19, 20). However, the role of pre-existing cross-reactive T-cells in an insufficient and failed immune response against novel influenza strains was inferred from the studies on Dengue virus and mouse LCMV (21, 22). This was further strengthened by several reports on the suppression of naive and follicular influenza-specific helper T-cells by the pre-existing cross-reactive memory (23, 24). However, new findings show that pre-existing influenza-specific memory, both cellular and humoral, is not always detrimental but on the contrary might be helpful in terms of vaccination efficacy and protection against natural infection (25, 26). One report showed that the pre-existing cross-reactive memory CD4 specific to highly conserved internal influenza virus proteins are sufficient to alleviate influenza infection in a human inoculation model (27). However, data on the role of pre-existing memory against highly variable hemagglutinin

(HA) and neuraminidase (NA) induced by vaccination are very limited.

The goal of the current study was to elucidate the generation of influenza-specific helper T-cells upon vaccination with novel, previously unexperienced strains and to unravel their role in the formation of humoral immunity against novel influenza strains.

# MATERIALS AND METHODS
## Study Cohort

A total of 15 healthy adult individuals between 24 and 64 years old were involved in the study. The including criteria were as follows: 18 years or older, no previous influenza vaccination with the strains from the current composition (seasonal influenza vaccine 2011/2012) and/or no confirmed influenza infections in the past three years, no acute or chronic diseases, no known allergy to vaccine components, no pregnancy, good general health condition, written informed consent.

## Vaccination and Sample Collection

The vaccination was performed intramuscularly by a study physician with the trivalent influenza vaccine (Mutagrip 2011/2012 Sanofi-Pasteur). The vaccine was composed of A/California/7/2009 (H1N1), A/Perth/16/2009 (H3N2), B/Brisbane/60/2008 according to WHO recommendation. 50 ml venous blood was drawn at day 0, 7, 14, and 21 post vaccination using Lithium-Heparin Vacutainers (BD Biosciences) and processed immediately.

## Hemagglutination Inhibition Assay

Influenza-specific antibody titers were measured by a standard hemagglutination inhibition (HAI) assay, using vaccine strains (s. vaccine composition) and turkey hen erythrocytes (28). Baseline (day 0) and post vaccination (day 21) sera were tested simultaneously in duplicates and the antibody titers estimated. Baseline seronegativity was defined by a HAI titer <10 (29). For statistical evaluation the combined vaccination efficacy for three vaccine components was calculated as the sum of the binary logarithm fold change ($\Delta LF$) between day 21 and baseline according to the formula:

$$\Delta LF = \sum_{c=1}^{3} \log_2 \left( \frac{titer\,(c, day21)}{titer\,(c, day0)} \right),$$

where the sum ranges over the three components $c$.

## PBMC Preparation

Peripheral blood mononuclear cells (PBMCs) were isolated by gradient centrifugation with Ficoll-Paque Plus (GE Healthcare). PBMCs were re-suspended in complete medium (RPMI/10%FCS/Penicillin/Streptomycin, all from Gibco).

## Flow Cytometric Assessment and Isolation of Influenza-Specific Helper T-Cells

Frequency, cytokine production and phenotype analysis of the influenza-specific helper T-cells was done after overnight PBMC stimulation with the vaccine (at least 10 μg/mL of HA from every strain). As negative and positive controls, PBMC were incubated alone or with staphylococcal enterotoxin B (1 μg/ml, Sigma-Aldrich). Brefeldin A was added after 2 h of stimulation (10 μg/mL, Sigma-Aldrich). At the end of the stimulation PBMC were harvested, stained for surface, and intracellular markers using FACS-Lysing and FACS-Perm Solution (BD Biosciences), and analyzed on BD Fortessa flow cytometer (BD Biosciences).

Influenza-specific helper T-cells were isolated after overnight PBMC stimulation with the vaccine (10 μg/mL of HA from every strain) and human anti-CD40 antibodies (clone HB14, Miltenyi Biotec). Live sorting was done on BD FACS Aria (BD Biosciences) with sorting strategy provided in **Figure S2**. The following subsets were enriched with high purity: naive (CD45RA+CCR7+), central memory (CM, CD45RA-CCR7+) and effector (Eff, CD45RA-CCR7-). Following antibodies were used for the cytometric analysis and sorting: CD3 eFluor 650 (HIT3a, eBioscience), CD4 QDot 565 (OKT4, Biolegend, in-house fluorochrome coupling), CD8 QDot 525 (RPT-T8, Biolegend, in-house fluorochrome coupling), CCR7 FITC (G043H7, Biolegend), CD45RA eFlour 605 (HI100, eBioscience), CD154 APC/Cy7 (24-31, Biolegend), CD69 Pe/Cy5 (FN50, Biolegend), TNFa Pacific Blue (Mab11, Biolegend), IFNg Alexa Fluor 700 (B27, Biolegend), IL2 Pe (MQ1-17H12, Biolegend), IL4 Pe/Cy7 (MP4-25D2, Biolegend), IL17 PerCP/Cy5.5 (BL168, Biolegend), CD19 V500 (HIB19, BD Biosciences), CD27 PerCP-Cy5.5 (M-T271, Biolegend), IgD FITC (IA6-2, BD Biosciences), CD20 eFluor 650 (2H7, eBioscience), CD38 Alexa Fluor 700 (HB-7, Biolegend), CD2/3/4/14/15/34/56/61/235a-biotin (as part of Pan B Cell Isolation Kit, Miltenyi Biotec), anti-biotin-Vio Blue (Bio3-18E7, Miltenyi Biotec). Peripheral blood plasmablasts were gated as CD27++CD38++CD20low/- cells among Lineage-CD19low/+ population (**Figure S1**). Absolute cell counts in peripheral blood were estimated as previously described (30). Detailed information on the sorted influenza-specific CD4 T-cells is provided in **Table S1**.

## Clonotype Analysis

The clonotype analysis was performed based on NGS-sequencing of the TCRβ chain of the FACS-enriched influenza-specific subsets. The detailed method description with primer sequences and amplification parameters can be found in the original publication (31, 32). Briefly, DNA was isolated using AllPrep DNA Micro Kit (QIagen) and the recombined TCRβ locus was amplified and processed using Illumina NGS platform. The raw sequencing data were deposited at Sequence Read Archive (SRA) with the following BioProject ID: PRJNA445234.

The raw sequences were processed with subsequent clone grouping on the nucleotide level using our free open-source clonotyping platform IMSEQ with analysis parameters provided in the supplementary Method Information (33). Detailed information on recovered sequencing reads is provided in **Table S1**. For the clonotype richness and overlap analysis, samples with less than 1,000 raw sequencing reads were discarded. In order to increase sensitivity of the clonotype analysis, clonotypes from the memory subsets at baseline (CM and Eff day 0) were grouped as a common pre-existing memory. The unique clones from the naive and common memory at

baseline were tracked into the memory subsets post vaccination and the cumulative frequencies of the corresponding clones were calculated. Clonotype richness was assessed as the number of unique clonotype after sample size normalization. For this reason, subsets were size-normalized to 40,000 raw sequencing reads (corresponding to the size of the smallest analyzed sample) and the unique clones grouped. The number of unique clones per normalized sample represented the value of clonotype richness.

## Flow Cytometry and Statistical Data Analysis

FACS data were analyzed with FlowJo 9.9.3 (TreeStar).

Statistical analysis was performed using GraphPad Prism with following hypotheses defined beforehand:

1. Serologically exposed and non-exposed cohorts show different kinetics of peripheral blood B- and influenza-specific CD4 T-cells,
2. Pre-existing influenza-specific T-cells define vaccination efficacy in the serologically non-exposed cohort,
3. Origin of influenza-specific CD4 T-cells post vaccination: baseline naive or cross-reactive memory,
4. Clonotype diversity/richness of the pre-existing influenza-specific CD4 T-cells define vaccination efficacy in the serologically non-exposed vaccinees.

Normality distribution was assessed by D'Agostino-Pearson omnibus or Shapiro-Wilk normality test. In case of normal distribution parametric $t$ test and Pearson correlation were calculated; otherwise Mann-Whitney test and Spearman correlation were performed. Multiple comparisons were adjusted using the Holm-Sidak approach. $P$-values <0.05 were considered significant and designated as following: <0.05 as *, <0.01 as ** and <0.001 as ***.

## RESULTS

First, we assessed the vaccination efficacy in the cohort of 15 healthy individuals anamnestically not exposed to the natural influenza or the seasonal vaccination in the previous 3 years. This way subjects with no recent definite contact with influenza were preselected. However, despite preselection strategy, further serology analysis showed preformed hemagglutination inhibiting (HI)-antibodies to one or several viral strains in 7 out of 15 study participants at baseline. The vaccinees were therefore stratified into HI-positive and -negative groups according to the baseline antibody titers (**Table 1**). Of note, there were no non-responders in the study. All individuals developed protective antibody titers upon vaccination.

## HI-Negative Donors Develop a Higher Plasmablast Response Post Vaccine Application

In order to determine any difference in the B-cell kinetics in two serological groups, we analyzed peripheral blood B-cells including plasmablasts (PB) at baseline and day 7, 14, and 21 post vaccination by flow cytometry. We did not observe any relevant changes in B-cell populations except PB. These were defined as

The Role of Pre-Existing Cross-Reactive Central Memory CD4 T-Cells in Vaccination with Previously Unseen...

161

**TABLE 1** | Humoral responses to seasonal influenza vaccine assessed as titers of neutralizing antibodies.

| Donor ID | Age | Gender | California D0 | Brisbane D0 | Perth D0 | California D21 | Brisbane D21 | Perth D21 | ΔLF |
|---|---|---|---|---|---|---|---|---|---|
| #30 | 26 | M | 1.00 | 1.00 | 1.00 | 8.32 | 4.91 | 4.32 | 14.55 |
| #37 | 56 | F | 4.32 | 3.32 | 6.32 | 5.32 | 3.32 | 7.32 | 2.00 |
| #38 | 30 | M | 1.00 | 1.00 | 1.00 | 1.00 | 6.32 | 3.32 | 7.64 |
| #39 | 59 | F | 1.00 | 1.00 | 1.00 | 1.00 | 6.32 | 6.32 | 10.64 |
| #40 | 61 | M | 1.00 | 1.00 | 1.00 | 4.32 | 7.91 | 4.32 | 13.55 |
| #41 | 57 | M | 1.00 | 3.32 | 1.00 | 6.32 | 5.32 | 5.91 | 12.23 |
| #42 | 64 | F | 1.00 | 1.00 | 1.00 | 1.00 | 5.32 | 11.32 | 14.64 |
| #43 | 64 | M | 1.00 | 5.32 | 1.00 | 5.32 | 6.32 | 6.32 | 10.64 |
| #45 | 26 | M | 7.32 | 5.32 | 1.00 | 8.32 | 9.32 | 5.32 | 9.32 |
| #47 | 29 | M | 1.00 | 1.00 | 1.00 | 5.32 | 7.91 | 9.32 | 19.55 |
| #51 | 26 | M | 1.00 | 1.00 | 1.00 | 7.91 | 4.32 | 6.91 | 16.14 |
| #52 | 24 | M | 7.32 | 6.32 | 1.00 | 7.32 | 6.32 | 4.32 | 3.32 |
| #53 | 26 | F | 1.00 | 1.00 | 1.00 | 9.91 | 7.32 | 7.32 | 21.55 |
| #54 | 62 | F | 1.00 | 4.32 | 4.32 | 6.32 | 6.32 | 10.32 | 13.32 |
| #55 | 29 | F | 5.32 | 4.32 | 4.32 | 7.32 | 7.32 | 7.91 | 8.58 |

*Neutralizing antibodies were assessed in HIA at baseline and day 21 post vaccination. Data are shown as binary logarithm of the corresponding dilution titers. ΔLF represents the summary serology change for three influenza strains included in the current vaccine composition.*

CD27++CD38++CD20low/- among CD19+/low population (**Figure S1**) and analyzed as relative frequencies and absolute counts per mL whole blood. Significant PB rise at day 7 post vaccination was present in both groups (**Figure 1**; HI-positive group $p < 0.01$; HI-negative group $p < 0.001$ and $p < 0.01$ analyzed as frequencies and counts, correspondingly). The HI-positive group showed less pronounced changes at day 7, and the HI-negative group had significantly higher PB ($p < 0.05$ for both frequencies and absolute counts). Though the analyses were done on the whole blood level without further determination of B-cell antigen specificity, the observed population reflects kinetics of the influenza-specific PB, as previously shown (34, 35).

## Influenza-Specific Central Memory CD4 T-Cells Influence the Vaccination Outcome in HI-Negative Individuals

In order to analyze the role of CD4 T-cells, peripheral blood samples from both groups were stimulated with the vaccine and analyzed by means of multiparameter flow cytometry using markers of antigen-specific stimulation (31, 36). Analyses were performed at baseline and day 7, 14, and 21 post vaccination as CD4 T-cell frequencies and absolute counts (**Figure S2**).

As anticipated, the HI-positive cohort showed pre-existing influenza-specific helper T-cells at baseline. This was also the case in the HI-negative individuals (**Figure 2A**). The kinetics analysis showed a significant increase of vaccine-specific CD4 T-cells in both groups with the peak at day 7 post vaccination (HI-positive group $p < 0.05$ for frequencies and absolute counts; HI-negative group $p < 0.001$ for frequencies and $p < 0.01$ for absolute counts) and a steady decline at later time points (**Figure 2A**). Of interest, the HI-negative subjects revealed a significantly higher magnitude of influenza-specific helper T-cells at the peak of vaccine-induced response as compared to HI-positive cohort.

While no differences between serological groups were found at baseline and decline, at day 7 the HI-negative group showed a significantly higher vaccine-specific response ($p < 0.01$ for frequencies and $p < 0.05$ for cell counts).

We next analyzed the differentiation status of influenza-specific CD4 T-cells before and after immunization. Using CCR7 and CD45RA the differentiation status of T-cells can be assessed with division into following subsets: naive (CD45RA+CCR7+), central memory (CM, CD45RA-CCR7+), effector (Eff, CD45RA-CCR7-), and terminally differentiated memory T-cells ($T_{EMRA}$, CD45RA+CCR7-). Our data showed that the majority of vaccine-specific T-cells at baseline were of memory phenotype (**Figures 2B–D**). In both serological groups, CM dominated over Eff. Surprisingly, both groups also revealed influenza-specific T-cells with naive phenotype at baseline (**Figure 2D**). Though in absolute minority as compared to memory subsets, naive cells were present in all participants.

The kinetics of vaccine-specific CM CD4 T-cells in the HI-positive group showed no significant changes. In the HI-negative group on the contrary, the changes were highly pronounced. Compared to baseline, influenza-specific CM CD4 T-cells showed a significant increase with the peak at day 7 with further decline (**Figure 2B**; $p < 0.001$ and $p < 0.01$ between baseline and day 7 and 14, respectively, for both frequencies and absolute counts; $p < 0.05$ between baseline and day 21 for frequency analysis).

Kinetics of vaccine-specific Eff CD4 T-cells resembled the pattern of unseparated influenza-specific T-cells with the peak at day 7 and a steady decline thereafter (**Figure 2C**; HI-positive group $p < 0.01$ and $p < 0.05$ for frequencies and counts; HI-negative group $p < 0.01$ for both analyses).

Unexpectedly, vaccine-specific T-cells with naive phenotype did not show any relevant changes in the course of immunization and were still present post vaccination (**Figure 2D**). These cells showed a truly naive nature as Boolean gating revealed low IL2

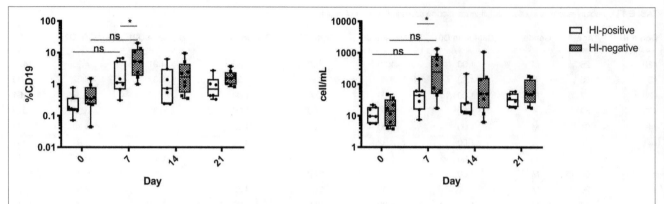

**FIGURE 1 |** Enhanced peripheral blood plasmablast response in the serologically naive group after vaccine application. Peripheral blood plasmablasts (PB) were defined as CD27++CD38+ cells among CD19+/low population as relative frequencies and absolute cell numbers per mL peripheral blood. Analyses were performed at baseline and different time points post vaccination in both HI-negative ($n = 8$) and HI-positive ($n = 7$) groups. Parametric $t$ tests with the Holm-Sidak approach for multiple comparisons were performed. The box plots show median with 25th to 75th percentiles and min to max range (whiskers). $P$-values are designated as following: <0.05 as *, <0.01 as ** and <0.001 as ***. The applied gating strategy is provided in **Figure S1**.

and no effector cytokine production. Memory influenza-specific T-cells on the contrary produced all measured effector cytokines (**Figures S3A,B**). Some donors revealed vaccine-specific $T_{EMRA}$ CD4 T-cells, however, at extremely low frequencies. This cell subset was therefore not analyzed further (**Figure S2**).

We further wondered, which factors influenced the establishment of influenza-specific humoral immunity. Thus, we performed a correlation analysis between the amount of influenza-specific helper T-cells, either complete or further separated based on different differentiation status, and the degree of humoral response. We found that in the HI-negative group the absolute counts of influenza-specific CM T-cells at baseline correlated significantly with the change in vaccine-specific antibody titer (**Figure 2E**; Pearson $R = 0.78$, adjusted $p = 0.02$). We could not identify other correlations in the HI-negative group; there were no correlations in the HI-positive group. Taken together, the data presented here show that the number of CM T-cells correlates with the vaccination efficacy in H-negative vaccinees.

## Influenza-Specific Helper T-Cells Post Vaccination Are Predominantly Recruited From the Pre-existing Memory

Both serological groups showed efficient vaccination as reflected by sufficient titers increase post vaccination (**Table 1**). The influenza-specific T- and B-cells in the HI-positive group were responsible for the sufficient cellular and humoral immunity resulting in increased HI-titers. In the HI-negative group, on the contrary, the role of the pre-existing cross-reactive memory T-cells in the vaccination process was not clear and for this reason we aimed to investigate to which extent these pre-existing T-cells contributed to the formation of influenza-specific T-cell memory as opposed to naive vaccine-specific T-cells.

For this purpose, subsets of vaccine-specific T-cells based on differentiation status were FACS-sorted at baseline and all analysis points post vaccination. The T-cell receptor (TCR) repertoires of all sorted populations were analyzed by sequencing

of the TCRβ chain on the nucleotide level. As T-cells originating from the same progenitor bear identical TCR on the cell surface, it can be used as a cellular identifier to track and thus elucidate the origin of T-cells with different phenotypic status, inter-subset dynamics and/or tissue distribution as previously demonstrated (31, 32). In order to define the origin of the influenza-specific CD4 T-cells post vaccination, unique clonotypes from the sorted baseline naive or pre-existing cross-reactive memory subsets (CM and Eff) were tracked post vaccination at memory subsets and the cumulative repertoire shares for the found clonotypes were calculated (schematically shown in **Figure 3A**). The analysis revealed that the influenza-specific clonotypes were predominantly recruited from the pre-existing cross-reactive memory and that these clonotypes constituted absolute majority of the vaccine-induced helper T-cells. Tracking naive clonotypes from day 0 in post vaccination repertoires revealed shared clonotypes of about 1% in only six out of 34 comparison pairs. The remaining pairs showed either neglectable clonotype share or could not reveal any single naive clonotype in post vaccination memory (**Figure 3B**). The pre-existing cross-reactive memory, on the contrary, contributed significantly higher to the post vaccination repertoires constituting up to 80% of the memory clonotypes ($p < 0.001$; **Figure 3B**). Based on these observations, we conclude, that the influenza-specific helper T-cells are predominantly recruited from the pre-existing cross-reactive memory and not the naive repertoires.

## Clonotype Diversity of Pre-existing Influenza-Specific CM T-Cells Correlates With the Serological Response to Vaccination

Clonotype richness/diversity is a prerequisite for an antigen-specific T-cell population to recognize broad array of pathogenic epitopes, since T-cells targeting numerous epitopes are more effective at combating the pathogens. To assess whether this feature of influenza-specific T-cells played a role in the vaccination efficacy we analyzed the correlation between the

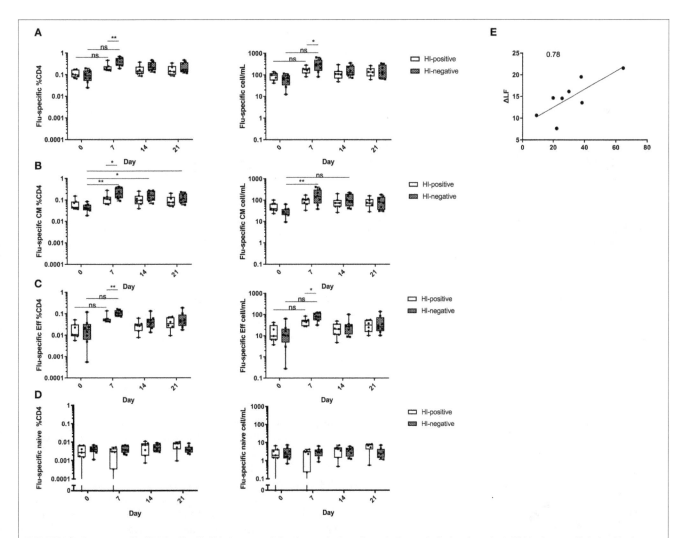

**FIGURE 2** | Influenza-specific CD4 T-cells with CM phenotype define the vaccination efficacy in the serologically naive cohort. **(A)** Vaccine-specific helper T-cells were analyzed in both serologically experienced (n = 7) and naive (n = 8) cohorts based on expression of CD154 and CD69, the cytokine-independent markers of antigen-specific CD4 T-helper activation. Influenza-specific helper T-cells were further analyzed based on CCR7 and CD45RA allowing discrimination of cell with CM **(B)**, Eff **(C)**, and naive phenotype **(D)**. CM helper T-cells were defined as CCR7+CD45RA-, Eff as CCR7-CD45RA- and naive as CCR7+CD45RA+. Relative frequencies among CD4 helper T-cells and absolute cell numbers per mL peripheral blood are shown. Parametric t tests with Holm-Sidak approach for multiple comparisons were performed. The box plots show median with 25th to 75th percentiles and min to max range (whiskers). P-values are designated as following: <0.05 as *, <0.01 as ** and <0.001 as ***. The applied gating strategy is provided in **Figure S2**. **(E)** Pearson correlation analysis of pre-existing vaccine-specific CD4 T-cells with CM phenotype in serologically unexperienced cohort at baseline (n = 8) analyzed as absolute cell numbers per mL peripheral blood and post-vaccination antibody titer increase. R, Pearson correlation coefficient. The line represents the best linear fit.

clonotype richness and the antibody titer change in the HI-negative group. As group size drastically influences diversity, the analyzed samples were first normalized to equal size. Next, sequence reads were grouped according to the clonal identity and the number of unique clones was defined as a measure of the sample richness. Our analyses revealed that the baseline richness of influenza-specific CM helper T-cells strongly correlated with serological outcome of vaccination in the HI-negative group (**Figure 4**; Pearson R = 0.91, adjusted p = 0.006). Clonotype diversity of further influenza-specific populations and time points revealed no correlation to the serology change. The detailed clonotype composition of CM T-helper cell at baseline in HI-negative group is presented in **Table S2**.

## DISCUSSION

Influenza results in the formation of a long-term immunity that can sometimes last lifelong (4, 37). Contacts with previously seen epitopes lead to memory activation and fast pathogen clearance. However, due to antigenic drift and shift new viral strains are constantly created that can escape pre-existing antibodies and T-cells. In this case the recruitment of naive T- and B-cells is necessary for the efficient eradication of novel viruses. Not all influenza virus components mutate with equal pace with HA and NA showing the highest mutation rate (38, 39). This results in a mixed immune response to both conserved and previously unseen viral epitopes. For several pathogens, including influenza, there are concerns that the pre-existing humoral and cellular

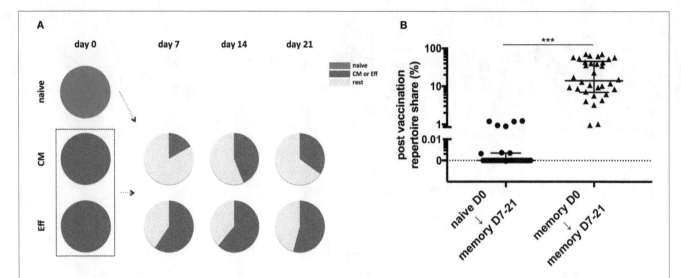

**FIGURE 3** | Post vaccination influenza-specific helper T-cell repertoires in the serologically unexposed group are formed predominantly from the pre-existing cross-reactive memory and not the naive T-cells. In the HI-negative cohort influenza-specific clonotypes from the baseline naive and memory subsets (CM and Eff) were tracked in the memory post vaccination and cumulative frequencies of the clonotypes with different origin (either naive or memory) were determined. **(A)** Schematic representation of the performed analysis. Single clonotypes from naive and common pre-existing memory were tracked in post vaccination subsets; cumulative frequencies of the corresponding clonotypes were estimated. **(B)** Cumulative frequencies of the influenza-specific clonotypes post-vaccination ($n = 40$) originating from either naive ($n = 6$) or pre-existing cross-reactive memory subsets ($n = 14$) at baseline. $^*p < 0.05$, $^{**}p < 0.01$, and $^{***}p < 0.001$. Detailed information on sorted cell populations and sequencing outcome is provided in **Table S1**.

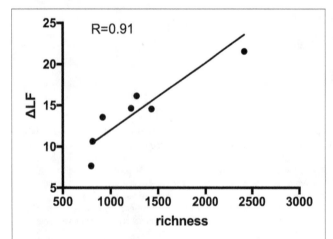

**FIGURE 4** | Clonotype richness of the cross-reactive vaccine-specific CM T-cells at baseline significantly correlates with the level of serological response to the previously unseen viral strains. Pearson correlation analysis between the clonotype richness of influenza-specific CM CD4 T-cell subsets ($n = 7$) at baseline and vaccination efficacy in the serologically unexperienced cohort. Clonotype richness of the influenza-specific T-cells was assessed as the number of unique clones per subset of normalized size (40,000 arbitrarily sampled raw sequencing reads according to the size of the smallest analyzed population). R, Pearson correlation coefficient. The line represents the best linear fit.

immunity can hamper the response against novel strains and skew the response against epitopes from previous encounters. This phenomenon known as original antigenic sin (OAS) was linked mostly to the pre-existing antibodies and described in numerous infections, including influenza (31, 40–44). One of the proposed mechanisms suggested the epitope masking by the pre-existing antibodies resulting in the inhibited recruitment of naive B-cells and skewed induction of memory B-cells from the previous encounters (45–47). The role of helper T-cells in the development of OAS in humans, however, was hardly addressed due to sampling and technological limitations. Original data from the Dengue virus and mouse LCMV studies pointed out on the cross-reactive T-cell memory among the reasons of the failed immunity (21, 22). Various animal studies confirmed this concept (40, 41, 48). However, new data revealed CD4+ memory specific to highly conserved internal influenza virus proteins as a protection correlate in human influenza infection (27).

Here, we analyzed the role of the pre-existing T-helper memory in the vaccination against previously unseen influenza strains. In order to exclude influence of immune senescence on the vaccination efficacy and decrease the chance of previous contacts with the vaccine strains, individuals younger than 65 were studied (49, 50). As the vaccine strains were previously circulating, we first applied anamnestic approach to exclude cases of overt infection as well as vaccination in the previous 3 years. As half of the study participants revealed vaccine-specific titers, these can be due to either subclinical/identified influenza or contacts with the virus for longer than the defined time window. Alternatively, this might reflect cross-reactive humoral immunity as broadly cross-reactive antibodies against numerous influenza strains were lately described (51, 52). Thus, final cohort definition relied on baseline serological status and serologically naive group was defined by absent vaccine-specific titers before vaccination.

The analysis of B-cell kinetics post vaccination revealed a strong increase of PB frequencies. Though the antigen specificity of the B-cell subsets was not assessed, the PB rise is most probably due to influenza-specific cells. It was previously shown, that up to 80% of PB at day 7 post vaccination are vaccine-specific (35). Furthermore, HI-positive cohort showed lower PB rise at the peak of response as compared to HI-negative one. This might be attributed to the pre-existing influenza-specific antibodies that dampen influenza-specific B-cell responses post vaccination (34). Still, even with lower PB increase the HI-positive group revealed protective antibody titers.

Using multiparameter flow cytometry and NGS-based clonotyping, we addressed the role of pre-existing helper T-cells in the early process of vaccine-specific memory formation. As MHC-class II tetramers are very limited and restrict cell analysis to a handful of epitopes and HLA-allele, we applied *ex vivo* stimulation and employed cytokine-independent analysis of antigen-specific helper T-cells (36, 53). Of notice, all subjects showed pre-existing memory T-cells at baseline, both serologically exposed and unexperienced, suggesting cross-reactive memory to conserved vaccine components and/or third-party antigens. As split vaccine was used for stimulation of influenza-specific T-cells, not only HA- and NA-specific but also T-cells with other specificities (including internal proteins NP and M1) were analyzed. The serology analysis utilizing HI-titers focused on antibodies targeting HA-antigens as these antibodies prevent hemagglutination induced by influenza hemagglutinins. However, even though present before vaccination and included into the analysis, the NP- and M1-specific T-cells (as well as other specificities against conserved antigens) are very unlikely to influence hemagglutinin-specific neutralizing titers as T- and B-cell-specific epitopes must be physically linked for efficient T-cell help (54, 55). In fact, it would be interesting to further clarify the influence of pre-existing NP- and M1-specific T-helper cell as cytotoxic T-cell with these specificities were associated with reduced influenza severity (13). Notably, memory T-helper cells specific to third-party microbial/environmental antigens were shown to be cross-reactive to influenza (as well as HIV) that were boosted after vaccination. As newborns showed only naive T-cells with these specificities it was linked to increased infection vulnerability (56).

On the clonal level we showed that in the serologically unexperienced group the vaccine-induced T-cells are recruited mostly from the pre-existing cross-reactive T-cell memory. Even though naive-derived T-cells also contributed to post vaccine-induced response, the clonotype share of naive-derived cells was neglectable as compared to pre-existing memory. To our knowledge this is the first report comparing contribution of pre-existing memory and naive T-cells in influenza vaccination. Our findings are in line with recent reports from animal LIV influenza vaccination showing that the pre-existing cross-reactive CD8 T-cell memory hampered recruitment of naive specificities (23, 57). Another study suggested that the subdominant heterotypic CD8 clonalities suppress naive precursors (58). Further mouse influenza studies revealed that cross-reactive memory specific to conserved epitopes inhibited expansion of naive specificities (25, 59). Another very recent report on whole blood clonotype analysis did not reveal significant clonotype changes after influenza vaccination suggesting that only a limited number of T-cells

was recruited in the course of vaccination which was not visible on a global scale (60). Our findings show that in serologically unexperienced individuals, the pre-existing cross-reactive T-cells provide sufficient help to naive B-cells. There is still a small hypothetical possibility, that even with lacking HI-titers low levels of HA-specific non-neutralizing antibodies were present at baseline stemming from the cross-reactive memory B-cells specific to close viral strains. These cross-reactive B-cells would eventually develop highly neutralizing antibodies through somatic hypermutation. However, regardless of the source of HI-titers, either naive of cross-reactive memory B-cells, the pre-existing T-cells are helpful in generating protective antibody titers with no or limited recruitment of naive T-cells.

We detected vaccine-specific T-cells with naive phenotype not only at baseline but also in follow-up, a phenomenon not unique to influenza. Recently, we reported on high frequencies of *A. fumigatus*-specific helper T-cells with naive phenotype (31). Even though *Aspergillus* represents a ubiquitous pathogen that constantly tackles the immune system, the substantial amount of fungus-specific T-cells still remain in the naive pool. This "dispensability" of naive T-cells might be another hint on sufficient help from the pre-formed T-cell memory.

Our analysis revealed that the pre-existing influenza-specific helper T-cells with CM phenotype at baseline strongly correlate with the serological response. To our knowledge this is the first report on the differentiation status of influenza-specific CD4 T-cells and vaccination efficacy. The post vaccination expansions of influenza-specific IFNg-producing T-helper cells as measured by Elispot were shown to tightly correlate with increase of neutralizing antibodies. However, no correlation was found between serology and the pre-existing cross-reactive T-cells at baseline (54, 61). Here, influenza-specific T-cells were analyzed independently of cytokine-producing capacities in with markers allowing analysis of differentiation status.

Another, yet unresolved question is to which extent the diversity of the antigen-specific T-cells is important for an efficient immune response. Few reports addressed the role of clonotype diversity of antigen-specific T-cells in immune response and specifically influenza vaccination (62, 63). As more diverse clonotypes cover higher array of antigens, this should more efficiently target a pathogen. We showed strong correlation between the richness of pre-existing influenza-specific CM helper T-cells and the humoral response to previously unseen influenza vaccine strains. To our knowledge this is the first report on the repertoire diversity of pre-existing influenza-specific T-cells and vaccination efficacy. In line with our results are the data showing impaired influenza-specific response by restricted diversity CD8 T-cells in mouse model (64). Another indication on the role of clonotype composition comes from the human CMV setting, showing inverse correlation between the breadth of CMV-specific clonotype and antibody titers (65). Our data are strongly corroborated by the analysis of circulating follicular T-helper cells (cTfh) in influenza vaccination that revealed strong correlation between an increased cTfh-clonality and rise of peripheral plasmablast cells post vaccination (62). However, no link between cTfh-clonality at baseline and vaccination efficacy was found. As baseline cTfh encompass limited specificities to previously encountered influenza strains, further T-helper subsets with differing specificities join cTfh-pool upon vaccination and provide efficient help to influenza-specific B-cells.

Although the role of pre-existing T-cells in the generation of sufficient humoral immunity needs further analysis, several authors suggest that the pre-existing memory T-cells can be of great practical importance in vaccination (66, 67). In mouse models, immunization with inactivated influenza viruses in the presence of cholera toxin was reported to increase cross-reactivity and enhance levels of neutralizing antibodies (68). Currently, numerous studies in humans try to piggyback cellular immunity to standard vaccines (diphtheria, tetanus, and pertussis) in order to improve vaccination efficacy in risk groups (69–71).

One limitation of the current study is the lack of patients with failed vaccination. Additional studies on a cohort with low or no response to vaccine in scenarios with or without pre-existing antibodies would help to elucidate the role of pre-existing immunity, either beneficial or detrimental, in this process.

Taken together, our study demonstrates an important role of pre-existing memory T-cells in the generation of vaccine-specific humoral immunity to previously unseen strains. While naive vaccine-specific T-cells could be detected prior and after vaccine application independently of serological status, these cells were not recruited in the formation of vaccine-specific cellular memory as demonstrated by NGS and multiparameter flow cytometry. Our findings suggest that T-cell memory from previous encounters with close influenza strains provides sufficient help to naive B-cells specific to previously unseen viral strains and that the extent of previous encounters is beneficial in terms of vaccine-induced antibody titers.

## AUTHOR CONTRIBUTIONS

Conceptualization: MN, AT, and NB; Methodology: MN, BS, AUN, AT, and NB; Software: US, FM, KJ, SR, and LK; Formal analysis: MN, FM, US, LG, SR, and LK; Investigation: MN, US, BS, JH and SK; Resources: BS, AUN, TW, PR, AT, JH, and NB; Data curation: FM, SR, and LK; Writing—original draft: MN; Visualization: MN, FM; Supervision: MN, PR, AT, NB; Funding acquisition: AUN, AT, SR, and NB.

## FUNDING

The project was funded from German Ministry of Education and Research (projects e:KID, Primage), OP EFRE NRW (project Osteosys EFRE-0800427), and the Mercator Research Center Ruhr (project MERCUR Pe-2013-0012). We acknowledge support from the German Research Foundation (DFG) and the Open Access Publication Fund of Charité - Universitätsmedizin Berlin.

## ACKNOWLEDGMENTS

The authors would like to thank Toralf Kaiser and Jenny Kirsch from the Flow Cytometry Unit of German Rheumatism Research Center and Dr. Désirée Kunkel from the Flow Cytometry and Mass Cytometry Core Unit of Berlin-Brandenburg Center for Regenerative Therapies, Charité University Medicine Berlin for excellent assistance with flow cytometry and cell sorting. We also would like to thank Ulrike Krueger and the staff of the NGS Core Unit of Berlin-Brandenburg Center for Regenerative Therapies for the assistance with NGS-based sequencing.

## REFERENCES

1. La Gruta NL, Turner SJ. T cell mediated immunity to influenza: mechanisms of viral control. *Trends Immunol.* (2014) 35:396–402. doi: 10.1016/j.it.2014.06.004
2. Rambal V, Müller K, Dang-Heine C, Sattler A, Dziubianau M, Weist B, et al. Differential influenza H1N1-specific humoral and cellular response kinetics in kidney transplant patients. *Med Microbiol Immunol.* (2014) 203:35–45. doi: 10.1007/s00430-013-0312-3
3. Rello J, Pop-Vicas A. Clinical review: primary influenza viral pneumonia. *Crit Care.* (2009) 13:235. doi: 10.1186/cc8183
4. Dormitzer PR, Galli G, Castellino F, Golding H, Khurana S, Del Giudice G, et al. Influenza vaccine immunology. *Immunol Rev.* (2011) 239:167–77. doi: 10.1111/j.1600-065X.2010.00974.x
5. Subbarao K, Joseph T. Scientific barriers to developing vaccines against avian influenza viruses. *Nat Rev Immunol.* (2007) 7:267–78. doi: 10.1038/nri2054
6. Bernstein E, Kaye D, Abrutyn E, Gross P, Dorfman M, Murasko DM. Immune response to influenza vaccination in a large healthy elderly population. *Vaccine.* (1999) 17:82–94. doi: 10.1016/S0264-410X(98)00117-0
7. Kunisaki KM, Janoff EN. Influenza in immunosuppressed populations: a review of infection frequency, morbidity, mortality, and vaccine responses. *Lancet Infect Dis.* (2009) 9:493–504. doi: 10.1016/S1473-3099(09)70175-6

8. Lu P Bridges CB, Euler GL, Singleton JA. Influenza vaccination of recommended adult populations, U.S., 1989-2005. *Vaccine.* (2008) 26:1786–93. doi: 10.1016/j.vaccine.2008.01.040

9. Altenburg AF, Rimmelzwaan GF, de Vries RD. Virus-specific T cells as correlate of (cross-)protective immunity against influenza. *Vaccine.* (2015) 33:500–6. doi: 10.1016/j.vaccine.2014.11.054

10. Lambert P, Liu M, Siegrist CA. Can successful vaccines teach us how to induce efficient protective immune responses? *Nat Med.* (2005) 11:S54–62. doi: 10.1038/nm1216

11. Rimmelzwaan GF, McElhaney JE. Correlates of protection: Novel generations of influenza vaccines. *Vaccine.* (2008) 26. doi: 10.1016/j.vaccine.2008.07.043

12. Saroja C, Lakshmi P, Bhaskaran S. Recent trends in vaccine delivery systems: a review. *Int J Pharm Investig.* (2011) 1:64–74. doi: 10.4103/2230-973X.82384

13. Sridhar S, Begom S, Bermingham A, Hoschler K, Adamson W, Carman W, et al. Cellular immune correlates of protection against symptomatic pandemic influenza. *Nat Med.* (2013) 19:1305–12. doi: 10.1038/nm.3350

14. Zinkernagel RM. On natural and artificial vaccinations. *Annu Rev Immunol.* (2003) 21:515–46. doi: 10.1146/annurev.immunol.21.120601.141045

15. Berlanda Scorza F, Tsvetnitsky V, Donnelly JJ. Universal influenza vaccines: Shifting to better vaccines. *Vaccine.* (2016) 34:2926–33. doi: 10.1016/j.vaccine.2016.03.085

16. Taubenberger JK, Morens DM. Influenza: the once and future pandemic. *Public Health Rep.* (2010) 125 (Suppl.):16–26. doi: 10.1177/00333549101250S305

17. Treanor J. Weathering the influenza vaccine crisis. *N Engl J Med.* (2004) 351:2037–40. doi: 10.1056/NEJMp048290

18. van de Sandt CE, Kreijtz JH, Rimmelzwaan GF. Evasion of influenza A viruses from innate and adaptive immune responses. *Viruses.* (2012) 4:1438–76. doi: 10.3390/v4091438

19. Henry C, Palm A-KE, Krammer F, Wilson PC. From original antigenic sin to the universal influenza virus vaccine. *Trends Immunol.* (2018) 39:70–9. doi: 10.1016/j.it.2017.08.003

20. Monto AS, Malosh RE, Petrie JG, Martin ET. The doctrine of original antigenic sin: separating good from evil. *J Infect Dis.* (2017) 215:1782–8. doi: 10.1093/infdis/jix173

21. Klenerman P, Zinkernagel RM. Original antigenic sin impairs cytotoxic T lymphocyte responses to viruses bearing variant epitopes. *Nature.* (1998) 394:482–5. doi: 10.1038/28860

22. Mongkolsapaya J, Dejnirattisai W, Xu X, Vasanawathana S, Tangthawornchaikul N, Chairunsri A, et al. Original antigenic sin and apoptosis in the pathogenesis of dengue hemorrhagic fever. *Nat Med.* (2003) 9:921–7. doi: 10.1038/nm887

23. Johnson LR, Weizman O, Rapp M, Way SS, Sun JC. Epitope-Specific vaccination limits clonal expansion of heterologous naive T cells during viral challenge. *Cell Rep.* (2016) 17:636–44. doi: 10.1016/j.celrep.2016.09.019

24. Olson MR, Chua BY, Good-Jacobson KL, Doherty PC, Jackson DC, Turner SJ. Competition within the virus-specific CD4 T-cell pool limits the T follicular helper response after influenza infection. *Immunol Cell Biol.* (2016) 94:729–40. doi: 10.1038/icb.2016.42

25. Di Piazza A, Richards KA, Knowlden ZAG, Nayak JL, Sant AJ. The role of CD4 T cell memory in generating protective immunity to novel and potentially pandemic strains of influenza. *Front Immunol.* (2016) 7:10. doi: 10.3389/fimmu.2016.00010

26. Linderman SL, Hensley SE. Antibodies with " original antigenic sin" properties are valuable components of secondary immune responses to influenza viruses. *PLoS Pathog.* (2016) 12:e1005806. doi: 10.1371/journal.ppat.1005806

27. Wilkinson TM, Li CK, Chui CS, Huang AK, Perkins M, Liebner JC, et al. Preexisting influenza-specific CD4+ T cells correlate with disease protection against influenza challenge in humans. *Nat. Med.* (2012) 18:276–82. doi: 10.1038/nm.2612

28. Meyer S, Adam M, Schweiger B, Ilchmann C, Eulenburg C, Sattinger E, et al. Antibody response after a single dose of an AS03-adjuvanted split-virion influenza A (H1N1) vaccine in heart transplant recipients. *Transplantation.* (2011) 91:1031–6. doi: 10.1097/TP.0b013e3182115be0

29. Allwinn R, Geiler J, Berger A, Cinatl J, Doerr HW. Determination of serum antibodies against swine-origin influenza A virus H1N1/09 by immunofluorescence, haemagglutination inhibition, and by neutralization

30. Stervbo U, Meier S, Mälzer JN, Baron U, Bozzetti C, Jürchott K, et al. Effects of aging on human leukocytes (part I): immunophenotyping of innate immune cells. *Age (Dordr).* (2015) 37:92. doi: 10.1007/s11357-015-9828-3

31. Bacher P, Heinrich F, Stervbo U, Nienen M, Vahldieck M, Iwert C, et al. Regulatory T cell specificity directs tolerance versus allergy against aeroantigens in humans. *Cell.* (2016) 167:1067–78.e16. doi: 10.1016/j.cell.2016.09.050

32. Dziubianau M, Hecht J, Kuchenbecker L, Sattler A, Stervbo U, Rödelsperger C, et al. TCR repertoire analysis by next generation sequencing allows complex differential diagnosis of T cell-related pathology. *Am J Transplant.* (2013) 13:2842–54. doi: 10.1111/ajt.12431

33. Kuchenbecker L, Nienen M, Hecht J, Neumann AU, Babel N, Reinert K, et al. IMSEQ-A fast and error aware approach to immunogenetic sequence analysis. *Bioinformatics.* (2014) 31:2963–71. doi: 10.1093/bioinformatics/btv309

34. Andrews SF, Kaur K, Pauli NT, Huang M, Huang Y, Wilson PC. High Preexisting serological antibody levels correlate with diversification of the influenza vaccine response. *J Virol.* (2015) 89:3308–17. doi: 10.1128/JVI.02871-14

35. Wrammert J, Smith K, Miller J, Langley WA, Kokko K, Larsen C, et al. Rapid cloning of high-affinity human monoclonal antibodies against influenza virus. *Nature.* (2008) 453:667–71. doi: 10.1038/nature06890

36. Frentsch M, Arbach O, Kirchhoff D, Moewes B, Worm M, Rothe M, et al. Direct access to CD4+ T cells specific for defined antigens according to CD154 expression. *Nat Med.* (2005) 11:1118–24. doi: 10.1038/nm1292

37. Dörner T, Radbruch A. Antibodies and B cell memory in viral immunity. *Immunity.* (2007) 27:384–92. doi: 10.1016/j.immuni.2007.09.002

38. Bhatt S, Holmes EC, Pybus OG. The genomic rate of molecular adaptation of the human influenza A virus. *Mol. Biol. Evol.* (2011) 28:2443–51. doi: 10.1093/molbev/msr044

39. Doherty PC, Turner SJ, Webby RG, Thomas PG. Influenza and the challenge for immunology. *Nat Immunol.* (2006) 7:449–55. doi: 10.1038/ni1343

40. Kim JH, Skountzou I, Compans R, Jacob J. Original antigenic sin responses to influenza viruses. *J Immunol.* (2009) 183:3294–301. doi: 10.4049/jimmunol.0900398

41. Morens DM, Burke DS, Halstead SB. The wages of original antigenic sin. *Emerg Infect Dis.* (2010) 16:1023–4. doi: 10.3201/eid1606.100453

42. Park MS, Kim J II, Park S, Lee I, Park MS. Original antigenic sin response to RNA viruses and antiviral immunity. *Immune Netw.* (2016) 16:261–70. doi: 10.4110/in.2016.16.5.261

43. Rehermann B, Shin E-C. Private aspects of heterologous immunity. *J Exp Med.* (2005) 201:667–70. doi: 10.1084/jem.20050220

44. Zompi S, Harris E. Original antigenic sin in dengue revisited. *Proc Natl Acad Sci USA.* (2013) 110:8761–2. doi: 10.1073/pnas.1306333110

45. Bergström JJE, Xu H, Heyman B. Epitope-Specific suppression of IgG responses by passively administered specific IgG: evidence of epitope masking. *Front Immunol.* (2017) 8:238. doi: 10.3389/fimmu.2017.00238

46. Henry Dunand CJ, Leon PE, Huang M, Choi A, Chromikova V, Ho IY, et al. Both neutralizing and non-neutralizing human H7N9 influenza vaccine-induced monoclonal antibodies confer protection. *Cell Host Microbe.* (2016) 19:800–13. doi: 10.1016/j.chom.2016.05.014

47. Zarnitsyna VI, Ellebedy AH, Davis C, Jacob J, Ahmed R, Antia R. Masking of antigenic epitopes by antibodies shapes the humoral immune response to influenza. *Philos Trans R Soc Lond B Biol Sci.* (2015) 370:20140248. doi: 10.1098/rstb.2014.0248

48. Alam S, Sant AJ. Infection with seasonal influenza virus elicits CD4 T cells specific for genetically conserved epitopes that can be rapidly mobilized for protective immunity to pandemic H1N1 influenza virus. *J Virol.* (2011) 85:13310–21. doi: 10.1128/JVI.05728-11

49. Centers for Disease Control and Prevention. *What You Should Know and Do this Flu Season If You Are 65 Years and Older.* cdc.gov/flu. (2017) Available online at: https://www.cdc.gov/flu/about/disease/65over.htm

50. Nichol KL, Nordin JD, Nelson DB, Mullooly JP, Hak E. Effectiveness of influenza vaccine in the community-dwelling elderly. *N Engl J Med.* (2007) 357:1373–81. doi: 10.1056/NEJMoa070844

51. Corti D, Voss J, Gamblin SJ, Codoni G, Macagno A, Jarrossay D, et al. A neutralizing antibody selected from plasma cells that binds to group

tests: how is the prevalence rate of protecting antibodies in humans? *Med Microbiol Immunol.* (2010) 199:117–21. doi: 10.1007/s00430-010-0143-4

1 and group 2 influenza A hemagglutinins. *Science.* (2011) 333:850–6. doi: 10.1126/science.1205669

52. Ellebedy AH, Krammer F, Li G-M, Miller MS, Chiu C, Wrammert J, et al. Induction of broadly cross-reactive antibody responses to the influenza HA stem region following H5N1 vaccination in humans. *Proc Natl Acad Sci USA.* (2014) 111:13133–8. doi: 10.1073/pnas.1414070111

53. Kern F, Surel IP, Brock C, Freistedt B, Radtke H, Scheffold A, et al. T-cell epitope mapping by flow cytometry. *Nat Med.* (1998) 4:975–8. doi: 10.1038/nm0898-975

54. Nayak JL, Fitzgerald TF, Richards KA, Yang H, Treanor JJ, Sant AJ. CD4+ T-cell expansion predicts neutralizing antibody responses to monovalent, inactivated 2009 pandemic influenza A(H1N1) virus subtype H1N1 vaccine. *J. Infect. Dis.* (2013) 207:297–305. doi: 10.1093/infdis/jis684

55. Sette A, Moutaftsi M, Moyron-Quiroz J, McCausland MM, Davies DH, Johnston RJ, et al. Selective CD4+ T cell help for antibody responses to a large viral pathogen: deterministic linkage of specificities. *Immunity.* (2008) 28:847–58. doi: 10.1016/j.immuni.2008.04.018

56. Su LF, Kidd BA, Han A, Kotzin JJ, Davis MM. Virus-specific CD4(+) memory-phenotype T cells are abundant in unexposed adults. *Immunity.* (2013) 38:373–83. doi: 10.1016/j.immuni.2012.10.021

57. Zehn D, Turner MJ, Lefrançois L, Bevan MJ. Lack of original antigenic sin in recall CD8(+) T cell responses. *J Immunol.* (2010) 184:6320–6. doi: 10.4049/jimmunol.1000149

58. Oberle SG, Hanna-El-Daher L, Chennupati V, Enouz S, Scherer S, Prlic M, et al. A minimum epitope overlap between infections strongly narrows the emerging T cell repertoire. *Cell Rep.* (2016) 17:627–35. doi: 10.1016/j.celrep.2016.09.072

59. Nayak JL, Alam S, Sant AJ. Cutting edge: heterosubtypic influenza infection antagonizes elicitation of immunological reactivity to hemagglutinin. *J Immunol.* (2013) 191:1001–5. doi: 10.4049/jimmunol.1203520

60. Sycheva AL, Pogorelyy MV, Komech EA, Minervina AA, Zvyagin IV, Staroverov DB, et al. Quantitative profiling reveals minor changes of T cell receptor repertoire in response to subunit inactivated influenza vaccine. *Vaccine.* (2018) 36:1599–605. doi: 10.1016/j.vaccine.2018.02.027

61. Nayak JL, Richards KA, Yang H, Treanor JJ, Sant AJ. Effect of influenza A(H5N1) vaccine prepandemic priming on CD4+ T-cell responses. *J Infect Dis.* (2015) 211:1408–17.doi: 10.1093/infdis/jiu616

62. Herati RS, Muselman A, Vella L, Bengsch B, Parkhouse K, Del Alcazar D, et al. Successful annual influenza vaccination induces a recurrent oligoclonotypic memory response in circulating T follicular helper cells. *Sci. Immunol.* (2017) 2:eaag2152. doi: 10.1126/sciimmunol.aag2152

63. Messaoudi I. Direct link between mhc polymorphism, T cell avidity, and diversity in immune defense. *Science.* (2002) 298:1797–800. doi: 10.1126/science.1076064

64. Yager EJ, Ahmed M, Lanzer K, Randall TD, Woodland DL, Blackman MA. Age-associated decline in T cell repertoire diversity leads to holes in the repertoire and impaired immunity to influenza virus. *J Exp Med.* (2008) 205:711–23. doi: 10.1084/jem.20071140

65. Wang GC, Dash P, McCullers JA, Doherty PC, Thomas PG. T cell receptor αβ diversity inversely correlates with pathogen-specific antibody levels in human cytomegalovirus infection. *Sci Transl Med.* (2012) 4:128ra42. doi: 10.1126/scitranslmed.3003647

66. Welsh RM, Che JW, Brehm MA, Selin LK. Heterologous immunity between viruses. *Immunol Rev.* (2010) 235:244–66. doi: 10.1111/j.0105-2896.2010.00897.x

67. Welsh RM, Fujinami RS. Pathogenic epitopes, heterologous immunity and vaccine design. *Nat Rev Microbiol.* (2007) 5:555–63. doi: 10.1038/nrmicro1709

68. Quan F-S, Compans RW, Nguyen HH, Kang S-M. Induction of heterosubtypic immunity to influenza virus by intranasal immunization. *J Virol.* (2008) 82:1350–9. doi: 10.1128/JVI.01615-07

69. Kim JH, Davis WG, Sambhara S, Jacob J. Strategies to alleviate original antigenic sin responses to influenza viruses. *Proc Natl Acad Sci USA.* (2012) 109:13751–6. doi: 10.1073/pnas.0912458109

70. Lu S. Heterologous prime-boost vaccination. *Curr Opin Immunol.* (2009) 21:346–51. doi: 10.1016/j.coi.2009.05.016

71. US National Institutes of Health. *ClinicalTrials.gov.* U.S. Natl. Institutes Heal., ClinicalTrials.gov Identifier: NCT02765126. (2016) Available online at: http://clinicaltrials.gov/

# 13

# Attenuation of Human Respiratory Viruses by Synonymous Genome Recoding

Cyril Le Nouën*, Peter L. Collins and Ursula J. Buchholz

*RNA Viruses Section, LID, NIAID, NIH, Bethesda, MD, United States*

**\*Correspondence:**
*Cyril Le Nouën*
*lenouenc@niaid.nih.gov*

Using computer algorithms and commercial DNA synthesis, one or more ORFs of a microbial pathogen such as a virus can be recoded and deoptimized by several strategies that may involve the introduction of up to thousands of nucleotide (nt) changes without affecting amino acid (aa) coding. The synonymous recoding strategies that have been applied to RNA viruses include: deoptimization of codon or codon-pair usage, which may reduce protein expression among other effects; increased content of immunomodulatory CpG and UpA RNA, which increase immune responses and thereby restrict viral replication; and substitution of serine and leucine codons with synonymous codons for which single-nt substitutions can yield nonsense codons, thus limiting evolutionary potential. This can reduce pathogen fitness and create potential live-attenuated vaccines that may have improved properties. The combined approach of genome recoding, synthetic biology, and reverse genetics offers several advantages for the generation of attenuated RNA viruses. First, synonymous recoding involves many mutations, which should reduce the rate and magnitude of de-attenuation. Second, increasing the amount of recoding can provide increased attenuation. Third, because there are no changes at the aa level, all of the relevant epitopes should be expressed. Fourth, attenuation frequently does not compromise immunogenicity, suggesting that the recoded viruses have increased immunogenicity per infectious particle. Synonymous deoptimization approaches have been applied to two important human viral pathogens, namely respiratory syncytial virus (RSV) and influenza A virus (IAV). This manuscript will briefly review the use of these different methods of synonymous recoding to generate attenuated RSV and IAV strains. It also will review the characterization of these vaccine candidates *in vitro* and in animal models, and describe several surprising findings with respect to phenotypic and genetic instability of some of these candidates.

Keywords: human respiratory virus, respiratory syncytial virus, influenza virus, vaccine, genome recoding, synonymous codon deoptimization, synthetic biology

## INTRODUCTION

The availability and affordability of large-scale commercial DNA synthesis opened the field of synthetic biology (1, 2). This technological advance allowed, in 2002, the rescue of an infectious poliovirus entirely from synthetic DNA (3). During the following years, synthetic biology and reverse genetics were combined to design and rescue viruses with extensive targeted modifications.

This resulted, in 2006, in the rescue of poliovirus strains with extensive codon deoptimization (CD) (4, 5). This exemplifies the approach of synonymous genome recoding, in which one or more ORFs of a microbial pathogen are modified at the nt level without altering coding at the aa level. Subsequently, synonymous genome recoding has been widely applied to reduce pathogen fitness and create potential live-attenuated vaccines.

Deoptimization by synonymous genome recoding offers several advantages for viral vaccine design. Genomes of recoded viruses may contain up to thousands of synonymous nucleotide mutations in one or several ORFs. Many of these likely contribute to attenuation, in aggregate this large number should impose a significant barrier against reversion to virulence, because any single-site reversion likely would yield only a small amount of de-attenuation (6–8). In principle, the level of attenuation can be modulated by adjusting the number of introduced mutations. Recoded vaccine candidates encode all viral proteins with the same aa sequence as the wt parent, and thus should induce innate, humoral, and cell-mediated responses against the same array of epitopes. Recoded viruses also can contain an increased number of CpG and UpA RNA dinucleotides that may increase host immune responses that restrict the virus and provide greater efficacy. Because synonymous recoding does not involve the lengthy development of specific attenuating mutations, it provides an expedited means of developing attenuated strains of a known or newly emerging pathogen.

Synonymous genome recoding has been applied to two important human respiratory viruses with negative-sense RNA genomes, namely respiratory syncytial virus (RSV) and influenza virus type A (IAV). RSV belongs to the *Pneumoviridae* family and is the most important viral agent of severe respiratory illness in infants and young children worldwide, and also is an important cause of respiratory illness in the frail elderly. Vaccines or antiviral drugs suitable for routine use are not yet available. A live-attenuated vaccine is a strategy of choice for the pediatric population because it is free of RSV disease enhancement that is associated with inactivated and subunit RSV vaccines in RSV-naïve recipients. The RSV genome consists of a single non-segmented negative-sense 15.2 kb RNA, containing 10 genes in the order 3′-NS1-NS2-N-P-M-SH-G-F-M2-L-5′. The M2 mRNA encodes two separate proteins, M2-1 and M2-2, from overlapping ORFs.

IAV belongs to the *Orthomyxoviridae* family, and contains eight RNA genome segments, each encoding one or two proteins: segment 1, PB2; 2, PB1 and PB1-F2; 3, PA, and PA-X protein; 4, HA; 5, NP; 6, NA; 7, M1, and M2; 8, NS1. Antigenic change of IAV is driven by point mutations in the HA and NA proteins as well as segment reassortment. Three types of vaccines are currently licensed for IAV: inactivated, live-attenuated, and recombinant HA protein. This review describes the current strategies of synonymous genome recoding used to generate attenuated RSV and IAV viruses and the characterization *in vitro* and *in vivo* of the resulting vaccine candidates.

# FOUR STRATEGIES FOR SYNONYMOUS GENOME RECODING

The four approaches used to deoptimize the different strains of IAV and RSV and the resulting number of silent nt mutations that have been introduced in these viruses ORFs are summarized in **Table 1**.

## Codon Deoptimization (CD)

Due to the degeneracy of the genetic code, most amino acids are encoded by more than one nucleotide triplet (synonymous codons). Some codons are used more or less frequently than one would expect based on random chance. This unequal frequency of usage of synonymous codons, referred to as codon bias [CB, (19)], can be found in many organisms including viruses (20, 21). CD involves recoding part or all of one or more ORFs to increase the content of synonymous codons that normally are under-represented in the genome of these organisms.

Several hypotheses that have been proposed to explain CB—as well as the effects of CD—involve mechanisms by which CB might affect protein expression (usually to increase expression), and indeed there is a significant association between CB and translation efficiency in *Escherichia. coli* (*E. coli*) and *Saccharomyces cerevisiae* (22). One hypothesis is that the codon usage of a virus is adapted to the host tRNA abundance, thereby enhancing viral translation and fitness (21, 23–25). Indeed, in several prokaryotes and unicellular eukaryotes there is a consistent correlation between tRNA abundance and the corresponding codon usage frequency (26). This correlation is more difficult to establish for multicellular eukaryotes. In humans, the tRNA abundance varies widely among different tissues. However, the tRNA abundance was statistically correlated to codon usage of highly expressed genes specific for those tissues (27, 28). Nt assignments involved in mRNA secondary structures, and an avoidance of GC content, also might sometimes contribute to CB (19, 29, 30). Of note, the codon bias of negative strand RNA viruses frequently differs from that of their host. A recent study suggests that this discrepancy is due to constraints of the viral replication machinery; in a VSV minigenome system, the purine/pyrimidine content of viral RNAs affected the stability of the viral nucleocapsids and the RNA synthesis activity of viral polymerase complex (31). CB also has been suggested to occur as a means of regulating protein folding: for example, underrepresented tRNAs can decrease the rate of polypeptide chain elongation and thereby improve the quality of protein folding (32). In addition, selective pressure to reduce the content of CpG and UpA RNA, which appear to stimulate innate and adaptive immune responses that would restrict the virus, may contribute to CB (14).

## Codon-Pair Deoptimization (CPD)

Just as codons may appear more or less frequently than expected, the usage of particular pairs of codons may be more or less frequent than expected which is called "codon pair bias" (CPB) (33). For example, in *E. coli*, two codon pairs encoding Leu-Ala [CTG-GCA and CTG-GCG] are highly overrepresented, while the synonymous codon pair CTG-GCC is under-represented.

**TABLE 1 |** Attenuation of influenza and respiratory syncytial virus by synonymous genome recoding.

| Virus | Deoptimization strategy | Virus strain | Gene(s) deoptimized | Number of silent mutations[j] | Main results | References |
|---|---|---|---|---|---|---|
| IAV | CD[a] | Seasonal H1N1 | PB2, PB1, PA, HA, NP, NA, M, NS[b] | 62, 77, 65, 46, 31, 47, 27, 18 | No effect on protein expression *in vitro* Virus attenuated in mammalian cells and in mice Immunogenicity in mice equivalent to wt | (9) |
| | | PR8 H1N1 | NS | 135 | Reduced NS1 and NEP protein expression *in vitro* Reduced virus replication *in vitro* Virus attenuated in mice Immunogenicity in mice equivalent to wt | (10) |
| | CPD | PR8 H1N1 | NP, HA, NA, PB1[c] | 314, 353, 265, 236 | Reduced protein expression of CPD ORFs *in vitro* Reduced virus replication *in vitro* Viruses attenuated in mice Immunogenicity equivalent to or higher than wt | (11, 12) |
| | | 2009 pH1N1[d] | HA, NA[e] | 346, 293 | Reduced rate of replication *in vitro* Final titers in the lung of ferrets equivalent to wt | (13) |
| | Increasing CpG or UpA content | PR8 H1N1 | NP | 86 (CpG-high virus), 73 (UpA-high virus) | Reduced virus replication *in vitro* Virus attenuated in mice Immunogenicity equivalent to wt | (14) |
| | Mutations in ser and leu codons[f] | 2009 pH1N1 | HA, PA[g] | 94, 111 | No effect on virus replication *in vitro* Virus attenuated in mice Immunogenicity equivalent to wt | (15) |
| RSV | CD | A2 | NS1, NS2, G[h] | 84, 82, Not indicated | Reduced protein expression of CD genes *in vitro* Reduced virus replication *in vitro* Virus attenuated in mice or cotton rats Immunogenicity equivalent to or higher than wt | (16, 17) |
| | CPD | A2 | NS1, NS2, N, P, M, SH, G, F, L[i] | 65, 60, 241, 143, 163, 23, 197, 422, 1,378 | Reduced protein expression of CPD genes Reduced virus replication *in vitro* Viruses attenuated in mice, hamsters, and African green monkeys Immunogenicity equivalent to wt | (18) |

[a] CD, codon deoptimization; CPD, codon-pair deoptimization.
[b] Recoded individually or in the combination of eight.
[c] Recoded individually and in combinations, notably NP-HA-PB1 (11) and HA-NA (12).
[d] 2009 pandemic (p)H1N1.
[e] Recoded in combination.
[f] Serine and leucine codons recoded into synonymous codons for which some single-nt substitutions result in nonsense codons.
[g] Recoded separately.
[h] Recoded in the combinations NS1-NS2 and NS1-NS2-G.
[i] Recoded in the combinations NS1-NS2-N-P-M-SH; G-F; L; and all genes except M2-1 and M2-2.
[j] Number of silent mutations introduced in each gene, respectively.

While this non-randomness was evident for pairs of codons, a bias was much less obvious in control analyses evaluating pairs of non-adjacent codons, and almost absent when pairs were separated by two or three intervening codons (33). CPB is thought to affect translation due to differences in the compatibility of different synonymous pairs of aminoacyl-tRNAs in the translating ribosome (33, 34). Buchan and al. suggested that structural features that regulate tRNA geometry within the ribosome may favor specific codon pairs and thus govern genomic codon pair patterns, driving enhanced translational fidelity and/or rate (35). As with CB, other factors may contribute to CPB, such as selection to reduce the content of CpG and UpA RNA thought to be immunostimulatory (36). CPD is achieved by rearranging synonymous codons to increase the frequency of codon-pairs that typically are under-represented, without changing the overall codon usage or nt content. The first CPD of an RNA virus involved poliovirus, in 2008 (37).

## Increasing the CpG and UpA Content

CpG and UpA RNAs typically are under-represented in RNA virus genomes, presumably due to selective pressure to reduce immune recognition by innate immunity sensors. CPD or CD of a viral genome frequently result in inadvertent increases in the CpG and UpA content of the recoded virus, which may account for the increased immunogenicity per PFU that sometimes is observed (11). For several RNA virus genomes, the content of CpG and UpA was deliberately increased while preserving the natural overall CPB and CB ratios (14, 38–40). The resulting

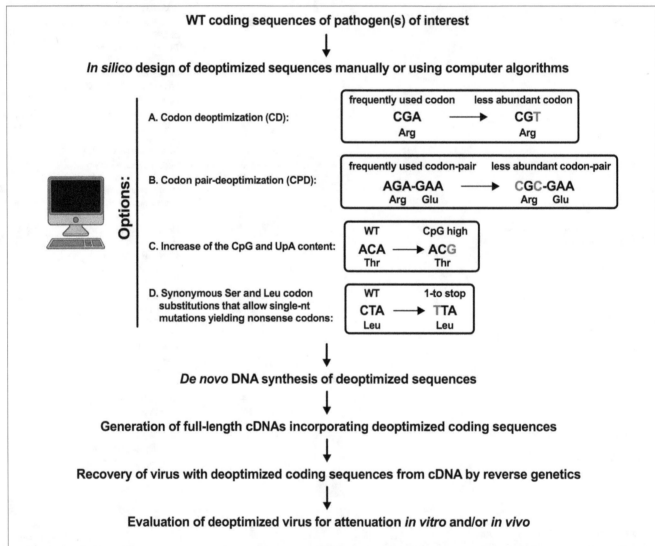

**FIGURE 1 |** Methodology used to generate genome scale deoptimized RSV or IAV viruses. Four strategies of deoptimization have been used to attenuate RSV and IAV: **(A)** codon deoptimization (CD), **(B)** codon-pair deoptimization (CPD), **(C)** increase of the CpG and UpA content and **(D)** synonymous Serine and Leucine codon substitutions that allow single-nt mutations yielding non-sense codons. An example is shown for each approach. The synonymous mutations generated by the deoptimization process are indicated in red. In **(A)**, the "A" to "T" mutation resulted in the introduction of an underrepresented Arg codon (10). In **(B)**, the CPD process (37) may yield CpG dinucleotides at codon boundaries that were shown to be significantly suppressed in wt viruses (36). In **(C)**, the program "Sequence Mutate" in the SSE package (43) introduces a synonymous mutation ("A" to "G") that resulted in the introduction of a CpG motif in the Thr amino acid. Finally in **(D)**, a synonymous mutation "C" to "T" generated a Leu codon "TTA" that by only a single-nucleotide change can generate a stop codon (TAA or TGA) (15).

viruses were substantially attenuated yet were as immunogenic as their wt parents, presumably due to greater stimulation of innate immune sensors by CpG and UpA resulting in increased immune responses and restriction of virus replication.

Note that CpG DNA can directly and very efficiently activate B cells but also Natural Killer cells, dendritic cells and monocytes/macrophages through TLR9 stimulation (41). While this is less clear for CpG RNA, synthetic CpG RNAs have been shown to stimulate human monocytes resulting in IL-6 and IL-12 production and costimulatory molecule up-regulation. However, this effect is not mediated through TLR3, 7/8, or 9 and the pathways remain to be defined (42). In addition, during virus replication, large amounts of viral mRNAs or double-stranded intermediates are produced that could be potentially be recognized by sensors of the innate immune response. Whether or not the increased CpG and UpA content in recoded viruses results in increased immunogenicity remains to be determined.

Recently, the host Zinc-finger antiviral protein (ZAP) was shown to inhibit a recoded CpG-rich version of HIV-1 by directly binding to regions of the viral RNA rich in CpG RNA. This suggests that ZAP is part of the cellular system for detecting non-self RNA containing CpG RNA (40).

## Synonymous Serine and Leucine Codon Substitutions That Allow Single-nt Mutations Yielding Nonsense Codons

Serine and leucine codons, which have the highest codon redundancy, can be recoded to increase the use of synonymous codons for which some of the possible single-nt changes result in nonsense mutations ("1-to-Stop" mutations) (15). This reduces the number of mutations at a given serine or leucine codon that can yield fit virus, and thus reduces evolutionary potential and viral fitness. This strategy has been applied to the pathogenic enterovirus Coxsackie B3 as well as to IAV (15).

## METHODOLOGY USED TO GENERATE DEOPTIMIZED RSV AND IAV VACCINE CANDIDATES

The methodologies that have been applied to RSV or IAV to generate deoptimized vaccine candidates are described in **Figure 1**. In all approaches, following identification of the gene(s) or portion(s) of the ORF(s) that will be targeted for deoptimization, silent mutations were first introduced *in silico,* manually (9, 10, 15) or using computer algorithms (11–14, 18), as described below. For each approach, packaging and splicing signals or replication/translation elements were excluded from the deoptimization process.

CD (**Figure 1A**) of the PR8 NS gene by Nogales and colleagues was done by introducing synonymous mutations to increase the abundance of codons that were under-represented in the natural coding sequences (10). Fan and colleagues used a different approach, as they changed the CB of a seasonal human H1N1 virus to an avian-like IAV CB (9). To do so, the authors first determined the segment specific CBs of the human H1N1 strain and the corresponding avian IAV sequences. This allowed to

determine the number of mutations that had to be introduced into the human H1N1 ORFs to change its CB to an avian IAV-like CB. Mutations were randomly distributed in the targeted ORF at sites that were highly conserved at the amino acid sequence level to reduce the possibility of introducing mutations into potential mutational hot spots, or disrupting potential critical RNA signals. The free energy of the resulting RNAs and the dinucleotide usage frequency were unchanged by these modifications.

CPD (**Figure 1B**) was done using a computer algorithm to enrich a given viral coding sequence for codon-pairs under-represented in a core set of human genes (37). First, the CPB of an ORF is defined by a codon pair score (CPS). This CPS is defined as the natural log of the ratio of the observed over the expected number of occurrences of each codon pair. The expected number of each codon pair was calculated so that it is independent both of the amino acid frequency and the codon bias (33). The CPB for an ORF was then determined as the arithmetic mean of all CPS. The CPD algorithm of Coleman and colleagues (37) shuffles the existing codons of an ORF to generate under represented codon pairs, while preserving the codon bias and the free energy of the folding of the recoded RNA.

The increase of the CpG and UpA content of IAV NP gene (**Figure 1C**) (14) was completed using the computer algorithm "Sequence Mutate" in the SSE package (43) while maintaining the mononucleotide composition through the introduction of compensatory substitutions elsewhere in the sequence. The CPB was not modified by this process.

Finally, Moratorio and colleagues introduced synonymous mutations that allow single-nt mutations yielding nonsense codons into the HA or PA gene of the 2009 pandemic H1N1 virus only in codons coding for two amino acids with the highest codon redundancy (Leu and Ser) to limit the overall change in nucleotide sequence to <5%. These Leu and Ser mutations did not affect the CB, CPB, CpG content or dinucleotide frequency (**Figure 1D**) (15).

In every case, the deoptimized sequences were synthetized *de novo* and cloned into plasmids that were used to rescue the deoptimized virus of interest by reverse genetics. The rescued viruses were then evaluated phenotypically *in vitro* and *in vivo.*

## SYNONYMOUS GENOME RECODING OF IAV

### Codon Deoptimization (CD)

CD was applied to the seasonal human H1N1 by converting its codon usage so that it was similar to that observed in avian influenza virus, in order to attenuate the virus for humans without reducing yield in embryonated chicken eggs, the substrate for vaccine production (9). All eight segments were codon-deoptimized alone or in combination. This attenuated the virus in mammalian cells and in mice, whereas replication in embryonated eggs remained comparable to wt. Surprisingly, CD did not affect protein expression (9), illustrating that its effects can be different than predicted.

CD also was applied to the laboratory-passaged H1N1 PR8 strain, involving only the NS gene (10). CD did not affect NS mRNA transcription in MDCK cells but, as expected, did reduce NS protein expression in MDCK and human airway A549 cells, and virus replication was reduced in A549 cells. The CD PR8 virus was attenuated in mice. Both the CD seasonal human H1N1 and the CD PR8 IAV retained their immunogenicity despite attenuation and conferred homologous and heterologous protection against IAV challenge in mice (9, 10).

## Codon-Pair Deoptimization (CPD)

The NP, HA, NA, and PB1 segments of the laboratory-passaged PR8 H1N1 strain were subjected to CPD alone or in several combinations (11, 12). PR8 that contained CPD NP, HA, NA, and PB1 alone or in various combinations replicated to about 10-fold lower titers than wt PR8 on MDCK cells. However, the replication of the PR8/CPD-HA-NA virus in human A549 cells was 1,000-fold lower than wt. As expected, translation of the CPD genes was reduced compared to other genes from the same virus (11). Surprisingly, in case of the CPD NA mRNA, transcription was also reduced, with the underlying mechanism being unclear (12).

Despite overall robust replication *in vitro*, PR8 viruses with various combinations of CPD NP, HA, PB1 genes were attenuated in mice, and the attenuation increased with increasing number of CPD genome segments (11). In mice, the PR8/CPD-NP-HA-PB1virus did not induce any disease symptoms or weight loss and was 3,000-fold reduced for replication compared to wt. In addition, it was a more potent inducer of IAV-specific antibodies than wt, and replication of challenge virus was below the level of detection in 80% of the mice (11). The virus PR8/CPD-HA-NA also was attenuated *in vivo*, replicating to 100- to 1,000-fold lower titers than wt in the lungs of mice, with the NA gene being the major contributor of attenuation (12). This virus also induced a strong antibody response that was equivalent to wt, and it efficiently protected against lethal challenge, with protection being durable for at least 7 months (12).

Since CPD of the HA and NA genes was so highly attenuating for the PR8 virus, the HA, and NA genes of the 2009 pandemic (p)H1N1 strain similarly were subjected to CPD in combination (13). The resulting virus had a reduced rate of replication in MDCK cells, but final titers were similar to those of its pH1N1 parent (13). In ferrets, the CPD-HA-NA virus was non-pathogenic. However, no significant difference in virus titers in the lung at day 3 pi was observed between this virus and its pH1N1 parent, suggesting that additional genes will need to be subjected to CPD to obtain additional attenuation (13). Thus, there can be strain-to-strain variability in the attenuation achieved by CPD.

## Increasing the CpG and UpA Content

Segment 5 (encoding NP) of IAV PR8 was recoded to increase the content of CpG or UpA RNA (14). Replication of the two resulting viruses (CpG-high or UpA-high) was delayed compared to wt in MDCK cells, with final titers that were about 10-fold reduced. Plaque size and infectivity were also reduced. The viruses replicated to 10-fold lower titers than their wt parent in mice, but cytokine production, CD4+, CD8+-T cell and antibody responses were comparable to those induced by wt virus, and the mutants were fully protective against wt challenge.

This suggested that CpG- and UpA-high IAV viruses may induce innate and adaptive immune responses disproportionate to their replication phenotypes (14).

## Synonymous Serine and Leucine Codon Substitutions That Allow Single-nt Mutations Yielding Nonsense Codons

Moratorio and colleagues recoded either the HA or PA gene of the 2009 pandemic H1N1 virus to replace serine and leucine codons with synonymous codons for which a number of single-nt substitutions could yield nonsense mutations (15). There was no effect of the recoding on virus replication in MDCK cells. However, both viruses exhibited an increase in nonsense mutations in the mutated genes compared to wt, that significantly reduced viral fitness. In addition, virus replication was reduced 10- to 100-fold in mice. Despite reduced replication, the antibody response was comparable to wt and these viruses induced complete protection against wt virus. The apparent greater immunogenicity per PFU was suggested to be due to immune stimulation by truncated proteins and by adjuvant effects of defective viruses (15). Thus, reducing the evolutionary potential of a virus provides a novel attenuation strategy.

## SYNONYMOUS GENOME RECODING OF RSV

### Codon-Deoptimization (CD)

CD was performed for the ORFs encoding the RSV interferon antagonist non-structural proteins 1 (NS1) and 2 (NS2) (16, 17, 44, 45) and the gene encoding the attachment glycoprotein G (17). As a result of CD, the level of NS1 and NS2 protein was reduced in Vero, BEAS-2B, and Hep-2 cells (16, 44) and the expression of G was reduced in Vero cells (17). CD of NS1 and NS2 did not affect virus replication in Hep-2 and Vero cells, but significantly reduced virus replication in the interferon competent bronchial airway BEAS-2B cells, as well as in differentiated normal human bronchial epithelium (NHBE) cells grown at the air-liquid interface (ALI) (16). The addition of the CD G further reduced virus replication on NHBE/ALI cells, probably due to the role of G in attachment to primary cells (17). Interestingly, while infection of human 293 cells with wt RSV induced a 50% reduction of STAT2 expression, RSV/CD-NS1-NS2 had no effect on STAT2 levels, indicating that this virus had lost the ability to inhibit this aspect of innate immunity. Compared to wt RSV-infected cells, NF-kB activation was reduced in RSV/CD-NS1-NS2- infected cells. The reduced activation of NF-kB by this virus may increase cell apoptosis thus contributing to the attenuated phenotype of this virus (16).

RSV/CD-NS1-NS2 and RSV/CD-NS1-NS2-G replicated to 10-fold lower titers in the lungs of mice compared to wt, but induced significantly higher level of antibodies, and animals were protected against challenge (16). The RSV/CD-NS1-NS2-G virus also was strongly attenuated in the upper and lower respiratory tract of cotton rats, but still induced high levels of antibodies and the vaccinated animals were completely protected against wt challenge (17).

## Codon-Pair Deoptimization (CPD)

Our group studied the effect of genome-scale CPD of RSV (18, 46). Four CPD RSV strains were designed in which one (L), two (G and F), six (NS1, NS2, N, P, M, and SH), and nine (all except M2-1 and M2-2) ORFs were subjected to CPD. All four CPD RSVs were temperature sensitive, which is a novel and unexplained effect, but as one possibility might indicate deficiencies in protein folding resulting from altered translation of CPD ORFs. The viruses grew less efficiently than wt *in vitro* and had reduced mRNA and protein synthesis. CPD of the surface glycoproteins G and F resulted in the strongest reduction in virus replication. The CPD RSVs exhibited a level of attenuation in mice and African Green monkeys comparable with that of two attenuated RSV strains presently in clinical trials (18).

The RSV bearing nine CPD ORFs was phenotypically and genetically stable when subjected to serial passage *in vitro* at progressively increasing temperature. Serial passage at increasing temperature of the RSV bearing the CPD L ORF (Min L) induced a partial loss of temperature-sensitivity and the acquisition of a broad array of mutations that were predominantly missense. Surprisingly, many of the mutations involved ORFs other than L, suggestive of changes affecting protein interactions to compensate for the reduced quantity of L protein. Unexpectedly, each of two compensatory missense mutations in the M2-1 protein had a major effect on restoring viral fitness, which differs from the expectation that individual mutations would have modest effects on viral fitness. The introduction of several of the compensatory mutations identified in the passaged viruses into Min L resulted in increased genetic stability, and the resulting virus was strongly attenuated *in vivo* but was comparable to wt RSV in immunogenicity and protective efficacy, yielding an improved vaccine candidate (46).

## BENEFITS, POTENTIAL LIMITS, AND FUTURE OF SYNONYMOUS GENOME RECODING

Genome scale deoptimization of RNA viruses resulted in the generation of vaccine candidates that in most cases were attenuated *in vitro,* and always attenuated in animal models. While this approach has many advantages that have been described above, the underlying mechanism and resultant effects of the deoptimization still need to be further explored.

Firstly, the extent of deoptimization tolerated by viruses differs widely from virus to virus. For example, while extensive CPD of RSV (up to 9 out the of 11 ORFs CPD) still readily generates a replicating virus, this is not the case for poliovirus or HIV, where extensive CPD or CD did not yield replicating virus. This renders the effect of deoptimization on viral genes hard to predict and implies that, in each case, phenotypes have to be evaluated experimentally. In addition, CD, CPD, and the increase of the CpG and UpA content in some cases resulted in the decrease of the specific infectivity of the recoded viruses. This effect varied depending of the virus and the genes that had been deoptimized and also has to be carefully evaluated on a case-by-case basis.

Most of the approaches described above share common features. For example, the increase of the CpG content was the intended effect in one approach (14), and an also a side effect of CPD. Translation efficiency is expected to be affected both by CD and CPD. With the exception of poliovirus, different deoptimization approaches have not been directly compared side by side using the same genes or portion of genes of a pathogen. This renders the comparison of the efficiency of the different strategies difficult. For poliovirus, both CD and CPD of the same region of the capsid-encoding ORF generated attenuated viruses (5, 37). Interestingly, while both approaches reduced the specific infectivity of the deoptimized viruses, CD reduced the specific infectivity 10-fold more than CPD, suggesting that CD might have a greater effect on the specific infectivity than CPD, at least for poliovirus.

A direct comparison of deoptimized vaccine candidates to those generated by traditional approaches (e.g., biological viruses attenuated by serial passage, recombinant viruses attenuated by gene or codon deletions or non-synonymous attenuating mutations) is also mostly lacking. Pre-clinical evaluation of CPD RSV vaccine candidates showed that the level of restriction of CPD RSVs in African green monkeys was similar to that of two live-attenuated pediatric RSV vaccine candidates presently in clinical trials in infants and young children (18).

Importantly, despite strong restriction of replication *in vivo*, the deoptimized viruses generally induced a strong immune response in vaccinated animals, usually at the level observed with wt virus. As mentioned above, large amounts of viral mRNAs or double-stranded intermediates are produced during virus replication that could be potentially be recognized by the innate immune sensors. It is tempting to speculate that the increased CpG and UpA content in the recoded viruses results in viral mRNAs and/or double double-stranded intermediates with increased immunogenicity. However, this hypothesis would need to be verified. A comprehensive evaluation of the activation and/or proliferation of immune cells (dendritic cells, CD4+, and CD8+ T cells) following stimulation with these viruses would be helpful to elucidate the basis of this strong immunogenicity. In addition, a comprehensive evaluation of the immune response of non-human primates would be informative. Evaluation of the attenuation and immunogenicity of deoptimized vaccine candidates in phase I studies will provide answers on the usefulness of these approaches. Finally, it would also be of interest to complete the reverse experiment by recoding viruses using the most used codon pairs or by further reducing the CpG and UpA content to investigate the resulting effect on virus replication and immunogenicity in animal models.

Overall, the data available to date encourage the further evaluation of these vaccine candidates in clinical trials. However, a more comprehensive understanding is needed of the mechanisms of attenuation conferred by the different strategies of deoptimization. De-attenuation appears to be rare, suggesting that these viruses are genetically stable (4, 5, 16, 17, 37, 47–51). However, an important limitation is that the de-optimized viruses generally have not been subjected to strong selective pressure that would favor the outgrowth of viruses with de-attenuating mutations. In the study in which strong selective pressure was applied to CPD RSV, the virus containing nine CPD ORFs was stable. However, selective pressure on the virus that contained only the CPD L ORF (Min L) resulted in a number of unexpected findings, including de-attenuating mutations outside the CPD ORF that presumably compensated for the low expression of the CPD genes. Importantly, those mutations were used to make a more stable and more immunogenic vaccine candidate. Thus, further studies will be needed to understand escape mechanisms from the restrictions imposed by CPD.

## CONCLUSION

While genome scale deoptimization of RNA viruses was initiated a decade ago, most of the vaccine candidates generated to date have been evaluated only in animal models.

These synonymous recoding strategies may prove useful for developing novel live-attenuated vaccines, such as for pediatric respiratory RSV vaccines as well as for emerging highly pathogenic viruses.

## AUTHOR CONTRIBUTIONS

All authors listed have made a substantial, direct and intellectual contribution to the work, and approved it for publication.

## ACKNOWLEDGMENTS

This research was supported by the Intramural Research Program of the National Institute of Allergy and Infectious Diseases (NIAID), National Institutes of Health (NIH).

## REFERENCES

1. Abil Z, Xiong X, Zhao H. Synthetic biology for therapeutic applications. *Mol Pharm.* (2015) 12:322–31. doi: 10.1021/mp500392q
2. Burbelo PD, Ching KH, Han BL, Klimavicz CM, Iadarola MJ. Synthetic biology for translational research. *Am J Transl Res.* (2010) 2:381–9.
3. Cello J, Paul AV, Wimmer E. Chemical synthesis of poliovirus cDNA: generation of infectious virus in the absence of natural template. *Science.* (2002) 297:1016–8. doi: 10.1126/science.1072266
4. Burns CC, Shaw J, Campagnoli R, Jorba J, Vincent A, Quay J, et al. Modulation of poliovirus replicative fitness in HeLa cells by deoptimization of synonymous codon usage in the capsid region. *J Virol.* (2006) 80:3259–72. doi: 10.1128/JVI.80.7.3259-3272.2006
5. Mueller S, Papamichail D, Coleman JR, Skiena S, Wimmer E. Reduction of the rate of poliovirus protein synthesis through large-scale codon deoptimization causes attenuation of viral virulence by lowering specific infectivity. *J Virol.* (2006) 80:9687–96. doi: 10.1128/JVI.00738-06
6. Lauring AS, Jones JO, Andino R. Rationalizing the development of live attenuated virus vaccines. *Nat Biotechnol.* (2010) 28:573–9. doi: 10.1038/nbt.1635
7. Hanley KA. The double-edged sword: How evolution can make or break a live-attenuated virus vaccine. *Evolution (NY).* (2011) 4:635–43. doi: 10.1007/s12052-011-0365-y
8. Bull JJ. Evolutionary reversion of live viral vaccines: can genetic engineering subdue it? *Virus Evol.* (2015) 1:vev005. doi: 10.1093/ve/vev005
9. Fan RL, Valkenburg SA, Wong CK, Li OT, Nicholls JM, Rabadan R, et al. Generation of live attenuated influenza virus by using codon usage bias. *J Virol.* (2015) 89:10762–73. doi: 10.1128/JVI.01443-15
10. Nogales A, Baker SF, Ortiz-Riano E, Dewhurst S, Topham DJ, Martinez-Sobrido L. Influenza A virus attenuation by codon deoptimization of the NS gene for vaccine development. *J Virol.* (2014) 88:10525–40. doi: 10.1128/JVI.01565-14
11. Mueller S, Coleman JR, Papamichail D, Ward CB, Nimnual A, Futcher B, et al. Live attenuated influenza virus vaccines by computer-aided rational design. *Nat Biotechnol.* (2010) 28:723–6. doi: 10.1038/nbt.1636
12. Yang C, Skiena S, Futcher B, Mueller S, Wimmer E. Deliberate reduction of hemagglutinin and neuraminidase expression of influenza virus leads to an ultraprotective live vaccine in mice. *Proc Natl Acad Sci USA.* (2013) 110:9481–6. doi: 10.1073/pnas.1307473110
13. Broadbent AJ, Santos CP, Anafu A, Wimmer E, Mueller S, Subbarao K. Evaluation of the attenuation, immunogenicity, and efficacy of a live virus vaccine generated by codon-pair de-optimization of the 2009 pandemic H1N1 influenza virus, in ferrets. *Vaccine.* (2015) 34:563–70. doi: 10.1016/j.vaccine.2015.11.054
14. Gaunt E, Wise HM, Zhang H, Lee LN, Atkinson NJ, Nicol MQ, et al. Elevation of CpG frequencies in influenza A genome attenuates

pathogenicity but enhances host response to infection. *Elife.* (2016) 5:e12735. doi: 10.7554/eLife.12735
15. Moratorio G, Henningsson R, Barbezange C, Carrau L, Borderia AV, Blanc H, et al. Attenuation of RNA viruses by redirecting their evolution in sequence space. *Nat Microbiol.* (2017) 2:17088. doi: 10.1038/nmicrobiol.2017.88
16. Meng J, Lee S, Hotard AL, Moore ML. Refining the balance of attenuation and immunogenicity of respiratory syncytial virus by targeted codon deoptimization of virulence genes. *MBio.* (2014) 5:e01704–14. doi: 10.1128/mBio.01704-14
17. Stobart CC, Rostad CA, Ke Z, Dillard RS, Hampton CM, Strauss JD, et al. A live RSV vaccine with engineered thermostability is immunogenic in cotton rats despite high attenuation. *Nat Commun.* (2016) 7:13916. doi: 10.1038/ncomms13916
18. Le Nouen C, Brock LG, Luongo C, McCarty T, Yang L, Mehedi M, et al. Attenuation of human respiratory syncytial virus by genome-scale codon-pair deoptimization. *Proc Natl Acad Sci USA.* (2014) 111:13169–74. doi: 10.1073/pnas.1411290111
19. Plotkin JB, Kudla G. Synonymous but not the same: the causes and consequences of codon bias. *Nat Rev Genet.* (2011) 12:32–42. doi: 10.1038/nrg2899
20. Goni N, Iriarte A, Comas V, Sonora M, Moreno P, Moratorio G, et al. Pandemic influenza A virus codon usage revisited: biases, adaptation and implications for vaccine strain development. *Virol J.* (2012) 9:263. doi: 10.1186/1743-422X-9-263
21. Wong EH, Smith DK, Rabadan R, Peiris M, Poon LL. Codon usage bias and the evolution of influenza A viruses. codon usage biases of influenza virus. *BMC Evol Biol.* (2010) 10:253. doi: 10.1186/1471-2148-10-253
22. Tuller T, Waldman YY, Kupiec M, Ruppin E. Translation efficiency is determined by both codon bias and folding energy. *Proc Natl Acad Sci USA.* (2010) 107:3645–50. doi: 10.1073/pnas.0909910107
23. Jenkins GM, Holmes EC. The extent of codon usage bias in human RNA viruses and its evolutionary origin. *Virus Res.* (2003) 92:1–7. doi: 10.1016/S0168-1702(02)00309-X
24. Hershberg R, Petrov DA. Selection on codon bias. *Annu Rev Genet.* (2008) 42:287–99. doi: 10.1146/annurev.genet.42.110807.091442
25. Aragones L, Guix S, Ribes E, Bosch A, Pinto RM. Fine-tuning translation kinetics selection as the driving force of codon usage bias in the hepatitis A virus capsid. *PLoS Pathog.* (2010) 6:e1000797. doi: 10.1371/journal.ppat.1000797
26. Ikemura T. Codon usage and tRNA content in unicellular and multicellular organisms. *Mol Biol Evol.* (1985) 2:13–34. doi: 10.1093/oxfordjournals.molbev.a040335
27. Dittmar KA, Goodenbour JM, Pan T. Tissue-specific differences in human transfer RNA expression. *PLoS Genet.* (2006) 2:e221. doi: 10.1371/journal.pgen.0020221

28. Quax TE, Claassens NJ, Soll D, van der Oost J. Codon bias as a means to fine-tune gene expression. *Mol Cell.* (2015) 59:149–61. doi: 10.1016/j.molcel.2015.05.035

29. Kozak M. Pushing the limits of the scanning mechanism for initiation of translation. *Gene.* (2002) 299:1–34. doi: 10.1016/S0378-1119(02)01056-9

30. Shabalina SA, Ogurtsov AY, Spiridonov NA. A periodic pattern of mRNA secondary structure created by the genetic code. *Nucleic Acids Res.* (2006) 34:2428–37. doi: 10.1093/nar/gkl287

31. Gumpper RH, Li W, Luo M. Constraints of Viral RNA synthesis on codon usage of negative-strand RNA virus. *J Virol.* (2019) 93:e01775–18. doi: 10.1128/JVI.01775-18

32. Gustafsson C, Govindarajan S, Minshull J. Codon bias and heterologous protein expression. *Trends Biotechnol.* (2004) 22:346–53. doi: 10.1016/j.tibtech.2004.04.006

33. Gutman GA, Hatfield GW. Nonrandom utilization of codon pairs in *Escherichia coli. Proc Natl Acad Sci USA.* (1989) 86:3699–703. doi: 10.1073/pnas.86.10.3699

34. Gamble CE, Brule CE, Dean KM, Fields S, Grayhack EJ. Adjacent codons act in concert to modulate translation efficiency in yeast. *Cell.* (2016) 166:679–90. doi: 10.1016/j.cell.2016.05.070

35. Buchan JR, Aucott LS, Stansfield I. tRNA properties help shape codon pair preferences in open reading frames. *Nucleic Acids Res.* (2006) 34:1015–27. doi: 10.1093/nar/gkj488

36. Kunec D, Osterrieder N. Codon pair bias is a direct consequence of dinucleotide bias. *Cell Rep.* (2015) 14:55–67. doi: 10.1016/j.celrep.2015.12.011

37. Coleman JR, Papamichail D, Skiena S, Futcher B, Wimmer E, Mueller S. Virus attenuation by genome-scale changes in codon pair bias. *Science.* (2008) 320:1784–7. doi: 10.1126/science.1155761

38. Tulloch F, Atkinson NJ, Evans DJ, Ryan MD, Simmonds P. RNA virus attenuation by codon pair deoptimisation is an artefact of increases in CpG/UpA dinucleotide frequencies. *Elife.* (2014) 3:e04531. doi: 10.7554/eLife.04531

39. Atkinson NJ, Witteveldt J, Evans DJ, Simmonds P. The influence of CpG and UpA dinucleotide frequencies on RNA virus replication and characterization of the innate cellular pathways underlying virus attenuation and enhanced replication. *Nucleic Acids Res.* (2014) 42:4527–45. doi: 10.1093/nar/gku075

40. Takata MA, Goncalves-Carneiro D, Zang TM, Soll SJ, York A, Blanco-Melo D, Bieniasz PD. CG dinucleotide suppression enables antiviral defence targeting non-self RNA. *Nature.* (2017) 550:124–7. doi: 10.1038/nature24039

41. Krieg AM. CpG motifs in bacterial DNA and their immune effects. *Annu Rev Immunol.* (2002) 20:709–60. doi: 10.1146/annurev.immunol.20.100301.064842

42. Sugiyama T, Gursel M, Takeshita F, Coban C, Conover J, Kaisho T, et al. CpG RNA: identification of novel single-stranded RNA that stimulates human CD14+CD11c+ monocytes. *J Immunol.* (2005) 174:2273–9. doi: 10.4049/jimmunol.174.4.2273

43. Simmonds P. SSE: a nucleotide and amino acid sequence analysis platform. *BMC Res Notes.* (2012) 5:50. doi: 10.1186/1756-0500-5-50

44. Rostad CA, Stobart CC, Gilbert BE, Pickles RJ, Hotard AL, Meng J, et al. A recombinant respiratory syncytial virus vaccine candidate attenuated by a low-fusion F protein is immunogenic and protective against challenge in cotton rats. *J Virol.* (2016) 90:7508–18. doi: 10.1128/JVI.00012-16

45. Rostad CA, Stobart CC, Todd SO, Molina SA, Lee S, Blanco JCG, et al. Enhancing the thermostability and immunogenicity of a respiratory syncytial virus (RSV) live-attenuated vaccine by incorporating unique RSV line19f protein residues. *J Virol.* (2018) 92:e01568–17. doi: 10.1128/JVI.01568-17

46. Le Nouen C, McCarty T, Brown M, Smith ML, Lleras R, Dolan MA, et al. Genetic stability of genome-scale deoptimized RNA virus vaccine candidates under selective pressure. *Proc Natl Acad Sci USA.* (2017) 114:E386–95. doi: 10.1073/pnas.1619242114

47. Bull JJ, Molineux IJ, Wilke CO. Slow fitness recovery in a codon-modified viral genome. *Mol Biol Evol.* (2012) 29:2997–3004. doi: 10.1093/molbev/mss119

48. Nougairede A, De Fabritus L, Aubry F, Gould EA, Holmes EC, de Lamballerie X. Random codon re-encoding induces stable reduction of replicative fitness of Chikungunya virus in primate and mosquito cells. *PLoS Pathog.* (2013) 9:e1003172. doi: 10.1371/journal.ppat.1003172

49. Vabret N, Bailly-Bechet M, Lepelley A, Najburg V, Schwartz O, Verrier B, et all. Large-scale nucleotide optimization of simian immunodeficiency virus reduces its capacity to stimulate type I interferon *in vitro. J Virol.* (2014) 88:4161–72. doi: 10.1128/JVI.03223-13

50. Ni YY, Zhao Z, Opriessnig T, Subramaniam S, Zhou L, Cao D, et al. Computer-aided codon-pairs deoptimization of the major envelope GP5 gene attenuates porcine reproductive and respiratory syndrome virus. *Virology.* (2014) 450–451:132–9. doi: 10.1016/j.virol.2013.12.009

51. Cheng BY, Ortiz-Riano E, Nogales A, de la Torre JC, Martinez-Sobrido L. Development of live-attenuated arenavirus vaccines based on codon deoptimization. *J Virol.* (2015) 89:3523–33. doi: 10.1128/JVI.03401-14

# 14

# Drug Repurposing Approaches for the Treatment of Influenza Viral Infection: Reviving Old Drugs to Fight Against a Long-Lived Enemy

*Andrés Pizzorno, Blandine Padey, Olivier Terrier*[*][†] *and Manuel Rosa-Calatrava*[*][†]

*Virologie et Pathologie Humaine–VirPath Team, Centre International de Recherche en Infectiologie (CIRI), INSERM U1111, CNRS UMR5308, ENS Lyon, Université Claude Bernard Lyon 1, Université de Lyon, Lyon, France*

**\*Correspondence:**
*Olivier Terrier*
*olivier.terrier@univ-lyon1.fr*
*Manuel Rosa-Calatrava*
*manuel.rosa-calatrava@univ-lyon1.fr*

[†]*These authors share co-last authorship*

Influenza viruses still constitute a real public health problem today. To cope with the emergence of new circulating strains, but also the emergence of resistant strains to classic antivirals, it is necessary to develop new antiviral approaches. This review summarizes the state-of-the-art of current antiviral options against influenza infection, with a particular focus on the recent advances of anti-influenza drug repurposing strategies and their potential therapeutic, regulatory and economic benefits. The review will illustrate the multiple ways to reposition molecules for the treatment of influenza, from adventitious discovery to *in silico*-based screening. These novel antiviral molecules, many of which targeting the host cell, in combination with conventional antiviral agents targeting the virus, will ideally enter the clinics and reinforce the therapeutic arsenal to combat influenza virus infections.

**Keywords: influenza virus, antivirals, antiviral resistance, drug repurposing, drug repositioning, drug discovery, drug combination, transcriptional profiling**

## INFLUENZA VIRUSES, A LONG-LIVED THREAT FOR POPULATIONS

*"A piece of bad news wrapped up in a protein,"* definition of a virus by Sir Peter Medawar.

Despite its apparent blandness for the collective mindset of an important portion of the society, the intrinsic morbidity and mortality as well as the related deaths because of bacterial superinfections or exacerbation of chronic illnesses, make of influenza infections a major and recurrent global public health concern. Indeed, human influenza type A and B viruses are responsible for annual flu epidemics marked by up to 1 billion infections, 3–5 million severe cases and 300,000–650,000 deaths worldwide, with an huge economic burden in terms of medical visits, hospitalizations, work/school absenteeism. and productivity loss (1–3). As members of the *Orthomyxoviridae* family, influenza viruses (type A, B, C, or D) are enveloped viruses harboring a negative-sense single-stranded RNA segmented genome. In such segmented nature of the viral genome resides the capacity of influenza viruses to form new reassortant strains following the concomitant infection of a host with more than one strain of human, and/or animal origin, a phenomenon so far observed only among type A influenza viruses [reviewed in (4)]. Owing to viral reassortment, the genetic baggage of progeny viruses does not exactly match that of one of the "parental" strains but a combination of both. Depending on the specific combination of genetic segments, and notably in the case of a human influenza strain acquiring the Hemagglutinin (HA) and/or Neuraminidase

(NA) major surface antigens from animal origin, reassortment events can result in an *antigenic shift*, defined as the generation of a new virus with antigenic properties drastically different from those of the circulating strains. Should this new variant be sufficiently antigenically different to escape the repertoire of pre-existing immunity in the population, it might rapidly disseminate and replace the circulating strains, hence triggering a global influenza pandemic. Although relatively rare–three veritable pandemics occurred during the 20th Century and one so far in the twenty-first century–the outbreak of pandemics is a quite unpredictable event that might entail potentially devastating effects [reviewed in (5)], particularly considering the contemporary state of affairs regarding global transportation and trade, migration, and the narrowing interface between rural and overcrowded urban areas.

Influenza vaccination constitutes the most effective strategy to prevent seasonal flu and its clinical complications, mainly among high-risk populations such as very young children, the elderly, pregnant women, immunocompromised patients as well as people with obesity, diabetes, or cardiorespiratory comorbidities (6, 7). Nevertheless, current flu vaccination still presents several limitations that make it fall short of expectations in terms of effectiveness. The short duration of vaccine-induced immunity coupled with the intrinsic *antigenic drift* of influenza viruses resulting from the gradual accumulation of point mutations in the antigenic sites of the HA (and to a lesser extent the NA) surface protein underscore the need of the annual reformulation of vaccine composition. Moreover, the length of the current vaccine manufacturing process (at least 6 months to produce sufficiently large vaccine quantities) demands continual strain selection to be done approximately 8 months before the next flu season (6, 8). Should an antigenic drift occur during this time window, the possibility of a mismatch between the vaccine composition and circulating strains might negatively affect protection. Even in the absence of seasonal mismatches or the emergence of pandemic strains, insufficient vaccine coverage and suboptimal uptake in specific target groups (i.e., the elderly or the immunocompromised) also compromise vaccine effectiveness. Furthermore, despite the recent progress made in the pursue of the "Holy Grail" of a universal influenza vaccine that can provide broader, long-lasting protection against both matching, and antigenically diverse influenza strains (9, 10), their clinical effectiveness remains to be evaluated, hence highlighting the need of complementary therapeutic approaches to manage influenza infections.

Besides vaccination, antiviral drugs represent the other pillar for the control of seasonal influenza epidemics and play a central role as major prophylactic and therapeutic agents in the event of a pandemic outbreak. In that regard, this review summarizes the state-of-the-art of current antiviral options against influenza infection, with a particular focus on the recent advances of anti-influenza drug repurposing strategies and their potential therapeutic, regulatory and economic benefits. This review presents examples of the multiple ways to reposition molecules for the treatment of influenza, from adventitious discovery to *in silico*-based screening. These novel antiviral candidates, many of which target the host cell, could also be used in combination with conventional virus-targeted antiviral agents in order to reinforce our very limited therapeutic arsenal against influenza virus infections.

## CURRENT ANTIVIRAL OPTIONS FOR TREATING INFLUENZA INFECTIONS

As mentioned above, antivirals are key players in pandemic preparedness programs, being the first choice for the treatment of infected patients as well as for preventive post-exposure prophylaxis of those potentially exposed to the new virus, especially during the initial pandemic period in which no vaccine is available. Antivirals are as well important in the normal seasonal setting. Although their use is mostly focused on the treatment of severely ill patients and the immunocompromised, some countries, including the USA and Japan, regularly resort to antivirals for the management of uncomplicated influenza in otherwise healthy patients (11, 12). To date, only two classes of antiviral agents are globally approved and available for the treatment of influenza infections: M2 ion-channel blockers and neuraminidase (NA) inhibitors. The first class includes adamantane derivatives, amantadine and rimantadine, which inhibit proton conductivity of the M2 ion channel of influenza A viruses hence preventing the viral uncoating step of the viral replication cycle. Nevertheless, although quite efficient in their early days, widespread dissemination of the S31N (and to a much lesser extent V27A) M2 resistance mutation in post-2006 H3N2 and post-2009 H1N1 circulating strains prompted the WHO to remove both amantadine and rimantadine from the list of recommended anti-influenza agents for clinical use, in 2009 (6). As a result, NA inhibitors stand as the only influenza antivirals currently recommended by the WHO (13).

NA inhibitors are competitive analogs of sialic acid, the preferred influenza receptor on the host cell's surface. By binding to the broadly conserved active site of the NA, NA inhibitors interfere with the sialidase enzymatic activity of the viral protein, which is essential for the release of newly formed progeny viruses from the infected cell, hence preventing the spread of infection to the rest of the respiratory tissue (14). Three NA inhibitors are currently licensed worldwide for the treatment of influenza A and B infections: oseltamivir, zanamivir, and peramivir. Oral oseltamivir (administered as its prodrug oseltamivir phosphate) is the most largely used of the three, whereas inhaled zanamivir is not recommended for very young children nor for individuals with underlying respiratory conditions, and intravenous peramivir is prioritized in hospitalized patients that cannot receive oral treatment (15). Additionally, inhaled laninamivir, a single-dose long lasting NA inhibitor, is approved in Japan for the prevention and treatment of influenza A and B in both adult and pediatric patients (16). It is important to note that some degree of skepticism is still present regarding the real efficacy of NA inhibitors, notably following the 2014's Cochrane clinical meta-analysis that reported only a minimal shortening of influenza symptoms in children and adults with uncomplicated influenza but not in hospitalized patients (17). Nevertheless, actual evidence-based consensus points to a moderate efficacy of NA inhibitor treatment in reducing symptom duration, pneumonia, hospitalization and mortality, especially when administered within 48 h from symptom onset (18, 19). Conversely, delayed treatment initiation is associated with compromised efficacy but may yet be beneficial in at-risk patients. Moreover, the emergence of NA inhibitor-resistant virus variants is a matter of concern, with particularly higher frequencies among children and the immunocompromised (20). The H275Y NA substitution is the main mutation responsible for both oseltamivir and peramivir resistance in H1N1 viruses while R292K and E119V are the most commonly reported in H3N2 viruses, these latter two also conferring reduced susceptibility to zanamivir and laninamivir (17, 21). Even if nowadays the prevalence of drug-resistance in circulating strains is quite low (≤1%), evidence form pre-2009 seasonal strains has proved that, given the appropriate conditions, resistance could rapidly disseminate to attain a prevalence of 90–100% (17, 21). In that regard, the relatively recent detection of localized clusters of NA inhibitor-resistant H1N1pdm09 viruses harboring the H274Y mutation combined or not with I222R/V NA substitutions (22, 23) strengthens the importance of continuous surveillance.

In addition to M2 ion channel blockers and NA inhibitors, two small molecules that target the viral RNA-dependent RNA polymerase, favipiravir and baloxavir marboxil, are undergoing clinical evaluation in the US and Europe but already obtained approval by Japanese Health authorities. Favipiravir is a nucleoside analog that acts as a competitive inhibitor of viral polymerase substrate, approved since 2014 for the treatment of influenza infections with newly emerging strains and/or resistant to other antiviral agents. However, despite the apparent high threshold for drug resistance (24) and broad-spectrum antiviral potential notably validated in the context of recent Ebola virus outbreaks (25), recent results of Phase II/III randomized trials on its therapeutic efficacy against uncomplicated influenza were not completely conclusive (26). Baloxavir marboxil is a selective inhibitor of the cap-dependent endonuclease activity of the influenza viral PA polymerase subunit (27), therefore interfering with the cap-snatching activity of the viral polymerase complex. In that regard, a very recent report disclosed for the first time the results of two randomized (Phases II and III) clinical trials evaluating the efficacy of a single-dose oral treatment with baloxavir marboxil in otherwise healthy outpatients with acute uncomplicated influenza, compared with placebo and a regular 5-day treatment with oseltamivir (28). Overall, baloxavir marboxil and oseltamivir moderately reduced the time to symptom alleviation compared to placebo, while the former outperformed the two others in reducing viral loads. These results prompted the US Food and Drug Administration (FDA) to approve Xofluza® (baloxavir marboxil) for the treatment of acute uncomplicated influenza in patients 12 years of age and older who have been symptomatic for no more than 48 h (29). Nevertheless, this first antiviral flu treatment with a novel mechanism of action approved by the FDA in nearly 20 years does not seem to escape the problem of all other virus-targeted anti-influenza agents. The emergence of virus variants (mostly due to the I38T/M PA amino acid substitutions) conferring significant levels of reduced susceptibility to baloxavir marboxil

was observed in up to 9.7% of the patients receiving the drug (28, 30).

Overall, **Table 1** summarizes the main characteristics of the abovementioned currently available antiviral options for influenza. Such limited therapeutic arsenal coupled with the recurrent risk of emerging drug-resistance highlights the obvious unmet need of novel approaches to complement existing therapies with new anti-influenza drugs.

## WHAT IS DRUG REPURPOSING?

*"The most fruitful basis for the discovery of a new drug is to start with an old drug,"* famously stated the 1998 Nobel Prize in Physiology and Medicine Laureate, Sir James Black.

Despite the enormous scientific and technological advances that the field of biomedical research has witnessed in the last 20–30 years, this scenario failed to efficiently translate into significant improvement on the success rate of the classic "from the bench to the bedside" target-centered, mechanistically biased *de novo* drug discovery process (38). Indeed, with an almost unchanged total number of 25–30 novel molecules out of the approximately 50 new drugs yearly approved by the FDA (39), biopharmaceutical experts estimate that only 12% of drug candidates that make it into Phase I clinical trials receive the final green light (40). In other words, of 5,000–10,000 compounds that come from classic drug discovery, only one is likely to be approved. The causes of this phenomenon are multifactorial, including the targeting of more intricate diseases, limitations of reductionist experimental models to reproduce biological complexity, increased regulatory stringency, tolerability issues, and unexpected side effects. Altogether, the total R&D process leading to the introduction of a new drug in the market demands on average 13–15 years and between U$S 1.5 and 2.6 billion (40–42).

In this context, drug repurposing stands as a worthwhile attractive alternative to fill part of this so-called innovation gap. Drug repurposing, also termed drug repositioning, defines the process of identifying and validating a new therapeutic indication for an existing or developmental drug (38, 42, 43). The basis of drug repurposing relies on bypassing long, risky and expensive preclinical and early clinical evaluation stages by focusing on available extensive human clinical, pharmacokinetics and safety data as the starting point for further development (**Figure 1**). An extended definition could also include not only already marketed drugs but also "sleeping" candidates that have seen their development abandoned in advanced phases of clinical evaluation (e.g., Phase II/III trials) due to non-satisfactory efficacy for their first intended medical use, which might find a second life in a novel therapeutic indication Noteworthy, repurposing arguably accounts for 30% of the new drug products approved by the FDA (44).

In practice, the concept of drug repurposing represents a broad term encompassing many different, though not mutually exclusive, experimental approaches to recognize potential new applications outside the scope of the original medical indication (42), including:

**TABLE 1 |** Currently approved drugs for the treatment of influenza viral infections.

| International non-proprietary name | Pharmaceutical brand names (examples) | Antiviral class | Antiviral activity | Clinical indication | Resistance reported | Discovery/ Reference |
|---|---|---|---|---|---|---|
| Amantadine hydrochloride | Mantadix Symmetrel Symadine Osmolex ER | M2 ion-channel blockers | Blocks influenza virus uncoating and entry into host cell | High risk old adults and children Prophylaxis Or treatment 24/48 post symptoms appearance | YES | 1963 (31) |
| Rimantadine hydrochloride | Roflual Flumandine | | | | | 1969 (32) |
| Oseltamivir phosphate | Tamiflu | NA inhibitors | Sialic acid structural analog, competitive inhibitor of the influenza viral neuraminidase substrate | Children, adolescent and adults 48 h from symptom onset | YES | 1998 (33) |
| Zanamivir | Relenza | | | Children and adults ≥5 years (prophylaxis) ≥7 years (treatment) 48 h from symptom onset | | 1993 (34) |
| Peramivir | Rapivab Peramiflu Rapiacta | | | Children, adolescent and adults intravenous peramivir is prioritized in hospitalized patients that cannot receive oral treatment 48 h from symptom onset | | 2000 (35) |
| Laninamivir octanoate | Inavir | | | Children and adults inhaled laninamivir Prevention adults and pediatric patients | | 2000 (36) |
| Favipiravir | Avigan | Polymerase inhibitor | Nucleoside analog, competitive inhibitor of viral RNA-dependent RNA polymerase substrate | Limited to cases in which other influenza antiviral drugs are ineffective or not sufficiently effective | YES | 2002 (37) |
| Baloxavir marboxil | Xofluza | | Selective inhibitor of the cap-dependent endonuclease activity of the influenza viral PA polymerase subunit | Treatment of acute uncomplicated influenza in patients 12 years of age and older who have been symptomatic for no more than 48 h | | 2018 (27) |

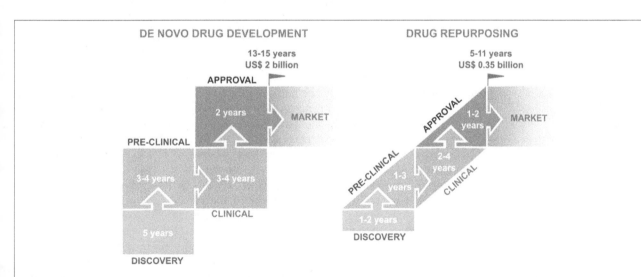

**FIGURE 1 |** From the bench to the bedside: comparison between *de novo* drug development and drug repurposing. *De novo* (classic) drug development constitutes a time-consuming and expensive process. From initial discovery to market, it generally takes 13–15 years and costs up to US$ 2 billion, with a very low success rate (10%). In contrast, drug repurposing approaches offer several advantages. Indeed, the time frame from discovery to market is shorter (5–11 years), less expensive (US$ 350 million), and with a higher success rate (30%), mostly because a large part of preclinical and clinical testings (e.g., safety, formulation, posology) have been already performed for the drug's initial therapeutic indication (41, 42).

## Serendipitous Observations

Some of the best-known success stories of drug repurposing have their starting point on serendipitous observations recorded in the context of either preclinical models of disease or pre-/post-approval clinical trials, leading to a subsequent rationalized evaluation and validation of the new treatment potential (41). Thalidomide and sildenafil are two examples of such key observations. The first one was initially introduced as an anti-nausea for pregnant women but had to be rapidly removed from the market due to its teratogenicity. Further research enabled this molecule as well as some derivatives to be repurposed for the treatment of leprosy and multiple myeloma (45). Sildenafil, on the other hand, never reached the market for its originally intended use in the treatment of hypertension but the observed side-effects on erectile dysfunction ended in its approval in under the commercial name of Viagra®. More recently, sildenafil found a third life under the commercial brand of Revatio® for the treatment of pulmonary hypertension (46).

## Target-Based Repurposing

Although serendipitous observation has historically proved its usefulness, the intrinsic necessity of the casual observation of an unintended and usually infrequent second benefit poses a significant hurdle for exploiting the full potential of drug repurposing, for which more controlled, systematic methodologies are needed. Target-based repurposing relies on having previous knowledge of the specific molecular or cellular determinant/function target recognized by the drug intended to be repurposed. If new research finds out that target is plays an important role in a condition or disease other than the original indication, there is a potential for repurposing. Of note, the target might but not necessarily has to play the same role in both conditions. For example, in the case of the previously mentioned favipiravir, the drug plays the same role as viral RNA polymerase inhibitor against both influenza and Ebola viruses. On the other hand, the Abelson tyrosine-protein kinase 2 (Abl2), target of the anticancer drug imatinib, has been found to be required for efficient fusion and release of severe acute respiratory syndrome coronavirus (SARS-CoV) and Middle East respiratory syndrome coronavirus (MERS-CoV) pseudovirions into the cytoplasm of the infected cell, a key step for viral replication (47).

An alternative scenario of target-based repurposing can happen when a particular drug of known mechanism of action is found to have a new molecular/cellular target, and this previously unrecognized second target is associated with a different disease. The molecule is therefore said to present *polypharmacology*-related features, meaning the capacity to act on multiple targets (48, 49). Polypharmacological phenomena includes both a single drug acting on multiple targets of a unique disease pathway, or a single drug acting on multiple targets pertaining to multiple disease pathways (50). In fact, polypharmacology is usually responsible for treatment toxicity or other undesirable adverse events, but some of these "side-effects" might also lead to drug repurposing, as further exemplified in the next sections. During the last decade, an increasing number of studies converged on proposing that many drugs, initially designed for a unique therapeutics target, are in fact expected to hit on average between 6 and 13 different targets (51, 52).

## Phenotypic Screening

One major limitation of the target-based drug repurposing model relies on its dependence on the existing scientific knowledge of the drug/disease mechanism(s) of action/pathology as well as on potential alternative targets, which is usually incomplete. In other words, we cannot fully anticipate the repurposing potential of a drug unless we have characterized its molecular/cellular target(s), or if we do not know that a given drug target plays an important role on a particular disease. Phenotypic screening of bioactive molecule libraries in different experimental cell-based or *in vivo* disease models without the need of *a priori* knowledge or consideration of the target and/or mechanism of action the candidate was designed to modulate can provide valuable contribution to overcome this constraint (53). Indeed, despite this approach has been questioned due to the fact that the expected altered phenotype readout as a surrogate of an exploitable biological effect induced by the drug candidate might account for an important number of false positive "hits," it is nonetheless true that the contribution of high-throughput phenotypic screening to first-in-class small molecule drug discovery exceeded that of target-based approaches (54, 55). In that regard, many well-annotated collections of small-molecule libraries could be readily made available through different collaborative and/or commercial partnerships in order to accelerate drug repurposing through hypothesis biased or unbiased phenotypic screening [reviewed in (54–57)].

## *In silico*-Assisted Repurposing

With the advent of big data and systems biology, computer-based approaches are gaining increasing acceptance in the field of drug discovery, and drug repurposing is not an exception. Besides the inclusion of constantly emerging "omics" (e.g., transcriptomic, proteomic, metabolomic) data to expand our current knowledge of drug/disease-associated mechanisms, *in silico* data mining and modeling tools have pushed our capacity to analyze data to the next level (58–60). These *in silico* methods include the screening of chemical, biological, and text databases, analysis of quantitative structure-activity relationships, pharmacophores, homology models, and other molecular modeling approaches as well as network analysis of biological functions, machine learning and almost any other analysis tools that include using a computer (61–64). In that regard, proper mining of biological, chemical and clinical datasets, has proved effective in unveiling novel relationships (65, 66). Moreover, another level of complexity can be added by combining, for example, epidemiologic information obtained in-house and/or from publicly available literature databases with *in vitro* experimental molecule screenings with the aim to identify novel indications, as in the case of digoxin and prostate cancer (67, 68). Indeed, the real power of computer-assisted drug repurposing resides on adopting an integrative strategy that combines the predictive and analytic capacity of *in silico* tools with some of the target biased or unbiased experimental evaluation/validation methods previously mentioned. This "systems pharmacology" approach

(69–71) across the boundaries of traditional disciplines would put researchers in a better-informed position to design more comprehensive repurposing strategies with more effective predictive capacity and, hopefully, improved candidate success rates.

## THE EMERGENCE OF DRUG REPURPOSING APPROACHES IN THE FIELD OF ANTIVIRAL DRUG DISCOVERY

These last 10 years, there has been a remarkable growing interest for drug repurposing in the field of antiviral drug discovery, fueled by the incontestable reality of many known viral infections still lacking specific treatment. This interest is inversely correlated with the very low number of classic antiviral molecules that have been market-approved these last 5 years, mostly for the treatment of hepatitis C virus or HIV-related pathologies (72). The best example of antiviral drug repurposing approaches are emerging viruses such as Ebola, Zika virus or MERS-CoV, for which there is an urgent and cost-effective need for therapeutics solutions. Indeed, to rapidly propose a solution in the context of a viral outbreak, one interesting approach consists to look at the available pharmacopeia used to treat pathogens. For example, chloroquine, a major antimalarial drug, has been proposed for the treatment of filoviral infections, and more largely for the treatment of other emerging pathogens, as it targets endosomal acidification, a pivotal step in the replication cycle of a large number of viruses (73, 74). Another interesting illustration is the previously cited example of favipiravir, which proved its repurposing potential for the treatment of Zika or Ebola viral infections (25, 43, 75).

## DRUG REPURPOSING FOR INFLUENZA VIRAL INFECTION

As mentioned before, the intrinsic ever-evolving nature of the virus, high transmissibility, host promiscuity, suboptimal vaccine efficacy, limited antiviral arsenal, and zoonotic, and pandemic potential are more than convincing factors to consider influenza viruses as attractive targets for drug repurposing. Despite many interesting omics-based approaches (76) or high-throughput screening of specific drug libraries, such as kinase inhibitors (77), no anti-influenza agent issued from drug repurposing has yet reached regulatory market approval. However, advances made during the last years forecast optimism. The following selected examples constitute a very good illustration of the diversity and capabilities of drug repurposing strategies for influenza infection. An exhaustive list of anti-influenza candidates issued from drug repurposing approaches is presented in **Table 2**.

The case of statins is arguably the best-known example of anti-influenza repurposing issued from clinical observations. In the early 2000s, clinicians observed that besides the cardioprotective activity of statins, these hydroxyl methylglutaryl-coenzyme A (HMG-CoA) reductase inhibitors approved for their use as cholesterol metabolism regulators could have pleiotropic anti-inflammatory and immunomodulatory effects, which could be of

benefit to improve survival of patients with severe influenza (78–80). Although many mouse and observational studies account for the protective role of statins in pneumonia, most *in vivo* studies reported so far failed to clearly demonstrate such a beneficial effect in the specific context of influenza infection (99–102). On the other hand, a few but not all observational studies highlighted an association between statin treatment with up to 41% reduction of 30-day all-cause mortality in patients hospitalized with laboratory-confirmed seasonal influenza (103–105). A randomized placebo-controlled Phase II clinical trial (NCT02056340) aimed at evaluating the potential effect of atorvastatin to reduce the severity of illness in influenza-infected patients is currently undergoing.

Nitazoxanide is another illustration of a serendipitous repurposing approach, and probably one of the most promising examples. Nitazoxanide is a thiazolide anti-infective initially licensed for the treatment of parasitic infections, for which anti-influenza properties were first documented by Rossignol et al. (81). Interestingly, the proposed mode of action of nitazoxanide toward influenza is clearly distinct to that for which it was designed in its initial indication, acting at the post-translational level by selectively blocking the maturation of the viral glycoprotein HA, with a consecutive impact on its intracellular trafficking and insertion into the host plasma membrane (81, 106). This drug presents potent antiviral activity against a large panel of circulating strains (82). The effectiveness of nitazoxanide in treating patients with non-complicated influenza was successful in a Phase IIb/III trial (107) and is currently being assessed in a Phase III clinical trial (NCT01610245).

BAY81-8781/LASAG (D, L-Lysine acetylsalicylate-glycine), a modified version of the anti-inflammatory drug acetylsalicylic acid (ASA) licensed for intravenous and inhalation delivery, is currently investigated as an anti-influenza treatment as a result of a mixed serendipitous and target-based repurposing strategy. It was initially shown that ASA had interesting antiviral effects against influenza viruses *in vitro* and *in vivo* via the inhibition of the NF-kB activating kinase IkkB, which negatively impacts influenza vRNP transport and release of infectious viral particles (108–110). However, due to the pharmacokinetic limitations of ASA, the LASAG modified version with improved stability and tolerability was developed. Like ASA, this molecule also demonstrates antiviral activity against several human and avian influenza viruses *in vitro*. In a mouse infection model, inhalation of LASAG resulted in reduced lung viral titers and protection of mice from lethal infection (85). More recently, a Phase II proof-of-concept study comparing LASAG *versus* placebo in patients with severe influenza (all patients receiving Tamiflu as standard of care treatment) demonstrated that aerosolized LASAG improved the time to symptom alleviation compared to placebo, despite the absence of a statistically significant reduction of viral load in LASAG-treated group (86).

Naproxen constitutes a nice example of *in-silico* & target-based strategy for the identification of new antivirals. Lejal et al. used a structure-based modeling approach to identify drugs of interest directed against the nucleoprotein (NP) of influenza A virus, using the X-ray structure of the RNA-free NP of H1N1 as prototype. An *in-silico* screening, focused of a defined specific

TABLE 2 | Drug repurposing approaches for the treatment of influenza viral infections.

| Name | Initial indication | Initial activity | Repurposing approach | Anti-influenza activity | Status | References |
|---|---|---|---|---|---|---|
| Statins (i.e., Atorvastatin) | Cholesterol modulators | HMG-CoA reductase inhibitor | Serendipity | Immunomodulator | Phase II (NCT02056340) | (78–80) |
| Nitazoxanide | Anti-parasitic Chronic hepatitis | Inhibition of the pyruvate: ferredoxin/flavodoxin oxidoreductase cycle | | HA maturation & transport inhibition | Phase III (NCT03336619) | (81, 82) |
| PPAR antagonists (i.e., Gemfibrozil) | Anti-hyperlipidemic | Hepatic glucogenesis inhibitor | Serendipity & Phenotypic screening | Immunomodulator | Preclinical | (83, 84) |
| LASAG (BAY81-87981) | Anti-inflammatory | NF-kB inhibitor | Serendipity & Target-based | NF-kB inhibition | Phase II (2012-004072-19) | (85, 86) |
| Celecoxib | Anti-inflammatory | COX-2 inhibitor | Target-based | Immunomodulator | Phase III (NCT02108366) | (87, 88) |
| Etanercept | Anti-inflammatory Rheumatoid arthritis | Anti-TNF-α agent | | Immunomodulator | Preclinical | (89) |
| Metformin | Approved Type 2 diabetes drug | Hepatic glucogenesis inhibitor | Phenotypic screening | Immunomodulator Autophagy induction | Preclinical | (78, 83) |
| Gemcitabine | Approved anti-cancer drug | Ribonucleotide reductase inhibitor | | Immunomodulator | Preclinical | (90) |
| Dapivirine | Phase III anti-HIV drug | Reverse transcriptase inhibitor | | vRNP transport inhibition | Preclinical | (91) |
| Trametinib | Approved anti-cancer drug | MEK1/2 inhibitor | | vRNP transport inhibition | Preclinical | (92) |
| Lisinopril | Approved anti-hypertensive drug | peptidyl dipeptidase inhibitor | In-silico assisted, target-based screening | NA inhibitor | Preclinical | (93) |
| Naproxen | Approved NSAID Phase I anticancer | COX-2 inhibitor | | NP-RNA binding inhibitor | Phase II (ISRCTN11273879) | (94) |
| Nalidixic acid | Approved antibiotic | Bacterial DNA replication inhibitor | | NA inhibitor | Preclinical | (95) |
| Dorzolamide | Approved anti-glaucoma drug | Carbonic anhydrase inhibitor | | NA inhibitor | Preclinical | (95) |
| Ruxolitinib | Approved for myelofibrosis treatment | JAK inhibitor | | Virion formation & vRNA incorporation inhibition | Preclinical | (96) |
| Midodrine | Approved anti-hypotensive drug | Adrenergic alpha agonist | In-silico assisted, phenotypic screening | Immunomodulator ? | Phase II (NCT01546506) | (97) |
| Diltiazem | Approved anti-hypertensive drug | Ca2+ channel inhibitor | | Immunomodulator ? | Phase II (NCT03212716) | (98) |

site of NP structure, has identified naproxen, a known inhibitor of inducible cyclooxygenase type 2 (COX-2) commonly used as non-steroidal anti-inflammatory drug. This identified molecule has shown antiviral properties against influenza A virus *in vitro* and *in vivo* (94). More recently, naproxen analogs with improved efficacy have been developed, showing high level of inhibition of both NP-RNA and NP-polymerase subunit PA complexes, without parallel inhibition of COX-2 (111, 112). Interestingly, in contrast to other examples of drug repurposing strategies, the example of naproxen remains virus-targeted and future works will determine if this drug will present the same Achille's heel than classic antivirals regarding selection of antiviral resistance.

The last two examples of this chapter are midodrine and diltiazem, that we identified as influenza antivirals in the context of an *in-silico* assisted strategy based on transcriptional profiling. An emerging approach in drug repurposing is based on signature matching, which consists of comparing a specific characteristic of a drug–its cellular signature–to that of a disease (42). This approach, mostly based on transcriptomic data, was successfully exploited to identify drug repurposing opportunities in a large range of therapeutics areas, and notably in the field of oncology and rare diseases (42). Our group was the first to transpose this approach to the field of viral infectious diseases, thanks to the development and democratization of DNA-microarray and more recently RNAseq techniques. In a proof-of-concept study using an *in vitro* model of infection, we postulated that host global gene expression profiling can be considered as a "fingerprint" or signature of any specific cell state, including during infection or drug treatment, and hypothesized that the screening of databases for compounds that counteract virogenomic signatures could enable rapid identification of effective antivirals (97). Among the molecules identified *in silico*, midodrine, an adrenergic alpha receptor agonist widely used to treat hypotension, demonstrated very interesting *in vitro* antiviral activities (97). These results prompted the Phase II clinical evaluation of midodrine (NCT01546506) for the treatment of uncomplicated seasonal flu in primary care centers.

Based on this previous proof-of-concept obtained from *in vitro* gene expression profiles, we further improved the strategy by analyzing upper respiratory tract clinical samples collected from a cohort of influenza A(H1N1)pdm09-infected patients and determined their respective transcriptomic signatures. We then performed an *in-silico* drug screening and identified a list of candidate bioactive molecules with signatures anti-correlated with those of the patient's acute infection state. The potential antiviral properties of selected market-approved molecules were firstly validated *in vitro*, and the most effective compounds were further compared to oseltamivir for the treatment of influenza A(H1N1)pdm09 virus infections in mice and in a physiological *in vitro* model of reconstituted human airway epithelia (MucilAir™). These results notably highlighted diltiazem, a calcium channel blocker used as an anti-hypertensive drug, as a very promising repurposed host-targeted inhibitor of influenza infection (98). An ongoing French multicenter randomized clinical trial is investigating the effect of diltiazem-oseltamivir bitherapy compared with standard oseltamivir

monotherapy for the treatment of severe influenza infections in intensive care units (FLUNEXT trial NCT03212716).

## VIRUS-TARGETED vs. HOST-TARGETED THERAPY, WHY NOT BOTH?

*"Two are better than one, because they have a good return for their labor"* Ecclesiastes 4:9-10.

The concept of antiviral combination therapy was originally pioneered for antiretroviral treatments, with the primary goal of preventing or at least delaying the emergence of drug resistance via the targeting of multiple steps of the viral cycle (113). Another expected complementary goal is to obtain additive or synergistic effects by combining drugs, a "double-trigger" effect, to increase effectiveness and/or reduce dosage. In the context of influenza infections, the combination of classic antivirals, mostly NA inhibitors, was explored by several research groups, including ours, with relatively mixed conclusions. For example, in a mouse model, the combination of oseltamivir with zanamivir was shown to be not superior to zanamivir monotherapy in the context of influenza A(H3N2) or A(H1N1)pdm09 infection (114). A clinical trial was conducted during the A(H1N1)pdm09 pandemic in 2009-2010 (COMBINA trial NCT00830323) and failed to demonstrate whether oseltamivir/zanamivir combination therapy improved or reduced the effectiveness of oseltamivir alone in the treatment of influenza infections in community patients (115). Other clinical investigations have shown a greater effectiveness of such combination therapy to reduce influenza transmissibility (116).

As most alternative antiviral strategies for the treatment of influenza infections, including those related to drug repurposing and targeting the host instead of viral determinants, an emerging trend consists to propose innovative therapies that combine classic antivirals with host-targeting drugs, which starts to show promising results (87). For example, Belardo et al. have demonstrated, in cell culture-based assays using different human and avian models, that the combination of NA inhibitors and nitazoxanide presents synergistic anti-influenza effects (117). Convincing results were also obtained using a combination treatment including naproxen. In a clinical trial enrolling hospitalized patients infected by influenza A(H3N2), combination therapy with naproxen, oseltamivir, and clarithromycin showed improved efficacy in terms of hospital stay duration and patient mortality, when compared to oseltamivir treatment alone (118). In the context of the evaluation of the antiviral activity of diltiazem in the reconstituted human airway epithelium model MucilAir™, our group demonstrated that the diltiazem-oseltamivir combination treatment conferred a greater reduction of apical viral titers than that was measured with the same-dose monotherapy, with a marked delay of viral production (98). An ongoing French multicenter randomized clinical trial is investigating the effect of diltiazem-oseltamivir bitherapy compared with standard oseltamivir monotherapy for the treatment of severe influenza infections in intensive care units (FLUNEXT trial NCT03212716).

Altogether, these results plead in favor of the use of drug repurposing for the improvement of the current standard of care anti-influenza therapy. In contrast to other technological domains, the innovation is not necessary chasing and replacing the established standard, and future works are still necessary to investigate the real impact of these novel "host & virus-targeted" multi-therapy approaches on the management and control of the emergence of viral resistance.

## CONCLUDING REMARKS

*"We do not need to find new drugs; rather we need to find the patients who can benefit from existing drugs"* the saying goes. Although somehow exaggerated, this statement summarizes pretty clearly the essence behind the drug repurposing initiative. Finding new indications for already-existing drugs has many benefits, mainly by improving cost-effectiveness, reducing risks, and shortening time to market (37, 41). The purpose of this review was to foster discussion on drug repurposing as an option to complete and implement our current anti-influenza therapeutic arsenal. We are facing an important need for the development of novel antiviral strategies that improve treatment effectiveness–especially in the case of severe diseases–and that are less prone to selection for antiviral resistance. In that regard, the identification and validation by different and complementary means of repurposed drugs is incontestably of great interest, notably in combination with current classic virus-targeted inhibitors. In addition, the deposition of data, including negative results, into public database should be encouraged, as it would facilitate efforts to repurpose licensed or orphaned drugs, and consecutively increase our chances to find new efficient antiviral drugs. With a growing number of academic groups and pharmaceutical companies working on this emerging field, we should most certainly see interesting progress and efficient novel anti-influenza therapies reaching regulatory market approval in a near future.

In the context of a globalized world facing major vicissitudes including population dynamics, climate change and the multiple emergence/re-emergence of zoonotic viruses, the effectiveness and reaction force of the classic *de novo* development of antivirals is challenged. Despite inherent limits, drug repurposing offers a very large palette of possibilities to rapidly and efficiently find new antiviral drugs.

## AUTHOR CONTRIBUTIONS

All authors listed have made a substantial, direct and intellectual contribution to the work, and approved it for publication.

## ACKNOWLEDGMENTS

This work was funded by grants from the French Ministry of Social Affairs and Health (DGOS), Institut National de la Santé et de la Recherche Médicale (INSERM), the Université Claude Bernard Lyon 1, the Région Auvergne Rhône-Alpes (CMIRA N° 14007029, and AccueilPro COOPERA N° 15458 grants).

## REFERENCES

1. Influenza (Seasonal). *World Health Organization*. Available online at: http://www.who.int/news-room/fact-sheets/detail/influenza-(seasonal) (Accessed October 28, 2018).
2. Iuliano AD, Roguski KM, Chang HH, Muscatello DJ, Palekar R, Tempia S, et al. Estimates of global seasonal influenza-associated respiratory mortality: a modelling study. *Lancet*. (2018) 391:1285–300. doi: 10.1016/S0140-6736(17)33293-2
3. Pelletier AJ, Mansbach JM, Camargo CA. Direct medical costs of bronchiolitis hospitalizations in the United States. *Pediatrics*. (2006) 118:2418–23. doi: 10.1542/peds.2006-1193
4. Medina RA, García-Sastre A. Influenza A viruses: new research developments. *Nat Rev Microbiol*. (2011) 9:590–603. doi: 10.1038/nrmicro2613
5. Krammer F, Smith GJD, Fouchier RAM, Peiris M, Kedzierska K, Doherty PC, et al. Influenza. *Nat Rev Dis Primers*. (2018) 4:3. doi: 10.1038/s41572-018-0002-y
6. Paules C, Subbarao K. Influenza. *Lancet*. (2017) 390:697–708. doi: 10.1016/S0140-6736(17)30129-0
7. Restivo V, Costantino C, Bono S, Maniglia M, Marchese V, Ventura G, et al. Influenza vaccine effectiveness among high-risk groups: a systematic literature review and meta-analysis of case-control and cohort studies. *Hum Vaccin Immunother*. (2017) 14:724–35. doi: 10.1080/21645515.2017.1321722
8. Buckland BC. The development and manufacture of influenza vaccines. *Hum Vaccin Immunother*. (2015) 11:1357–60. doi: 10.1080/21645515.2015.1026497
9. Paules CI, Marston HD, Eisinger RW, Baltimore D, Fauci AS. The pathway to a universal influenza vaccine. *Immunity*. (2017) 47:599–603. doi: 10.1016/j.immuni.2017.09.007
10. Khurana S. Development and regulation of novel influenza virus vaccines: a United States young scientist perspective. *Vaccines*. (2018) 6:E24. doi: 10.3390/vaccines6020024
11. Nguyen-Van-Tam JS, Venkatesan S, Muthuri SG, Myles PR. Neuraminidase inhibitors: who, when, where? *Clin Microbiol Infect*. (2015) 21:222–5. doi: 10.1016/j.cmi.2014.11.020
12. Sugaya N. Widespread use of neuraminidase inhibitors in Japan. *J Infect Chemother*. (2011) 17:595–601. doi: 10.1007/s10156-011-0288-0
13. WHO. *WHO Guidelines for Pharmacological Management of Pandemic (H1N1) Influenza and Other Influenza Viruses*. WHO (2009). Available online at: http://www.who.int/csr/resources/publications/swineflu/h1n1_use_antivirals_20090820/en/ (Accessed January 24, 2019).
14. Moscona A. Neuraminidase inhibitors for influenza. *N Engl J Med*. (2005) 353:1363–73. doi: 10.1056/NEJMra050740
15. McKimm-Breschkin JL. Influenza neuraminidase inhibitors: antiviral action and mechanisms of resistance. *Influenza Other Respir Viruses*. (2013) 7:25–36. doi: 10.1111/irv.12047
16. Sunagawa S, Higa F, Cash HL, Tateyama M, Uno T, Fujita J. Single-dose inhaled laninamivir: registered in Japan and its potential role in control of influenza epidemics. *Influenza Other Respir Viruses*. (2013) 7:1–3. doi: 10.1111/j.1750-2659.2012.00351.x
17. Jefferson T, Jones MA, Doshi P, Del Mar CB, Hama R, Thompson MJ, et al. Neuraminidase inhibitors for preventing and treating influenza in healthy adults and children. *Cochrane Database Syst Rev*. (2014) CD008965. doi: 10.1002/14651858.CD008965.pub4

18. Dobson J, Whitley RJ, Pocock S, Monto AS. Oseltamivir treatment for influenza in adults: a meta-analysis of randomised controlled trials. *Lancet.* (2015) 385:1729–37. doi: 10.1016/S0140-6736(14)62449-1

19. Venkatesan S, Myles PR, Leonardi-Bee J, Muthuri SG, Al Masri M, Andrews N, et al. Impact of outpatient neuraminidase inhibitor treatment in patients infected with influenza A(H1N1)pdm09 at high risk of hospitalization: an individual participant data metaanalysis. *Clin Infect Dis.* (2017) 64:1328–34. doi: 10.1093/cid/cix127

20. Li TCM, Chan MCW, Lee N. Clinical implications of antiviral resistance in influenza. *Viruses.* (2015) 7:4929–44. doi: 10.3390/v7092850

21. Kamali A, Holodniy M. Influenza treatment and prophylaxis with neuraminidase inhibitors: a review. *Infect Drug Resist.* (2013) 6:187–98. doi: 10.2147/IDR.S36601

22. Takashita E, Meijer A, Lackenby A, Gubareva L, Rebelo-de-Andrade H, Besselaar T, et al. Global update on the susceptibility of human influenza viruses to neuraminidase inhibitors, 2013-2014. *Antiviral Res.* (2015) 117:27–38. doi: 10.1016/j.antiviral.2015.02.003

23. Hurt AC, Hardie K, Wilson NJ, Deng Y-M, Osbourn M, Gehrig N, et al. Community transmission of oseltamivir-resistant A(H1N1)pdm09 influenza. *N Engl J Med.* (2011) 365:2541–2. doi: 10.1056/NEJMc1111078

24. Cheung PPH, Watson SJ, Choy K-T, Fun Sia S, Wong DDY, Poon LLM, et al. Generation and characterization of influenza A viruses with altered polymerase fidelity. *Nat Commun.* (2014) 5:4794. doi: 10.1038/ncomms5794

25. Sissoko D, Laouenan C, Folkesson E, M'Lebing A-B, Beavogui A-H, Baize S, et al. Experimental treatment with favipiravir for ebola virus disease (the JIKI Trial): a historically controlled, single-arm proof-of-concept trial in Guinea. *PLoS Med.* (2016) 13:e1001967. doi: 10.1371/journal.pmed.1001967

26. McKimm-Breschkin JL, Jiang S, Hui DS, Beigel JH, Govorkova EA, Lee N. Prevention and treatment of respiratory viral infections: presentations on antivirals, traditional therapies and host-directed interventions at the 5th ISIRV Antiviral Group conference. *Antiviral Res.* (2018) 149:118–42. doi: 10.1016/j.antiviral.2017.11.013

27. Noshi T, Kitano M, Taniguchi K, Yamamoto A, Omoto S, Baba K, et al. *In vitro* characterization of baloxavir acid, a first-in-class cap-dependent endonuclease inhibitor of the influenza virus polymerase PA subunit. *Antiviral Res.* (2018) 160:109–17. doi: 10.1016/j.antiviral.2018. 10.008

28. Hayden FG, Sugaya N, Hirotsu N, Lee N, de Jong MD, Hurt AC, et al. Baloxavir marboxil for uncomplicated influenza in adults and adolescents. *N Engl J Med.* (2018) 379:913–23. doi: 10.1056/NEJMoa1716197

29. *Roche Announces FDA Approval of Xofluza (baloxavir marboxil) for Influenza.* Available online at: https://www.roche.com/de/media/releases/ med-cor-2018-10-24.htm (Accessed October 28, 2018).

30. Omoto S, Speranzini V, Hashimoto T, Noshi T, Yamaguchi H, Kawai M, et al. Characterization of influenza virus variants induced by treatment with the endonuclease inhibitor baloxavir marboxil. *Sci Rep.* (2018) 8:9633. doi: 10.1038/s41598-018-27890-4

31. Jackson GG, Muldoon RL, Akers LW. Serological evidence for prevention of influenzal infection in volunteers by an anti-influenzal drug adamantanamine hydrochloride. *Antimicrob Agents Chemother.* (1963) 161:703–7.

32. Rabinovich S, Baldini JT, Bannister R. Treatment of influenza. The therapeutic efficacy of rimantadine HCl in a naturally occurring influenza A2 outbreak. *Am J Med Sci.* (1969) 257:328–35.

33. Kim CU, Lew W, Williams MA, Wu H, Zhang L, Chen X, et al. Structure-activity relationship studies of novel carbocyclic influenza neuraminidase inhibitors. *J Med Chem.* (1998) 41:2451–60. doi: 10.1021/jm980162u

34. von Itzstein M, Wu WY, Kok GB, Pegg MS, Dyason JC, Jin B, et al. Rational design of potent sialidase-based inhibitors of influenza virus replication. *Nature.* (1993) 363:418–23. doi: 10.1038/363418a0

35. Babu YS, Chand P, Bantia S, Kotian P, Dehghani A, El-Kattan Y, et al. BCX-1812 (RWJ-270201): discovery of a novel, highly potent, orally active, and selective influenza neuraminidase inhibitor through structure-based drug design. *J Med Chem.* (2000) 43:3482–3486. doi: 10.1021/jm0002679

36. Yamashita M, Tomozawa T, Kakuta M, Tokumitsu A, Nasu H, Kubo S. CS-8958, a prodrug of the new neuraminidase inhibitor R-125489, shows long-acting anti-influenza virus activity. *Antimicrob Agents Chemother.* (2009) 53:186–92. doi: 10.1128/AAC.00333-08

37. Furuta Y, Takahashi K, Fukuda Y, Kuno M, Kamiyama T, Kozaki K, et al. *In vitro* and *in vivo* activities of anti-influenza virus compound T-705. *Antimicrob Agents Chemother.* (2002) 46:977–81. doi: 10.1177/095632020301400502

38. Strittmatter SM. Overcoming drug development bottlenecks with repurposing: old drugs learn new tricks. *Nat Med.* (2014) 20:590–1. doi: 10.1038/nm.3595

39. Drug Innovation. *Novel Drug Approvals for 2018.* (2018) Available online at: https://www.fda.gov/Drugs/DevelopmentApprovalProcess/ DrugInnovation/ucm592464.htm (Accessed October 28, 2018).

40. *Chart Pack: Biopharmaceuticals in Perspective, Summer 2018.* Phrma (2018). Available online at: http://www.phrma.org/report/chart-pack-biopharmaceuticals-in-perspective-summer-2018 (Accessed October 28, 2018).

41. Ashburn TT, Thor KB. Drug repositioning: identifying and developing new uses for existing drugs. *Nat Rev Drug Discov.* (2004) 3:673–83. doi: 10.1038/nrd1468

42. Pushpakom S, Iorio F, Eyers PA, Escott KJ, Hopper S, Wells A, et al. Drug repurposing: progress, challenges and recommendations. *Nat Rev Drug Discov.* (2018). doi: 10.1038/nrd.2018.168. [Epub ahead of print].

43. Devillers J. Repurposing drugs for use against Zika virus infection. *SAR QSAR Environ Res.* (2018) 29:103–15. doi: 10.1080/1062936X.2017.1411642

44. Hernandez JJ, Pryszlak M, Smith L, Yanchus C, Kurji N, Shahani VM, et al. Giving drugs a second chance: overcoming regulatory and financial hurdles in repurposing approved drugs as cancer therapeutics. *Front Oncol.* (2017) 7:273. doi: 10.3389/fonc.2017.00273

45. Rehman W, Arfons LM, Lazarus HM. The rise, fall and subsequent triumph of thalidomide: lessons learned in drug development. *Ther Adv Hematol.* (2011) 2:291–308. doi: 10.1177/2040620711413165

46. Ghofrani HA, Osterloh IH, Grimminger F. Sildenafil: from angina to erectile dysfunction to pulmonary hypertension and beyond. *Nat Rev Drug Discov.* (2006) 5:689–702. doi: 10.1038/nrd2030

47. Coleman CM, Sisk JM, Mingo RM, Nelson EA, White JM, Frieman MB. Abelson kinase inhibitors are potent inhibitors of severe acute respiratory syndrome coronavirus and middle east respiratory syndrome coronavirus fusion. *J Virol.* (2016) 90:8924–33. doi: 10.1128/JVI.01429-16

48. Hopkins AL. Network pharmacology: the next paradigm in drug discovery. *Nat Chem Biol.* (2008) 4:682–90. doi: 10.1038/nchembio.118

49. Hopkins AL. Drug discovery: predicting promiscuity. *Nature.* (2009) 462:167–8. doi: 10.1038/462167a

50. Reddy AS, Zhang S. Polypharmacology: drug discovery for the future. *Expert Rev Clin Pharmacol.* (2013) 6:41–7. doi: 10.1586/ecp.12.74

51. Medina-Franco JL, Giulianotti MA, Welmaker GS, Houghten RA. Shifting from the single- to the multitarget paradigm in drug discovery. *Drug Discov Today.* (2013) 18:495–501. doi: 10.1016/j.drudis.2013.01.008

52. Naveja JJ, Dueñas-González A, Medina-Franco JL. Chapter 12 - drug repurposing for epigenetic targets guided by computational methods. In: *Epi-Informatics,* ed J. L. Medina-Franco (Boston: Academic Press), 327–57. doi: 10.1016/B978-0-12-802808-7.00012-5

53. Moffat JG, Vincent F, Lee JA, Eder J, Prunotto M. Opportunities and challenges in phenotypic drug discovery: an industry perspective. *Nat Rev Drug Discov.* (2017) 16:531–43. doi: 10.1038/nrd.2017.111

54. Swinney DC, Anthony J. How were new medicines discovered? *Nat Rev Drug Discov.* (2011) 10:507–19. doi: 10.1038/nrd3480

55. Bastos LFS, Coelho MM. Drug repositioning: playing dirty to kill pain. *CNS Drugs.* (2014) 28:45–61. doi: 10.1007/s40263-013-0128-0

56. Loregian A, Palù G. How academic labs can approach the drug discovery process as a way to synergize with big pharma. *Trends Microbiol.* (2013) 21:261–4. doi: 10.1016/j.tim.2013.03.006

57. Jones LH, Bunnage ME. Applications of chemogenomic library screening in drug discovery. *Nat Rev Drug Discov.* (2017) 16:285–96. doi: 10.1038/nrd.2016.244

58. Knox C, Law V, Jewison T, Liu P, Ly S, Frolkis A, Pon A, et al. DrugBank 3.0: a comprehensive resource for "omics" research on drugs. *Nucleic Acids Res.* (2011) 39:D1035–41. doi: 10.1093/nar/gkq1126

59. Ferrero E, Dunham I, Sanseau P. *In silico* prediction of novel therapeutic targets using gene–disease association data. *J Transl Med.* (2017) 15:182. doi: 10.1186/s12967-017-1285-6

60. Hurle MR, Yang L, Xie Q, Rajpal DK, Sanseau P, Agarwal P. Computational drug repositioning: from data to therapeutics. *Clin Pharmacol Ther.* (2013) 93:335–41. doi: 10.1038/clpt.2013.1

61. Ekins S, Mestres J, Testa B. *In silico* pharmacology for drug discovery: methods for virtual ligand screening and profiling. *Br J Pharmacol.* (2007) 152:9–20. doi: 10.1038/sj.bjp.0707305

62. Tari LB, Patel JH. Systematic drug repurposing through text mining. *Methods Mol Biol.* (2014) 1159:253–67. doi: 10.1007/978-1-4939-0709-0_14

63. Cichonska A, Rousu J, Aittokallio T. Identification of drug candidates and repurposing opportunities through compound-target interaction networks. *Expert Opin Drug Discov.* (2015) 10:1333–45. doi: 10.1517/17460441.2015.1096926

64. Sidders B, Karlsson A, Kitching L, Torella R, Karila P, Phelan A. Network-based drug discovery: coupling network pharmacology with phenotypic screening for neuronal excitability. *J Mol Biol.* (2018) 430:3005–15. doi: 10.1016/j.jmb.2018.07.016

65. Chatterjee S, Szustakowski JD, Nanguneri NR, Mickanin C, Labow MA, Nohturfft A, et al. Identification of novel genes and pathways regulating SREBP transcriptional activity. *PLoS ONE.* (2009) 4:5197. doi: 10.1371/journal.pone.0005197

66. Oprea TI, Nielsen SK, Ursu O, Yang JJ, Taboureau O, Mathias SL, et al. Associating drugs, targets and clinical outcomes into an integrated network affords a new platform for computer-aided drug repurposing. *Mol Inform.* (2011) 30:100–11. doi: 10.1002/minf.201100023

67. Chiang AP, Butte AJ. Systematic evaluation of drug-disease relationships to identify leads for novel drug uses. *Clin Pharmacol Ther.* (2009) 86:507–510. doi: 10.1038/clpt.2009.103

68. Platz EA, Yegnasubramanian S, Liu JO, Chong CR, Shim JS, Kenfield SA, et al. A novel two-stage, transdisciplinary study identifies digoxin as a possible drug for prostate cancer treatment. *Cancer Discov.* (2011) 1:68–77. doi: 10.1158/2159-8274.CD-10-0020

69. Allarakhia M. Open-source approaches for the repurposing of existing or failed candidate drugs: learning from and applying the lessons across diseases. *Drug Des Devel Ther.* (2013) 7:753–66. doi: 10.2147/DDDT. S46289

70. van der Graaf PH, Benson N. Systems pharmacology: bridging systems biology and pharmacokinetics-pharmacodynamics (PKPD) in drug discovery and development. *Pharm Res.* (2011) 28:1460–4. doi: 10.1007/s11095-011-0467-9

71. Zhou W, Wang Y, Lu A, Zhang G. Systems pharmacology in small molecular drug discovery. *Int J Mol Sci.* (2016) 17:246. doi: 10.3390/ijms17020246

72. Mercorelli B, Palù G, Loregian A. Drug repurposing for viral infectious diseases: how far are we? *Trends Microbiol.* (2018) 26:865–76. doi: 10.1016/j.tim.2018.04.004

73. Akpovwa H. Chloroquine could be used for the treatment of filoviral infections and other viral infections that emerge or emerged from viruses requiring an acidic pH for infectivity. *Cell Biochem Funct.* (2016) 34:191–6. doi: 10.1002/cbf.3182

74. Al-Bari MAA. Targeting endosomal acidification by chloroquine analogs as a promising strategy for the treatment of emerging viral diseases. *Pharmacol Res Perspect.* (2017) 5:e00293. doi: 10.1002/prp2.293

75. Pires de Mello CP, Tao X, Kim TH, Vicchiarelli M, Bulitta JB, Kaushik A, et al. Clinical regimens of favipiravir inhibit zika virus replication in the hollow-fiber infection model. *Antimicrob Agents Chemother.* (2018) 62:e00967–18. doi: 10.1128/AAC.00967-18

76. Ludwig S. Will omics help to cure the flu? *Trends Microbiol.* (2014) 22:232–3. doi: 10.1016/j.tim.2014.03.003

77. Perwitasari O, Yan X, O'Donnell J, Johnson S, Tripp RA. Repurposing kinase inhibitors as antiviral agents to control influenza a virus replication. *Assay Drug Dev Technol.* (2015) 13:638–49. doi: 10.1089/adt.2015.0003.drrr

78. Fedson DS. Treating influenza with statins and other immunomodulatory agents. *Antiviral Res.* (2013) 99:417–35. doi: 10.1016/j.antiviral.2013.06.018

79. Fedson DS. Clinician-initiated research on treating the host response to pandemic influenza. *Hum Vaccin Immunother.* (2018) 14:790–5. doi: 10.1080/21645515.2017.1378292

80. Mehrbod P, Omar AR, Hair-Bejo M, Haghani A, Ideris A. Mechanisms of action and efficacy of statins against influenza. *Biomed Res Int.* (2014) 2014:872370. doi: 10.1155/2014/872370

81. Rossignol JF, La Frazia S, Chiappa L, Ciucci A, Santoro MG. Thiazolides, a new class of anti-influenza molecules targeting viral hemagglutinin at the post-translational level. *J Biol Chem.* (2009) 284:29798–808. doi: 10.1074/jbc.M109.029470

82. Tilmanis D, van Baalen C, Oh DY, Rossignol J-F, Hurt AC. The susceptibility of circulating human influenza viruses to tizoxanide, the active metabolite of nitazoxanide. *Antiviral Res.* (2017) 147:142–8. doi: 10.1016/j.antiviral.2017.10.002

83. Moseley CE, Webster RG, Aldridge JR. Peroxisome proliferator-activated receptor and AMP-activated protein kinase agonists protect against lethal influenza virus challenge in mice. *Influenza Other Respir Viruses.* (2010) 4:307–11. doi: 10.1111/j.1750-2659.2010.00155.x

84. Budd A, Alleva L, Alsharifi M, Koskinen A, Smythe V, Müllbacher A, et al. Increased survival after gemfibrozil treatment of severe mouse influenza. *Antimicrob Agents Chemother.* (2007) 51:2965–8. doi: 10.1128/AAC.00219-07

85. Droebner K, Haasbach E, Dudek SE, Scheuch G, Nocker K, Canisius S, et al. Pharmacodynamics, pharmacokinetics, and antiviral activity of BAY 81-8781, a novel NF-κB inhibiting anti-influenza drug. *Front Microbiol.* (2017) 8:2130. doi: 10.3389/fmicb.2017.02130

86. Scheuch G, Canisius S, Nocker K, Hofmann T, Naumann R, Pleschka S, et al. Targeting intracellular signaling as an antiviral strategy: aerosolized LASAG for the treatment of influenza in hospitalized patients. *Emerg Microbes Infect.* (2018) 7:21. doi: 10.1038/s41426-018-0023-3

87. Davidson S. Treating influenza infection, from now and into the future. *Front Immunol.* (2018) 9:1946. doi: 10.3389/fimmu.2018.01946

88. Carey MA, Bradbury JA, Rebolloso YD, Graves JP, Zeldin DC, Germolec DR. Pharmacologic inhibition of COX-1 and COX-2 in influenza A viral infection in mice. *PLoS ONE.* (2010) 5:e11610. doi: 10.1371/journal.pone.0011610

89. Shi X, Zhou W, Huang H, Zhu H, Zhou P, Zhu H, et al. Inhibition of the inflammatory cytokine tumor necrosis factor-alpha with etanercept provides protection against lethal H1N1 influenza infection in mice. *Crit Care.* (2013) 17:R301. doi: 10.1186/cc13171

90. Denisova OV, Kakkola L, Feng L, Stenman J, Nagaraj A, Lampe J, et al. Obatoclax, saliphenylhalamide, and gemcitabine inhibit influenza a virus infection. *J Biol Chem.* (2012) 287:35324–32. doi: 10.1074/jbc.M112.392142

91. Hu Y, Zhang J, Musharrafieh RG, Ma C, Hau R, Wang J. Discovery of dapivirine, a nonnucleoside HIV-1 reverse transcriptase inhibitor, as a broad-spectrum antiviral against both influenza A and B viruses. *Antiviral Res.* (2017) 145:103–13. doi: 10.1016/j.antiviral.2017.07.016

92. Schräder T, Dudek SE, Schreiber A, Ehrhardt C, Planz O, Ludwig S. The clinically approved MEK inhibitor Trametinib efficiently blocks influenza A virus propagation and cytokine expression. *Antiviral Res.* (2018) 157:80–92. doi: 10.1016/j.antiviral.2018.07.006

93. Rohini K, Shanthi V. Hyphenated 3D-QSAR statistical model-drug repurposing analysis for the identification of potent neuraminidase inhibitor. *Cell Biochem Biophys.* (2018) 76:357–76. doi: 10.1007/s12013-018-0844-7

94. Lejal N, Tarus B, Bouguyon E, Chenavas S, Bertho N, Delmas B, et al. Structure-based discovery of the novel antiviral properties of naproxen against the nucleoprotein of influenza A virus. *Antimicrob Agents Chemother.* (2013) 57:2231–42. doi: 10.1128/AAC.02335-12

95. Bao J, Marathe B, Govorkova EA, Zheng JJ. Drug repurposing identifies inhibitors of oseltamivir-resistant influenza viruses. *Angew Chem Int Ed Engl.* (2016) 55:3438–41. doi: 10.1002/anie.201511361

96. Watanabe T, Kawakami E, Shoemaker JE, Lopes TJS, Matsuoka Y, Tomita Y, et al. Influenza virus-host interactome screen as a platform for antiviral drug development. *Cell Host Microbe.* (2014) 16:795–805. doi: 10.1016/j.chom.2014.11.002

97. Josset L, Textoris J, Loriod B, Ferraris O, Moules V, Lina B, et al. Gene expression signature-based screening identifies new broadly effective influenza a antivirals. *PLoS ONE.* (2010) 5:13169. doi: 10.1371/journal.pone.0013169

98. Pizzorno A, Terrier O, Nicolas de Lamballerie C, Julien T, Padey B, Traversier A, et al. Repurposing of drugs as novel influenza inhibitors from clinical gene expression infection signatures. *Front Immunol.* (2019) 10:60. doi: 10.3389/fimmu.2019.00060

99. Kumaki Y, Morrey JD, Barnard DL. Effect of statin treatments on highly pathogenic avian influenza H5N1, seasonal and H1N1pdm09

virus infections in BALB/c mice. *Future Virol.* (2012) 7:801–18. doi: 10.2217/fvl.12.71

100. Salomon R, Hoffmann E, Webster RG. Inhibition of the cytokine response does not protect against lethal H5N1 influenza infection. *Proc Natl Acad Sci USA.* (2007) 104:12479–81. doi: 10.1073/pnas.0705289104

101. Belser JA, Szretter KJ, Katz JM, Tumpey TM. Simvastatin and oseltamivir combination therapy does not improve the effectiveness of oseltamivir alone following highly pathogenic avian H5N1 influenza virus infection in mice. *Virology.* (2013) 439:42–6. doi: 10.1016/j.virol.2013.01.017

102. Radigan KA, Urich D, Misharin AV, Chiarella SE, Soberanes S, Gonzalez A, et al. The effect of rosuvastatin in a murine model of influenza A infection. *PLoS ONE.* (2012) 7:e35788. doi: 10.1371/journal.pone.0035788

103. Enserink M. Infectious disease. Old drugs losing effectiveness against flu; could statins fill gap? *Science.* (2005) 309:1976–7. doi: 10.1126/science.309.5743.1976a

104. Vandermeer ML, Thomas AR, Kamimoto L, Reingold A, Gershman K, Meek J, et al. Association between use of statins and mortality among patients hospitalized with laboratory-confirmed influenza virus infections: a multistate study. *J Infect Dis.* (2012) 205:13–9. doi: 10.1093/infdis/jir695

105. Brett SJ, Myles P, Lim WS, Enstone JE, Bannister B, Semple MG, et al. Pre-admission statin use and in-hospital severity of 2009 pandemic influenza A(H1N1) disease. *PLoS ONE.* (2011) 6:e18120. doi: 10.1371/journal.pone.0018120

106. Rossignol J-F. Nitazoxanide: a first-in-class broad-spectrum antiviral agent. *Antiviral Res.* (2014) 110:94–103. doi: 10.1016/j.antiviral.2014.07.014

107. Haffizulla J, Hartman A, Hoppers M, Resnick H, Samudrala S, Ginocchio C, et al. Effect of nitazoxanide in adults and adolescents with acute uncomplicated influenza: a double-blind, randomised, placebo-controlled, phase 2b/3 trial. *Lancet Infect Dis.* (2014) 14:609–18. doi: 10.1016/S1473-3099(14)70717-0

108. Mazur I, Wurzer WJ, Ehrhardt C, Pleschka S, Puthavathana P, Silberzahn T, et al. Acetylsalicylic acid (ASA) blocks influenza virus propagation via its NF-kappaB-inhibiting activity. *Cell Microbiol.* (2007) 9:1683–94. doi: 10.1111/j.1462-5822.2007.00902.x

109. Yin MJ, Yamamoto Y, Gaynor RB. The anti-inflammatory agents aspirin and salicylate inhibit the activity of I(kappa)B kinase-beta. *Nature.* (1998) 396:77–80. doi: 10.1038/23948

110. Wurzer WJ, Ehrhardt C, Pleschka S, Berberich-Siebelt F, Wolff T, Walczak H, et al. NF-kappaB-dependent induction of tumor necrosis factor-related apoptosis-inducing ligand (TRAIL) and Fas/FasL is crucial for efficient influenza virus propagation. *J Biol Chem.* (2004) 279:30931–7. doi: 10.1074/jbc.M403258200

111. Tarus B, Chevalier C, Richard C-A, Delmas B, Di Primo C, Slama-Schwok A. Molecular dynamics studies of the nucleoprotein of influenza A virus:

role of the protein flexibility in RNA binding. *PLoS ONE.* (2012) 7:e30038. doi: 10.1371/journal.pone.0030038

112. Dilly S, Fotso Fotso A, Lejal N, Zedda G, Chebbo M, Rahman F, et al. From naproxen repurposing to naproxen analogues and their antiviral activity against influenza A virus. *J Med Chem.* (2018) 61:7202–17. doi: 10.1021/acs.jmedchem.8b00557

113. Chaudhuri S, Symons JA, Deval J. Innovation and trends in the development and approval of antiviral medicines: 1987–2017 and beyond. *Antiviral Res.* (2018) 155:76–88. doi: 10.1016/j.antiviral.2018.05.005

114. Pizzorno A, Abed Y, Rhéaume C, Boivin G. Oseltamivir-zanamivir combination therapy is not superior to zanamivir monotherapy in mice infected with influenza A(H3N2) and A(H1N1)pdm09 viruses. *Antiviral Res.* (2014) 105:54–8. doi: 10.1016/j.antiviral.2014.02.017

115. Escuret V, Cornu C, Boutitie F, Enouf V, Mosnier A, Bouscambert-Duchamp M, et al. Oseltamivir-zanamivir bitherapy compared to oseltamivir monotherapy in the treatment of pandemic 2009 influenza A(H1N1) virus infections. *Antiviral Res.* (2012) 96:130–7. doi: 10.1016/j.antiviral.2012.08.002

116. Carrat F, Duval X, Tubach F, Mosnier A, Van der Werf S, Tibi A, et al. Effect of oseltamivir, zanamivir or oseltamivir-zanamivir combination treatments on transmission of influenza in households. *Antivir Ther.* (2012) 17:1085–90. doi: 10.3851/IMP2128

117. Belardo G, Cenciarelli O, La Frazia S, Rossignol JF, Santoro MG. Synergistic effect of nitazoxanide with neuraminidase inhibitors against influenza A viruses *in vitro*. *Antimicrob Agents Chemother.* (2015) 59:1061–9. doi: 10.1128/AAC.03947-14

118. Hung IFN, To KKW, Chan JFW, Cheng VCC, Liu KSH, Tam A, et al. Efficacy of clarithromycin-naproxen-oseltamivir combination in the treatment of patients hospitalized for influenza A(H3N2) infection: an open-label randomized, controlled, phase IIb/III trial. *Chest.* (2017) 151:1069–80. doi: 10.1016/j.chest.2016.11.012

# 15

# Systems Immunology Characterization of Novel Vaccine Formulations for *Mycoplasma hyopneumoniae* Bacterins

*Anneleen M. F. Matthijs [1], Gaël Auray [2,3], Virginie Jakob [4], Obdulio García-Nicolás [2,3], Roman O. Braun [2,3], Irene Keller [5,6], Rémy Bruggman [5], Bert Devriendt [7], Filip Boyen [8], Carlos A. Guzman [9], Annelies Michiels [1], Freddy Haesebrouck [8], Nicolas Collin [4], Christophe Barnier-Quer [4], Dominiek Maes [1†] and Artur Summerfield [2,3*†]*

[1] Department of Reproduction, Obstetrics and Herd Health, Faculty of Veterinary Medicine, Ghent University, Merelbeke, Belgium, [2] Institute of Virology and Immunology, Mittelhäusern, Switzerland, [3] Department of Infectious Diseases and Pathobiology, Vetsuisse Faculty, University of Bern, Bern, Switzerland, [4] Vaccine Formulation Laboratory, University of Lausanne, Epalinges, Switzerland, [5] Interfaculty Bioinformatics Unit, Swiss Institute of Bioinformatics, University of Bern, Bern, Switzerland, [6] Department of Biomedical Research, University of Bern, Bern, Switzerland, [7] Laboratory of Veterinary Immunology, Department of Virology, Parasitology and Immunology, Faculty of Veterinary Medicine, Ghent University, Merelbeke, Belgium, [8] Department of Pathology, Bacteriology and Avian Diseases, Faculty of Veterinary Medicine, Ghent University, Merelbeke, Belgium, [9] Department of Vaccinology and Applied Microbiology, Helmholtz Centre for Infection Research, Brunswick, Germany

*Correspondence:
Artur Summerfield
artur.summerfield@vetsuisse.unibe.ch

†These authors have contributed
equally to this work

We characterized five different vaccine candidates and a commercial vaccine in terms of safety, immunogenicity and using a systems vaccinology approach, with the aim to select novel vaccine candidates against *Mycoplasma hyopneumoniae*. Seven groups of six *M. hyopneumoniae*-free piglets were primo- and booster vaccinated with the different experimental bacterin formulations, the commercial vaccine Hyogen® as a positive control or PBS as a negative control. The experimental bacterin was formulated with cationic liposomes + c-di-AMP (Lipo_AMP), cationic liposomes + Toll-like receptor (TLR) 2/1, TLR7, and TLR9 ligands (TLR ligands; Lipo_TLR), micro-particles + TLR ligands (PLGA_TLR), squalene-in-water emulsion + TLR ligands (SWE_TLR), or DDA:TDB liposomes (Lipo_DDA:TDB). Lipo_DDA:TDB and Lipo_AMP were the most potent in terms of serum antibody induction, and Lipo_DDA:TDB, Lipo_AMP, and SWE_TLR significantly induced Th1 cytokine-secreting T-cells. Only PLGA_TLR appeared to induce Th17 cells, but was unable to induce serum antibodies. The transcriptomic analyses demonstrated that the induction of inflammatory and myeloid cell blood transcriptional modules (BTM) in the first 24 h after vaccination correlated well with serum antibodies, while negative correlations with the same modules were found 7 days post-vaccination. Furthermore, many cell cycle and T-cell BTM upregulated at day seven correlated positively with adaptive immune responses. When comparing the delivery of the identical TLR ligands with the three formulations, we found SWE_TLR to be more potent in the induction of an early innate immune response, while the liposomal formulation more strongly promoted late cell cycle and T-cell BTM. For the PLGA formulation we found signs of a delayed and weak perturbation of these BTM. Lipo_AMP was found to be the most potent vaccine at inducing a BTM profile similar to that correlating with adaptive immune response in this and other studies. Taken together, we identified four promising vaccine candidates able to induce *M. hyopneumoniae*-specific antibody and T-cell responses. In addition, we have adapted a systems vaccinology approach developed for human to pigs and demonstrated its capacity in identifying early immune signatures in the blood relating to adaptive immune responses. This approach represents an important step in a more rational design of efficacious vaccines for pigs.

Keywords: *Mycoplasma hyopneumoniae*, bacterins, safety, immune responses, transcriptomics

# INTRODUCTION

*Mycoplasma hyopneumoniae (M. hyopneumoniae)* is the primary cause of enzootic pneumonia (EP), a chronic respiratory disease in pigs. The disease causes severe economic losses in swine-producing countries worldwide due to a reduced average daily weight gain of the pigs, a higher feed conversion ratio and an increased use of antimicrobial agents (1–3). Control of the disease can be achieved by optimizing management and housing conditions combined with medication and vaccination (2).

Vaccination with inactivated, adjuvanted whole-cell bacterins is practiced worldwide to control EP (4). However, current commercial vaccines only offer partial protection, have a limited effect on the transmission of the microorganism and cannot prevent colonization (5–7). Most commercial bacterins are based on the J-strain, a low virulent *M. hyopneumoniae* strain isolated in the UK in the sixties (8–10), and contain adjuvants including aluminum hydroxide, carbopol, mineral oil or biodegradable oil (4). The main effects of vaccination are a reduction in clinical symptoms, lung lesions, medication use, and performance losses (11, 12). Those effects may vary between pig herds (2), which could be partially explained by antigenic and pathogenic differences between the strains circulating in the herd and the vaccine strain (10).

The immune mechanisms leading to protection against *M. hyopneumoniae* infection are complex and not yet fully elucidated. *M. hyopneumoniae*-specific serum antibody concentrations induced by vaccination are not correlated with the severity of lung lesions in *M. hyopneumoniae*-infected pigs (5, 13), indicating that systemic antibodies play only a minor role in protective immunity. However, local mucosal antibodies (IgA) are considered important to prevent and control *M. hyopneumoniae*-induced pneumonia, as the adherence of the microorganism to the ciliated epithelium of the respiratory tract is the first step in the pathogenesis (14). Also, several studies suggest that systemic cell-mediated immune responses play a major role in disease protection (14–17).

Based on this knowledge, innovative bacterin formulations that include virulent *M. hyopneumoniae* strains formulated with adjuvants specifically designed to promote cellular immune responses could improve vaccine efficacy. Therefore, we developed three different vaccine formulations to deliver a cocktail of TLR 2/1, TLR 7, and TLR 9 ligands previously shown to potently activate porcine antigen presenting cells including dendritic cells (DC), monocytes and B cells (18, 19). The formulations included a liposomal, a micro-particle and an oil-in-water formulation. In addition, we developed a liposomal formulation to deliver a cyclic di-nucleotide targeting the STING pathway (20) as an alternative immunostimulant, and another cationic liposomal formulation to deliver a Mincle ligand, also previously found to be efficacious (21). All formulations were based on the *M. hyopneumoniae* strain F7.2C, a highly virulent field strain isolated in Belgium in 2000 (22, 23), and shown to be antigenically different from the J-strain (23).

Overall, the aim of this study was to assess the safety of these five novel bacterin formulations and characterize the immune responses induced by the formulations, compared to a commercial vaccine in order to select new promising vaccine candidates. To this end, *M. hyopneumoniae*-specific T cell responses and antibody responses were measured in pigs. For T cells, we focussed on Th1 and Th17 based on their known role in protective immunity against *Mycoplasma* infection, as identified in mouse models (24). Next to that, we employed a systems immunology approach to understand how different formulations modulate the immune system toward potent immunogenicity. This analysis employed "blood transcriptional modules" (BTM) defined for peripheral blood cells in human (25), which were adapted to pigs. This technique sheds light into the black box of the immune response by identifying pathways and networks of genes related to adaptive immune responses as previously demonstrated for human and sheep (25–34). Also, this approach has been shown to possess more discriminative power for analyses of peripheral blood leukocytes during vaccination when compared to gene sets based on canonical pathways (25). Our work has demonstrated the possibilities of such novel approaches in vaccinology and identified vaccine candidates for further exploration.

# MATERIALS AND METHODS

## Vaccines

The vaccine strain *M. hyopneumoniae* F7.2C was grown in modified Friis medium (35) for 5 days at 37°C. The culture,

---

**Abbreviations:** EP, enzootic pneumonia; CCU, color changing units; PLGA, poly(lactic-co-glycolic acid); SWE, squalene-in-water emulsion; DDA, dimethyl dioctadecylammonium; DPPC:DC-Chol, 1,2-dipalmitoyl-sn-glycero-3-phosphocholine and dimethylaminoethane carbamoyl cholesterol; TDB, trehalose 6,6-dibehenate; c-di-AMP, cyclic diadenylate monophosphate; PAM, Pam3Cys-SK4; CpG, CpG ODN SL03; PS, particle size; Pdi, polydispersity index; ZP, zeta potential; IM, intramuscularly; ID, intradermally; ISR, injection site reaction; ADG, average daily gain; BAL, bronchoalveolar lavage; GSEA, gene set enrichment analysis; FDR, false discovery rate; DEG, differentially expressed genes; BTM, blood transcriptional modules.

containing $5 \times 10^8$ color changing units (CCU)/ml, was inactivated by incubation with 4 mM binary ethyleneimine (BEI) under agitation at 37°C for 24 h. Subsequently, the BEI was neutralized by incubating the inactivated culture with 4 mM sodium thiosulfate under agitation at 37°C for 24 h. Inactivated bacteria were pelleted at 15,000 g for 40 min at 4°C and washed three times in 50 ml sterile phosphate buffered saline (PBS). The final pellet was resuspended in sterile PBS.

For this study, five adjuvant formulations were developed based on the association of particle-based delivery systems [liposomes, poly(lactic-co-glycolic acid) [PLGA] microparticles and a squalene-in-water emulsion (SWE)] with different immune stimulators. These included the Mincle agonist trehalose 6,6-dibehenate (TDB, Avanti, Alabaster, AL, USA), the STING ligand cyclic diadenylate monophosphate (c-di-AMP, produced at the Helmholtz Center for Infection Research, Braunschweig, Germany) and a combination of TLR ligands: TLR1/2 ligand Pam3Cys-SK4 (PAM, EMC Microcollections, Tübingen, Germany), TLR9 ligand CpG ODN SL03 (CpG, Eurofins Genomics, Les Ulis, France), and TLR7/8 ligand resiquimod (Chemdea, Ridgewood, NJ, USA).

Two cationic liposome formulations were produced, based on the thin lipid film method (36), and followed by extrusion: TDB was combined with dimethyl dioctadecylammonium (DDA) bromide to form Lipo_DDA:TDB, and c-di-AMP was encapsulated into 1,2-dipalmitoyl-sn-glycero-3-phosphocholine and dimethylaminoethane-carbamoyl-cholesterol (DPPC:DC-Chol) cationic liposomes (37) to obtain Lipo_AMP. The TLR ligand selection was combined in different delivery systems: PLGA micro-particles, cationic liposomes and SWE. Cationic liposomes (DPPC:DC-Chol) and PLGA cationic micro-particles (combined to ethylaminoethyl-dextran) were produced with the thin lipid film and the double emulsion (W/O/W) methods (38), respectively. Pam3Cys-SK4 and resiquimod were encapsulated into both types of particles and CpG was later adsorbed to their surface to form the Lipo_TLR and PLGA_TLR formulations. Finally, for the SWE_TLR formulation, SWE [a squalene-based formulation developed and produced by the Vaccine Formulation Laboratory, and composed of 3.9% (w/v) squalene, 0.5% (w/v) Tween 80 and 0.5% (w/v) Span 85 (39)] was mixed with the same immune stimulators (PAM, CpG, and resiquimod).

For each formulation we measured the following physico-chemical characteristics: particle size (PS), polydispersity index (Pdi), and zeta potential (ZP), by means of dynamic light scattering for the liposomes and SWE, and laser diffraction for the micro-particles (Zetasizer Nano ZS and Mastersizer 3000, Malvern, UK). The amounts of immune-stimulators loaded into the Lipo_AMP and Lipo_TLR formulations were indirectly determined by the use of nanodrop (for c-di-AMP) and fluorescently labeled immune-stimulator (CpG-FITC and Pam-Rhodamine, Invivogen, San Diego, CA, USA) methods. The free immune-stimulators were separated from the liposomes by filtration using the Vivaspin® 500 centrifugal concentrator (PED membrane, MWCO 100 kDa, Sartorius, Göttingen, Germany) and then quantified as mentioned above (**Supplementary Table 1**) Antigen was mixed with the final product, and PS and ZP of the formulations were monitored over a period of 1 month.

The composition of each experimental vaccine is given in **Table 1**. The commercial vaccine employed was Hyogen® (CEVA Santé Animale, Libourne Cedex, France) representing a mineral oil emulsion with *Escherichia coli* J5 non-toxic LPS as immunostimulant and inactivated *M. hyopneumoniae* field isolate BA 2940-99 as antigen.

## Animal Experiment

The study was performed after approval by the Ethical Committee for Animal Experiments of the Faculty of Veterinary Medicine, Ghent University (approval number EC2016/91). Forty-two *M. hyopneumoniae*-free Rattlerlow-Seghers piglets (RA-SE Genetics NV, Ooigem, Belgium) were enrolled in the study. All animals were purchased from a herd that has been free of *M. hyopneumoniae* for many years based on repeated serological testing, nested PCR testing on tracheobronchial swabs, and absence of clinical signs and pneumonia lesions in the slaughter house. The piglets were weaned at 28 days of age and transported 4 days later to the experimental facilities of the Faculty of Veterinary Medicine, Ghent University, Belgium. They were housed in stables with absolute air filters for impending particles (HEPA U15) on both incoming and outgoing ventilation shafts and fed *ad libitum* with a non-antimicrobial-supplemented diet. On the day of arrival at the experimental facilities, the piglets were randomly allocated into six vaccination groups and one control group of six piglets each. Due to practical reasons, the piglets were vaccinated, sampled and euthanized over 2 consecutive days. After an acclimatization period of 6 days, the piglets of the vaccination groups were primo-vaccinated (D0; 39–40 days of age) intramuscularly (IM) into the right side of the neck with 2 mL vaccine. Additionally, group Lipo_DDA:TDB was vaccinated intradermally (ID) into the left side of the neck with 0.2 mL vaccine. The rationale for the ID injection of formulation Lipo_DDA:TDB was based on a previous report showing that CAF01, a liposome-based adjuvant containing similar immunomodulators, was able to induce mucosal immunity when administered this way (40). The piglets of the control group were injected IM into the right side of the neck with 2 mL sterile PBS. Two weeks later (D14), the piglets of the vaccination groups were booster vaccinated IM with 2 mL vaccine (all groups). The control group received 2 mL PBS IM. On D28 all piglets were euthanized.

## Safety Parameters

The piglets were observed daily for at least 15 min from D-6 until D28 of the study. On the days of vaccine administration, the piglets were observed twice: shortly before (D0; D14) and 4 h after vaccination (D0+4h; D14+4h). For each piglet, clinical findings regarding body condition (skinny), behavior (depressed, unconscious), respiration (sneezing, coughing, abdominal breathing), digestion (diarrhea, vomiting), lameness and other remarkable findings were recorded. At necropsy (D28), lungs were macroscopically examined for the presence of lesions according to Hannan et al. (41). Subsequently, bronchoalveolar lavage (BAL) fluid was collected from one lung part by flushing the head bronchus with 20 mL sterile PBS, as previously described (15). From the BAL fluid, DNA was extracted using a commercial kit (DNeasy® Blood & Tissue

**TABLE 1 |** Composition of the experimental *M. hyopneumoniae* bacterins and their route of administration.

| Vaccine formulation | Dose (mL) | Delivery system | Immune-stimulators (µg/dose) | Antigen dose (CCU) | Administration route | |
|---|---|---|---|---|---|---|
| | | | | | Primo | Booster |
| Lipo_AMP | 2 | DPPC:DC-Chol liposomes | C-di.AMP (100) | $10^9$ | IM | IM |
| Lipo_TLR | 2 | DPPC:DC-Chol liposomes | Pam3Cys-SK4/CpG ODN SL03/resiquimod (80/80/80) | $10^9$ | IM | IM |
| PLGA_TLR | 2 | PLGA micro-particles (combined to ethylaminoethyl-dextran) | Pam3Cys-SK4/CpG ODN SL03/resiquimod (80/80/80) | $10^9$ | IM | IM |
| SWE_TLR | 2 | squalene-in-water emulsion | Pam3Cys-SK4/CpG ODN SL03/resiquimod (80/80/80) | $10^9$ | IM | IM |
| Lipo_DDA:TDB | IM 2 ID 0.2 | DDA liposomes | TDB (500) | IM $10^9$ ID $2\times10^8$ | IM+ID | IM |

*CCU, color changing units; IM, intramuscular; ID, intradermal; DPPC:DC-Chol, 1,2-dipalmitoyl-sn-glycero-3-phosphocholine and dimethylaminoethane-carbamoyl-cholesterol; c-di-AMP, bis-(3',5')-cyclic dimeric adenosine monophosphate; PLGA, poly(lactic-co-glycolic acid); DDA, dimethyl dioctadecylammonium; TDB, trehalose 6,6'-dibehenate.*

kit, Qiagen, Venlo, The Netherlands) and a nested PCR for the detection of *M. hyopneumoniae* DNA was performed according to Stärk et al. (42).

The pigs were weighed on the day of primo-vaccination (D0) and at euthanasia (D28). Average daily gain (ADG) in g/pig/day was calculated according to Sacristán et al. (43).

Rectal body temperature was measured shortly before and 4 h after vaccine administration, then daily until 4 days post-vaccine administration, and on D7, 10, 21, 24, and 28 of the study. This was based on the guidelines on safety evaluation of veterinary vaccines written in the European Pharmacopeia 8.0.

Injection site reactions (ISR) were evaluated shortly before vaccination, 4 h after vaccination and then daily from D1 to D28 using the scoring system explained in **Supplementary Table 2**. Scores could range from 0 to 3 with 0 = normal, 1 = mild, 2 = moderate, and 3 = severe. At euthanasia (D28), tissue samples from the injection site were collected from all study animals for histopathological examination. All IM and ID injection sites were marked with a permanent pen upon vaccination. Out of the marked area a tissue sample of approximately 2 cm² with a depth of 5 cm (IM injection site) or 3 cm (ID injection site) was removed in an angle of 90° to the skin. A tissue sample with a dimension of 2 × 2 × 3 cm from the left side of the neck was collected as described above from the pigs of the control group to serve as a control for the ID injection sites. The tissues were fixed immediately after sampling in 10% neutral formalin. After fixation, tissue blocks were sectioned from the samples, embedded in paraffin and histological slides were stained with hematoxylin and eosin. Each injection site sample was evaluated using light microscopy and an overall score ranging from 0 to 3 (0 = not detected, 1 = mild, 2 = moderate, and 3 = severe) was given. This score took into account the presence and degree of hemorrhage, blood resorption, necrosis, inflammation (acute and chronic), angiogenesis, and proliferation of connective tissue.

## Serology

Before primo-vaccination (D0), on D7, on the day of booster vaccination (D14) and at euthanasia (D28), serum samples were collected and analyzed for the presence of antibodies against *M. hyopneumoniae* with a commercial blocking ELISA (IDEIA™

*Mycoplasma hyopneumoniae* EIA kit, Oxoid Limited, Hampshire, UK) according to the manufacturer's instructions. Samples with optical density (OD) lower than 50% of the average OD of the buffer control were considered positive. Samples with OD-values equal or bigger than 50% of the average OD of the buffer control were classified as negative.

Immunoglobulin (Ig) G and IgA isotypes of the *M. hyopneumoniae*-specific antibodies in serum were determined with an in-house indirect ELISA. Briefly, Nunc Maxisorb® flat-bottom 96 well plates (eBioscience, San Diego, CA, USA) were coated overnight at room temperature with Tween 20-extracted *M. hyopneumoniae* antigens (44). After blocking with PBS containing 0.05% Tween 20 and 1% BSA for 2 h at 37°C, plates were washed three times with PBS + 0.05% Tween 20 and serum diluted 1:200 and 1:100 was added for the detection of IgG and IgA, respectively. After incubating for 30 min at 37°C, plates were washed again, and peroxidase-labeled goat anti-porcine polyclonal IgG diluted 1:60,000 and IgA diluted 1:20,000 (Bethyl Laboratories, Montgomery, TX, USA) were added. Plates were incubated again for 30 min at 37°C, washed and 3,3'5,5'-tetramethylbenzidin substrate (Sigma-Aldrich, Saint Louis, MO, USA) was added. After incubating for 10 min, the reaction was stopped with 2 N HCl and the OD was measured at 450 nm. All samples were tested in duplicate. To relatively quantify the antibody levels a standard curve was made using two-fold serial dilutions of a positive reference serum corresponding to defined arbitrary units (1:800 dilution defined as 1 unit). The interpolation from the standard curve employed non-linear regression with least square fits using Graphpad Prism 7.0 (GraphPad Software Inc., San Diego, CA, USA).

## *M. hyopneumoniae*-Specific Antibodies in Bronchoalveolar Lavage (BAL) Fluid

The BAL fluid collected on D28 was analyzed undiluted for the presence of *M. hyopneumoniae*-specific IgA antibodies using peroxidase-labeled goat anti-porcine polyclonal IgA (Bethyl Laboratories, Montgomery, TX, USA) diluted 1:80,000 in an in-house indirect ELISA as described above. A cut-off was calculated as mean OD-value from the control animals plus three times the SD and established at an OD-value of 0.098. Samples with OD-values higher than the cut-off were considered positive and samples equal to or below the cut-off were considered negative.

## T Cell Assays

Shortly before the booster vaccination on D14 and on the day of euthanasia (D28), blood samples were taken from each animal to assess the primary and secondary T cell-specific responses against *M. hyopneumoniae*. For each animal, samples were restimulated in triplicate cultures and analyzed separately. Briefly, peripheral blood mononuclear cells (PBMCs) were isolated using a ficoll-plaque density gradient (1.077 g/L, GE Healthcare Bio-sciences Corp., Piscataway, NJ, USA) and plated in 12-well plates at $5 \times 10^6$ cells/well in 1 ml of AIM-V medium (Gibco™, ThermoFisher Scientific, Waltham, MA, USA). Subsequently, the cells were restimulated *in vitro* overnight (18 h) with $6.25 \times 10^7$ CCU/mL of *M. hyopneumoniae* F7.2C bacterin. For the last 4 h of stimulation, we added Brefeldin A (eBioscience, San Diego, CA, USA) in each well to inhibit cytokine release and allow intra-cellular detection of cytokines by flow cytometry (FCM). Concanavalin A stimulation (10 µg/mL, Sigma-Aldrich, Saint Louis, MO, USA) was employed as a positive control. Cells were then harvested and the cytokine production of T cell populations was determined by FCM, using a 5-step 6-color staining protocol. Cells were first incubated with the LIVE/DEAD™ Fixable Aqua Dead Cell Stain Kit (Invitrogen™, ThermoFisher Scientific, Waltham, MA, USA) according to the manufacturer's instructions. The cells were then incubated with anti-CD4 (clone 74-12-4, Southern Biotech, Birmingham, AL, USA) and anti-CD8β (clone PG164A, WSU, Pullman, WA, USA) antibodies, and subsequently with the corresponding secondary antibodies: anti-mouse IgG2b AlexaFluor 488 (Molecular Probes, Eugene, OR, USA) and anti-mouse IgG2a PE-Cy7 (Abcam, Cambridge, UK), respectively. Following surface staining, cells were fixed and permeabilized using the BD Cytofix/Cytoperm™ Fixation/Permeabilization Solution kit (Becton Dickinson, Franklin Lakes, NJ, USA) according to the manufacturer's instructions. Cells were finally incubated with directly coupled anti-human TNF-α AlexaFluor 647 (clone MAb11, BioLegend, San Diego, CA, USA), anti-pig IFN-γ PerCP-Cy5.5 (clone P2G10, Becton Dickinson, Franklin Lakes, NJ, USA), and anti-human IL-17A PE (clone SCPL1362, Becton Dickinson, Franklin Lakes, NJ, USA). Flow cytometry acquisition was performed on a CytoFLEX flow cytometer (Beckman Coulter, Brea, CA, USA) and the results were further analyzed with the FlowJo™ software (Tree Star Inc., Ashland, OR, USA).

## Vaccine-Induced Transcriptional Responses

Blood samples were collected on D0, D1, and D7 for RNA preparation (2.5 ml in PAXgene® Blood RNA Tubes, Becton Dickinson, Franklin Lakes, NJ, USA). RNA was extracted using the Paxgene® Blood RNA kit (Qiagen, Venlo, The Netherlands) and the RNA quality was controlled with a Fragment Analyzer. All samples were found to have good quality [RNA integrity number (RIN) > 8] and were sequenced using an Illumina® HiSeq 3000 sequencer (Illumina, San Diego, CA,

USA). The quality of the reads was assessed using FastQC v. 0.11.2[1] The reads were mapped to the *Sus scrofa* reference genome (Sscrofa_11.1) with HISAT2 v. 2.1.0 (45). Feature Counts from Subread v. 1.5.3 was employed to count the number of reads overlapping with each gene, as specified in the Ensembl annotation build 91. The RNAseq data are available in the European Nucleotide Archive[2] under the accession number PRJEB30361.

The Bioconductor package DESeq2 v. 1.18.1 was used to test for differential gene expression between the different time points for each vaccine separately (46). Our specific interest was to identify genes where the change between two time points was different in vaccinated animals compared to the controls. Therefore, a two-factorial model was used, including the factors time point and group (vaccine vs. control), and their interaction. The genes were then ranked based on the P-values for the interaction term for a "ranked gene set enrichment analysis" (GSEA) (47) using the BTM as defined by Li et al. (48).

The BTM were adapted to the pig by replacing human genes with their pig homologs. This step involved extensive manual curation. The final lists of genes for each module can be found in the **Data Sheet 1**.

To compare the module activity of the different vaccines, all modules with a false discovery rate (FDR) $q < 0.1$ were used. In GSEA, a cut-off of 0.25 is recommended but in this study a cut-off of 0.1 was selected to reduce the amount of BTM changing over time. Heat maps were created reflecting the modular activity calculated as the negative natural logarithm of the P-value. For negative enriched BTM, this was multiplied with −1 to obtain a positive value. The rationale of this was to obtain a value reflecting both the enrichment of a module and its statistical significance.

## Correlation Analyses of BTM and Vaccine-Induced Adaptive Immune Responses

To get more insight in the immunomodulation toward a potent immune response, BTM were correlated with the vaccine-induced adaptive immune responses (antibodies, *M. hyopneumoniae*-specific INFγ+TNF+ CD4 T cells and CD8 T cells). To this end, single-sample (ss) GSEA scores were first calculated to transform a single sample's gene expression profile to a gene set (BTM) enrichment profile[3] as described in Barbie et al. (49). Subsequently, the time-dependent changes in ssGSEA values for each BTM were determined as the ratio of D1:D0, D7:D0, and D1:D7 ssGSEA values. These ratios were then correlated to the immune response values using Pearson's correlation coefficient. In order to obtain sufficient values, the data from all vaccinated animals (controls excluded) was used. Only correlation coefficients with $P < 0.05$ were considered.

---

[1] http://www.bioinformatics.babraham.ac.uk/projects/fastqc/
[2] www.ebi.ac.uk/ena
[3] http://software.broadinstitute.org/cancer/software/genepattern/modules/docs/ssGSEAProjection/4

## Statistical Analyses

Fisher's exact tests were performed to analyse differences in the number of animals with ISR and histopathological findings (irrespective of type) at the injection site between the control group and the vaccinated groups. A Bonferroni correction for multiple tests was applied. Rectal temperature values were averaged for the following periods: D1-3, D4-14, D15-17, and D18-28 to distinguish between systemic reactions shortly after vaccination (D1-3; D15-17) and systemic reactions developed later on (D4-14; D18-28). Rectal temperature and ADG were not normally distributed according to the Shapiro-Wilk's test, and Mann-Whitney U tests were run to analyse differences between the control and vaccinated groups in ADG, rectal temperature measured 4 h after vaccination (D0+4h; D14+4h) and during the following periods: D1-3, D4-14, D15-17, D18-28. The Bonferroni method was applied to correct for multiple comparisons. For the quantitative antibody ELISA and T cell data, a two-way ANOVA was employed using the factors vaccine and time. Tukey's or Dunnett's tests were used to correct for multiple comparisons, respectively. Statistical analyses of clinical variables were conducted in SPSS 24 for Windows (IBM, Armonk, NY, USA) and for immune response data using GraphPad Prism 7.0 (GraphPad Software Inc., San Diego, CA, USA). Significance is indicated as $*P \leq 0.05$; $**P < 0.01$; $***P < 0.001$.

## RESULTS

### Safety of the Vaccines

To evaluate the safety of the vaccines the general health, ADG and rectal temperature of the piglets was closely monitored. Diarrhea, which sometimes resulted in skinny pigs, was the most frequent clinical finding observed in all groups (Lipo_DDA:TDB: 2/6; Hyogen and PLGA_TLR: 4/6; control, Lipo_TLR, SWE_TLR: 5/6; Lipo_AMP: 6/6; **Supplementary Figure 1B**). As it was mostly seen during the acclimatization period and started the day after arrival, it was diagnosed as post-weaning diarrhea. All pigs were treated once with 5 mg enrofloxacin per kg body weight (Floxadil® 50 mg/mL, Emdoka, Hoogstraten, Belgium) IM in the hind leg and responded well on treatment. Arthritis (swollen joints) was also observed (control, Lipo_AMP, Lipo_TLR, PLGA_TLR: 1/6; Hyogen: 3/6) and cases occurred during the whole study period (**Supplementary Figure 1C**). Bursitis was recorded for one pig in groups Lipo_TLR, SWE_TLR and Hyogen, and lameness for one pig in groups Lipo_AMP and Lipo_DDA:TDB (**Supplementary Figures 1D–E**). Behavior and respiration were normal throughout the entire study, except for one pig of the PLGA_TLR group that showed severe abdominal breathing following blood sampling on D14. At necropsy (D28), none of the pigs had macroscopic lung lesions and no *M. hyopneumoniae* DNA was detected in BAL fluid. The vaccinated groups did not differ in ADG compared to the control group (data not shown). Four hours after primo- and booster vaccination (D0+4h, D14+4h), rectal temperatures of groups SWE_TLR and Hyogen were significantly higher compared to the control group ($P \leq 0.05$). Rectal temperatures from Lipo_AMP and Lipo_TLR were also increased over the physiological threshold (>40°C) 4 h after primo- and

booster vaccination. However, this increase was only statistically significant compared to the control group at D0+4h and D14+4 for groups Lipo_TLR and Lipo_AMP, respectively ($P \leq 0.05$). A slight increase, although not statistically significant, was observed for PLGA_TLR 4 h after primo-vaccination. Group means were back to normal 1 day after vaccination and all remained within normal physiological levels during the remainder of the trial (**Supplementary Figure 1F**).

The presence and severity of ISR was recorded daily and a histopathological examination of each injection site was performed at the end of the study (D28). No ISR were seen in the control group and group PLGA_TLR. Overall mild and transient ISR were observed in one pig of group SWE_TLR, and in two pigs of each of the groups Lipo_AMP, Lipo_TLR, and Hyogen. In the group Lipo_DDA:TDB three pigs showed a moderate but transient ISR at the IM injection site. However, at the ID injection site, all pigs showed a prolonged mild to moderate ISR which lasted until the end of the study in 4/6 pigs. A more detailed overview of the duration of the ISR and their severity is given in **Supplementary Table 3**. Histopathological examination of the injection site at D28 revealed an overall severe foreign body reaction with chronic inflammation, angiogenesis, and proliferation of connective tissue in 5/6 ID injection site samples from group Lipo_DDA:TDB. Mild (moderate for one pig in group SWE_TLR) focal chronic inflammation was observed in all IM injected groups. Mild to moderate hemorrhage was also observed in all IM injected groups. This was probably caused by the sampling itself as it was most of the time located at the borders of the collected tissue. The results of the histopathological examination of the injection sites are represented in **Supplementary Table 4**.

## *M. hyopneumoniae*-Specific Antibody Responses

According to the commercial blocking ELISA (Oxoid; **Supplementary Table 5**), all pigs from the control group remained serologically negative for *M. hyopneumoniae* throughout the study. On day 28 of the study, all the animals from groups Lipo_AMP, Lipo_TLR, SWE_TLR, Lipo_DDA:TDB, and Hyogen were seropositive. From the PLGA_TLR group, only two out of six pigs seroconverted at D28.

To quantify serum IgG levels in arbitrary units we used an in-house indirect ELISA with a positive reference serum as a standard (**Figure 1**). At D28, groups Lipo_AMP, SWE_TLR, Lipo_DDA:TDB, and Hyogen were statistically different from the control group. The Lipo_DDA:TDB formulation induced the highest IgG response, followed by the Hyogen and Lipo_AMP formulations. Group Lipo_TLR was not significantly higher than the control group, although we could detect *M. hyopneumoniae*-specific IgG antibodies in all animals from this group. In the PLGA_TLR group, only one animal appeared to react. No *M. hyopneumoniae*-specific IgA antibodies were observed for any of the groups at any time point in the serum. Only one animal from the SWE_TLR group was positive for *M. hyopneumoniae*-specific IgA in BAL fluid on D28 (**Supplementary Table 3**).

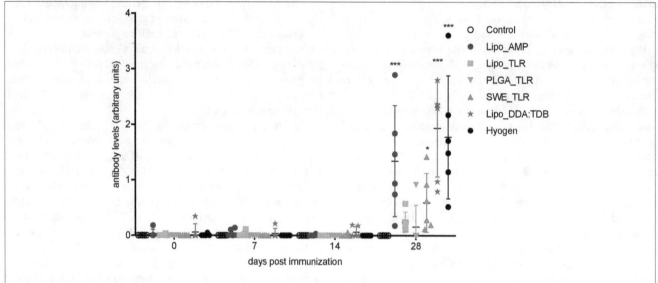

**FIGURE 1 |** Serum antibody levels following vaccination of pigs with vaccine candidates. *M. hyopneumoniae*-specific IgG antibodies induced by the five novel vaccines and one commercial vaccine listed in the legend were determined by indirect ELISA. Six animals per group received two injections in 14 days interval. Individual animals are shown. Significance was calculated using two-way ANOVA followed by Tukey's test (*$P < 0.05$; **$P < 0.01$; ***$P < 0.001$).

## T Cell Responses

The results of the *M. hyopneumoniae*-specific T cell responses after primo-vaccination (D14) are presented in **Figures 2A–C**. No significant group differences were found for the percentage of cytokine-producing T cells in the peripheral blood compartment. Nevertheless, as antigen-specific T cells are transient in the blood, a negative result cannot be interpreted as a lack of T cell response. In fact, a few animals appeared to respond (defined as being above the 99% confidence interval (CI) of the control group) indicating some degree of T cell priming in certain groups. This was found in particular in the groups SWE_TLR, Lipo_DDA:TDB and Hyogen with three animals above this threshold for the TNF$^+$IFN-$\gamma^+$ double positive CD4 (Th1) cells (**Figure 2A**). For the CD8$^+$ TNF$^+$IFN-$\gamma^+$ T cells, two animals were above the threshold in the PLGA_TLR, SWE_TLR, and Hyogen groups (**Figure 2C**).

At D28, the SWE_TLR and Lipo_DDA:TDB groups were significantly higher than the control group for the percentage of CD4$^+$ TNF$^+$IFN-$\gamma^+$ T cells (**Figure 2D**) and the PLGA_TLR group was significantly higher than the control group for the percentage of CD4$^+$IL17A$^+$ (Th17) cells (**Figure 2E**). For the percentage of CD8$^+$ TNF$^+$IFN-$\gamma^+$ T cells, groups Lipo_AMP and lipo_DDA:TDB were significantly higher compared to the control animals (**Figure 2D**). Despite the lack of statistical significance, other vaccines also appeared to have induced specific T cell immunity in some animals. For the CD4$^+$ TNF$^+$IFN-$\gamma^+$ cells, three animals were above the 99% CI threshold in the Lipo_AMP group and two in the Hyogen group. For the CD8$^+$ TNF$^+$IFN-$\gamma^+$ cells, two pigs were above the 99% CI threshold in the Lipo_TLR group, five in the SWE_TLR group and three in the Hyogen group (**Figures 2D–F**).

When focusing on TNF$^-$IFN-$\gamma^+$-producing T cells, we found a high level of non-specific responses at both D14 and D28 in the unvaccinated group which "masked" the

vaccine induced responses (**Supplementary Figure 2**). Only Lipo_DDA:TDB induced a significant level of CD4$^+$ TNF$^+$IFN-$\gamma^-$-producing T cells at D28 (**Supplementary Figure 3**).

In conclusion, the vaccines SWE_TLR and Lipo_DDA:TDB induced a statistically significant Th1 driven T cell response. In the groups receiving the Hyogen and Lipo_AMP formulations, despite a trend suggesting stimulation of Th1 responses, the differences were not statistically significant in the current setting. Interestingly, the PLGA_TLR formulation was the only vaccine candidate which significantly induced a Th17 response, although only 3/6 animals in this group were above the threshold.

## Blood Transcriptional Modules Correlating to Vaccine-Induced Adaptive Immune Responses

In order to shed light on the immunological perturbations associated with adaptive immune responses, changes in transcriptional modules expression were correlated to the immune responses shown in **Figures 1, 2**.

For the early transcriptional responses (determined as modular changes between D0 and D1), a total of seven inflammatory, eight myeloid cell, three DC/antigen presentation and one IFN type I BTM correlated positively with the antibody response. Interestingly, none of these modules correlated with the CD4 T cell response, but some with the CD8 T cell response. For the late transcriptional responses (determined as modular changes between D1 and D7), a negative correlation was found for many BTM belonging to the families of modules reflecting innate immune responses. This was found again mainly for the antibody and CD8 T cell responses (**Figure 3**).

Main positive correlations of the CD4 T cell response were the D0 to D7 changes in cell cycle BTM (**Figure 4**). For the change of

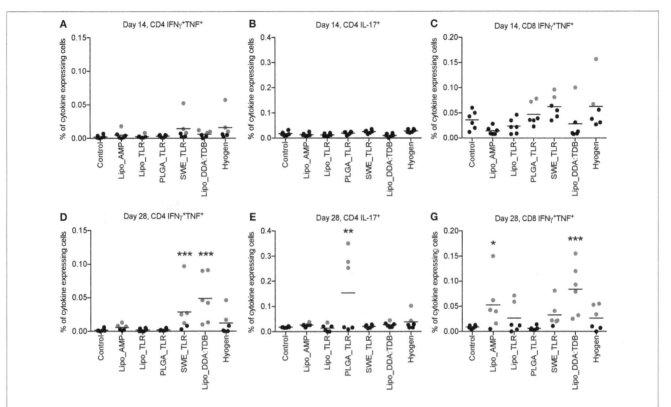

FIGURE 2 | *M. hyopneumoniae*-specific T cell responses induced following vaccination of pigs with vaccine candidates. Six animals per group were prime-boost vaccinated on D0 and D14. At D14 and D28, *M. hyopneumoniae*-specific T cells induced by the tested vaccines listed in the legend were determined by *in vitro* restimulation of PBMC from vaccinated animals followed by intracellular cytokine staining and multicolor flow cytometry. Following doublet exclusion, live cells were gated and the percentage of $IFN\gamma^+TNF^+$ double positive $CD4^+$ **(A,D)** and $CD8\beta^+$ **(C,F)** T cells as well as $IL-17A^+$ CD4 T cells **(B,E)** was determined. The mean values obtained from triplicate cultures for individual animals are shown. Positive animals are marked in red (defined as being above the 99% CI of the control group). Significance was calculated using two-way ANOVA followed by Dunnett's test (*$P < 0.05$; **$P < 0.01$; ***$P < 0.001$). PBMC, peripheral blood mononuclear cells.

cell cycle BTM between D1 and D7, we also found many modules correlating with antibody and T cell responses.

T/NK cell BTM upregulation between D0 and D7 correlated well with CD8 T cell responses. The induction of these BTM also correlated with antibody levels between D1 and D7 (**Figure 4**).

## Transcriptional Profiling of Vaccines

To better understand differences in the induction of immune responses between the vaccines, we next performed a transcription profiling. From the reads obtained, we first calculated the differentially expressed genes (DEG) using DSeq2, and then employed a two-factorial model, including the factors time point and group (vaccine vs. control), to identify genes differing between two time points in vaccinated animals compared to the controls. Next, we used ranked GSEA analyses using BTM as gene sets and ranked DEG between D0 and D1, D0 and D7, and D1 and D7 of each vaccine group. All data are shown in **Figures 5–8** and **Supplementary Figures 4, 5**, and summarized in **Table 2**.

### Inflammatory Responses

From D0 to D1, the Lipo_AMP formulation induced the highest number of inflammatory BTM, followed by the groups SWE_TLR and Lipo_DDA:TDB (**Figure 5**). Interestingly, in the PLGA_TLR group, no inflammatory BTM were induced and some even showed a downregulation. For the D0 to D7 comparison, again groups Lipo_AMP and SWE_TLR showed the highest upregulation of these BTM. For the D1 to D7 comparison, we found a downregulation of inflammatory modules in the Lipo_AMP, Lipo_TLR, and the Hyogen groups but not in the Lipo_DDA:TDB group, which still had BTM related to platelet activation overexpressed. In the PLGA_TLR group, eight BTM were upregulated indicating a delayed innate immune response. In summary, the three vaccines which induced significant T cell responses in terms of IFNγ/TNF secreting cells as well as antibody responses were those with the strongest positive early upregulation of inflammatory BTM, confirming the results obtained using the correlation analysis (**Figure 3**).

### IFN Type I Responses

With respect to IFN type I BTM, only vaccines which contained IFN inducers such as c-di-AMP (Lipo_AMP) and CpG (Lipo_TLR, SWE_TLR) induced an early IFN type I BTM response. The PLGA_TLR formulation contained the same TLR cocktail as SWE_TLR and Lipo_TLR, but was unable to induce such responses (**Figure 5**).

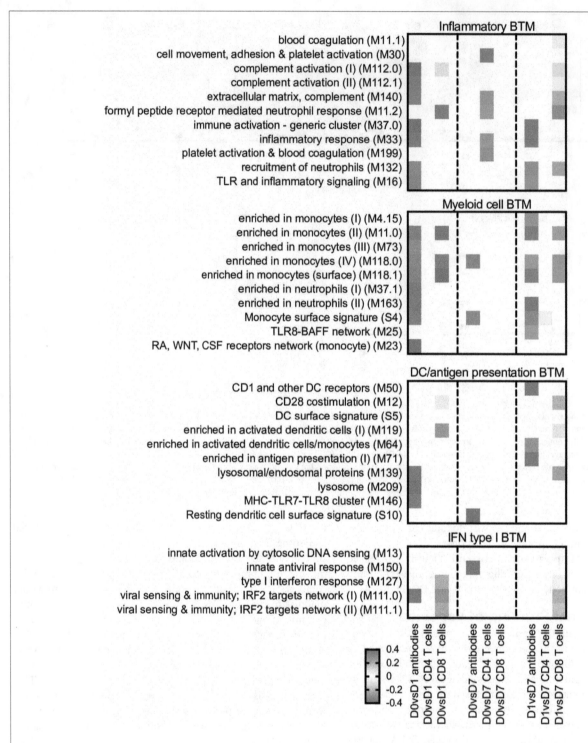

**FIGURE 3 |** Innate immune response BTM correlating with adaptive immune responses. Time-dependent changes in scores for BTM were determined using ssGSEA and then correlated to antibodies, *M. hyopneumoniae*-specific INFγ$^+$TNF$^+$ CD4 T cells and CD8 T cells. Pearson correlation coefficients for the BTM changes from D0 to D1 (D0 vs. D1), from D0 to D7 (D0 vs. D7), and from D1 to D7 (D1 vs. D7) are shown as heat maps. A $P < 0.05$ was used as cut-off. Red colors indicate positive and blue negative correlations. The BTM were grouped into inflammatory, myeloid cell, DC/antigen presentation and IFN type I BTM as previously described (34). BTM, blood transcriptional modules.

## Myeloid and DC/Antigen Presentation Responses

All vaccines with the exception of PLGA_TLR induced an early (D0 to D1) myeloid cell response (**Figure 6**). The number of BTM being modulated was the highest in the Lipo_AMP group, followed by the groups SWE_TLR, Lipo_DDA:TDB, and Hyogen (the latter two being very similar). The PLGA_TLR

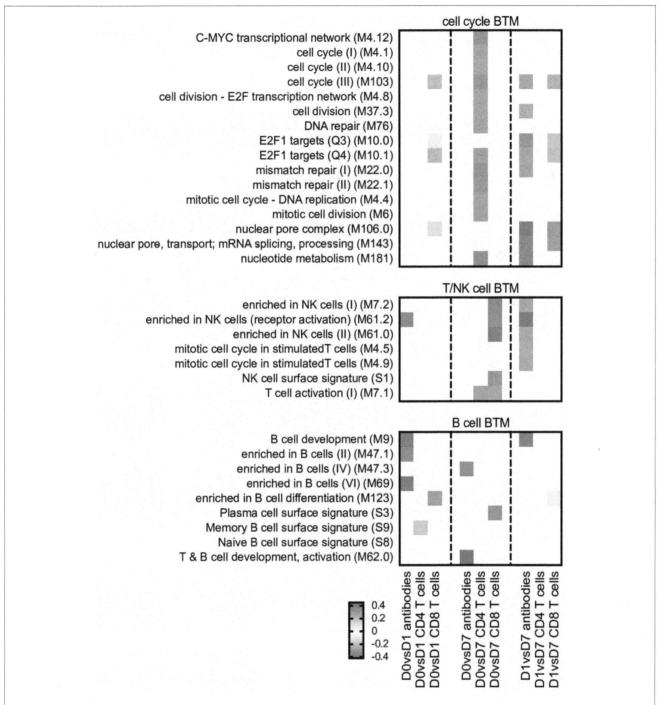

FIGURE 4 | Cell cycle and lymphocyte BTM correlating with adaptive immune responses. Time-dependent changes in scores for BTM were determined using ssGSEA and then correlated to antibodies, *M. hyopneumoniae*-specific INFγ⁺ TNF⁺ CD4 T cells and CD8 T cells. Pearson correlation coefficients for the BTM changes from D0 to D1 (D0 vs. D1), from D0 to D7 (D0 vs. D7) and from D1 to D7 (D1 vs. D7) are shown as heat maps. A $P < 0.05$ was used as cut-off. Red colors indicate positive and blue negative correlations. The BTM were grouped into cell cycle, T/NK cell and B cell BTM as previously described (34). BTM, blood transcriptional modules.

formulation actually had a negative influence on myeloid cell BTM response. Only Lipo_AMP, Lipo_TLR, and Hyogen induced a clear downregulation of these BTM from D1 to D7. This was interesting considering that a late D1 to D7 downregulation of myeloid cell BTM was found to strongly correlate with antibody and CD8 T cell responses (**Figure 3**). In

summary, the vaccines which induced good adaptive immune responses were also those which induced an early induction of many myeloid cell BTM.

The Lipo_AMP formulation was found to be the most potent to induce BTM relating to DC and antigen presentation from D0 to D1. Similar to the myeloid cell BTM, DC/antigen

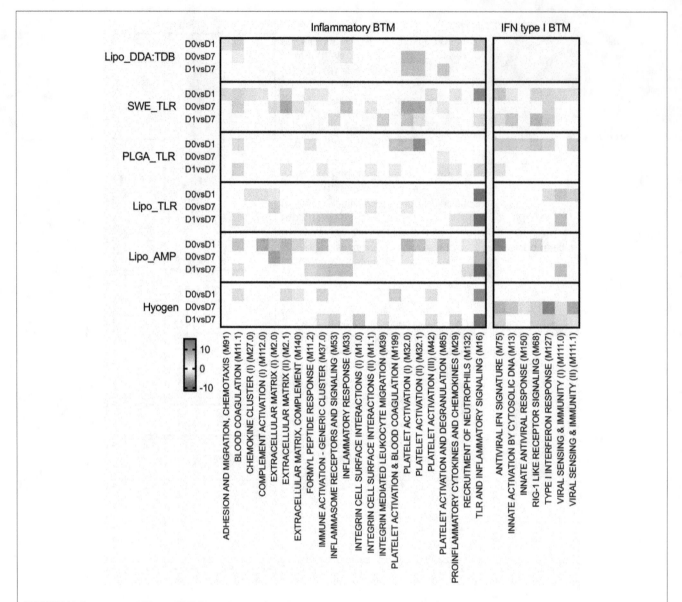

**FIGURE 5 |** Inflammatory and IFN type I BTM induced by vaccines. The heat maps show the vaccine-dependent induction of BTM activity determined for D0 to D1 (D0 vs. D1), for D0 to D7 (D0 vs. D7), and for D1 to D7 (D1 vs. D7) changes in the modules. The values shown were calculated by −log(P-value)*1 for positively enriched BTM and as −log(P-value)* −1 for negatively enriched BTM. A cut-off of an FDR of $q < 0.1$ was employed. Red colors indicate BTM upregulation and blue downregulation. BTM, blood transcriptional modules.

presentation BTM were downregulated from D1 to D7 by the formulations Lipo_AMP and Lipo_TLR, and to a lower extent by the Hyogen vaccine.

## Cell Cycle/Proliferation

The Lipo_DDA:TDB and SWE_TLR vaccines were found to downregulate, while PLGA_TLR upregulated cell cycle BTM from D0 to D1 (**Figure 7**). The two liposomal formulations Lipo_AMP and Lipo_TLR had a clear positive effect on these BTM at later time points (D0 to D7 and D1 to D7). Interestingly, the correlation analyses demonstrated a clear association between the late (D0 or D1 to D7) upregulation of these BTM and adaptive immune responses (**Figure 4**).

## B Cell BTM and T/NK Cell BTM

The Lipo_AMP, SWE_TLR, and Hyogen vaccines had an overall negative effect on the early expression (D0 to D1) of B-cell BTM (**Figure 8**). The SWE_TLR and Hyogen formulations were those to strongly induce these BTM at later time points (D1 to D7). Common BTM between the strong vaccines in terms of antibody responses were plasma cells and immunoglobulin (M156.0 and M156.1), which were overexpressed from D1 to D7. However, these BTM were not found significant in the correlation analyses (**Figure 4**).

For the T cell/NK cell BTM, a variable early downregulation by the more immunogenic vaccines Lipo_AMP, SWE_TLR, Lipo_DDA:TDB, and Hyogen was found. Only the liposomal

**TABLE 2 |** Overview of the immune responses induced by the *M. hyopneumoniae* bacterins.

| Vaccine formulation | Ab response (D28) | Th1 response (D14/D28) | Th17 response (D14/D28) | Early inflam. BTM | Early IFN type I BTM | Early myeloid cell/DC BTM | Late cell cycle BTM | Late T/NK-cell BTM | Late Ig BTM |
|---|---|---|---|---|---|---|---|---|---|
| Lipo_AMP | ++ | + | – | +++ | + | +++ | ++ | ++ | ++ |
| Lipo_TLR | + | + | – | + | + | + | ++ | ++ | ++ |
| PLGA_TLR | – | – | + | – | – | – | – | – | – |
| SWE_TLR | + | ++ | – | ++ | ++ | ++ | – | – | +++ |
| Lipo_DDA:TDB | ++ | +++ | – | + | – | ++ | – | – | ++ |
| Hyogen | ++ | + | – | + | – | ++ | – | – | ++ |

*Six animals per group were prime-boost vaccinated on D0 and D14. Ab, antibody; Th, T helper; BTM, blood transcriptional modules; early, upregulation from D0 to D1; late, upregulation from D1 to D7; –, none to weak; +, moderate; ++, strong; +++, very strong.*

formulations Lipo_AMP and Lipo_TLR induced a late D0/D1 to D7 upregulation of these modules, although many of those modules correlated to antibody and T cell responses (**Figure 4**).

## DISCUSSION

The present study assessed the safety and performed a detailed immunological profiling of five novel *M. hyopneumoniae* bacterin formulations. We included as well the commercial vaccine Hyogen® in our study. Hyogen® is a recently developed bacterin based on a virulent *M. hyopneumoniae* field isolate with a TLR4 ligand as immunostimulant, and in that way comparable with our experimental bacterin formulations.

In terms of side effects, formulations Lipo_AMP, Lipo_TLR, and SWE_TLR induced a significant but transient increase in rectal body temperature shortly (4 h) after vaccination. This was also observed for the Hyogen® vaccine, and comparable observations were made by Llopart et al. (50) after two shot vaccination against *M. hyopneumoniae* with the commercial vaccine Mypravac suis® (HIPRA, Amer, Spain). Fever beginning a few hours after vaccination and persisting for 24 to 36 h is the result of an excessive induction of pro-inflammatory cytokines by the vaccine (51, 52). Systemic reactions of such kind are commonly reported and considered as "normal toxicity" associated with vaccination (52).

Overall, the ISR occasionally observed in all IM vaccinated groups and at the IM injection site of group Lipo_DDA:TDB were mild and resolved quickly. Transient redness and swelling at vaccination sites were also reported in other *M. hyopneumoniae* vaccination studies (53–55). Such local reactions often occur after parenteral administration of adjuvanted vaccines and are tolerated in terms of safety (52). Microscopically, mild focal chronic inflammation was observed in all IM injected groups, including the control group, indicating that these findings were probably caused by the tissue damage due to needle insertion and injection of fluid, and not by the administered vaccine formulation. Nevertheless, prolonged mild to moderate ISR were observed in all pigs from group Lipo_DDA:TDB at the ID injection site and histopathological examination of this injection site at D28 of the study showed a severe foreign body granuloma in five pigs. Local reactions of such kind could result in carcass trim losses at slaughter and are therefore considered to be a

relevant adverse side effect of vaccination (51, 56). The transient ISR at the IM injection site of this vaccine group suggests that the prolonged and rather severe ISR is at least partially due to the ID administration. However, this cannot be stated with certainty as there was no control group ID injected with sterile PBS.

Two weeks after booster vaccination, the commercial vaccine Hyogen® as well as the vaccines Lipo_DDA:TDB and Lipo_AMP induced a strong humoral response. Vaccine formulations SWE_TLR and Lipo_TLR generated a moderate serological response, whereas for the PLGA_TLR formulation only two animals seroconverted. Nevertheless, as we do not know the antigen payload of the Hyogen® vaccine, we cannot directly compare its efficacy to the experimental vaccines. Although systemic antibodies are considered to play a minor role in protection against EP (5, 13), high levels of serum antibodies induced by vaccination can be an easy and practical tool to confirm successful vaccination in the field (57). It can also be expected that high levels of IgG will only be induced with significant induction of Th cell activation. We only found IgA antibodies in BAL fluid of one pig injected with the SWE_TLR vaccine. This is not surprising considering the parenteral vaccine administration, and is in line with previous studies showing IgA in BAL fluid of vaccinated pigs only after challenge (13, 14). Future studies are required to investigate the potential of adjuvants to induce both local and systemic immune responses after mucosal application of the vaccine. For example, this has been achieved for inactivated viruses using nanoparticle-based delivery (58, 59). Nevertheless, the absence of detectable IgA antibodies in BAL fluid from vaccinated pigs does not exclude priming of the immune system for such responses as vaccinated animals had higher mucosal IgA responses compared to unvaccinated animals following challenge (13, 14). Although we did not measure *M. hyopneumoniae*-specific IgG in BAL fluid, it can reach the alveolar lumen by transudation from the blood and might also play a role in protection against disease. In fact, the implementation of the human parenterally-administered conjugate vaccine against type B *Haemophilus influenza* resulted in a reduction of carriage and a reduced risk of horizontal transmission. This was hypothesized to be due to such IgG (60, 61).

Circulating *M. hyopneumoniae*-specific TNF⁺IFN-γ⁺ CD4 and CD8 T cells were identified in particular in the SWE_TLR,

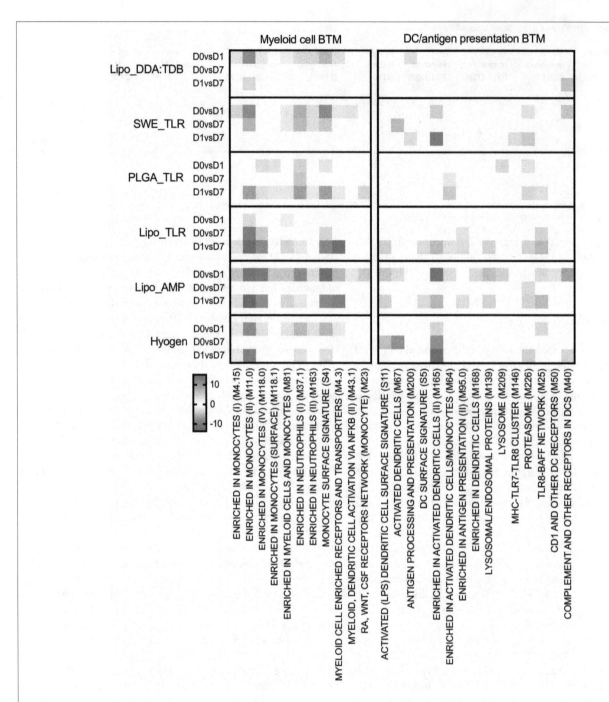

**FIGURE 6 |** Myeloid cell and DC/antigen presentation BTM induced by vaccines. The heat maps show the vaccine-dependent induction of BTM activity determined for D0 to D1 (D0 vs. D1), for D0 to D7 (D0 vs. D7), and for D1 to D7 (D1 vs. D7) changes in the modules. The values shown were calculated by −log(P-value)*1 for positively enriched BTM and as −log(P-value)* −1 for negatively enriched BTM. A cut-off of an FDR of $q < 0.1$ was employed. Red colors indicate BTM upregulation and blue downregulation. BTM, blood transcriptional modules.

Lipo_DDA:TDB, and Lipo_AMP groups. However, also in the Lipo_TLR and Hyogen groups a few animals appeared to have such cells. Such Th1 response is expected to promote cell-mediated immunity via activation of NK cells and macrophages, as well as by inducing antigen-specific cytotoxic immunity (CD8 cells) (62). While such responses could participate in protection against *M. hyopneumoniae,* pro-inflammatory CD4 Th responses

might also mediate lung damage and clinical disease (63). While the classical effector functions of CD8 T cells are likely irrelevant for the immune response against a *Mycoplasma* species that is not an intracellular organism, mouse models indicate that CD8 T cells are suspected to dampen inflammatory responses mediated by CD4[+] Th cells (24, 64). Furthermore, CD8 T cells contribute to Th1 responses, which based on mouse models could

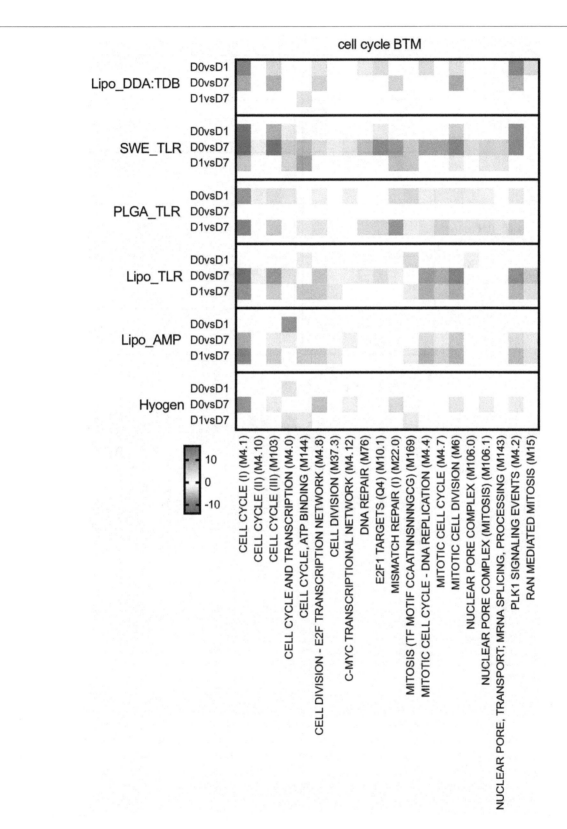

**FIGURE 7 |** Cell cycle BTM induced by vaccines. The heat maps show the vaccine-dependent induction of BTM activity determined for D0 to D1 (D0 vs. D1), for D0 to D7 (D0 vs. D7), and for D1 to D7 (D1 vs. D7) changes in the modules. The values shown were calculated by −log(P-value)*1 for positively enriched BTM and as −log(P-value)* −1 for negatively enriched BTM. A cut-off of an FDR of $q < 0.1$ was employed. Red colors indicate BTM upregulation and blue downregulation. BTM, blood transcriptional modules.

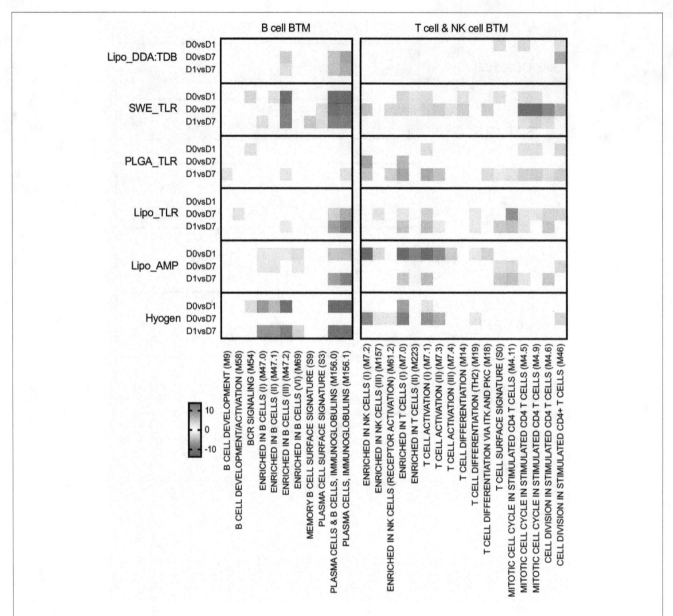

**FIGURE 8 |** B cell and T/NK cell BTM induced by vaccines. The heat maps show the vaccine-dependent induction of BTM activity determined for D0 to D1 (D0 vs. D1), for D0 to D7 (D0 vs. D7), and for D1 to D7 (D1 vs. D7) changes in the modules. The values shown were calculated by −log(P-value)*1 for positively enriched BTM and as −log(P-value)* −1 for negatively enriched BTM. A cut-off of an FDR of $q < 0.1$ was employed. Red colors indicate BTM upregulation and blue downregulation. BTM, blood transcriptional modules.

be protective against *Mycoplasma* infection. Based on this their induction by the present vaccines could be viewed as positive.

In this study, the PLGA_TLR formulation was the best at inducing a Th17 response, although in only three of six animals a response was detected. The lack of detection of IL-17-producing Th cells does not mean a lack of priming, as activated/memory T cells could have left the blood circulation. Nevertheless, future studies are required to confirm the ability of this formulation to induce Th17 responses. It has been suggested that Th17 cells may play a major role in the protection of the lung mucosa against respiratory pathogens by recruiting other immune cells to the inflamed mucosa for pathogen clearance (65) and by promoting

IgA secretion into the airway lumen (66). Similar to other species, porcine IL-17-producing cell differentiation can be induced *in vitro* by TGF-β in the presence of IL-6 and/or IL-1β (67), and *in vivo* during several extracellular bacterial infections (68–70).

In addition to these classical vaccinology readouts we also applied a transcriptomics-based approach to obtain a more precise profile of the type of immune response induced by our vaccine candidates, and to better understand the immune modulatory effector functions needed for induction of a protective immune response after vaccination. We identified a number of BTM correlating to adaptive immune responses which have been previously reported in human and sheep studies (25, 26, 28–30, 34). This was an early upregulation of monocytes BTM, such as S4, M11.0, M118.0, and M118.1, neutrophil BTM such as M163 and M37.1, modules related to inflammation and pathogen sensing such as M16, M146, and M37.0, and BTM related to antigen presentation such as M147, M139, and M209. Interestingly, many of these modules strongly negatively correlated with the antibody and CD8 T cell responses from D1 to D7. This suggests that a strong innate immune response in the first 24 h followed immediately by a down-regulation is associated with the initiation of a stronger adaptive immune response. This inverse correlation was also seen at later time points in a previous study using sheep (34). Similar to previous reports (25, 28, 29, 34) a few cell cycle, B cell, and T/NK cell BTM upregulated in the first 24 h after vaccination negatively correlated with adaptive immune responses. While these correlations were mainly found for the antibody responses, most of the modules correlating to CD4 T cell responses were found to be cell cycle BTM upregulated between D0 and D7. This was also reported by Qi et al. (30) who found a strong association of cell cycle and DNA repair BTM to virus-specific T cells (common BTM are M4.4, M4.12, M103, M76, M22.0, M22.1). The upregulation of T/NK cell modules between D0 and D7 positively correlated to CD8 T cell responses, as well as to the antibody responses between D1 and D7. Altogether, these results confirm the importance of early innate immune responses in the myeloid and DC cell compartment within the first 24 h for a potent vaccine-induced adaptive immune response. Clearly, the upregulation of myeloid cell and DC/antigen presentation BTM could partially reflect changes in cell population, i.e., those that are caused by enhanced hematopoiesis following stimulation of the innate immune system (71). Nevertheless, in a previous study we were unable to identify a significant increase in the circulation of monocytes, indicating that the BTM changes reflect more than changes in cell populations (34). This study also demonstrates that the main upregulated BTM from D0 or D1 to D7 correlating to adaptive immune responses are cell cycle and T/NK cell BTM. This could reflect the first recirculation of activated T cells leaving the lymph nodes that drain the site of vaccine injection.

After obtaining this information, we went back and analyzed which BTM were actually induced by the vaccines. While all vaccines, with the exception of the PLGA_TLR formulation, induced early upregulation of inflammatory, myeloid cell and DC/antigen presentation BTM, the Lipo_AMP vaccine appeared to be the most potent in stimulating these early innate immune responses. When it came to the later upregulation of cell cycle and T/NK cell BTM, this was only a feature of the Lipo_AMP and the Lipo_TLR vaccines. This was surprising considering that the Lipo_TLR was not found to be a particularly potent formulation. Furthermore, the more potent vaccines, such as Lipo_DDA:TDB and SWE_TLR, actually induced a downregulation of these BTM. While this requires further investigations, our current interpretation is that there could be differences in the kinetics of activated lymphocyte recirculation, which would have required more frequent sampling to detect. Furthermore, it should again be noted that T cell recirculation and the presence of memory

T cells in the circulation is a dynamic process. Therefore, a lack of antigen-specific T cells in the peripheral blood cannot be interpreted as a lack of priming. On the other hand, the BTM profile induced by the PLGA_TLR vaccine was in line with its rather poor immunogenicity.

Overall, our data demonstrate the potency of cationic liposome formulations as delivery system to induce potent B and T cell responses using inactivated *M. hyopneumoniae* as antigen. Cationic liposomes may have the advantage of a more targeted delivery of the immunostimulant and antigen to DC, and also have been shown to enhance the retention time in lymph nodes (72, 73). This may favor strong T cell responses. Although we did not specifically address the requirement of an immunostimulant for liposomal vaccines, it is well-described that immunogenicity of liposomal vaccines can be enhanced (72). Our data indicate that both AMP and TDB appear to be good candidate molecules for the *M. hyopneumoniae* vaccine. The transcriptomic profile of the Lipo_AMP vaccine was particularly impressive as it corresponded best to a BTM profile known to correlate with adaptive immune responses. From all experimental formulations, Lipo_DDA:TDB induced the highest antibody and Th1 responses. Unfortunately, this formulation caused a prolonged ISR after ID administration. Applying this vaccine only via the IM route could resolve this safety issue, but it would be probably associated with a loss of immunogenicity (74). In contrast, the PLGA-based MP formulation did not appear to be suitable to induce good antibody and Th1 responses, possibly in part due to a delayed TLR ligand delivery to innate immune cells. Nevertheless, the fact that this vaccine induced IL17-producing Th cells at least in some animals is interesting and should be kept in mind for future investigations. The present work also identified the SWE_TLR as an interesting vaccine candidate, as it induced a robust Th1 response and IgA in BAL fluid of one animal. This vaccine has the advantage of being easy to produce. Moreover, O/W formulations are known to have a much better safety profile as W/O vaccines (72). Future studies are required to address which immunostimulant is best suited for a SWE adjuvant in the pig. This will require the use of a selection of identical antigens.

In conclusion, the present study identified promising *M. hyopneumoniae* bacterin formulations to be selected for future challenge experiments, based on their ability to induce strong innate immune responses and robust Th1 or Th17 responses. We also demonstrated the utility of transcriptome-based systems immunology analyses to unravel the mechanistic events leading to the stimulation of adaptive immune responses after vaccine injection. While the present study was not designed to identify the effects of formulation and immunostimulants but rather to select the most promising candidates from five novel vaccines, the information provided on these vaccine formulations will also be very valuable for other vaccines and future adjuvant research.

## AUTHOR CONTRIBUTIONS

AMM, GA, OG-N, ROB, BD, and AM performed the animal experimentation, acquisition and analyses of data. VJ, CG, CB-Q, and NC designed, produced, and characterized the vaccines. IK, RB, and AS performed the bioinformatic analyses. DM, CB-Q, FB, FH, and AS designed and supervised the overall project.

## FUNDING

This study was financially supported by the European H2020 Project SAPHIR (Project No. 633184). BD is supported by a postdoctoral grant of the Research Foundation—Flanders (FWO-Vlaanderen).

## ACKNOWLEDGMENTS

We are grateful to Muriel Fragnière and Tosso Leeb from the Next Generation Sequencing Platform of the University of Bern, and Corinne Hug from the Institute of Virology and Immunology for the RNA preparation and sequencing. We would like to thank as well Dr. Ilias Chantziaras from the Porcine Health Management Unit of the University of Ghent for his statistical advice.

## REFERENCES

1. Rautiainen E, Virtala AM, Wallgren P, Saloniemi H. Varying effects of infections with *Mycoplasma hyopneumoniae* on the weight gain recorded in three different multisource fattening pig herds. *J Vet Med Ser B*. (2000) 47:461–9. doi: 10.1046/j.1439-0450.2000.00370.x

2. Maes D, Segales J, Meyns T, Sibila M, Pieters M, Haesebrouck F. Control of *Mycoplasma hyopneumoniae* infections in pigs. *Vet Microbiol*. (2008) 126:297–309. doi: 10.1016/j.vetmic.2007.09.008

3. Martínez J, Peris B, Gómez EA, Corpa JM. The relationship between infectious and non-infectious herd factors with pneumonia at slaughter and productive parameters in fattening pigs. *Vet J*. (2009) 179:240–6. doi: 10.1016/j.tvjl.2007.10.006

4. Maes D, Sibila M, Kuhnert P, Segalés J, Haesebrouck F, Pieters M. Update on *Mycoplasma hyopneumoniae* infections in pigs: knowledge gaps for improved disease control. *Transbound Emerg Dis*. (2018) 65:110–24. doi: 10.1111/tbed.12677

5. Thacker EL, Thacker BJ, Boettcher TB, Jayappa H. Comparison of antibody production, lymphocyte stimulation, and protection induced by four commercial *Mycoplasma hyopneumoniae* bacterins. *J Swine Health Prod*. (1998) 6:107–12.

6. Meyns T, Dewulf J, De Kruif A, Calus D, Haesebrouck F, Maes D. Comparison of transmission of *Mycoplasma hyopneumoniae* in vaccinated and non-vaccinated populations. *Vaccine*. (2006) 24:7081–6. doi: 10.1016/j.vaccine.2006.07.004

7. Villarreal I, Meyns T, Dewulf J, Vranckx K, Calus D, Pasmans F, et al. The effect of vaccination on the transmission of *Mycoplasma hyopneumoniae* in pigs under field conditions. *Vet J*. (2011) 188:48–52. doi: 10.1016/j.tvjl.2010.04.024

8. Goodwin R, Whittlestone P. Production of enzootic pneumonia in pigs with an agent grown in tissue culture from the natural disease. *Br J Exp Pathol*. (1963) 44:291.

9. Stakenborg T, Vicca J, Butaye P, Maes D, Peeters J, De Kruif A, et al. The diversity of *Mycoplasma hyopneumoniae* within and between herds using pulsed-field gel electrophoresis. *Vet Microbiol*. (2005) 109:29–36. doi: 10.1016/j.vetmic.2005.05.005

10. Villarreal I, Vranckx K, Calus D, Pasmans F, Haesebrouck F, Maes D. Effect of challenge of pigs previously immunised with inactivated vaccines containing homologous and heterologous *Mycoplasma hyopneumoniae* strains. *BMC Vet Res*. (2012) 8:2. doi: 10.1186/1746-6148-8-2

11. Jensen C, Ersbøll AK, Nielsen JP. A meta-analysis comparing the effect of vaccines against *Mycoplasma hyopneumoniae* on daily weight gain in pigs. *Prev Vet Med*. (2002) 54:265–78. doi: 10.1016/S0167-5877(02)00005-3

12. Haesebrouck F, Pasmans F, Chiers K, Maes D, Ducatelle R, Decostere A. Efficacy of vaccines against bacterial diseases in swine: what can we expect? *Vet Microbiol*. (2004) 100:255–68. doi: 10.1016/j.vetmic.2004.03.002

13. Djordjevic S, Eamens G, Romalis L, Nicholls P, Taylor V, Chin J. Serum and mucosal antibody responses and protection in pigs vaccinated against *Mycoplasma hyopneumoniae* with vaccines containing a denatured membrane antigen pool and adjuvant. *Austr Veter J*. (1997) 75:504–11. doi: 10.1111/j.1751-0813.1997.tb14383.x

14. Thacker EL, Thacker BJ, Kuhn M, Hawkins PA, Waters WR. Evaluation of local and systemic immune responses induced by intramuscular injection of a *Mycoplasma hyopneumoniae* bacterin to pigs. *Am J Vet Res*. (2000) 61:1384–9. doi: 10.2460/ajvr.2000.61.1384

15. Marchioro SB, Maes D, Flahou B, Pasmans F, Sacristán RDP, Vranckx K, et al. Local and systemic immune responses in pigs intramuscularly injected with an inactivated *Mycoplasma hyopneumoniae* vaccine. *Vaccine*. (2013) 31:1305–11. doi: 10.1016/j.vaccine.2012.12.068

16. Seo HW, Han K, Oh Y, Park C, Choo EJ, Kim S-H, et al. Comparison of cell-mediated immunity induced by three commercial single-dose *Mycoplasma hyopneumoniae* bacterins in pigs. *J Vet Med Sci*. (2013) 75:245–7. doi: 10.1292/jvms.12-0292

17. Martelli P, Saleri R, Cavalli V, De Angelis E, Ferrari L, Benetti M, et al. Systemic and local immune response in pigs intradermally and intramuscularly injected with inactivated *Mycoplasma hyopneumoniae* vaccines. *Vet Microbiol*. (2014) 168:357–64. doi: 10.1016/j.vetmic.2013.11.025

18. Auray G, Keller I, Python S, Gerber M, Bruggmann R, Ruggli N, et al. Characterization and transcriptomic analysis of porcine blood conventional and plasmacytoid dendritic cells reveals striking species-specific differences. *J Immunol*. (2016) 197:4791–806. doi: 10.4049/jimmunol.1600672

19. Braun RO, Python S, Summerfield A. Porcine B cell subset responses to toll-like receptor ligands. *Front Immunol*. (2017) 8:1044. doi: 10.3389/fimmu.2017.01044

20. Libanova R, Becker PD, Guzmán CA. Cyclic di-nucleotides: new era for small molecules as adjuvants. *Microb Biotechnol*. (2012) 5:168–76. doi: 10.1111/j.1751-7915.2011.00306.x

21. Tandrup Schmidt S, Foged C, Korsholm KS, Rades T, Christensen D. Liposome-based adjuvants for subunit vaccines: formulation strategies for subunit antigens and immunostimulators. *Pharmaceutics*. (2016) 8:E7. doi: 10.3390/pharmaceutics8010007

22. Vicca J, Stakenborg T, Maes D, Butaye P, Peeters J, De Kruif A, et al. Evaluation of virulence of *Mycoplasma hyopneumoniae* field isolates. *Vet Microbiol*. (2003) 97:177–90. doi: 10.1016/j.vetmic.2003.08.008

23. Calus D, Baele M, Meyns T, De Kruif A, Butaye P, Decostere A, et al. Protein variability among *Mycoplasma hyopneumoniae* isolates. *Vet Microb.* (2007) 120:284–91. doi: 10.1016/j.vetmic.2006.10.040

24. Dobbs NA, Odeh AN, Sun X, Simecka JW. The multifaceted role of T cell-mediated immunity in pathogenesis and resistance to *Mycoplasma* respiratory disease. *Curr Trends Immunol.* (2009) 10:1–19.

25. Li S, Rouphael N, Duraisingham S, Romero-Steiner S, Presnell S, Davis C, et al. Molecular signatures of antibody responses derived from a systems biology study of five human vaccines. *Nat Immunol.* (2014) 15:195–204. doi: 10.1038/ni.2789

26. Matsumiya M, Harris SA, Satti I, Stockdale L, Tanner R, O'shea MK, et al. Inflammatory and myeloid-associated gene expression before and one day after infant vaccination with MVA85A correlates with induction of a T cell response. *BMC Infect Dis.* (2014) 14:314. doi: 10.1186/1471-2334-14-314

27. Hagan T, Nakaya HI, Subramaniam S, Pulendran B. Systems vaccinology: enabling rational vaccine design with systems biological approaches. *Vaccine.* (2015) 33:5294–301. doi: 10.1016/j.vaccine.2015.03.072

28. Nakaya HI, Hagan T, Duraisingham SS, Lee EK, Kwissa M, Rouphael N, et al. Systems analysis of *Immunity* to influenza vaccination across multiple years and in diverse populations reveals shared molecular signatures. *Immunity.* (2015) 43:1186–98. doi: 10.1016/j.immuni.2015.11.012

29. Nakaya HI, Clutterbuck E, Kazmin D, Wang L, Cortese M, Bosinger SE, et al. Systems biology of immunity to MF59-adjuvanted versus nonadjuvanted trivalent seasonal influenza vaccines in early childhood. *Proc Natl Acad Sci USA.* (2016) 113:1853–8. doi: 10.1073/pnas.1519690113

30. Qi Q, Cavanagh MM, Le Saux S, Wagar LE, Mackey S, Hu J, et al. Defective T memory cell differentiation after varicella zoster vaccination in older individuals. *PLoS Pathog.* (2016) 12:e1005892. doi: 10.1371/journal.ppat.1005892

31. Hou J, Wang S, Jia M, Li D, Liu Y, Li Z, et al. A systems vaccinology approach reveals temporal transcriptomic changes of immune responses to the yellow fever 17D vaccine. *J Immunol.* (2017) 199:1476–89. doi: 10.4049/jimmunol.1700083

32. Kazmin D, Nakaya HI, Lee EK, Johnson MJ, Van Der Most R, Van Den Berg RA, et al. Systems analysis of protective immune responses to RTS,S malaria vaccination in humans. *Proc Natl Acad Sci USA.* (2017) 114:2425–30. doi: 10.1073/pnas.1621489114

33. Li S, Sullivan NL, Rouphael N, Yu T, Banton S, Maddur MS, et al. Metabolic phenotypes of response to vaccination in humans. *Cell.* (2017) 169:862–877.e17. doi: 10.1016/j.cell.2017.04.026

34. Braun RO, Brunner L, Wyler K, Auray G, Garcia-Nicolas O, Python S, et al. System immunology-based identification of blood transcriptional modules correlating to antibody responses in sheep. *NPJ Vaccines.* (2018) 3:41. doi: 10.1038/s41541-018-0078-0

35. Calus D, Maes D, Vranckx K, Villareal I, Pasmans F, Haesebrouck F. Validation of ATP luminometry for rapid and accurate titration of *Mycoplasma hyopneumoniae* in Friis medium and a comparison with the color changing units assay. *J Microbiol Methods.* (2010) 83:335–40. doi: 10.1016/j.mimet.2010.09.001

36. Christensen D, Foged C, Rosenkrands I, Nielsen HM, Andersen P, Agger EM. Trehalose preserves DDA/TDB liposomes and their adjuvant effect during freeze-drying. *Biochim Biophys Acta Biomembr.* (2007) 1768:2120–9. doi: 10.1016/j.bbamem.2007.05.009

37. Barnier-Quer C, Elsharkawy A, Romeijn S, Kros A, Jiskoot W. Adjuvant effect of cationic liposomes for subunit influenza vaccine: influence of antigen loading method, cholesterol and immune modulators. *Pharmaceutics.* (2013) 5:392–410. doi: 10.3390/pharmaceutics5030392

38. Singh M, Briones M, Ott G, O'hagan D. Cationic microparticles: a potent delivery system for DNA vaccines. *Proc Natl Acad Sci.* (2000) 97:811–6. doi: 10.1073/pnas.97.2.811

39. Ventura R, Brunner L, Heriyanto B, De Boer O, O'hara M, Huynh C, et al. Technology transfer of an oil-in-water vaccine-adjuvant for strengthening pandemic influenza preparedness in Indonesia. *Vaccine.* (2013) 31:1641–5. doi: 10.1016/j.vaccine.2012.07.074

40. Dietrich J, Andreasen LV, Andersen P, Agger EM. Inducing dose sparing with inactivated polio virus formulated in adjuvant CAF01. *PLoS ONE.* (2014) 9:e100879. doi: 10.1371/journal.pone.0100879

41. Hannan P, Bhogal B, Fish J. Tylosin tartrate and tiamutilin effects on experimental piglet pneumonia induced with pneumonic pig lung homogenate containing mycoplasmas, bacteria and viruses. *Res Vet Sci.* (1982) 33:76–88. doi: 10.1016/S0034-5288(18)32364-6

42. Stärk KD, Nicolet J, Frey J. Detection of *Mycoplasma hyopneumoniae* by air sampling with a nested PCR assay. *Appl Environ Microbiol.* (1998) 64:543–8.

43. Sacristán RDP, Sierens A, Marchioro S, Vangroenweghe F, Jourquin J, Labarque G, et al. Efficacy of early *Mycoplasma hyopneumoniae* vaccination against mixed respiratory disease in older fattening pigs. *Vet Rec.* (2014) 174:197. doi: 10.1136/vr.101597

44. Bereiter M, Young T, Joo H, Ross R. Evaluation of the ELISA and comparison to the complement fixation test and radial immunodiffusion enzyme assay for detection of antibodies against *Mycoplasma hyopneumoniae* in swine serum. *Vet Microbiol.* (1990) 25:177–92. doi: 10.1016/0378-1135(90)90075-7

45. Kim D, Langmead B, Salzberg SL. HISAT: a fast spliced aligner with low memory requirements. *Nat Methods.* (2015) 12:357. doi: 10.1038/nmeth.3317

46. Love MI, Huber W, Anders S. Moderated estimation of fold change and dispersion for RNA-seq data with DESeq2. *Genome Biol.* (2014) 15:550. doi: 10.1186/s13059-014-0550-8

47. Subramanian A, Tamayo P, Mootha VK, Mukherjee S, Ebert BL, Gillette MA, et al. Gene set enrichment analysis: a knowledge-based approach for interpreting genome-wide expression profiles. *Proc Natl Acad Sci USA.* (2005) 102:15545–50. doi: 10.1073/pnas.0506580102

48. Li S, Nakaya HI, Kazmin DA, Oh JZ, Pulendran B. Systems biological approaches to measure and understand vaccine immunity in humans. *Semin Immunol.* (2013) 25:209–18. doi: 10.1016/j.smim.2013.05.003

49. Barbie DA, Tamayo P, Boehm JS, Kim SY, Moody SE, Dunn IF, et al. Systematic RNA interference reveals that oncogenic KRAS-driven cancers require TBK1. *Nature.* (2009) 462:108–12. doi: 10.1038/nature08460

50. Llopart D, Casal J, Clota J, Navarra I, March R, Riera P, et al. Evaluation of the field efficacy and safety of a *Mycoplasma hyopneumoniae* vaccine in finishing pigs. *PIG J.* (2002) 49:70–83.

51. Roth JA. Mechanistic bases for adverse vaccine reactions and vaccine failures. *Adv Vet Med.* (1999) 41:681–700. doi: 10.1016/S0065-3519(99)80053-6

52. Meyer EK. Vaccine-associated adverse events. *Vet Clin Small Anim Pract.* (2001) 31:493–514. doi: 10.1016/S0195-5616(01)50604-X

53. Jones GF, Rapp-Gabrielson V, Wilke R, Thacker EL, Thacker BJ, Gergen L, et al. Intradermal vaccination for *Mycoplasma hyopneumoniae.* *J Swine Health Product.* (2005) 13:19–27.

54. Galliher-Beckley A, Pappan L, Madera R, Burakova Y, Waters A, Nickles M, et al. Characterization of a novel oil-in-water emulsion adjuvant for swine influenza virus and *Mycoplasma hyopneumoniae* vaccines. *Vaccine.* (2015) 33:2903–8. doi: 10.1016/j.vaccine.2015.04.065

55. Beffort L, Weiß C, Fiebig K, Jolie R, Ritzmann M, Eddicks M. Field study on the safety and efficacy of intradermal versus intramuscular vaccination against *Mycoplasma hyopneumoniae.* *Vet Rec.* (2017) 181:348. doi: 10.1136/vr.104466

56. Spickler AR, Roth JA. Adjuvants in veterinary vaccines: modes of action and adverse effects. *J Vet Int Med.* (2003) 17:273–81. doi: 10.1111/j.1939-1676.2003.tb02448.x

57. Xiong Q, Wei Y, Xie H, Feng Z, Gan Y, Wang C, et al. Effect of different adjuvant formulations on the immunogenicity and protective effect of a live *Mycoplasma hyopneumoniae* vaccine after intramuscular inoculation. *Vaccine.* (2014) 32:3445–51. doi: 10.1016/j.vaccine.2014.03.071

58. Binjawadagi B, Dwivedi V, Manickam C, Ouyang K, Wu Y, Lee LJ, et al. Adjuvanted poly(lactic-co-glycolic) acid nanoparticle-entrapped inactivated porcine reproductive and respiratory syndrome virus vaccine elicits cross-protective immune response in pigs. *Int J Nanomedicine.* (2014) 9:679–94. doi: 10.2147/IJN.S56127

59. Dhakal S, Renu S, Ghimire S, Shaan Lakshmanappa Y, Hogshead BT, Feliciano-Ruiz N, et al. Mucosal immunity and protective efficacy of intranasal inactivated influenza vaccine is improved by chitosan nanoparticle delivery in pigs. *Front Immunol.* (2018) 9:934. doi: 10.3389/fimmu.2018.00934

60. Kauppi M, Eskola J, Käyhty H. Anti-capsular polysaccharide antibody concentrations in saliva after immunization with *Haemophilus influenzae* type b conjugate vaccines. *Pediatr Infect Dis J.* (1995) 14:286–94. doi: 10.1097/00006454-199504000-00008

61. Wenger JD. Epidemiology of *Haemophilus influenzae* type b disease and impact of *Haemophilus influenzae* type b conjugate vaccines in

the United States and Canada. *Pediatr Infect Dis J.* (1998) 17:S132–6. doi: 10.1097/00006454-199809001-00008

62. Schroder K, Hertzog PJ, Ravasi T, Hume DA. Interferon-γ: an overview of signals, mechanisms and functions. *J Leukocyte Biol.* (2004) 75:163–89. doi: 10.1189/jlb.0603252

63. Jones HP, Simecka JW. T lymphocyte responses are critical determinants in the pathogenesis and resistance to *Mycoplasma* respiratory disease. *Front Biosci.* (2003) 8:930–45. doi: 10.2741/1098

64. Jones HP, Tabor L, Sun X, Woolard MD, Simecka JW. Depletion of CD8+ T cells exacerbates CD4+ Th cell-associated inflammatory lesions during murine *Mycoplasma* respiratory disease. *J Immunol.* (2002) 168:3493–501. doi: 10.4049/jimmunol.168.7.3493

65. Liang SC, Long AJ, Bennett F, Whitters MJ, Karim R, Collins M, et al. An IL-17F/A heterodimer protein is produced by mouse Th17 cells and induces airway neutrophil recruitment. *J Immunol.* (2007) 179:7791–9. doi: 10.4049/jimmunol.179.11.7791

66. Jaffar Z, Ferrini ME, Herritt LA, Roberts K. Cutting edge: lung mucosal Th17-mediated responses induce polymeric Ig receptor expression by the airway epithelium and elevate secretory IgA levels. *J Immunol.* (2009) 182:4507–11. doi: 10.4049/jimmunol.0900237

67. Kiros TG, Van Kessel J, Babiuk LA, Gerdts V. Induction, regulation and physiological role of IL-17 secreting helper T-cells isolated from PBMC, thymus, and lung lymphocytes of young pigs. *Vet Immunol Immunopathol.* (2011) 144:448–54. doi: 10.1016/j.vetimm.2011.08.021

68. Luo Y, Van Nguyen U, De La Fe Rodriguez PY, Devriendt B, Cox E. F4+ ETEC infection and oral immunization with F4 fimbriae elicits an IL-17-dominated immune response. *Vet Res.* (2015) 46:121. doi: 10.1186/s13567-015-0264-2

69. De Witte C, Devriendt B, Flahou B, Bosschem I, Ducatelle R, Smet A, et al. *Helicobacter suis* induces changes in gastric inflammation and acid secretion markers in pigs of different ages. *Vet Res.* (2017) 48:34. doi: 10.1186/s13567-017-0441-6

70. Mullebner A, Sassu EL, Ladinig A, Frombling J, Miller I, Ehling-Schulz M, et al. *Actinobacillus pleuropneumoniae* triggers IL-10 expression in tonsils to mediate colonisation and persistence of infection in pigs. *Vet Immunol Immunopathol.* (2018) 205:17–23. doi: 10.1016/j.vetimm.2018.10.008

71. Guilliams M, Mildner A, Yona S. Developmental and functional heterogeneity of monocytes. *Immunity.* (2018) 49:595–613. doi: 10.1016/j.immuni.2018.10.005

72. Bonam SR, Partidos CD, Halmuthur SKM, Muller S. An overview of novel adjuvants designed for improving vaccine efficacy. *Trends Pharmacol Sci.* (2017) 38:771–93. doi: 10.1016/j.tips.2017.06.002

73. Bookstaver ML, Tsai SJ, Bromberg JS, Jewell CM. Improving vaccine and immunotherapy design using biomaterials. *Trends Immunol.* (2018) 39:135–50. doi: 10.1016/j.it.2017.10.002

74. Combadiere B, Liard C. Transcutaneous and intradermal vaccination. *Hum Vaccines.* (2011) 7:811–27. doi: 10.4161/hv.7.8.16274

# 16

# Evaluation of the Antiviral Activity of Sephin1 Treatment and its Consequences on eIF2α Phosphorylation in Response to Viral Infections

Maxime Fusade-Boyer[1], Gabriel Dupré[1], Pierre Bessière[1], Samira Khiar[2], Charlotte Quentin-Froignant[1,3], Cécile Beck[4], Sylvie Lecollinet[4], Marie-Anne Rameix-Welti[5,6], Jean-François Eléouët[7], Frédéric Tangy[2], Barbora Lajoie[8], Stéphane Bertagnoli[1], Pierre-Olivier Vidalain[9], Franck Gallardo[3] and Romain Volmer[1]*

[1] Université de Toulouse, ENVT, INRA, UMR 1225, Toulouse, France, [2] Viral Genomics and Vaccination Unit, CNRS UMR-3569, Institut Pasteur, Paris, France, [3] NeoVirTech SAS, Institute for Advanced Life Science Technology, Toulouse, France, [4] UMR 1161 Virology, INRA, ANSES, Ecole Nationale Vétérinaire d'Alfort, ANSES Animal Health Laboratory, EURL for Equine Diseases, Maisons-Alfort, France, [5] UMR INSERM U1173 2I, UFR des Sciences de la Santé Simone Veil—UVSQ, Montigny-le-Bretonneux, France, [6] AP-HP, Laboratoire de Microbiologie, Hôpital Ambroise Paré, Boulogne-Billancourt, France, [7] Unité de Virologie et Immunologie Moléculaires (UR892), INRA, Université Paris-Saclay, Jouy-en-Josas, France, [8] Laboratoire de Génie Chimique CNRS, INPT, UPS Université de Toulouse III, Faculté des Sciences Pharmaceutiques, Toulouse, France, [9] Laboratoire de Chimie et Biochimie Pharmacologiques et Toxicologiques, Equipe Chimie & Biologie, Modélisation et Immunologie pour la Thérapie, CNRS UMR 8601, Université Paris Descartes, Paris, France

*Correspondence:
Romain Volmer
r.volmer@envt.fr

The guanabenz derivative Sephin1 has recently been proposed to increase the levels of translation initiation factor 2 (eIF2α) phosphorylation by inhibiting dephosphorylation by the protein phosphatase 1—GADD34 (PPP1R15A) complex. As phosphorylation of eIF2α by protein kinase R (PKR) is a prominent cellular antiviral pathway, we evaluated the consequences of Sephin1 treatment on virus replication. Our results provide evidence that Sephin1 downregulates replication of human respiratory syncytial virus, measles virus, human adenovirus 5 virus, human enterovirus D68, human cytomegalovirus, and rabbit myxoma virus. However, Sephin1 proved to be inactive against influenza virus, as well as against Japanese encephalitis virus. Sephin1 increased the levels of phosphorylated eIF2α in cells exposed to a PKR agonist. By contrast, in virus-infected cells, the levels of phosphorylated eIF2α did not always correlate with the inhibition of virus replication by Sephin1. This work identifies Sephin1 as an antiviral molecule in cell culture against RNA, as well as DNA viruses belonging to phylogenetically distant families.

Keywords: PKR, GADD34, PPP1R15A, virus, antiviral, eIF2α, host, broad-spectrum

## INTRODUCTION

Most clinically available antiviral drugs act by directly targeting viral components to inhibit a critical step in the viral life cycle, such as entry, replication, or viral egress (1). These molecules have several advantages, as they can be very potent inhibitors and should have minor side effects because they are, in theory, virus specific. However, viruses evolve constantly and the selective pressure of the treatment can give rise to mutants that are resistant to these drugs. This is illustrated for example by the emergence of influenza virus strains resistant to viral neuraminidase inhibitors (2).

By contrast, antiviral molecules targeting host functions that are necessary for the virus life cycle are less likely to lead to the emergence of resistant viral mutants (3). Moreover, broad-spectrum antiviral molecules can be developed if the targeted host cell function regulates the replication of a wide range of viruses. Numerous host factors have been identified as required for viral replication through whole-genome genetic screens, providing impetus to develop antiviral molecules targeting these host factors (4). The numerous pathways experimentally identified as potential targets for antiviral therapy include viral entry or egress, viral assembly, viral protein synthesis or maturation, and the immune response against viruses (3, 5, 6). Currently, approved drugs targeting the host include the widely used type I interferons, which boost the antiviral innate immune response, ribavirin, which modulates the pool of intracellular nucleosides and is reported to modulate the innate immune response, and finally maraviroc, inhibiting human immunodeficiency virus entry by targeting C-C chemokine receptor type 5 (CCR5) (1). In an effort to limit toxicity, it is necessary to target a host cell function that is not crucial to the cell physiology and/or that is more specific to infected cells.

The phosphorylation of serine 51 of the $\alpha$ subunit of eukaryotic translation initiation factor 2 (eIF2$\alpha$) inhibits initiation of protein translation in response to various cellular stresses (7). Four protein kinases have been shown to specifically phosphorylate eIF2$\alpha$. The protein kinase RNA-like endoplasmic reticulum kinase (PERK) phosphorylates eIF2$\alpha$ in response to endoplasmic reticulum stress, due to the accumulation of unfolded proteins in the endoplasmic reticulum or to perturbations of the endoplasmic reticulum membrane lipid composition (8, 9). The haem-regulated inhibitor kinase (HRI) phosphorylates eIF2$\alpha$ in response to iron deficiency and has been demonstrated to regulate the differentiation of red blood cells (10). The general control non-derepressible-2 (GCN2) phosphorylates eIF2$\alpha$ in response to amino-acid deficiency (11). Finally, the interferon-induced double-stranded RNA-activated protein kinase (PKR) phosphorylates eIF2$\alpha$ in response to the accumulation of viral RNA harboring a double-stranded or other nucleic acids secondary structures produced during viral replication (12). Increased eIF2$\alpha$ phosphorylation attenuates translation of most mRNAs and is a physiological response to adapt to the various cellular stresses described above. Activation of PKR is for example an antiviral response aiming at reducing the translation of viral proteins in infected cells. The importance of PKR in antiviral defense is illustrated by the broad-array of viral countermeasures selected during evolution to inhibit PKR activation or eIF2$\alpha$ phosphorylation (12). It should however be noted that increased eIF2$\alpha$ phosphorylation seems to benefit to some viruses, including viruses belonging the *Togaviridae* family (13), *Reoviridae* family (14), and hepatitis C virus (15), most likely because translation of their mRNAs relies on secondary structures from which initiation can proceed even in the presence of high levels of eIF2$\alpha$ phosphorylation (12). As a consequence, developing means to increase eIF2$\alpha$ phosphorylation could be an antiviral intervention only for viruses whose mRNA translation is inhibited by increased eIF2$\alpha$ phosphorylation.

Dephosphorylation of eIF2$\alpha$ allows the cell to resume initiation of protein translation and is achieved by a binary complex between the catalytic phosphatase subunit PP1 and a regulatory subunit composed of either GADD34 (or PPP1R15A) (16) or CReP (or PPP1R15B) (17). The regulatory subunits GADD34 and CReP target the phosphatase PP1 specifically to the phosphorylated eIF2$\alpha$ substrate. CReP is constitutively expressed. By contrast, GADD34 expression is induced by eIF2$\alpha$ phosphorylation and therefore should be specifically expressed in stressed cells. GADD34 thus provides a negative feedback on eIF2$\alpha$ phosphorylation (8).

The guanabenz derivative Sephin1 was shown to increase eIF2$\alpha$ phosphorylation in cells stimulated with drugs causing PERK activation via the accumulation of unfolded proteins in the endoplasmic reticulum lumen (18). Sephin1 was described as a specific inhibitor of GADD34, although the identity of its target is currently subject of debate [see section Discussion and (19–21)]. We reasoned that inhibition of GADD34 could have antiviral effects by potentiating eIF2$\alpha$ phosphorylation in infected cells. Moreover, given that GADD34 is induced in cells with increased eIF2$\alpha$ phosphorylation, a GADD34 inhibitor should specifically act in stressed cells, such as infected cells, thus enhancing drug selectivity.

In the current work, we provide evidence that Sephin1 exhibited antiviral effects against specific viruses belonging to various viral families. In addition, Sephin1 increased eIF2$\alpha$ phosphorylation in response to activators of PKR, suggesting that Sephin1 may act by increasing eIF2$\alpha$ phosphorylation in virus-infected cells.

## MATERIALS AND METHODS

### Reagents and Cellular Treatments

Cells were treated for 16 h with 2.5 µg/ml tunicamycin (Sigma, USA) or with 1 µg/ml of intracellularly delivered Poly(I:C) (HMW)/LyoVec (Invivogen, France). Sephin1 was purchased from Tocris (United-Kingdom) or synthesized according to the protocol described in Das et al. (18). Purity was verified by nuclear magnetic resonance. Sodium arsenite (Sigma, USA) was added to cells in culture at a final concentration of 500 µM for 1 h before lysis. Cells were treated for 24 h with 1,000 U/ml of bacterially produced recombinant human interferon $\alpha$ A (PBL assay science, USA).

### Cells and Viruses

Human HEK293, HEK293T, human ARPE-19, and rabbit RK13 cells were grown at 37°C in DMEM containing glutamate supplemented with 10% FBS, 1x penicillin-streptomycin. Human HEp-2 cells were grown at 37°C in MEM containing glutamate supplemented with 10% FBS, 1x Penicillin-Streptomycin. Wild-type mouse embryonic fibroblasts (MEF WT) and MEF in which the endogenous eIF2$\alpha$ gene has been genetically replaced by a nonphosphorylable (S51A) allele (MEF S51A) have been described previously and were kindly provided by David Ron, University of Cambridge, United Kingdom (22, 23). Human respiratory syncytial virus (hRSV), derived from the strain Long, genetically modified to express firefly luciferase or the fluorescent protein mCherry were previously described and used to infect HEp-2 cells (24). Enterovirus D68, kindly provided by Caroline Tapparel, Université de Genève, Switzerland (25), was used to infect human RD cells cultured at 33°C, as previously described (26). Human adenovirus serotype 5 (hAdV), belonging to serotype 5, genetically modified to express the bacterial partitioning system-based AnchOR3 was used to infect human HEK cells, as recently described (27). Measles virus strain Schwartz genetically modified to express the firefly luciferase (28) was used to infect human HEKT cells, as previously described (29). Myxoma virus strain T1 was used to infect RK13 cells as previously described (30). Human cytomegalovirus (hCMV) derived from the TB40/E strain and genetically modified to express the bacterial partitioning system-based AnchOR3 was used to infect human ARPE-19 cells, as recently described (31). The AnchOR3 system is distributed by NeoVirTech SAS, France and is available upon request. Influenza A/Puerto Rico/8/1934 (H1N1) and A/turkey/Italy/977/1999(H7N1) were used to infect A549 or MDCK cells, as previously described (32, 33). Japanese encephalitis virus genotype 3 strain Nakayama (34) was used to infect HEK293T cells. Briefly, HEK293T cells were infected with JEV at a MOI of 0.01 for 48 h and JEV RNAs in cell supernatants were quantified by real-time RT-PCR as described in Yang et al. (35). Theiler's murine encephalomyelitis virus (TMEV) genetically modified to express a mutant L protein and the fluorescent protein Cherry (36) was used to infect MEF WT and MEF S51A. Cellular viability was measured with Vita-Blue Cell Viability Reagent (Biomake) according to the manufacturer's protocol. This assay is based on a fluorescent dehydrogenase enzymes substrate, which correlates with cellular metabolic activity.

## Western-Blot Analyses

Cells were lysed as previously described (37) and used for western-blot analyses. Phosphorylated eIF2α was detected with a polyclonal rabbit antibody (ab32157, Abcam, United-Kingdom) or (44-728G, ThermoFischer Scientific, USA). Total eIF2α was detected with a polyclonal rabbit antibody (Proteintech, USA).

## Quantification of Virus Replication

Myxoma virus titers were determined by standard plaque assay on RK13 cells, as described in Camus-Bouclainville et al. (30). Enterovirus D68 and influenza virus titers were determined by the tissue culture infectious dose 50 ($TCID_{50}$) method, as described in Soubies et al. (38). We measured replication of luciferase expressing virus 24 h post-infection by lysing cells and measuring light emission on a Clariostar (BMG Labtech) plate reader using the Luciferase assay System kit (Promega) according to the manufacturer's instructions. We measured replication of TMEV expressing the fluorescent protein Cherry by measuring fluorescence using a Clariostar (BMG Labtech) plate reader. hRSV expressing Cherry was detected in paraformaldehyde fixed HEp-2 cells by immunofluorescence and imaged using a confocal microscope. Replication of hAdV and hCMV expressing AnchOR3 protein was quantified by measuring GFP foci using automated microscopy, as described in Komatsu et al. (27) and Mariamé et al. (31).

## Rabbit Infections and Treatments

Rabbit infections and treatments were described in a protocol approved by the Ethical committee Science et Santé Animale (SSA 115) and the French Ministry of Research (protocol reference number 2015112009419390). Rabbits were infected by injection of 50 plaque-forming units of myxoma virus wild-type strain in the dermis of the right ear. The myxoma virus wild-type strain LH 3082 used for the *in vivo* infection was isolated in 2008 from the eyelid of a rabbit found dead in a farm in the South West of France. Sephin1 was solubilized in DMSO at a concentration of 1 mg/ml and further diluted in pineapple juice to administer either at 5 mg/kg (first experience), or 100 mg/kg (second experiment) by a single daily oral administration. Control animals received equivalent volumes of DMSO in pineapple juice. Animals were monitored daily for clinical signs and conjonctival swabs were performed at the indicated days post-infection to monitor for virus replication as recommended (39).

## RESULTS

### Consequences of Sephin1 Treatment on eIF2α Phosphorylation in Cells Stimulated With Known Stimulators of eIF2α Kinases

To determine the levels of eIF2α phosphorylation, we performed western-blot analysis using antibodies against phosphorylated eIF2α and against total eIF2α. In order to verify the specificity of these antibodies, we treated cells with sodium arsenite, a well-known potent inducer of eIF2α phosphorylation that mainly activates HRI (40). High levels of phosphorylated eIF2α were detected in sodium arsenite treated cells (**Figure 1A**, lanes 7), demonstrating the specificity of these antibodies and the position of the band corresponding to phosphorylated eIF2α, indicated with an asterisk. To evaluate the consequences of Sephin1 treatment on eIF2α phosphorylation, we exposed HEKT cells to the glycosylation inhibitor, tunicamycin, a known inducer of ER stress causing the accumulation of unfolded proteins in the ER. The accumulation of unfolded proteins in the ER leads to the activation of PERK, which phosphorylates eIF2α. As expected, eIF2α phosphorylation was increased in cells treated with tunicamycin (**Figure 1A**, lanes 1 vs. 5). Co-treatment with Sephin1 increased tunicamycin-induced eIF2α phosphorylation (**Figure 1A**, lanes 5 vs. 6), in agreement with previously published results (18). We next evaluated if Sephin1 could also potentiate eIF2α phosphorylation in the context of viral infections by stimulating cells with intracellularly delivered Poly(I:C), a synthetic RNA mimicking viral RNA and known to stimulate PKR (41). Poly(I:C) induced eIF2α phosphorylation (**Figure 1A**, lanes 1 vs. 3), which was further increased in cells treated simultaneously with Sephin1 (**Figure 1A**, lanes 3 vs. 4). Upon interferon α-pretreatment, which is known to upregulate PKR expression, we observed increased eIF2α phosphorylation in Poly(I:C)-treated HEK293T cells (**Supplementary Figure 1**,

## A   HEK293T cells

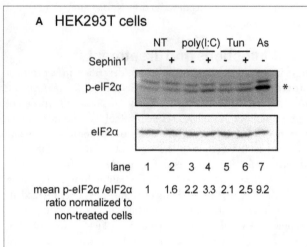

## B   RD cells

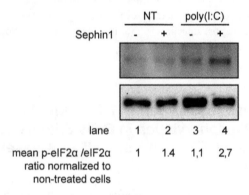

## C   HEp-2 cells

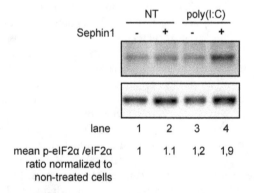

**FIGURE 1 |** Consequences of Sephin1 treatment on eIF2α phosphorylation. **(A)** HEK293T cells were either left untreated (NT), treated for 16 h with intracellularly delivered poly(I:C), which stimulates PKR or with tunicamycin (Tun), which stimulates PERK, in the presence or absence of 50 μM Sephin1. The asterisk indicates the position of phosphorylated eIF2α, as revealed in cells stimulated with sodium arsenite (As), a potent inducer of eIF2α phosphorylation. **(B)** RD cells and **(C)** HEp-2 cells were either left untreated (NT) or treated for 16 h with intracellularly delivered poly(I:C), in the presence or absence of 50 μM Sephin1. The mean fold increase of the phosphorylated eIF2α phosphorylation/total eIF2α ratio normalized to non-treated cells calculated from three independent experiments is shown below the photographs.

lanes 3 vs. 7). Simultaneous treatment with Sephin1 further increased eIF2α phosphorylation in Poly(I:C)-treated cells (**Supplementary Figure 1**, lanes 7 vs. 8). Sephin1 treatment also increased eIF2α phosphorylation in RD cells (**Figure 1B**) and in HEp-2 cells (**Figure 1C**) treated overnight with intracellularly delivered Poly(I:C). Altogether, these results suggest that Sephin1 could boost PKR-mediated eIF2α phosphorylation, possibly by inhibiting GADD34-mediated dephosphorylation of eIF2α.

# Evaluation of the Antiviral Properties of Sephin1 Against RNA Viruses

Human respiratory syncytial virus (hRSV) is a negative strand RNA virus belonging to the *Pneumoviridae* family. hRSV is a common cause of acute lower respiratory disease in infants and young children. Current antiviral therapies against hRSV are limited to an expensive humanized monoclonal antibody used as a prophylactic treatment and to ribavirin, which has limited efficacy and relatively high toxicity (42). There is therefore a need to develop new antiviral therapies. In order to test if Sephin1 was able to inhibit hRSV replication, we infected HEp-2 cells with a genetically engineered hRSV expressing the Firefly luciferase, used to quantify virus replication (24). Following virus adsorption for 1 h, cells were treated with increasing doses of Sephin1. Measurement of luciferase activity 24 h post-infection revealed a dose dependent inhibition of hRSV replication by Sephin1 (**Figure 2A**). A 30-fold inhibition of replication was observed when Sephin1 was used at 50 μM, which is the highest dose used in the experiments. Cellular viability was measured with a fluorescent dehydrogenase enzymes substrate, which reveals cellular metabolic activity. Cellular viability did not decrease significantly following Sephin1 treatment for 24 h and remained above 80% in HEp-2 cells treated with 50 μM Sephin1 (**Figure 2B**). Fluorescence and bright-field microscopic analysis of HEp-2 cells infected with a genetically engineered hRSV expressing the fluorescent protein Cherry (24) confirmed that treatment with 50 μM Sephin1 for 24 h led to a significant reduction of virus replication and was not associated with significant changes in cellular morphology or density (**Figure 2C**).

We further documented the antiviral spectrum of Sephin1 by testing its antiviral potential against measles virus. Measles virus is a negative strand RNA virus belonging to the *Paramyxoviridae* family currently causing large outbreaks due to suboptimal vaccination coverage in many countries (43). To evaluate the antiviral properties of Sephin1 against measles virus, we infected human HEK293T cells with a genetically engineered measles virus expressing the Firefly luciferase (28). Following virus adsorption for 1 h, cells were treated with increasing doses of Sephin1. Measurement of luciferase activity 24 h post-infection revealed a dose dependent inhibition of measles virus replication in HEK293T cells by Sephin1 (**Figure 3A**). A 10-fold inhibition of replication was observed when Sephin1 was used at 40 μM, which is the highest dose used in these experiments. Cellular viability remained above 75% in HEK293T cells treated for 24 h with 40 μM Sephin1 (**Figure 3B**).

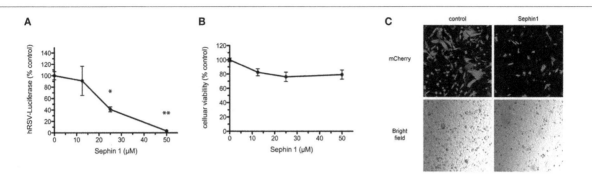

**FIGURE 2 |** Evaluation of the antiviral properties of Sephin1 against hRSV. **(A)** HEp-2 cells were infected with a recombinant strain of hRSV expressing luciferase and incubated with increasing doses of Sephin1 or DMSO alone. After 24 h, luciferase expression was determined. **(B)** Viability of HEp-2 cells incubated with increasing doses of Sephin1 or DMSO alone was determined after 24 h of incubation using the cellular viability assay Vita-Blue. **(C)** HEp-2 cells were infected with a recombinant strain of hRSV expressing mCherry and incubated with increasing doses of Sephin1 or DMSO alone. After 24 h, cells were fixed and imaged using a confocal microscope. Data represent mean ± SEM from representative experiments, repeated at least three times. *$p < 0.05$, **$p < 0.01$ by one-way analysis of variance, followed by Bonferroni comparison test comparing the Sephin1-treated group at the indicated concentration to the vehicle-treated control group.

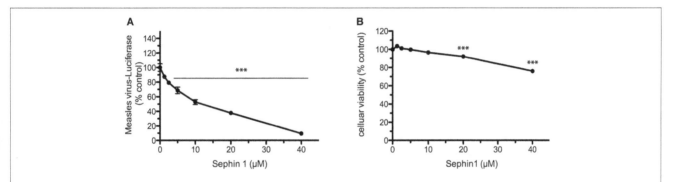

**FIGURE 3 |** Evaluation of the antiviral properties of Sephin1 against measles virus. **(A)** HEK293T cells were infected with a recombinant strain of measles virus expressing luciferase and incubated with increasing doses of Sephin1 or DMSO alone. After 24 h, luciferase expression was determined. Data represent mean values from a representative experiment, repeated at least three times. **(B)** Viability of HEK293T cells incubated with increasing doses of Sephin1 or DMSO alone was determined after 24 h incubation using the cellular viability assay Vita-Blue. Data represent mean ± SEM from representative experiments, repeated at least three times. ***$p < 0.001$ by one-way analysis of variance, followed by Bonferroni comparison test comparing the Sephin1-treated groups at the indicated concentrations to the vehicle-treated control group.

We next tested the antiviral properties of Sephin1 against enterovirus D68. Enterovirus D68 is a positive strand RNA virus belonging to the *Picornaviridae* family and causing upper respiratory tract infections in children (44). To mimic physiological temperatures found in the human upper tract, we infected human RD cells grown at 33°C with enterovirus D68 (26). Cells were infected at a low MOI to allow multiple cycles of infection. Following virus adsorption for 1 h, cells were treated with 50 μM Sephin1 and supernatants collected at the indicated time post-infection to quantify viral load by standard tissue culture infectious dose 50 (TCID$_{50}$) method. Treatment with 50 μM Sephin1 caused a more than 10-fold reduction of enterovirus ED68 titers (**Figure 4A**). Inhibition of enterovirus ED68 was readily detected at 24 h post-infection and persisted throughout the experiment up to 72 h post-infection, even though Sephin1 was added via a single treatment in the culture medium at 1 h post-infection. RD cells viability did not decrease significantly following 50 μM Sephin1 treatment for 24 h and remained above 90% (**Figure 4B**), consistent with

cellular viability results observed in Sephin1-treated HEp-2 cells and HEK293T cells.

We further tested the antiviral potential of Sephin1 against influenza A virus. We infected human A549 cells with the influenza A/Puerto Rico/8/1934 (H1N1) strain at a low multiplicity of infection. Following 1 h adsorption, A549 cells were treated with 50 μM Sephin1 or control cells treated with vehicle only. Viral titers in the supernatants were determined by standard plaque assay. We did not observe any inhibitory effect of Sephin1 on influenza virus replication (**Figure 5**). Similar results were obtained when experiments were performed on the canine MDCK cell line or when experiments were performed with the avian influenza A/turkey/Italy/977/1999(H7N1) virus strain (data not shown).

To assess the antiviral potential of Sephin1 against a virus belonging to the *Flaviviridae* family, we infected HEK293T cells with Japanese encephalitis virus. Sephin 1 had no effect on the replication of Japanese encephalitis virus, as determined by quantifying viral genomes in the supernatants by quantitative

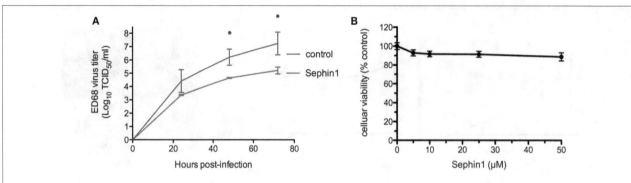

**FIGURE 4 |** Evaluation of the antiviral properties of Sephin1 against enterovirus ED68. **(A)** RD cells were infected with enterovirus ED68 and incubated at 33°C in the presence of 50 μM Sephin1 or DMSO alone (control). Viral titers were determined from supernatants harvested at the indicated times post-infection. **(B)** Viability of RD cells incubated with increasing doses of Sephin1 or DMSO alone was determined after 24 h of incubation using the cellular viability assay Vita-Blue. Data represent mean ± SEM from representative experiments, repeated at least three times. *$p < 0.05$ by one-way analysis of variance, followed by Bonferroni comparison test comparing the Sephin1-treated groups at the indicated concentrations to the vehicle-treated control group.

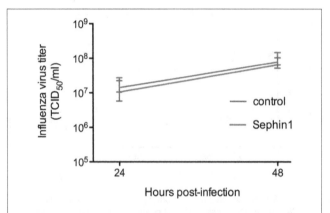

**FIGURE 5 |** Evaluation of the antiviral properties of Sephin1 against influenza virus. A549 cells were infected with influenza A/Puerto Rico/8/1934 (H1N1) strain and incubated in the presence of 50 μM Sephin1 or DMSO alone (control). Viral titers were determined from supernatants harvested at the indicated times post-infection. Data represent mean ± SEM from a representative experiment, repeated at least three times.

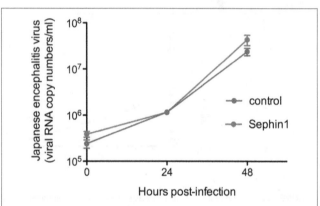

**FIGURE 6 |** Evaluation of the antiviral properties of Sephin1 against Japanese encephalitis virus. HEK293T cells were infected with Japanese encephalitis virus and incubated in the presence of 50 μM Sephin1 or DMSO alone (control). Viral titers were determined by quantitative RT-PCR from supernatants harvested at the indicated times post-infection. Data represent mean ± SEM from a representative experiment, repeated at least three times.

RT-PCR (**Figure 6**). We thus identified viruses that are not inhibited by Sephin1, demonstrating that although Sephin1 has a broad antiviral spectrum, it is not active against all viruses.

## Evaluation of the Antiviral Properties of Sephin1 Against DNA Viruses

In order to test if Sephin1 could inhibit phylogenetically distant viruses, we analyzed its antiviral potential against human Adenovirus (hAdV), a DNA virus belonging to the *Adenoviridae* family causing respiratory tract infections in humans. A genetically modified hAdV expressing the bacterial partitioning system-based AnchOR3 was used to infect HEK293 cells. The AnchOR3 system allows for the real-time detection of viral DNA replication in living cells through the detection of GFP foci and is therefore used to monitor DNA virus replication

in real-time by fluorescent microscopy (27). Cells were treated with increasing doses of Sephin1 or vehicle only and infected immediately with AnchOR3 hAdV. Measurement of GFP fluorescent foci by automated microscopy 24 h post-infection revealed a dose dependent inhibition of hAdV replication by Sephin1 (**Figure 7A**). A four-fold inhibition of replication was observed when Sephin1 was used at 50 μM, which is the highest dose used in the experiments. Cellular viability did not decrease significantly following Sephin1 treatment for 24 h and remained above 80% in HEK293 cells treated with 50 μM Sephin1 (**Figure 7B**).

We next analyzed the antiviral potential of Sephin1 against myxoma virus, a DNA virus of the *Poxviridae* family, which contains pathogens of major importance in human and veterinary medicine. Myxoma virus is responsible for Myxomatosis in European rabbits, a disease of medical

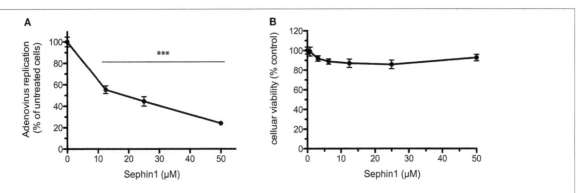

**FIGURE 7 |** Evaluation of the antiviral properties of Sephin1 against human Adenovirus. **(A)** HEK293 cells were infected with a recombinant strain of hAdV expressing ANCHOR3 and incubated with increasing doses of Sephin1 or DMSO alone. After 24 h, virus replication was determined by automated counting of GFP foci. **(B)** Viability of HEK293 cells incubated with increasing doses of Sephin1 or DMSO alone was determined after 24 h incubation using the cellular viability assay Vita-Blue. Data represent mean ± SEM from representative experiments, repeated at least three times. ***$p < 0.001$ by one-way analysis of variance, followed by Bonferroni comparison test comparing the Sephin1-treated groups at the indicated concentrations to the vehicle-treated control group.

importance in veterinary medicine, worsened due to the emergence of strains causing respiratory diseases in rabbits (39). Following myxoma virus adsorption for 1 h, rabbit RK13 cells were treated with 50 μM Sephin1. Cells and supernatants were harvested at 24, 72, and 120 h post-infection and subjected to three freeze-thaw cycles to detect free viral particles, as well as cell-associated virus particles (30). Virus titration by standard plaque-assay revealed that Sephin1 significantly inhibited myxoma virus replication (**Figure 8A**). Cellular viability did not decrease significantly following Sephin1 treatment of RK13 cells for 24 h (**Figure 8B**).

Finally, we evaluated the antiviral of Sephin1 against human cytomegalovirus (hCMV), a DNA virus belonging to the *Herpesviridae* family. hCMV is widespread in the human population and causes severe diseases following congenital infection. A genetically modified hCMV expressing the AnchOR3 system to detect viral DNA replication by the accumulation of GFP foci was used to infect the human retinal pigment cell line ARPE-19 (31). Sephin1 had a dose-dependent inhibitory effect on hCMV replication in the human ARPE-19 cell line, reaching a five-fold inhibition at 50 μM (**Figure 9A**). At this dose Sephin1 caused a 40% reduction in cellular viability, indicating that Sephin1 is associated with moderate toxicity at 50 μM in the ARPE-19 cell line (**Figure 9B**). Altogether these results provide evidence that Sephin1 has antiviral activity against respiratory viruses belonging to phylogenetically distant families.

## Evaluation of the Contribution of eIF2α Phosphorylation to the Antiviral Effects of Sephin1

To test if the antiviral effect of Sephin1 correlated with increased eIF2α phosphorylation, we performed western-blot analyses of virus-infected cells. eIF2α phosphorylation was increased in cells infected with hRSV (**Figure 10A**, compare lanes 1 and 3). However, treatment with 50 μM Sephin1 did not increase eIF2α

phosphorylation in hRSV-infected cells (**Figure 10A**, compare lanes 3 and 4). eIF2α phosphorylation was not increased in cells infected with measles virus (**Figure 10B**, compare lanes 1 and 3) or in cells infected with myxoma virus (**Figure 10C**, compare lanes 1 and 3), even when cells were treated with 50 μM Sephin1 (**Figures 10B,C**, compare lanes 3 and 4). Thus, the antiviral activity of Sephin1 does not correlate with increased eIF2α phosphorylation, raising the possibility that some antiviral effects of Sephin1 could be independent of eIF2α phosphorylation.

To test if Sephin1 could inhibit virus replication independently of eIF2α phosphorylation, we compared wild-type mouse embryonic fibroblasts (MEF WT) and mouse embryonic in which the endogenous eIF2α gene has been genetically replaced by a nonphosphorylable (S51A) allele (MEF S51A) (22). These cells were infected with Theiler's murine encephalomyelitis virus (TMEV), a positive strand RNA virus belonging to the *Picornaviridae* family. We used a genetically modified virus, which has a deleted L protein, rendering the virus highly susceptible to the antiviral effects of PKR and expressing the fluorescent protein Cherry, used as a reporter to quantify virus replication (36). Following virus adsorption for 1 h, cells were either treated with vehicle only or treated with 50 μM Sephin1. Virus replication was evaluated by measuring Cherry fluorescence using a fluorescent microplate reader. Sephin1 reduced Cherry fluorescence in MEF WT cells, indicating that it inhibited TMEV-Cherry replication in MEF WT cells (**Figure 10D**). Surprisingly, Cherry fluorescence was higher in Sephin1-treated MEF S51A cells compared to non-treated S51A cells, indicating that Sephin1 treatment increased TMEV replication in cells expressing nonphosphorylable eIF2α (**Figure 10E**). It is currently unclear how Sephin1 could increase TMEV replication in cells expressing nonphosphorylable eIF2α. This result nevertheless demonstrates that eIF2α phosphorylation is required for the antiviral effects of Sephin1 against TMEV.

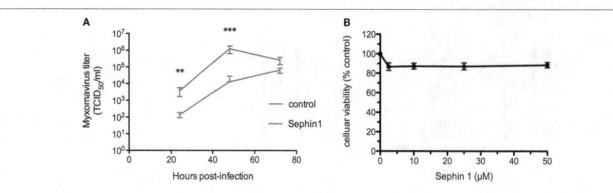

**FIGURE 8 |** Evaluation of the antiviral properties of Sephin1 against myxoma virus. **(A)** RK13 cells were infected with myxoma virus and incubated in the presence of 50 μM Sephin1 or DMSO alone (control). Viral titers were determined from crude lysates harvested at the indicated times post-infection. **(B)** Viability of RK13 cells incubated with increasing doses of Sephin1 or DMSO alone was determined after 24 h incubation using the cellular viability assay Vita-Blue. Data represent mean ± SEM from representative experiments, repeated at least three times. **$p < 0.001$, ***$p < 0.001$ by one-way analysis of variance, followed by Bonferroni comparison test comparing the Sephin1-treated groups at the indicated concentrations to the vehicle-treated control group.

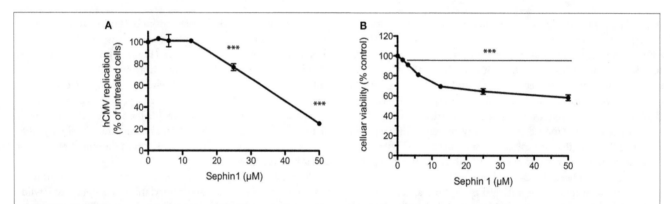

**FIGURE 9 |** Evaluation of the antiviral properties of Sephin1 against human cytomegalovirus. **(A)** ARPE-19 cells were infected with a recombinant strain of hCMV expressing ANCHOR3 and incubated with increasing doses of Sephin1 or DMSO alone. After 72 h, virus replication was determined by automated counting of GFP foci. **(B)** Viability of ARPE-19 cells incubated with increasing doses of Sephin1 or DMSO alone was determined after 72 h incubation using the cellular viability assay Vita-Blue. Data represent mean ± SEM from representative experiments, repeated at least three times. ***$p < 0.001$ by one-way analysis of variance, followed by Bonferroni comparison test comparing the Sephin1-treated groups at the indicated concentrations to the vehicle-treated control group.

## Sephin1 Is Showing Some Antiviral Effect *in vivo*, Which Is However Limited by Toxic Side Effects

In order to evaluate if Sephin1 could exert antiviral activity *in vivo*, we evaluated its therapeutic potential in European rabbits infected with myxoma virus. European rabbits are the natural hosts of myxoma virus. Rabbits were inoculated with 50 plaque-forming units of myxoma virus strain LH 3082 by intradermal inoculation in the right ear lobe. Sephin1 was administered by oral gavage once daily at a dose of 5 mg/kg. Treatment with Sephin1 began straight after virus inoculation. Control rabbits were treated similarly with vehicle. Except for two rabbits in the control group and one rabbit in the Sephin1-treated group, no other infected rabbits developed clinical signs of myxomatosis over the period of observation. Sephin1 appeared to be well-tolerated at a daily dose of 5mg/kg, as Sephin1-treated rabbits were clinically indistinguishable from the control rabbits. Conjonctival swabs were performed on day 0, 5, 9, and 11 to monitor for virus replication by q-PCR (**Figure 11**). Levels of

viral DNA increased in non-treated control animals over the observation period, indicating efficient virus replication in the rabbits. The levels of virus replication were much higher for the three rabbits showing clinical signs, indicated by arrows in **Figure 11**. We observed a significant reduction in virus replication at day 11 post-infection in the Sephin1-treated group compared to the control group, demonstrating that Sephin1 can exert an antiviral activity *in vivo*. However, the antiviral activity of Sephin1 given orally at 5 mg/kg daily was modest. We therefore repeated the experiment in order to administer Sephin1 at a higher dosage. In this second *in vivo* experiment, rabbits were infected as previously. Sephin1 was administered by oral gavage once daily at a dose of 100 mg/kg beginning straight after inoculation. When used at 100 mg/kg, acute toxicity was observed as soon as 2 days post-infection in the Sephin1 treated rabbits, which developed anorexia and presented ruffled fur. For ethical reasons, in compliance with the guidelines from the animal care and use committee, we euthanized the animals and terminated the experiment. Altogether these results suggest

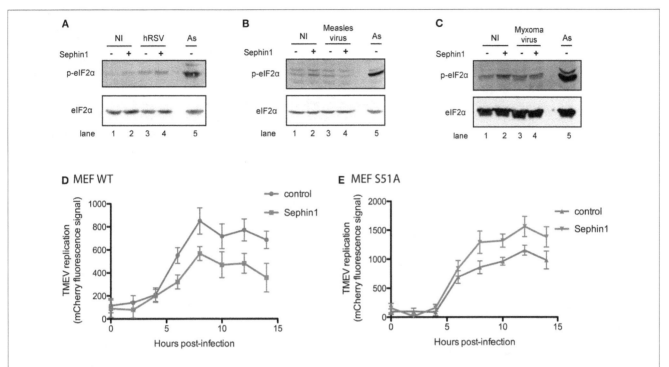

**FIGURE 10 |** Evaluation of the contribution of eIF2α phosphorylation to the antiviral effects of Sephin1. Cells were either left non-infected (NI) or infected with the indicated viruses, in the presence or absence of 50 μM Sephin1. Sodium arsenite (As), a potent inducer of eIF2α phosphorylation, was used as a positive control for detection of eIF2α phosphorylation by western-blot. **(A)** Analysis of eIF2α phosphorylation in HEp-2 cells infected with hRSV. **(B)** Analysis of eIF2α phosphorylation in HEK293T cells infected with measles virus. **(C)** Analysis of eIF2α phosphorylation in RK13 cells infected with myxoma virus. **(D)** Consequences of Sephin1 treatment on TMEV replication in WT mouse embryonic fibroblasts (MEF WT). **(E)** Consequences of Sephin1 treatment on TMEV replication in mouse embryonic fibroblasts expressing a non-phosphorylable (S51A) allele of eIF2α (MEF S51A). TMEV replication was determined by measuring mCherry fluorescence. Data represent mean ± SEM from representative experiments, repeated at least three times.

that although Sephin1 has some antiviral activity *in vivo* at 5 mg/kg, increasing the dosage to reach higher concentrations and possibly better antiviral activity is currently not possible due to the existence of major side effects.

## DISCUSSION

Negative strand RNA viruses, positive strand RNA viruses, as well as DNA viruses were inhibited by Sephin1 treatment in cell culture. Our results thus provide evidence that Sephin1 treatment has antiviral properties against a broad range of viruses belonging to phylogenetically distant viral families. A four to 100-fold inhibition of viral replication was obtained when Sephin1 was used at 50 μM. At this dose, cellular viability remained above 75% in all cell lines tested, with the exception of ARPE-19 cells, which had a 40% decrease in viability. This result demonstrates that, although the molecule had to be used at a high dose to reach a significant antiviral effect, inhibition of virus replication could not be attributable to alterations in cellular viability.

Secondary structures found in the RNA of some positive strand RNA viruses, such as viruses belonging to the *Togaviridae* family, *Reoviridae* family and hepatitis C virus, allow translation of these RNAs to proceed normally, or in some cases better, in the presence of high levels of eIF2α phosphorylation (12). It is therefore expected that Sephin1 would have no antiviral

effect against these viruses. In the case of influenza virus, the lack of antiviral activity of Sephin1 might be attributable to the tight inhibition of PKR activation by the viral protein NS1 (45). This inhibition is mediated by the binding of NS1 to PKR (46). Influenza A viruses with mutant NS1 proteins unable to bind to PKR are highly attenuated in wild-type mice, but replicate to high levels in PKR deficient mice (46). By contrast, wild-type influenza viruses replicate to similar levels in wild-type mice and in PKR deficient mice (46, 47). These observations suggest that PKR is an important antiviral pathway against influenza viruses, which is very efficiently counteracted by wild-type NS1 protein. The lack of activity of Sephin1 observed in cell culture may be due to the absence of PKR activation and eIF2α phosphorylation in influenza virus infected cells, as previously described (48). Similarly, the lack of antiviral activity of Sephin1 against Japanese encephalitis virus could be due to the tight inhibition of PKR activation by the viral protein NS2A (49). In the absence of eIF2α phosphorylation and consequent expression of GADD34, it is anticipated that Sephin1 would have no effect.

GADD34 has been shown to stimulate type I interferon production in response to the synthetic viral RNA analog poly(I:C) and in response to infection with Chikungunya virus, a member of the *Togaviridae* family (50). Activation of PKR by poly(I:C) and in response to Chikungunya virus infection leads to eIF2α phosphorylation, which inhibits initiation of

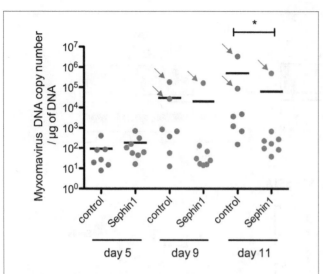

**FIGURE 11** | Evaluation of the antiviral potential of Sephin1 against myxoma virus *in vivo*. Rabbits were inoculated with 50 plaque-forming units of myxoma virus. Eight rabbits were treated with Sephin1 by oral gavage once daily at a dose of 5 mg/kg. Seven rabbits were administered vehicle only. Myxoma virus DNA was detected by q-PCR from conjonctival swabs performed at the indicated days post-infection. Rabbits exhibiting clinical signs are indicated with an arrow. *$p < 0.05$ by the two-tailed Mann–Whitney test.

protein translation, including translation of type I interferons. GADD34 expression and subsequent dephosphorylation of eIF2α resume initiation of protein translation and consequently allow translation of type I interferons (50). Inhibition of GADD34 is therefore a double-edged sword. On one hand, increased eIF2α phosphorylation caused by inhibition of GADD34 can potentiate the antiviral effects by causing a tighter inhibition of viral protein translation. On the other hand, a prolonged increase of eIF2α phosphorylation caused by inhibition of GADD34 can inhibit the translation of host proteins involved in antiviral defense, such as type I interferons and antiviral effector proteins. The potential beneficial effects of GADD34 inhibition are difficult to predict. For viruses, such as members of the *Togaviridae*, which are able to translate their proteins in the presence of high levels of eIF2α phosphorylation, inhibition of GADD34 will likely be detrimental to the host because of a reduction in the translation of host proteins involved in antiviral defense. For viruses, which are unable to translate their proteins in the presence of high levels of eIF2α phosphorylation, the consequences of GADD34 inhibition on viral replication are to our knowledge not predictable, and therefore most likely need to be experimentally tested.

Inhibition of myxoma virus and measles virus by Sephin1 was not associated with increased levels of eIF2α phosphorylation. We thus did not observe a strict correlation between the antiviral effects of Sephin1 and eIF2α phosphorylation. One tentative explanation is that viral inhibition leads to a reduction in the levels of viral PKR activators in Sephin1-treated cells compared to infected non-treated cells. However, these observations also raise the possibility that Sephin1 does not act by targeting GADD34-PP1 mediated dephosphorylation of eIF2α. Indeed, contradicting the initial description (18) and follow-up work

(21), Sephin1 and its derivative guanabenz were recently shown to lack any effect on GADD34-PP1 mediated dephosphorylation of eIF2α (19, 20, 51). We cannot rule out that Sephin1 mediates its effects independently of GADD34. However, we observed increased phosphorylation of eIF2α in cells stimulated with the PERK activator tunicamycin and in cells stimulated with the PKR activator poly(I:C). Moreover, the lack of antiviral activity of Sephin1 against Theiler's murine encephalomyelitis virus (TMEV) in MEF cells expressing a nonphosphorylable (S51A) allele demonstrates that eIF2α phosphorylation is required for the antiviral effects of Sephin1 against TMEV. Whether these effects are due to a specific inhibition of GADD34 by Sephin1 remains to be investigated.

We observed a modest antiviral effect of Sephin1 administered by oral gavage once daily at a dose of 5 mg/kg against myxoma virus in rabbits. At 5 mg/kg, no toxic side effects were detected by clinical examination of the rabbits. However, when we administered Sephin1 by oral gavage once daily at a dose of 100 mg/kg, major clinical signs were detected, indicating that at this dosage Sephin1 caused acute toxicity. GADD34 knock-out mice were viable and did not show any clinical signs under normal breeding conditions (52). This finding suggests that the toxic side effects of Sephin1 observed in rabbits are unlikely due to inhibition of GADD34, but rather point to Sephin1-induced alterations in physiology that are independent of GADD34. Ongoing studies to identify the causes of toxicity could provide information for the development of new treatment regimens, including new formulations and modes of administration. In addition, Sephin1 can be the scaffold of structure-activity relationship studies to identify new variants with increased efficiency or decreased *in vivo* toxicity, and thus exhibiting an improved selectivity index to consider these new variants as promising therapeutic antiviral candidates. In this chemical series, this is already well exemplified by the development of Sephin1 itself, which is derived from guanabenz to eliminate some unwanted binding to the α2- adrenergic receptor (18).

The prominent role of the PKR eIF2α pathway in antiviral defense is well-established. Direct stimulators of PKR will stimulate eIF2α phosphorylation in all cells exposed to the drug, therefore likely leading to unwanted side effects in non-infected cells. By contrast, GADD34 expression is stress-inducible and drugs targeting GADD34 should therefore be active only in cells that have increased levels of eIF2α phosphorylation, including virus-infected cells, thus increasing selectivity. GADD34 inhibitors would most likely be most effective in complement with other molecules, such as drugs targeting viral PKR antagonists or drugs thought to affect viral protein folding, such as nitazoxanide (53) or iminosugars (54), which could potentiate PERK-mediated eIF2α phosphorylation in infected cells.

## AUTHOR CONTRIBUTIONS

MF-B, GD, PB, SK, CQ-F, CB, SL, SB, P-OV, FG, and RV performed the experiments and analyzed the data. CB, SL, M-AR-W, J-FE, FT, BL, and FG provided reagents and analyzed

Evaluation of the Antiviral Activity of Sephin1 Treatment and its Consequences on eIF2α Phosphorylation...

219

the data. RV drafted the manuscript. All the authors contributed to the critical review and revision of the manuscript.

## FUNDING

This work was supported by the French Ministry of Agriculture.

## ACKNOWLEDGMENTS

The authors thank David Ron, University of Cambridge, United Kingdom, for the kind gift of wild-type mouse embryonic fibroblasts and mouse embryonic in which the endogenous eIF2α gene has been genetically replaced by a nonphosphorylable (S51A) allele, Caroline Tapparel, Université de Genève, Switzerland, for the kind gift of enterovirus D68 and Thomas Michiels, Université Catholique de Louvain, de Duve Institute, Bruxelles, Belgium for the kind gift of Theiler's murine encephalomyelitis virus genetically modified to express a mutant L protein and the fluorescent protein Cherry.

## REFERENCES

1. Chaudhuri S, Symons JA, Deval J. Innovation and trends in the development and approval of antiviral medicines: 1987–2017 and beyond. *Antiviral Res.* (2018) 155:76–88. doi: 10.1016/j.antiviral.2018.05.005
2. Li TCM, Chan MCW, Lee N. Clinical implications of antiviral resistance in influenza. *Viruses* (2015) 7:4929–44. doi: 10.3390/v7092850
3. Kaufmann SHE, Dorhoi A, Hotchkiss RS, Bartenschlager R. Host-directed therapies for bacterial and viral infections. *Nat Rev Drug Discov.* (2018) 17:35–56. doi: 10.1038/nrd.2017.162
4. Puschnik AS, Majzoub K, Ooi YS, Carette JE. A CRISPR toolbox to study virus-host interactions. *Nat Rev Microbiol.* (2017) 15:351–64. doi: 10.1038/nrmicro.2017.29
5. Schor S, Einav S. Combating intracellular pathogens with repurposed host-targeted drugs. *ACS Infect Dis.* (2018) 4:88–92. doi: 10.1021/acsinfecdis.7b00268
6. McKimm-Breschkin JL, Jiang S, Hui DS, Beigel JH, Govorkova EA, Lee N. Prevention and treatment of respiratory viral infections: presentations on antivirals, traditional therapies and host-directed interventions at the 5th ISIRV Antiviral Group conference. *Antiviral Res.* (2018) 149:118–42. doi: 10.1016/j.antiviral.2017.11.013
7. Sonenberg N, Hinnebusch AG. Regulation of translation initiation in eukaryotes: mechanisms and biological targets. *Cell* (2009) 136:731–45. doi: 10.1016/j.cell.2009.01.042
8. Walter P, Ron D. The unfolded protein response: from stress pathway to homeostatic regulation. *Science* (2011) 334:1081–6. doi: 10.1126/science.1209038
9. Volmer R, Ron D. Lipid-dependent regulation of the unfolded protein response. *Curr Opin Cell Biol.* (2015) 33:67–73. doi: 10.1016/j.ceb.2014.12.002
10. Han A-P, Yu C, Lu L, Fujiwara Y, Browne C, Chin G, et al. Heme-regulated eIF2α kinase (HRI) is required for translational regulation and survival of erythroid precursors in iron deficiency. *EMBO J.* (2001) 20:6909–18. doi: 10.1093/emboj/20.23.6909
11. Ron D, Walter P. Signal integration in the endoplasmic reticulum unfolded protein response. *Nat Rev Mol Cell Biol.* (2007) 8:519–29. doi: 10.1038/nrm2199
12. Dauber B, Wolff T. Activation of the antiviral kinase PKR and viral countermeasures. *Viruses* (2009) 1:523–44. doi: 10.3390/v1030523
13. Ventoso I, Sanz MA, Molina S, Berlanga JJ, Carrasco L, Esteban M. Translational resistance of late alphavirus mRNA to eIF2α phosphorylation: a strategy to overcome the antiviral effect of protein kinase PKR. *Genes Dev.* (2006) 20:87–100. doi: 10.1101/gad.357006
14. Rojas M, Arias CF, López S. Protein kinase R is responsible for the phosphorylation of eIF2α in rotavirus infection. *J Virol.* (2010) 84:10457–66. doi: 10.1128/JVI.00625-10
15. Robert F, Kapp LD, Khan SN, Acker MG, Kolitz S, Kazemi S, et al. Initiation of protein synthesis by hepatitis C virus is refractory to reduced eIF2 GTP met-tRNAiMet ternary complex availability. *MBoC* (2006) 17:4632–44. doi: 10.1091/mbc.e06-06-0478
16. Novoa I, Zeng H, Harding HP, Ron D. Feedback inhibition of the unfolded protein response by GADD34-mediated dephosphorylation of eIF2α. *J Cell Biol.* (2001) 153:1011–22. doi: 10.1083/jcb.153.5.1011
17. Jousse C, Oyadomari S, Novoa I, Lu P, Zhang Y, Harding HP, et al. Inhibition of a constitutive translation initiation factor 2alpha phosphatase, CReP, promotes survival of stressed cells. *J Cell Biol.* (2003) 163:767–75. doi: 10.1083/jcb.200308075
18. Das I, Krzyzosiak A, Schneider K, Wrabetz L, D'Antonio M, Barry N, et al. Preventing proteostasis diseases by selective inhibition of a phosphatase regulatory subunit. *Science* (2015) 348:239–42. doi: 10.1126/science.aaa4484
19. Crespillo-Casado A, Chambers JE, Fischer PM, Marciniak SJ, Ron D. PPP1R15A-mediated dephosphorylation of eIF2α is unaffected by Sephin1 or Guanabenz. *Elife* (2017) 6:26109. doi: 10.7554/eLife.26109
20. Crespillo-Casado A, Claes Z, Choy MS, Peti W, Bollen M, Ron D. A Sephin1-insensitive tripartite holophosphatase dephosphorylates translation initiation factor 2α. *J Biol Chem.* (2018) 293:7766–76. doi: 10.1074/jbc.RA118.002325
21. Carrara M, Sigurdardottir A, Bertolotti A. Decoding the selectivity of eIF2α holophosphatases and PPP1R15A inhibitors. *Nat Struct Mol Biol.* (2017) 24:708–16. doi: 10.1038/nsmb.3443
22. Scheuner D, Song B, McEwen E, Liu C, Laybutt R, Gillespie P, et al. Translational control is required for the unfolded protein response and in vivo glucose homeostasis. *Mol Cell* (2001) 7:1165–76. doi: 10.1016/S1097-2765(01)00265-9
23. Sekine Y, Zyryanova A, Crespillo-Casado A, Fischer PM, Harding HP, Ron D. Mutations in a translation initiation factor identify target of a memory-enhancing compound. *Science* (2015) 348:1027–30. doi: 10.1126/science.aaa6986
24. Rameix-Welti M-A, Le Goffic R, Hervé P-L, Sourimant J, Rémot A, Riffault S, et al. Visualizing the replication of respiratory syncytial virus in cells and in living mice. *Nat Commun.* (2014) 5:5104. doi: 10.1038/ncomms6104
25. Royston L, Essaidi-Laziosi M, Pérez-Rodríguez FJ, Piuz I, Geiser J, Krause K-H, et al. Viral chimeras decrypt the role of enterovirus capsid proteins in viral tropism, acid sensitivity and optimal growth temperature. *PLoS Pathog.* (2018) 14:e1006962. doi: 10.1371/journal.ppat.1006962
26. Oberste MS, Maher K, Schnurr D, Flemister MR, Lovchik JC, Peters H, et al. Enterovirus 68 is associated with respiratory illness and shares biological features with both the enteroviruses and the rhinoviruses. *J Gen Virol.* (2004) 85:2577–84. doi: 10.1099/vir.0.79925-0
27. Komatsu T, Quentin-Froignant C, Carlon-Andres I, Lagadec F, Rayne F, Ragues J, et al. In vivo labelling of adenovirus DNA identifies chromatin anchoring and biphasic genome replication. *J Virol.* (2018). doi: 10.1128/JVI.00795-18. [Epub ahead of print].
28. Komarova AV, Combredet C, Meyniel-Schicklin L, Chapelle M, Caignard G, Camadro J-M, et al. Proteomic analysis of virus-host interactions in an infectious context using recombinant viruses. *Mol Cell Proteomics* (2011) 10:M110.007443. doi: 10.1074/mcp.M110.007443
29. Lucas-Hourani M, Munier-Lehmann H, Helynck O, Komarova A, Desprès P, Tangy F, et al. High-throughput screening for broad-spectrum chemical inhibitors of RNA viruses. *J Vis Exp.* (2014). doi: 10.3791/51222

30. Camus-Bouclainville C, Fiette L, Bouchiha S, Pignolet B, Counor D, Filipe C, et al. A Virulence factor of myxoma virus colocalizes with NF-κB in the nucleus and interferes with inflammation. *J Virol.* (2004) 78:2510–6. doi: 10.1128/JVI.78.5.2510-2516.2004

31. Mariamé B, Kappler-Gratias S, Kappler M, Balor S, Gallardo F, Bystricky K. Real-time visualization and quantification of human Cytomegalovirus replication in living cells using the ANCHOR DNA labeling technology. *J Virol.* (2018) 92:e00571-18. doi: 10.1128/JVI.00571-18

32. Volmer R, Mazel-Sanchez B, Volmer C, Soubies SM, Guérin J-L. Nucleolar localization of influenza A NS1: striking differences between mammalian and avian cells. *Virol J.* (2010) 7:63. doi: 10.1186/1743-422X-7-63

33. Soubies SM, Hoffmann TW, Croville G, Larcher T, Ledevin M, Soubieux D, et al. Deletion of the C-terminal ESEV domain of NS1 does not affect the replication of a low-pathogenic avian influenza virus H7N1 in ducks and chickens. *J Gen Virol.* (2013) 94:50–8. doi: 10.1099/vir.0.045153-0

34. Ruget A-S, Beck C, Gabassi A, Trevennec K, Lecollinet S, Chevalier V, et al. Japanese encephalitis circulation pattern in swine of northern Vietnam and consequences for swine's vaccination recommendations. *Transbound Emerg Dis.* (2018) 65:1485–92. doi: 10.1111/tbed.12885

35. Yang D-K, Kweon C-H, Kim B-H, Lim S-I, Kim S-H, Kwon J-H, et al. TaqMan reverse transcription polymerase chain reaction for the detection of Japanese encephalitis virus. *J Vet Sci.* (2004) 5:345–51.

36. Jacobs S, Wavreil F, Schepens B, Gad HH, Hartmann R, Rocha-Pereira J, et al. Species specificity of type III interferon activity and development of a sensitive luciferase-based bioassay for quantitation of mouse IFN-λ. *J Interferon Cytokine Res.* 38:469–79. doi: 10.1089/jir.2018.0066

37. Bertolotti A, Zhang Y, Hendershot LM, Harding HP, Ron D. Dynamic interaction of BiP and ER stress transducers in the unfolded-protein response. *Nat Cell Biol.* (2000) 2:326–32. doi: 10.1038/35014014

38. Soubies SM, Volmer C, Croville G, Loupias J, Peralta B, Costes P, et al. Species-specific contribution of the four C-terminal amino acids of influenza A virus NS1 protein to virulence. *J Virol.* (2010) 84:6733–47. doi: 10.1128/JVI.02427-09

39. Bertagnoli S, Marchandeau S. Myxomatosis. *Rev Off Int Epizoot* (2015) 34:549–56. 539–47.

40. McEwen E, Kedersha N, Song B, Scheuner D, Gilks N, Han A, et al. Heme-regulated inhibitor kinase-mediated phosphorylation of eukaryotic translation initiation factor 2 inhibits translation, induces stress granule formation, and mediates survival upon arsenite exposure. *J Biol Chem.* (2005) 280:16925–33. doi: 10.1074/jbc.M412882200

41. Gilfoy FD, Mason PW. West nile virus-induced interferon production is mediated by the double-stranded RNA-dependent protein kinase PKR. *J Virol.* (2007) 81:11148–58. doi: 10.1128/JVI.00446-07

42. Turner TL, Kopp BT, Paul G, Landgrave LC, Hayes D, Thompson R. Respiratory syncytial virus: current and emerging treatment options. *Clinicoecon Outcomes Res.* (2014) 6:217–25. doi: 10.2147/CEOR.S60710

43. Bester JC. Measles and measles vaccination: a review. *JAMA Pediatr.* (2016) 170:1209–15. doi: 10.1001/jamapediatrics.2016.1787

44. Holm-Hansen CC, Midgley SE, Fischer TK. Global emergence of enterovirus D68: a systematic review. *Lancet Infect Dis.* (2016) 16:e64–75. doi: 10.1016/S1473-3099(15)00543-5

45. Marc D. Influenza virus non-structural protein NS1: interferon antagonism and beyond. *J Gen Virol.* (2014) 95:2594–611. doi: 10.1099/vir.0.069542-0

46. Schierhorn KL, Jolmes F, Bespalowa J, Saenger S, Peteranderl C, Dzieciolowski J, et al. Influenza A virus virulence depends on two amino acids in the N-terminal domain of its NS1 protein to facilitate inhibition of the RNA-dependent protein kinase PKR. *J Virol.* (2017) 91:e00198-17. doi: 10.1128/JVI.00198-17

47. Abraham N, Stojdl DF, Duncan PI, Méthot N, Ishii T, Dubé M, et al. Characterization of transgenic mice with targeted disruption of the catalytic domain of the double-stranded RNA-dependent protein kinase, PKR. *J Biol Chem.* (1999) 274:5953–62.

48. Min J-Y, Li S, Sen GC, Krug RM. A site on the influenza A virus NS1 protein mediates both inhibition of PKR activation and temporal regulation of viral RNA synthesis. *Virology* (2007) 363:236–43. doi: 10.1016/j.virol.2007. 01.038

49. Tu Y-C, Yu C-Y, Liang J-J, Lin E, Liao C-L, Lin Y-L. Blocking double-stranded RNA-activated protein kinase PKR by Japanese encephalitis virus nonstructural protein 2A. *J Virol.* (2012) 86:10347–58. doi: 10.1128/JVI.00525-12

50. Clavarino G, Cláudio N, Couderc T, Dalet A, Judith D, Camosseto V, et al. Induction of GADD34 is necessary for dsRNA-dependent interferon-β production and participates in the control of Chikungunya virus infection. *PLoS Pathog.* (2012) 8:e1002708. doi: 10.1371/journal.ppat. 1002708

51. Choy MS, Yusoff P, Lee IC, Newton JC, Goh CW, Page R, et al. Structural and functional analysis of the GADD34:PP1 eIF2α phosphatase. *Cell Rep.* (2015) 11:1885–91. doi: 10.1016/j.celrep.2015.05.043

52. Novoa I, Zhang Y, Zeng H, Jungreis R, Harding HP, Ron D. Stress-induced gene expression requires programmed recovery from translational repression. *EMBO J.* (2003) 22:1180–7. doi: 10.1093/emboj/cdg112

53. Piacentini S, Frazia SL, Riccio A, Pedersen JZ, Topai A, Nicolotti O, et al. Nitazoxanide inhibits paramyxovirus replication by targeting the Fusion protein folding: role of glycoprotein-specific thiol oxidoreductase ERp57. *Sci Rep.* (2018) 8:10425. doi: 10.1038/s41598-018-28172-9

54. Miller JL, Tyrrell BE, Zitzmann N. Mechanisms of antiviral activity of iminosugars against dengue virus. *Adv Exp Med Biol.* (2018) 1062:277–301. doi: 10.1007/978-981-10-8727-1_20

# Therapeutic Synergy Between Antibiotics and Pulmonary Toll-Like Receptor 5 Stimulation in Antibiotic-Sensitive or -Resistant Pneumonia

Laura Matarazzo, Fiordiligie Casilag, Rémi Porte [†], Frederic Wallet, Delphine Cayet, Christelle Faveeuw, Christophe Carnoy* and Jean-Claude Sirard*

*Univ. Lille, CNRS, Inserm, CHU Lille, Institut Pasteur de Lille, U1019 - UMR8204 - CIIL - Center for Infection and Immunity of Lille, Lille, France*

*\*Correspondence:*
*Christophe Carnoy*
*christophe.carnoy@univ-lille.fr*
*Jean-Claude Sirard*
*jean-claude.sirard@inserm.fr*

Bacterial infections of the respiratory tract constitute a major cause of death worldwide. Given the constant rise in bacterial resistance to antibiotics, treatment failure is increasingly frequent. In this context, innovative therapeutic strategies are urgently needed. Stimulation of innate immune cells in the respiratory tract [via activation of Toll-like receptors (TLRs)] is an attractive approach for rapidly activating the body's immune defenses against a broad spectrum of microorganisms. Previous studies of the TLR5 agonist flagellin in animal models showed that standalone TLR stimulation does not result in the effective treatment of pneumococcal respiratory infection but does significantly improve the therapeutic outcome of concomitant antibiotic treatment. Here, we investigated the antibacterial interaction between antibiotic and intranasal flagellin in a mouse model of pneumococcal respiratory infection. Using various doses of orally administered amoxicillin or systemically administered cotrimoxazole, we found that the intranasal instillation of flagellin (a dose that promotes maximal lung pro-inflammatory responses) induces synergistic rather than additive antibacterial effects against antibiotic–susceptible pneumococcus. We next set up a model of infection with pneumococcus that is resistant to multiple antibiotics in the context of influenza superinfection. Remarkably, the combination of amoxicillin and flagellin effectively treated superinfection with the amoxicillin-resistant pneumococcus since the bacterial clearance was increased by more than 100-fold compared to standalone treatments. Our results also showed that, in response to flagellin, the lung tissue generated an innate immune response even though it had been damaged by the influenza virus and pneumococcal infections. In conclusion, we demonstrated that the selective boosting of lung innate immunity is a conceptually advantageous approach for improving the effectiveness of antibiotic treatment and fighting antibiotic-resistant bacteria.

Keywords: flagellin, Toll-like receptor 5, antibiotic, resistance, *Streptococcus pneumoniae*, pneumonia, superinfection

# INTRODUCTION

Pneumonia constitutes a major cause of death, morbidity and health resource use worldwide. The main causative agents identified in adult patients hospitalized for community-acquired pneumonia (CAP) are viruses (in 27–30% of cases, the most common being rhinovirus, influenza and coronavirus) and bacteria (14–23% of cases, with a marked predominance of *Streptococcus pneumoniae* infections) (1–3). When faced with overt clinical signs of bacterial pneumonia, the standard of care is antibiotic treatment. The combination of a constant rise in antibiotic resistance in recent decades with a decline in the discovery of new drugs has led to an increase in treatment failure and mortality (4). In 2017, the World Health Organization's Global Action Plan highlighted the urgent need to control the emergence of antibiotic resistance (5). Given this context, a number of new anti-infectious treatment strategies are being developed.

The modulation of innate immunity [by targeting immune receptors, such as Toll-like receptors (TLRs)] is a promising approach (6, 7). Indeed, innate immunity is highly conserved in evolution, and this system constitutes the first line of defense against invading pathogens. Moreover, innate immunity triggers a broad range of antimicrobial defense mechanisms and immune cells—thereby greatly reducing the risk of resistance in the pathogens. Moreover, activation of TLR signaling has been associated with a favorable outcome in infections with antibiotic-resistant bacteria or colonization resistance by such pathogens (8–10). These observations support that stimulation and effector activities of innate immunity are not influenced by the antibiotic resistance mechanisms carried by bacteria. Flagellin is the main protein component of the bacterial flagellum and is a natural agonist of TLR5; the latter is expressed at the surface of a many different cell types, including mucosal epithelial cells and immune cells such as dendritic cells, macrophages, and lymphocytes (11). Various studies in animal models have highlighted the antimicrobial potency of flagellin against a wide variety of bacterial infections [such as intestinal infections caused by *Salmonella enterica*, *Enterococcus faecium*, *Clostridium difficile,* and *Escherichia coli* (8, 12–14), respiratory infections caused by *Pseudomonas aeruginosa* and *S. pneumoniae* (15, 16)], and viral and fungal infections (17–19). Although most studies have demonstrated the protective effect of flagellin administered before or during exposure to a microbial pathogen, the protein's immunostimulatory efficacy in therapeutic context has not been extensively characterized. Using a mouse model of *S. pneumoniae* lung infection, we recently demonstrated that combination treatment with mucosally administered flagellin and an orally or intraperitoneally administered low-dose (i.e., subtherapeutic) antibiotic is more effective than the antibiotic alone (i.e., with a lower bacterial load in the lung, and a lower mortality rate). Furthermore, the combination treatment was also effective in a model of post-flu pneumococcal superinfection (20). The effectiveness of these combination therapies depends on TLR5 signaling as demonstrated using TLR5-deficient animals and TLR5-mutated recombinant flagellin (20). Our studies highlighted that the airway epithelium is the main

TLR5-specific signaling compartment (21–23). Taken as a whole, these observations are the first to highlight the added value of respiratory delivery of flagellin as an immunomodulatory biologic for the adjunct treatment of bacterial pneumonia (i.e., in addition to the standard of care).

Our working hypothesis was that simultaneous treatment with an antibiotic and intranasal, i.e., respiratory flagellin constitutes a "double hit" against the pathogen. A combination of two drugs may result in independent actions or specific (i.e., additive, synergistic, or antagonistic) effects that define the biological outcome (24–26). An interaction between two drugs is considered to be synergistic when the measured effect of the combination treatment exceeds the predicted cumulative value of the two components given separately. Synergy increases treatment efficacy, and is expected to limit the emergence of drug resistance. Furthermore, synergy allows the physician to decrease the dose level or the frequency of dosing, which thereby dampens adverse drug reactions and may even enable the rehabilitation of neglected drugs. Conversely, an antagonistic combination treatment has a smaller effect than the predicted cumulative value of the two components given separately. Most studies of potentially synergistic antimicrobial agents are performed in *in vitro* systems such as bacterial cultures, using checkerboard assays and increasing doses of each drug (25, 27). Unlike antibiotics that directly affect the bacteria, immunomodulatory biologic activity requires sentinel cells for detection, downstream signaling and thus the production of antimicrobial effectors and the recruitment and/or activation of innate immune cells. At present, there are no comprehensive *in vitro* models of this complicated physiological system.

In the present study, we quantified the nature and magnitude of the interactions between antibiotics and intranasal instillation of flagellin with regard to antibacterial effectiveness in a murine model of *S. pneumoniae* respiratory infections. Furthermore, we wanted to assess the efficacy of this novel therapeutic strategy against infection with antibiotic-resistant bacteria, which represents major public health issues today. To this aim, we investigated the combination's effect on antibiotic-resistant *S. pneumoniae* in a relevant model of post-flu pneumococcal pneumonia, and characterized the immune response induced by the flagellin-mediated protection.

# MATERIALS AND METHODS

## Bacterial Strains and Cultures

Serotype 1 *S. pneumoniae* (Sp1; clinical isolate E1586) was obtained from the National Reference Laboratory—Ministry of Health, Uruguay (15). Serotype 3 *S. pneumoniae* (Sp3; strain 104491) was provided by the Institut Pasteur (Paris, France); it is a multidrug-resistant clinical isolate from a human bronchial secretion, and is resistant to amoxicillin (AMX), cefotaxime, doxycycline, erythromycin, chloramphenicol, streptomycin, and cotrimoxazole (SXT). Working stocks were prepared as described previously (15, 28). Briefly, fresh colonies grown on blood-agar plates were incubated in Todd Hewitt Yeast Broth (THYB) (Sigma-Aldrich, Saint-Louis, MO) at 37°C until the $OD_{600nm}$ reached 0.7–0.9 units. Cultures were stored at −80°C in THYB + glycerol 12% (vol./vol.) for up to 3 months. For infection, working stocks were thawed and washed with sterile Dulbecco's Phosphate-Buffered Saline (PBS, Gibco, Grand Island, NY) and diluted to the appropriate concentration. The number of bacteria (as colony forming units [CFUs]) was confirmed by plating serial dilutions onto 5% sheep blood agar plates.

## Mouse Models of Infection

Female BALB/cJ mice, female Swiss mice, and male C57BL/6J mice (6–8 weeks old) (Janvier Laboratories, Saint Berthevin, France, or Envigo, Huntingdon, UK) were maintained in individually ventilated cages and handled in a vertical laminar flow cabinet (class II A2, ESCO, Hatboro, PA). All experiments complied with institutional regulations and ethical guidelines (C59-350009, Institut Pasteur de Lille; Protocol 2015121722429127). Prior to intranasal infection, the mice were anesthetized via the intraperitoneal injection of 1.25 mg (50 mg/kg) ketamine plus 0.25 mg (10 mg/kg) xylazine in 250 μl of PBS. For primary infections with Sp1, $2–4 \times 10^6$ CFU were inoculated intranasally in 30 μl PBS, as described previously (20). The influenza infection model was developed in our laboratory on the C57BL/6J mice (29, 30). The Sp3 pneumococcal superinfection model was therefore performed in these animals. Briefly, mice were first infected intranasally with 30 μl PBS containing 50 plaque-forming units (PFUs) of the pathogenic, murine-adapted H3N2 influenza A virus strain Scotland/20/74, as described previously (30, 31). Seven days later, animals were infected intranasally with $10^3$ CFU of Sp3 in 30 μl PBS. For the determination of bacterial counts in lung and spleen, mice were sacrificed at selected times via the intraperitoneal injection of 5.47 mg of sodium pentobarbital in 100 μl PBS. Tissues were collected and homogenized with an UltraTurrax homogenizer (IKA-Werke, Staufen, Germany), and viable counts were determined by plating serial dilutions onto blood agar plates and incubating them at 37°C for 12–24 h.

## Flagellin and Antibiotic Administration

The recombinant flagellin $FliC_{\Delta 174–400}$ came from S. enterica serovar Typhimurium FliC and was produced with an histidine tag, as described previously (20, 32). The protein $FliC_{\Delta 174–400}$ was certified to be immunologically active in reporter cells and in mouse assays, and the residual lipopolysaccharide concentration was determined to be <20 pg per μg of flagellin (20). For flagellin treatment, $FliC_{\Delta 174–400}$ (1 ng to 25 μg in 30 μl PBS) was administrated intranasally under light anesthesia via isoflurane inhalation (Axience, Pantin, France). Control animals received intranasal PBS alone. Mice were treated either intragastrically with AMX [5–350 μg of amoxicillin trihydrate (Sigma-Aldrich) in 200 μl water per animal] or intraperitoneally with SXT—a combination of the antibiotics sulfamethoxazole and trimethoprim (Bactrim® Roche, Basel, Switzerland) at total doses of 1 mg (0.84 mg sulfamethoxazole and 0.16 mg trimethoprim) or 4 mg (3.34 mg sulfamethoxazole and 0.66 mg trimethoprim) in 200 μl PBS per animal.

## Testing for Synergy and Proportional Effects

The treatments' effects on S. pneumoniae lung infection were quantified as the percentage bacterial growth ($\%_{growth}$), corresponding to the ratio of the mean bacterial load in the lungs of infected, treated mice to the load in infected, non-treated (control) mice. For example, the effect of treatment A was calculated as follows: $\%_{growth[A]} = (mean\ CFU_{[A]}/mean\ CFU_{[control]}) \times 100$. The predicted additive effect (or predicted $\%_{growth}$) of a combination treatment was calculated as described previously (33). Briefly, the predicted $\%_{growth}$ of a treatment combining compounds A and B is the product of the experimentally defined $\%_{growth}$ values for each standalone treatment (predicted$\%_{growth[A+B]} = \%_{growth[A]} \times \%_{growth[B]}$). If the experimental $\%_{growth}$ for the combination treatment is lower or higher than the predicted $\%_{growth}$, then the two drugs are synergistic or antagonistic, respectively. When the experimental and predicted $\%_{growth}$ values are identical, the two drugs' effects are additive.

## Transcriptional Analysis by RT-qPCR

Total lung RNA was extracted with the NucleoSpin RNA Plus kit (Macherey-Nagel, Duren, Germany) and reverse-transcribed with the High-Capacity cDNA Archive Kit (Applied Biosystems, Foster City, CA). The cDNA was amplified using SYBR green-based real-time PCR on a Quantstudio 12K PCR system (Applied Biosystems). Relative mRNA levels ($2^{-\Delta\Delta CT}$) were determined by comparing first the PCR cycle thresholds ($C_q$) for the gene of interest and the reference genes Actb and B2m ($\Delta C_q$), and then the $\Delta C_q$ values for infected mice treated with the AMX+flagellin combination treatment and with AMX alone (control group) ($\Delta\Delta Cq$). All the primers used in the study (listed in **Table 1**) were validated for efficacy.

## Cell Analysis by Flow Cytometry

Bronchoalveolar lavage (BAL) fluid samples were obtained after intratracheal injection of $3 \times 1$ ml of PBS supplemented with 5% fetal calf serum (FCS). Lungs were perfused with PBS, excised and finely minced then digested in a solution of RPMI 1640 medium (Gibco) containing 1 mg/ml collagenase VIII (Sigma-Aldrich) and 80 μg/ml DNase I (Sigma-Aldrich) for 20 min at 37°C. After washes, red blood cells were removed using a lysis solution (Pharmlyse, BD Bioscience). Lung cell homogenates were then suspended in a 20% percoll gradient and centrifuged at 2,000 rpm without brake at room temperature for 10 min. The cell pellets were washed with PBS supplemented with 2% FCS and cells were filtrated before antibody labeling. BAL and lung cells were stained with anti-CD45-allophycocyanin-cyanine 7 (clone 30F11), anti-CD11b-Brilliant Violet 785 (clone M1.70), anti-SiglecF-AlexaFluor 647 (clone E50-2440), anti-Ly6C-peridinin chlorophyll protein-cyanine 5.5 (clone HK1.4), anti- Ly6G-phycoerythrin (clone 1A8), anti-CD11c-phycoerythrin-cyanine 7 (clone HL3), and CCR2-Brillant Violet 421 (clone SA203G11) antibodies. Dead cells were excluded from the analysis using propidium iodide. The antibodies were purchased from BD Biosciences (San Jose, CA) or BioLegend (San Diego, CA). Data

**TABLE 1 |** Sequences of the primers used for qPCR assays.

| Target gene | Forward primer (F) | Reverse primer (R) |
| --- | --- | --- |
| Actb | CGTCATCCATGGCGAACTG | GCTTCTTTGCAGCTCCTTCGT |
| B2m | TGGTCTTTCTGGTGCTTGTC | GGGTGGCGTGAGTATACTTGAA |
| Ccl20 | TTTTGGGATGGAATTGGACAC | TGCAGGTGAAGCCTTCAACC |
| Cxcl1 | CTTGGTTCAGAAAATTGTCCAAAA | CAGGTGCCATCAGAGCAGTCT |
| Cxcl2 | CCCTCAACGGAAGAACCAAA | CACATCAGGTACGATCCAGGC |
| Il1b | AATCTATACCTGTCCTGTGTAATGAAAGAC | TGGGTATTGCTTGGGATCCA |
| Il6 | GTTCTCTGGGAAATCGTGGAAA | AAGTGCATCATCGTTGTTCATACA |
| S100a9 | CACCCTGAGCAAGAAGGAAT | TGTCATTTATGAGGGCTTCATTT |

were collected on a BD LSR Fortessa and analyzed with the BD FACSDiva software.

## Cytokine and Chemokine Production

Concentration of CCL20, CXCL1, CXCL2, IL-6, IL-1β, and TNF was determined in BAL fluids and lung homogenates by enzyme-linked immunosorbent assay (ELISA kit from eBioscience, R&D Systems or Becton Dickinson). BAL fluids were obtained by intratracheal injection of $2 \times 1$ ml PBS supplemented with protease inhibitors (Roche). Lungs were perfused with PBS and collected in T-PER reagent (Pierce) supplemented with protease inhibitors and debris were eliminated by centrifugation. All samples were stored at $-20°C$.

## Statistical Analysis

The results were described as the mean ± standard error of the mean (SEM) or the median (range), as indicated. Intergroup differences were analyzed using the Mann-Whitney test and the log rank test. All analyses were performed with Prism software (version 5.0, GraphPad Software, La Jolla, CA). The threshold for statistical significance was set to $p < 0.05$.

## RESULTS

## Determination of the Minimum Dose of Intranasal Flagellin for the Full Activation of Respiratory Tract Innate Immune Responses

In earlier research, we had shown that the intranasal administration of a combination of flagellin FliC$_{\Delta174-400}$ and low-dose antibiotics improved the therapeutic outcome of lung infection with the antibiotic-susceptible Sp1 [minimum inhibitory concentration (MIC)$_{AMX}$ = 0.016 µg/ml] (20). Given the difficulty of performing in vitro checkerboard assays with immunomodulators, we therefore sought to evaluate the nature of antibiotic-flagellin interactions in vivo. We first defined the dose of flagellin that promoted saturating immune responses in Sp1-infected mice (**Figure 1**). Intranasally administered flagellin was associated with the production of various innate immunity-related components, including chemokines (CXCL1, CXCL2, and CCL20), inflammatory cytokines (IL-1β and IL-6), and antimicrobial peptides (S100A9), along with the recruitment of neutrophils to the airways

(15, 16, 20, 21, 23, 28). Mice were treated simultaneously with oral AMX (0.2 mg/kg) and intranasal flagellin FliC$_{\Delta174-400}$ (at doses of 0.4 µg to 1 mg/kg, i.e., 1 ng to 25 µg per animal). Immune responses were analyzed by monitoring the lung transcription of inflammatory genes associated with TLR5 signaling and by comparing mRNA levels to animals that received AMX alone. The results showed that doses from 1 to 25 µg per animal saturated the upregulation of transcriptional response for Cxcl1, Cxcl2, Ccl20, Il1b, and Il6 genes. Ultimately, the dose of 2.5 µg of FliC$_{\Delta174-400}$ was selected as a saturating immunostimulatory dose in the context of pneumococcal infection and lung inflammation.

## The Combination of Antibiotics and Respiratory Instillation of Flagellin Displays Synergistic Therapeutic Activity Against *S. pneumoniae* Infection

The next set of experiments was designed to characterize the therapeutic interaction between intranasal flagellin FliC$_{\Delta174-400}$ and oral AMX. Mice were infected with Sp1 and treated 12 h later with either a single intranasal instillation of flagellin (2.5 µg), a single intragastric administration of suboptimal AMX doses of 5 µg (0.2 mg/kg) or 40 µg (1.6 mg/kg) or the combination treatment. To define the treatments' efficacy, lung bacterial counts were measured at 12 h post-treatment. The results showed that flagellin alone had mostly no antibacterial effect, whereas 5 and 40 µg doses of AMX alone were, respectively, associated with 5- and 7-fold smaller bacterial loads, relative to untreated mice (**Figure 2A**). The combination treatment (AMX + FliC$_{\Delta174-400}$) induced a 10-fold relative decrease in bacterial counts for 5 µg of AMX and a 82-fold relative decrease for 40 µg of AMX—showing that AMX-flagellin combination treatment is more effective than the corresponding dose of AMX or flagellin as monotherapy (**Figure 2A**). The nature of the interactions between flagellin and antibiotics was further analyzed by comparing the bacterial growth upon treatment. The %$_{growth}$ values for the combination treatment (8.4% for flagellin + AMX 5 µg and 1.2% for flagellin + AMX 40 µg) were much lower than the corresponding predicted %$_{growth}$ values for additive effects, calculated as %$_{growth[AMX]}$ × %$_{growth[flagellin]}$ (19.2% for flagellin + AMX 5 µg and 12.3% for flagellin + AMX 40 µg) (**Figure 2B**).

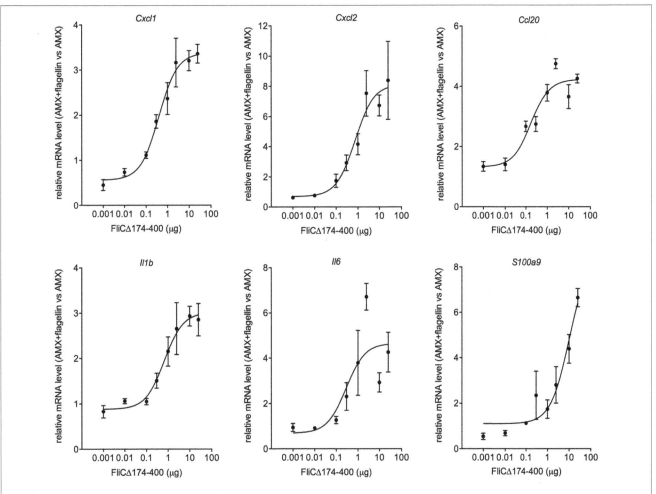

**FIGURE 1 |** The effect of the flagellin dose on the transcriptional response of immune system-related genes. BALB/c mice ($n = 4$ per group) were infected intranasally with $2 \times 10^6$ Sp1 and treated 12 h later with the antibiotic amoxicillin (AMX; 5 μg, intragastric administration) combined with the intranasal administration of various doses of flagellin FliC$_{\Delta174-400}$ (0.001, 0.1, 0.3, 1, 2.5, 10, and 25 μg in 30 μl of PBS) or vehicle only (PBS). Lungs were collected 2 h post-treatment, and RNA was extracted and reverse-transcribed. Gene expression was analyzed using quantitative PCR assays. The relative expression level for each gene is expressed against that of the reference genes *Actb* and *B2m* and the reference condition AMX+PBS (arbitrarily set to a value of 1). The data are quoted as the mean ± SEM.

This experiment indicated strong synergy between the two compounds.

Similar experiments were carried out with the combination of the antibiotic SXT and flagellin (**Figures 2C,D**). The antibiotic SXT was administered intraperitoneally at doses of 1 and 4 mg (40 and 160 mg/kg, respectively). Flagellin (2.5 μg) significantly improved the therapeutic outcome of SXT treatment, as evidenced by CFU counts in the mice's lungs 12 h after administration of the treatments (**Figure 2C**). The experimental %$_{growth}$ values for the combination treatment were lower than the corresponding predicted %$_{growth}$ values (14 vs. 23.5% for SXT 1 mg, and 0.88 vs. 7.3% for SXT 4 mg)—reflecting a synergy between flagellin and SXT (**Figure 2D**).

Taken as a whole, these results show that antibiotics + flagellin had a strong synergistic effect on pneumococcal lung infection in mice. Furthermore, the synergy seems to be independent of the type of antibiotic, since it was

observed with a compound that inhibits bacterial cell wall (AMX) and a pair of compounds that inhibits folic acid synthesis (SXT).

## A Model of Pneumonia With Antibiotic-Resistant *S. pneumoniae* in a Post-influenza Context

Next, we looked at whether the combination treatment's effect on an antibiotic-sensitive *S. pneumoniae* strain was also exerted on antibiotic-resistant bacteria. To this end, a mouse model of infection with a Sp3 strain that is resistant to a wide range of antibiotics including AMX (MIC$_{AMX}$ = 2 μg/ml, i.e., 125-fold higher than for Sp1) was developed. We found that the Sp3 strain failed to induce a lethal infection and other signs of disease (weight loss) in naïve mice—even at high doses of challenge ($10^6$ or $10^7$ bacteria per animal) (**Figures 3A,B**). Given that the influenza virus infection increases susceptibility to bacterial

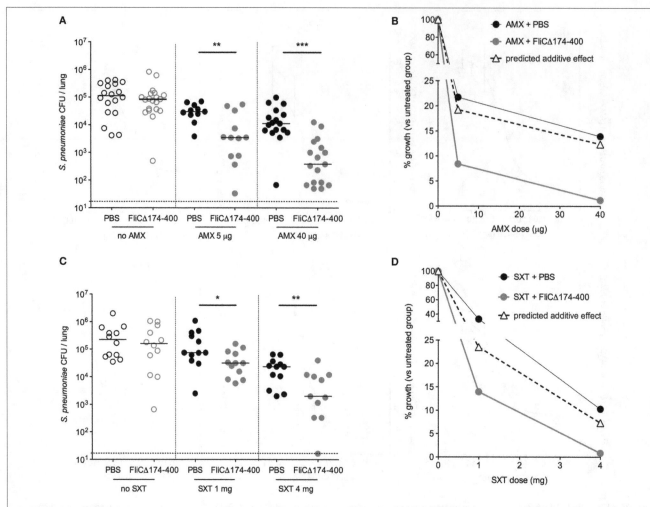

**FIGURE 2 |** Synergy between intranasal flagellin and antibiotics in the treatment of a pneumococcal lung infection. Swiss mice ($n$ = 12–20) were infected intranasally with $4 \times 10^6$ pneumococcus Sp1. The animals were treated 12 h later with the intragastric administration of amoxicillin (AMX; 5 or 40 μg) **(A,B)**, the intraperitoneal injection of cotrimoxazole that is the combination of the two antibiotics sulfamethoxazole and trimethoprim (SXT; 1 or 4 mg) **(C,D)**, and the intranasal administration of flagellin FliC$_{\Delta 174-400}$ (2.5 μg in 30 μl of PBS) or PBS only. Lungs were collected at 12 h post-treatment, homogenized, and plated with serial dilution onto blood agar plates. **(A,C)** Bacterial counts in the lungs of mice. Each symbol represents an individual animal. Colony-forming unit (CFU) counts for individual mice are shown. The solid line represents the median value, and the dashed line represents the detection threshold. Data from flagellin-treated mice were compared with those from PBS-treated mice in a Mann–Whitney test (*$p < 0.05$, **$p < 0.01$, and ***$p < 0.001$). **(B,D)** The treatments' effects on bacterial growth were quantified as the percentage of residual growth (% $_{growth}$) in treated mice (antibiotic + PBS or antibiotic + FliC$_{\Delta 174-400}$) vs. untreated mice (PBS). The predicted additive effect was calculated as % $_{growth[antibiotic]} \times$ % $_{growth[flagellin]}$. The values were plotted according to the dose of antibiotic.

infections even after it has been eliminated (34–37), Sp3 infection was assessed in mice that had already been exposed to the virus. Briefly, mice were infected first with an intranasal, sublethal dose of H3N2 virus (50 PFU) and then infected 7 days later with $10^3$ CFU of Sp3. This bacterial superinfection induced significant weight loss and was 100% lethal (**Figures 3A,B**). The bacterial counts increased gradually over time, and reached $10^7$ CFU per lung 24 h post-infection (**Figure 3C**). Sp3 was also detected in the spleen—indicating a translocation and systemic dissemination of the bacteria—from 24 h post-infection onwards (**Figure 3C**). In conclusion, the antibiotic-resistant Sp3 strain induced effective pneumonia when animals had been previously exposed to experimental flu.

## An Amoxicilin + Flagellin Combination Is Effective Against Amoxicillin-Resistant *S. pneumoniae*

In order to test the efficacy of an antibiotic+flagellin combination treatment in the post-influenza Sp3 superinfection model, mice were treated with AMX alone, flagellin FliC$_{\Delta 174-400}$ alone, or a combination of both compounds 12 h after the bacterial infection (**Figure 4A**). Due to the high level of AMX resistance, the doses of antibiotic used were 100 μg (4 mg/kg) and 350 μg (14 mg/kg). Using this regimen, the serum concentration levels of AMX in naïve animals were expected to be close to $1 \times$ MIC and $4 \times$ MIC, respectively (Professor Charlotte Kloft, personal communication). Flagellin treatment alone decreased bacterial

Therapeutic Synergy Between Antibiotics and Pulmonary Toll-Like Receptor 5 Stimulation...

227

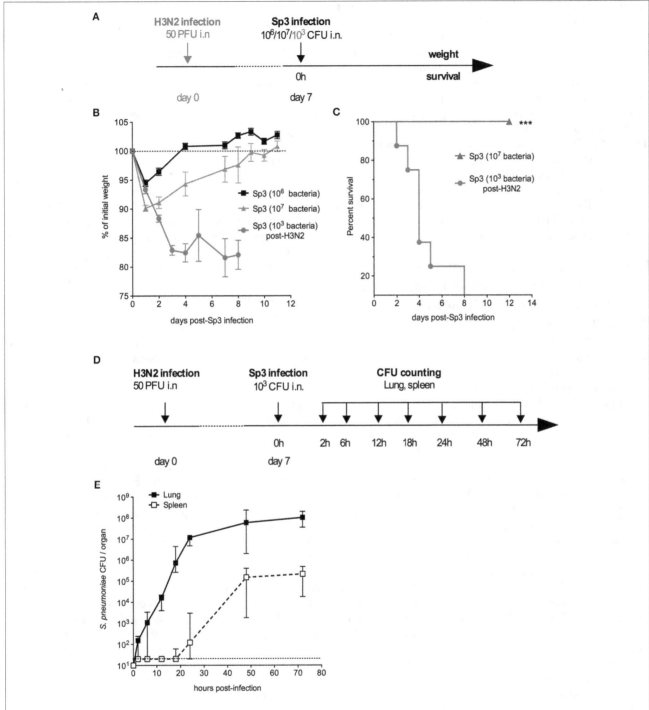

**FIGURE 3** | A murine model of pneumonia due to antibiotic-resistant pneumococcus. **(A–C)** C57BL/6J mice (*n* = 5–8) were infected intranasally with $10^6$ or $10^7$ antibiotic-resistant pneumococcus Sp3 in 30 μl of PBS or with 50 PFUs of H3N2 virus in 30 μl of PBS followed 7 days later by intranasal administration of $10^3$ Sp3. **(B)** Body weight was monitored after Sp3 infection and expressed as a percentage of the initial weight. The data are quoted as the mean ± SEM. **(C)** Survival was monitored daily for 12 days. Data were compared in a log-rank test. ***$p$ < 0.001. **(D,E)** C57BL/6J mice were infection intranasally with 50 PFUs of H3N2 virus in 30 μl of PBS followed 7 days later by intranasal administration of $10^3$ Sp3. **(E)** Bacterial counts in the lung and spleen of mice (*n* = 5). Tissues were collected at the indicated times post-Sp3 infection, and plated in serial dilutions on blood-agar plates. The values correspond to the median (range) CFU count. The dashed line represents the detection threshold.

counts in the lungs by 5.6-fold, whereas AMX treatments decreased bacterial counts by 3.7-fold (for a dose of 100 μg) and 74.6-fold (for a dose of 350 μg). When AMX was combined with flagellin, bacterial counts were of 5,526- and 5,485-fold lower for the 100 and 350 μg doses of antibiotic, respectively. These results show a significant therapeutic advantage for the combination treatment, relative to standalone AMX or flagellin treatments (**Figure 4B**). We also determined CFU counts in the spleen; both AMX and AMX + flagellin treatments (either with 100 or 350 µg of the antibiotic) were able to prevent systemic dissemination of the infection (data not shown). Comparison of %$_{growth}$ for the observed effect of the combination treatment vs. predicted additive effect (0.7 vs. 8.9% for AMX 100 µg, and 0.02 vs. 0.9% for AMX 350 µg) demonstrated the synergy of the combination in the context of superinfection and antibiotic resistance (**Figure 4C**). After two administrations of treatments 12 and 36 h after Sp3 superinfection, the flagellin + AMX combination was found to significantly improve the survival of mice, relative to standalone treatments (**Figure 4D**). These data strongly suggest that flagellin + AMX have synergistic therapeutic effects to control the antibiotic-resistant pneumococcal infections in relevant pathophysiological contexts.

## The Respiratory Administration of Flagellin During Amoxicillin Treatment Stimulates Innate Immunity in the Context of Pneumococcal Post-influenza Superinfection

Since infection by influenza virus induces major changes in lung integrity and immune cell populations, we investigated the immunomodulatory impact of flagellin on post-flu respiratory infections by the antibiotic-resistant Sp3 strain. To this end, C57BL/6 mice were infected with influenza A virus at day 0 and then challenged with antibiotic-resistant Sp3 at day 7. Treatments with oral AMX (100 µg) combined or not with intranasal flagellin (2.5 µg) were administered 12 h after Sp3 infection. Lungs were collected 2 h post-treatment for transcriptional analysis using RT-qPCR assays, as described in **Figure 1**. We observed that despite the superinfection, flagellin still enhanced the transcription of *Cxcl1, Cxcl2, Ccl20, Il1b, Il6,* and *S100a9* genes, i.e., surrogate markers of TLR5-mediated lung stimulation (**Figure 5A**). We next quantified the cytokine/chemokine production after 6 h of treatment both in the BAL fluids and lung protein extracts. Delivery of flagellin in the lung of AMX-treated pneumococcal superinfection significantly increased levels of CCL20, CXCL1, CXCL2, and Tumor-necrosis factor (TNF) both in the lungs (**Figure 5B**) and in the BAL fluids (**Figure 5C**) in AMX+flagellin-treated mice compared with AMX+PBS-treated mice. We also observed increased IL-6 production in both compartments although it was not statistically significant. Production of IL-1β (or pro- IL-1β) was detected only in the lung tissue and was increased in flagellin-treated mice. Finally, we used flow cytometry to evaluate immune cell populations in BAL fluids and lung tissue collected 12 h post-treatment. The analysis showed that the neutrophil counts were higher in mice having receiving the combination treatment (i.e., TLR5 stimulation and AMX) than in mice having receiving AMX alone both in the lung tissues (**Figure 5D**) and the BAL fluids (**Figure 5E**). Interestingly, the innate response to combination treatment was also detectable in blood since the production of the inflammatory mediators were significantly augmented at 2 h (for IL-6, CCL20, CXCL1, and CXCL2) and

6 h (CCL20 and CXCL1) compared to AMX alone treatment (**Supplementary Figure 1**). The blood cytokine production then diminished to an undetectable or very low level at 12 h. Thus, these observations showed that the mucosal delivery of flagellin does not induce sustained systemic inflammation. Overall, the innate immune response to flagellin was effectively stimulated in the context of the influenza immunological imprinting, the superinfection challenge, and the antibiotic treatment.

## DISCUSSION

Our present results demonstrated the synergistic efficacy of a combination of an antibiotic (AMX or SXT) and the local administration of the immunomodulatory biologic flagellin against respiratory infections caused by *S. pneumoniae*. Of note, the efficacy of combined antibiotic + flagellin treatment, previously demonstrated in inbred BALB/c and C57BL/6 mice by Porte et al. (20), was here extended to outbred Swiss mice, showing genetic background independence of the protection. Remarkably, flagellin was able to trigger lung innate immune responses in the context of inflammation (i.e., airways damaged by bacterial pneumonia and flu). Immunostimulation in the lung was a dose-dependent process that was saturating by microgram-per-animal levels of flagellin. The synergy appeared to be independent of the antibiotic dose level and the antibiotic's target, since AMX acts on the bacterial cell wall and SXT inhibits DNA synthesis. The present study is also the first to have demonstrated that stimulating innate immunity can treat severe pneumonia induced by antibiotic-resistant pathogenic bacteria; this may open up new avenues for the treatment of pneumonia in the context of growing antimicrobial resistance.

It has been demonstrated that intranasal administration of flagellin activates TLR5-dependent local innate responses with broad-spectrum antibacterial activity (11, 15, 16, 20, 21, 23). The pulmonary response includes the production of various antimicrobial peptides (i.e., cathelicidin antimicrobial peptide and the β-defensins), cytokines (TNF, IL-1β, and IL-6), and chemokines (i.e., CCL20, CXCL1, CXCL2, CXCL5, and CXCL8). This cytokine and chemokine production is in line with the observed recruitment of phagocytes (and especially neutrophils) in the lung following the intranasal administration of flagellin to naïve mice (15, 23, 38). Flagellin intranasal administration specifically triggers TLR5-mediated transcription in the lungs from 2 to 30 h after a pneumococcus infection or from 7 to 14 days after an influenza infection (20). Here, we demonstrated that the lung innate immune signature induced by intranasal instillation of flagellin is still effective in a highly inflammatory context with associated lung damage (pneumococcal post-influenza superinfection), and is not influenced by antibiotic treatment (**Figure 5**). Interestingly, earlier reports indicated that influenza infections promote the partial but sustained desensitization of TLR-mediated lung innate responses and a reduction in TLR expression (39). Our observations demonstrate that, in the physiopathological context of superinfection, flagellin is still able to trigger sufficient levels of innate defense and exert synergy with antibiotics (**Figure 4**).

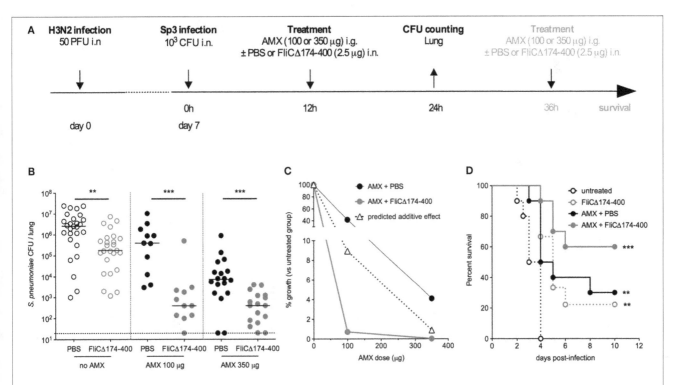

**FIGURE 4 |** Synergy between amoxicillin and intranasal administration of flagellin in the treatment of pneumonia with antibiotic-resistant pneumococcus. **(A)** C57BL/6J mice ($n = 12–28$) were infected intranasally first with 50 PFUs of H3N2 virus in 30 µl of PBS and then 7 days later with $10^3$ antibiotic-resistant pneumococcus Sp3 in 30 µl of PBS. Mice were treated 12 h after Sp3 infection via the intranasal administration of flagellin FliC$_{\Delta174–400}$ (2.5 µg in 30 µl of PBS), the intragastric administration of amoxicillin (AMX; 100 or 350 µg), or combination of both. Lungs were collected 24 h post-infection, homogenized, and plated in serial dilutions onto blood agar plates to measure the bacterial load. For survival experiment, mice received a second dose of the same treatment at 36 h post-Sp3 infection. **(B)** Lung bacterial counts. Colony-forming unit (CFU) counts for individual mice are shown, and the solid line represents the median value. The dashed line represents the detection threshold. Data from flagellin-treated and control (PBS-treated) mice were compared in a Mann-Whitney test (**$p < 0.01$, and ***$p < 0.001$). **(C)** The treatments' effects on bacterial growth were quantified as the percentage of residual growth (%$_{growth}$) in treated mice (AMX+PBS or AMX+FliC$_{\Delta174–400}$) vs. untreated mice (the PBS group). The predicted additive effect was calculated as %$_{growth[AMX]}$ × %$_{growth[flagellin]}$. The values were plotted according to the dose of AMX. **(D)** Survival was monitored daily for 12 days. Data from the treated groups were compared with data from an untreated group in a log-rank test (**$p < 0.01$, and ***$p < 0.001$).

Airway epithelial cells have been identified as an important component for detection of flagellin and TLR5 signaling at homeostasis (21, 22). These sentinel cells not only sense danger signals introduced in the conducting airways but also produce factors to directly impair the colonization and growth of pathogens or indirectly mobilize phagocytic and immune cells to clear infection. More generally, airway epithelium TLR signaling represent a key driving force in antibacterial defense (40). Recently, Anas et al. demonstrated an essential contribution of epithelial signaling in the respiratory tract in response to flagellin in the context of infection with *Pseudomonas aeruginosa* (41). Our data showed that several antimicrobial peptides (S100A9), cytokines (IL-1β and TNF), and chemokines (CCL20, CXCL1, and CXCL2) that were associated to epithelial responses are also upregulated after the administration of the combination treatment in the post-flu superinfection model, suggesting that the epithelium is also an important flagellin-specific driving force in the lung damaged by viral and bacterial infections. Targeting epithelium is a serious benefit for immunostimulation since it allows reducing the dose and bypassing systemic adverse effects.

Our data contribute to highlight the therapeutic potential of the association of two drugs with distinct modes of action:

an antibiotic with a direct effect on bacteria, and a TLR5-specific stimulator of innate immunity with indirect antibacterial activity mobilizing both multiple phagocytic host cells and various antimicrobial factors such as antibacterial peptides, and chemokines and cytokines that mobilize and activate immune cells. Besides pathogen killing, the multitargeting of innate immunity by flagellin could impact on bacterial fitness and thereby increase susceptibility to the antibiotic. The innate immune response induced by TLR5 signaling may also modify the distribution of antibiotic in lung tissues while the antibiotic, by damaging the pathogen, could also enhance the immune signaling. In addition, the pharmacokinetics of the antibiotic and the immunostimulator, i.e., a short-term dose-dependent effect for the antibiotic, and an immediate and long-lasting impact of the immunostimulator due to cell mobilization, are likely complementary. Finally, flagellin, by modulating innate immunity in the respiratory tract, has been shown to enhance the mucosal and systemic adaptive immunity (22, 23). Such property may be of interest to elicit anti-pathogen immune memory and prevent recurrent/relapse infections.

As an opportunistic bacterium, *S. pneumoniae* frequently colonizes the upper respiratory tract and thus represents

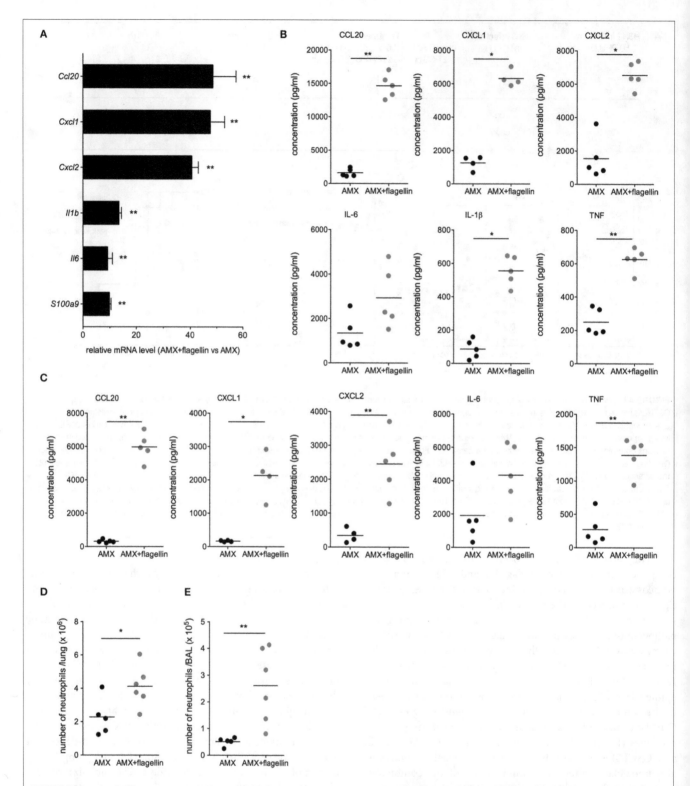

**FIGURE 5 |** Lung innate immune response during flagellin treatment in post-flu superinfection with antibiotic-resistant pneumococcus. C57BL/6J mice ($n = 4$–6) were infected intranasally first with 50 PFUs of H3N2 virus in 30 μl of PBS and then 7 days later with $10^3$ antibiotic-resistant pneumococcus Sp3 in 30 μl of PBS. Mice were treated 12 h after Sp3 infection with the antibiotic amoxicillin (AMX; 100 μg, intragastric administration) and the intranasal administration of flagellin FliC$_{\Delta 174-400}$ (2.5 μg in 30 μl of PBS) or PBS only. **(A)** Lungs were collected 2 h after treatment, and homogenized. After RNA extraction, expression levels of selected genes were then analyzed using RT-qPCR assays. The relative expression level for each gene is expressed against that of the reference genes *Actb* and *B2m* and the reference condition AMX+PBS (arbitrarily set to a value of 1). The data represent the mean ± SEM. Lungs **(B)** and BAL fluids **(C)** were collected 6 h after treatment and cytokine

*(Continued)*

Therapeutic Synergy Between Antibiotics and Pulmonary Toll-Like Receptor 5 Stimulation...

231

**FIGURE 5 |** and chemokine levels were measured by ELISA. Data from AMX+flagellin-treated and AMX+PBS-treated mice were compared in a Mann-Whitney test and are represented as individual values and mean. Lungs **(D)** and BALs **(E)** were collected 12 h after treatment. Lungs and BAL cell suspensions were stained using a mixture of antibodies specific for surface markers before flow cytometry analysis. Neutrophils were defined as CD45$^+$CD11b$^+$Ly6G$^+$ cells after exclusion of dead cells and alveolar macrophages (CD45$^+$SiglecF$^+$CD11c$^+$ cells) from the analysis. Numbers of neutrophils in the lung parenchyma **(D)** and BAL fluids **(E)** are shown for individual animal and the line represents the mean. Data from AMX+flagellin group were compared to those of AMX+PBS group in a Mann-Whitney test. Statistical significance is indicated as follows: $^*p < 0.05$, and $^{**}p < 0.01$.

the prime cause of bacterial-associated CAP (42). However, other microorganisms can cause CAP and healthcare-associated pneumonia; they include Gram-positive bacteria such as *Staphylococcus aureus*, Gram-negative bacteria like *P. aeruginosa*, *Klebsiella pneumoniae*, *Haemophilus influenzae*, mycoplasma (*M. pneumoniae*) and intracellular bacteria (*Legionella pneumophila*) (1). The diagnosis and treatment of CAP is complicated by the broad variety of causative agents, and the progression of antibacterial resistance. In this context, immunomodulators such as flagellin are of great interest because they activate a large number of antimicrobial immune mechanisms. Indeed, flagellin has already demonstrated its ability to protect against various pathogens including Gram-negative and Gram-positive bacteria (8, 12–16, 20). Furthermore, our present results showed that the therapeutic synergy between antibiotic and intranasal flagellin is independent of the antibiotic's mechanism of action—suggesting that flagellin can potentially be combined with various antibiotics for a wide range of clinical situations. The synergistic effects of the combined therapy have been determined to be independent of capsule antigenicity (serotype 1 or 3) of pneumococcus, suggesting that the general innate immune protecting mechanisms triggered by flagellin could potentially be effective against a large variety of serotypes.

Given the progression of antibiotic resistance, a model of infection by antibiotic-resistant bacteria would constitute an important tool for developing alternative anti-infectious approaches. We first attempted to develop such a model in immunocompetent animals. The multidrug-resistant clinical isolate of pneumococcus Sp3 was unable to induce a lethal infection, even at high doses. Acquisition of antibiotic resistance is often associated with a loss of bacterial fitness (43), which might explain the Sp3's very low virulence in naïve mice. It is now becoming clear that many cases of bacterial pneumonia result from co-infections or consecutive infections (especially influenza virus infections) (37). As shown by **Figures 3D,E, 4**, influenza virus infection creates a favorable environment for colonization and invasion by the low-virulence antibiotic-resistant pneumococcus Sp3 strain. Our data demonstrated that the flagellin+AMX combination treatment effectively reduces the bacterial burden caused by the Sp3 strain in the lung, and improves the survival rate among treated mice. Our proof-of-concept findings may be transposable to the clinic for patients with co-infections and superinfections, which are relevant physiopathological causes of hospitalization and complicated pneumonia.

Antibiotics constitute the current standard of care for bacterial pneumonia, and the growing threat of antibiotic resistance

is a major public health concern. When defining the dosing regiments of antibiotics used to treat a patient, the physician must take account of the antibiotic' pharmacokinetic and pharmacodynamic characteristics. The relationship between *in vivo* exposure to the drug and *in vitro* susceptibility of the bacteria conditions not only the treatment's clinical outcome (i.e., clearance of the infection) but also adverse effects or drug toxicity (44). Thus, the maximum dose of antibiotic that can be administered to a patient may not be enough to totally clear highly resistant bacteria. Our data suggest that the antibacterial efficacy of these antibiotic dose levels can be synergistically enhanced by the effect of flagellin on lung innate immunity.

Taken as a whole, the present results suggest that the selective boosting of innate lung immunity by flagellin improves the therapeutic outcome of antibiotic treatment. In humans, this approach might be a useful generic alternative to the treatment of bacterial pneumonia, thereby reducing the antibiotic dose and regimen as well as the emergence of antibiotic resistance. Moreover, such strategy promotes multitarget inhibition through multiple innate immune effectors that should be more resistant to the development of resistance and may restore some antibacterial activity to antibiotic in the context of antibiotic resistance. Characterization of flagellin's contribution to the lung antibacterial defenses at the molecular and cellular level and the protein's synergy with antibiotics is likely to open up new avenues for the immunotherapy of respiratory tract infections.

## AUTHOR CONTRIBUTIONS

LM performed all animal, RT-qPCR, and flow cytometry experiments. FC, RP, DC, and CF provided LM with technical assistance. FW analyzed the bacterial species and antibiotic resistance. LM, CC, and J-CS designed experiments and wrote the manuscript. J-CS and CC supervised the experimental work as a whole.

## FUNDING

The study was funded by INSERM, Institut Pasteur de Lille, Université de Lille, Inserm-Transfert (grant: CoPoC Innatebiotic

R12041ES), and the Era-Net Joint Programming Initiative on Antimicrobial Resistance and the Agence Nationale de la Recherche (grant ANR-15-JAMR-0001-01). LM is a fellow of the Innovation Pharmaceutique et Recherche program.

## ACKNOWLEDGMENTS

We thank Dr. Aneesh Vijayan for technical assistance in the production and quality control of recombinant proteins. We also thank the BICeL flow cytometry core facility and the animal facility at the Institut Pasteur de Lille for technical assistance.

## REFERENCES

1. Ieven M, Coenen S, Loens K, Lammens C, Coenjaerts F, Vanderstraeten A, et al. Aetiology of lower respiratory tract infection in adults in primary care: a prospective study in 11 European countries. *Clin Microbiol Infect.* (2018) 24:1158–63. doi: 10.1016/j.cmi.2018.02.004

2. Jain S, Self WH, Wunderink RG, Fakhran S, Balk R, Bramley AM, et al. Community-acquired pneumonia requiring hospitalization among U.S. adults. *N Engl J Med.* (2015) 373:415–27. doi: 10.1056/NEJMoa1500245

3. Quinton LJ, Mizgerd JP. Dynamics of lung defense in pneumonia: resistance, resilience, and remodeling. *Annu Rev Physiol.* (2015) 77:407–30. doi: 10.1146/annurev-physiol-021014-071937

4. Schäberle TF, Hack IM. Overcoming the current deadlock in antibiotic research. *Trends Microbiol.* (2014) 22:165–7. doi: 10.1016/j.tim.2013.12.007

5. WHO. *Global Action Plan on Antimicrobial Resistance [Internet].* WHO. Available online at: http://www.who.int/antimicrobial-resistance/publications/global-action-plan/en/ (accessed August 23, 2018).

6. Savva A, Roger T. Targeting toll-like receptors: promising therapeutic strategies for the management of sepsis-associated pathology and infectious diseases. *Front Immunol.* (2013) 4:387. doi: 10.3389/fimmu.2013.00387

7. Hancock REW, Nijnik A, Philpott DJ. Modulating immunity as a therapy for bacterial infections. *Nat Rev Microbiol.* (2012) 10:243–54. doi: 10.1038/nrmicro2745

8. Kinnebrew MA, Ubeda C, Zenewicz LA, Smith N, Flavell RA, Pamer EG. Bacterial flagellin stimulates Toll-like receptor 5-dependent defense against vancomycin-resistant Enterococcus infection. *J Infect Dis.* (2010) 201:534–43. doi: 10.1086/650203

9. Brandl K, Plitas G, Mihu CN, Ubeda C, Jia T, Fleisher M, et al. Vancomycin-resistant enterococci exploit antibiotic-induced innate immune deficits. *Nature.* (2008) 455:804–7. doi: 10.1038/nature07250

10. Abt MC, Buffie CG, Sušac B, Becattini S, Carter RA, Leiner I, et al. TLR-7 activation enhances IL-22-mediated colonization resistance against vancomycin-resistant enterococcus. *Sci Transl Med.* (2016) 8:327ra25. doi: 10.1126/scitranslmed.aad6663

11. Vijayan A, Rumbo M, Carnoy C, Sirard J-C. Compartmentalized antimicrobial defenses in response to flagellin. *Trends Microbiol.* (2018) 26:423–35. doi: 10.1016/j.tim.2017.10.008

12. Vijay-Kumar M, Aitken JD, Sanders CJ, Frias A, Sloane VM, Xu J, et al. Flagellin treatment protects against chemicals, bacteria, viruses, and radiation. *J Immunol.* (2008) 180:8280–5. doi: 10.4049/jimmunol.180.12.8280

13. Jarchum I, Liu M, Lipuma L, Pamer EG. Toll-like receptor 5 stimulation protects mice from acute *Clostridium difficile* colitis. *Infect Immun.* (2011) 79:1498–503. doi: 10.1128/IAI.01196-10

14. Andersen-Nissen E, Hawn TR, Smith KD, Nachman A, Lampano AE, Uematsu S, et al. Cutting edge: Tlr5-/- mice are more susceptible to *Escherichia coli* urinary tract infection. *J Immunol.* (2007) 178:4717–20. doi: 10.4049/jimmunol.178.8.4717

15. Muñoz N, Van Maele L, Marqués JM, Rial A, Sirard J-C, Chabalgoity JA. Mucosal administration of flagellin protects mice from *Streptococcus pneumoniae* lung infection. *Infect Immun.* (2010) 78:4226–33. doi: 10.1128/IAI.00224-10

16. Yu F, Cornicelli MD, Kovach MA, Newstead MW, Zeng X, Kumar A, et al. Flagellin stimulates protective lung mucosal immunity: role of cathelicidin-related antimicrobial peptide. *J Immunol.* (2010) 185:1142–9. doi: 10.4049/jimmunol.1000509

17. Zhang B, Chassaing B, Shi Z, Uchiyama R, Zhang Z, Denning TL, et al. Viral infection. Prevention and cure of rotavirus infection via TLR5/NLRC4-mediated production of IL-22 and IL-18. *Science.* (2014) 346:861–5. doi: 10.1126/science.1256999

18. Hossain MS, Ramachandiran S, Gewirtz AT, Waller EK. Recombinant TLR5 agonist CBLB502 promotes NK cell-mediated anti-CMV immunity in mice. *PLoS ONE.* (2014) 9:e96165. doi: 10.1371/journal.pone.0096165

19. Liu X, Gao N, Dong C, Zhou L, Mi Q-S, Standiford TJ, et al. Flagellin-induced expression of CXCL10 mediates direct fungal killing and recruitment of NK cells to the cornea in response to *Candida albicans* infection. *Eur J Immunol.* (2014) 44:2667–79. doi: 10.1002/eji.201444490

20. Porte R, Fougeron D, Muñoz-Wolf N, Tabareau J, Georgel A-F, Wallet F, et al. A toll-like receptor 5 agonist improves the efficacy of antibiotics in treatment of primary and influenza virus-associated pneumococcal mouse infections. *Antimicrob Agents Chemother.* (2015) 59:6064–72. doi: 10.1128/AAC.01210-15

21. Janot L, Sirard J-C, Secher T, Noulin N, Fick L, Akira S, et al. Radioresistant cells expressing TLR5 control the respiratory epithelium's innate immune responses to flagellin. *Eur J Immunol.* (2009) 39:1587–96. doi: 10.1002/eji.200838907

22. Van Maele L, Fougeron D, Janot L, Didierlaurent A, Cayet D, Tabareau J, et al. Airway structural cells regulate TLR5-mediated mucosal adjuvant activity. *Mucosal Immunol.* (2014) 7:489–500. doi: 10.1038/mi.2013.66

23. Fougeron D, Van Maele L, Songhet P, Cayet D, Hot D, Van Rooijen N, et al. Indirect Toll-like receptor 5-mediated activation of conventional dendritic cells promotes the mucosal adjuvant activity of flagellin in the respiratory tract. *Vaccine.* (2015) 33:3331–41. doi: 10.1016/j.vaccine.2015.05.022

24. Foucquier J, Guedj M. Analysis of drug combinations: current methodological landscape. *Pharmacol Res Perspect.* (2015) 3:e00149. doi: 10.1002/prp2.149

25. Rao GG, Li J, Garonzik SM, Nation RL, Forrest A. Assessment and modelling of antibacterial combination regimens. *Clin Microbiol Infect.* (2017) 24:689–96. doi: 10.1016/j.cmi.2017.12.004

26. Doern CD. When does 2 plus 2 equal 5? A review of antimicrobial synergy testing. *J Clin Microbiol.* (2014) 52:4124–8. doi: 10.1128/JCM.01121-14

27. Norden CW, Wentzel H, Keleti E. Comparison of techniques for measurement of *in vitro* antibiotic synergism. *J Infect Dis.* (1979) 140:629–33. doi: 10.1093/infdis/140.4.629

28. Van Maele L, Carnoy C, Cayet D, Ivanov S, Porte R, Deruy E, et al. Activation of Type 3 innate lymphoid cells and interleukin 22 secretion in the lungs during *Streptococcus pneumoniae* infection. *J Infect Dis.* (2014) 210:493–503. doi: 10.1093/infdis/jiu106

29. Paget C, Ivanov S, Fontaine J, Renneson J, Blanc F, Pichavant M, et al. Interleukin-22 is produced by invariant natural killer T lymphocytes during influenza A virus infection: potential role in protection against lung epithelial damages. *J Biol Chem.* (2012) 287:8816–29. doi: 10.1074/jbc.M111.304758

30. Paget C, Ivanov S, Fontaine J, Blanc F, Pichavant M, Renneson J, et al. Potential role of invariant NKT cells in the control of pulmonary inflammation and CD8+ T cell response during acute influenza A virus H3N2 pneumonia. *J Immunol.* (2011) 186:5590–602. doi: 10.4049/jimmunol.1002348

31. De Santo C, Arscott R, Booth S, Karydis I, Jones M, Asher R, et al. Invariant NKT cells modulate the suppressive activity of IL-10-secreting neutrophils differentiated with serum amyloid A. *Nat Immunol.* (2010) 11:1039–46. doi: 10.1038/ni.1942

32. Nempont C, Cayet D, Rumbo M, Bompard C, Villeret V, Sirard J-C. Deletion of flagellin's hypervariable region abrogates antibody-mediated neutralization

and systemic activation of TLR5-dependent immunity. *J Immunol.* (2008) 181:2036–43. doi: 10.4049/jimmunol.181.3.2036

33. Planer JD, Hulverson MA, Arif JA, Ranade RM, Don R, Buckner FS. Synergy testing of FDA-approved drugs identifies potent drug combinations against *Trypanosoma cruzi. PLoS Negl Trop Dis.* (2014) 8:e2977. doi: 10.1371/journal.pntd.0002977

34. McNamee LA, Harmsen AG. Both influenza-induced neutrophil dysfunction and neutrophil-independent mechanisms contribute to increased susceptibility to a secondary *Streptococcus pneumoniae* infection. *Infect Immun.* (2006) 74:6707–21. doi: 10.1128/IAI.00789-06

35. Kudva A, Scheller EV, Robinson KM, Crowe CR, Choi SM, Slight SR, et al. Influenza A inhibits Th17-mediated host defense against bacterial pneumonia in mice. *J Immunol.* (2011) 186:1666–74. doi: 10.4049/jimmunol.1002194

36. Rynda-Apple A, Robinson KM, Alcorn JF. Influenza and bacterial superinfection: illuminating the immunologic mechanisms of disease. *Infect Immun.* (2015) 83:3764–70. doi: 10.1128/IAI.00298-15

37. McCullers JA. The co-pathogenesis of influenza viruses with bacteria in the lung. *Nat Rev Microbiol.* (2014) 12:252–62. doi: 10.1038/nrmicro3231

38. Honko AN, Mizel SB. Mucosal administration of flagellin induces innate immunity in the mouse lung. *Infect Immun.* (2004) 72:6676–9. doi: 10.1128/IAI.72.11.6676-6679.2004

39. Didierlaurent A, Ferrero I, Otten LA, Dubois B, Reinhardt M, Carlsen H, et al. Flagellin promotes myeloid differentiation factor 88-dependent development of Th2-type response. *J Immunol.* (2004) 172:6922–30. doi: 10.4049/jimmunol.172.11.6922

40. Leiva-Juárez MM, Kolls JK, Evans SE. Lung epithelial cells: therapeutically inducible effectors of antimicrobial defense. *Mucosal Immunol.* (2018) 11:21–34. doi: 10.1038/mi.2017.71

41. Anas AA, van Lieshout MHP, Claushuis TAM, de Vos AF, Florquin S, de Boer OJ, et al. Lung epithelial MyD88 drives early pulmonary clearance of *Pseudomonas aeruginosa* by a flagellin dependent mechanism. *Am J Physiol Lung Cell Mol Physiol.* (2016) 311:L219–228. doi: 10.1152/ajplung.00078.2016

42. Donkor ES. Understanding the pneumococcus: transmission and evolution. *Front Cell Infect Microbiol.* (2013) 3:7. doi: 10.3389/fcimb.2013.00007

43. Andersson DI, Hughes D. Antibiotic resistance and its cost: is it possible to reverse resistance? *Nat Rev Microbiol.* (2010) 8:260–71. doi: 10.1038/nrmicro2319

44. de Velde F, Mouton JW, de Winter BCM, van Gelder T, Koch BCP. Clinical applications of population pharmacokinetic models of antibiotics: challenges and perspectives. *Pharmacol Res.* (2018) 134:280–8. doi: 10.1016/j.phrs.2018.07.005

# Permissions

# List of Contributors

**Franziska Voß, Thomas P. Kohler, Mohammed R. Abdullah, Malek Saleh and Sven Hammerschmidt**
Department of Molecular Genetics and Infection Biology, Center for Functional Genomics of Microbes, Interfaculty Institute of Genetics and Functional Genomics, University of Greifswald, Greifswald, Germany

**Tanja Meyer and Stephan Michalik**
Department of Functional Genomics, Center for Functional Genomics of Microbes, Interfaculty Institute of Genetics and Functional Genomics, University Medicine Greifswald, Greifswald, Germany

**Fred J. van Opzeeland, Saskia van Selm and Marien I. de Jonge**
Section Pediatric Infectious Diseases, Laboratory of Medical Immunology, Radboud Center for Infectious Diseases, Radboud Institute for Molecular Life Sciences, Radboud University Medical Center, Nijmegen, Netherlands

**Frank Schmidt**
Department of Functional Genomics, Center for Functional Genomics of Microbes, Interfaculty Institute of Genetics and Functional Genomics, University Medicine Greifswald, Greifswald, Germany
ZIK-FunGene, Department of Functional Genomics, Interfaculty Institute for Genetics and Functional Genomics, University Medicine Greifswald, Greifswald, Germany

**Yi Yang, Catherine R. Back, Ayla A. Wahid and Jean M. H. van den Elsen**
Department of Biology and Biochemistry, University of Bath, Bath, United Kingdom

**Melissa A. Gräwert and Dmitri I. Svergun**
Hamburg Unit, European Molecular Biology Laboratory, Deutsches Elektronen-Synchrotron, Hamburg, Germany

**Harriet Denton, Rebecca Kildani, Joshua Paulin and Kevin J. Marchbank**
Institute of Cellular Medicine, Newcastle University, Newcastle-upon-Tyne, United Kingdom

**Kristin Wörner and Wolgang Kaiser**
Dynamic Biosensors GmbH, Martinsried, Germany

**Asel Sartbaeva**
Department of Chemistry, University of Bath, Bath, United Kingdom

**Andrew G. Watts**
Department of Pharmacy and Pharmacology, University of Bath, Bath, United Kingdom

**Olivier Terrier and Aurélien Traversier**
Virologie et Pathologie Humaine—VirPath Team, Centre International de Recherche en Infectiologie, INSERM U1111, CNRS UMR5308, ENS Lyon, Université Claude Bernard Lyon 1, Université de Lyon, Lyon, France

**Marie-Eve Hamelin, Chantal Rhéaume, Guy Boivin and Andrés Pizzorno**
Virologie et Pathologie Humaine—VirPath Team, Centre International de Recherche en Infectiologie, INSERM U1111, CNRS UMR5308, ENS Lyon, Université Claude Bernard Lyon 1, Université de Lyon, Lyon, France
Research Center in Infectious Diseases of the CHU de Quebec and Laval University, Quebec City, QC, Canada

**Magali Roche and Claire Nicolas de Lamballerie**
Virologie et Pathologie Humaine—VirPath Team, Centre International de Recherche en Infectiologie, INSERM U1111, CNRS UMR5308, ENS Lyon, Université Claude Bernard Lyon 1, Université de Lyon, Lyon, France
Viroscan3D SAS, Lyon, France

**Thomas Julien, Blandine Padey and Manuel Rosa-Calatrava**
Virologie et Pathologie Humaine—VirPath Team, Centre International de Recherche en Infectiologie, INSERM U1111, CNRS UMR5308, ENS Lyon, Université Claude Bernard Lyon 1, Université de Lyon, Lyon, France
VirNext, Faculté de Médecine RTH Laennec, Université Claude Bernard Lyon 1, Université de Lyon, Lyon, France

**Séverine Croze**
ProfileXpert, SFR-Est, CNRS UMR-S3453, INSERM US7, Université Claude Bernard Lyon 1, Université de Lyon, Lyon, France

**Vanessa Escuret and Bruno Lina**
Virologie et Pathologie Humaine—VirPath Team, Centre International de Recherche en Infectiologie, INSERM U1111, CNRS UMR5308, ENS Lyon, Université Claude Bernard Lyon 1, Université de Lyon, Lyon, France
Laboratoire de Virologie, Centre National de Référence des virus Influenza Sud, Institut des Agents Infectieux, Groupement Hospitalier Nord, Hospices Civils de Lyon, Lyon, France

**Julien Poissy**
Pôle de Réanimation, Hôpital Roger Salengro, Centre Hospitalier Régional et Universitaire de Lille, Université de Lille 2, Lille, France

**Catherine Legras-Lachuer**
Viroscan3D SAS, Lyon, France
Ecologie Microbienne, UMR CNRS 5557, USC INRA 1364, Université Claude Bernard Lyon 1, Université de Lyon, Villeurbanne, France

**Julien Textoris**
Service d'Anesthésie et de Réanimation, Hôpital Edouard Herriot, Hospices Civils de Lyon, Lyon, France
Pathophysiology of Injury-Induced Immunosuppression (PI3), EA 7426 Hospices Civils de Lyon, bioMérieux, Université Claude Bernard Lyon 1, Hôpital Edouard Herriot, Lyon, France

**Stéphane Cauchi and Camille Locht**
Univ. Lille, U1019, UMR 8204, CIIL–Centre for Infection and Immunity of Lille, Lille, France
CNRS UMR8204, Lille, France
Inserm U1019, Lille, France
CHU Lille, Lille, France
Institut Pasteur de Lille, Lille, France

**Aneesh Thakur, Fabrice Rose and Camilla Foged**
Department of Pharmacy, Faculty of Health and Medical Sciences, University of Copenhagen, Copenhagen, Denmark

**Katayoun Saatchi, Tullio Esposito, Zeynab Nosrati and Urs O. Häfeli**
Faculty of Pharmaceutical Sciences, The University of British Columbia, Vancouver, BC, Canada

**Cristina Rodriguez-Rodríguez**
Faculty of Pharmaceutical Sciences, The University of British Columbia, Vancouver, BC, Canada
Department of Physics and Astronomy, The University of British Columbia, Vancouver, BC, Canada

**Peter Andersen and Dennis Christensen**
Department of Infectious Disease Immunology, Statens Serum Institut, Copenhagen, Denmark

**Zhidong Hu and Ling Gu**
Shanghai Public Health Clinical Center, Key Laboratory of Medical Molecular Virology of MOE/MOH, Fudan University, Shanghai, China

**Chun-Ling Li, Douglas B. Lowrie and Xiao-Yong Fan**
School of Laboratory Medicine and Life Science, Wenzhou Medical University, Wenzhou, China

**Tsugumine Shu**
ID Pharma, Ibaraki, Japan

**Laurie Gauthier and Dominic Arpin**
Département de Chimie, Université du Québec à Montréal, Montreal, QC, Canada
Quebec Network for Research on Protein Function, Engineering and Applications, PROTEO, Quebec, QC, Canada
Département des Sciences Biologiques, Université du Québec à Montréal, Montreal, QC, Canada
Faculté de Médecine Vétérinaire, Centre de Recherche en Infectiologie Porcine et Avicole (CRIPA), Université de Montréal, St-Hyacinthe, QC, Canada

**Soultan Al-Halifa**
Département de Chimie, Université du Québec à Montréal, Montreal, QC, Canada
Quebec Network for Research on Protein Function, Engineering and Applications, PROTEO, Quebec, QC, Canada

**Steve Bourgault**
Département de Chimie, Université du Québec à Montréal, Montreal, QC, Canada
Quebec Network for Research on Protein Function, Engineering and Applications, PROTEO, Quebec, QC, Canada
Faculté de Médecine Vétérinaire, Centre de Recherche en Infectiologie Porcine et Avicole (CRIPA), Université de Montréal, St-Hyacinthe, QC, Canada

**Denis Archambault**
Département des Sciences Biologiques, Université du Québec à Montréal, Montreal, QC, Canada
Faculté de Médecine Vétérinaire, Centre de Recherche en Infectiologie Porcine et Avicole (CRIPA), Université de Montréal, St-Hyacinthe, QC, Canada

**Aude Remot, Emilie Doz and Nathalie Winter**
INRA, Universite de Tours, UMR Infectiologie et Sante Publique, Nouzilly, France

**Jorge A. Soto, Nicolás M. S. Gálvez, Claudia A. Rivera, Christian E. Palavecino, Pablo F. Céspedes, Emma Rey-Jurado and Susan M. Bueno**
Departamento de Genética Moleculary Microbiología, Facultad de Ciencias Biológicas, Millennium Institute of Immunology and Immunotherapy, Pontificia Universidad Católica de Chile, Santiago, Chile

**Alexis M. Kalergis**
Departamento de Genética Moleculary Microbiología, Facultad de Ciencias Biológicas, Millennium Institute of Immunology and Immunotherapy, Pontificia Universidad Católica de Chile, Santiago, Chile
Departamento de Endocrinología, Facultad de Medicina, Pontificia Universidad Católica de Chile, Santiago, Chile

**Valentina Bernasconi, Ajibola Omokanye, Karin Schön and Nils Lycke**
Mucosal Immunobiology and Vaccine Center, Department of Microbiology and Immunology, Institute of Biomedicine, Sahlgrenska Academy, University of Gothenburg, Gothenburg, Sweden

**Beatrice Bernocchi, Minh Quan Lê and Rodolphe Carpentier**
Lille Inflammation Research International Center – U995, University of Lille, INSERM and CHU Lille, Lille, France

**Liang Ye**
Institute of Virology, University Medical Center Freiburg, Freiburg, Germany

**Xavier Saelens**
VIB-UGent Center for Medical Biotechnology, Ghent, Belgium
Department of Biomedical Molecular Biology, Ghent University, Ghent, Belgium

**Peter Staeheli**
Institute of Virology, University Medical Center Freiburg, Freiburg, Germany
Faculty of Medicine, University of Freiburg, Freiburg, Germany

**Didier Betbeder**
Lille Inflammation Research International Center – U995, University of Lille, INSERM and CHU Lille, Lille, France
Faculté des Sciences du Sport, University of Artois, Arras, France

**Caroline N. Jones, Felix Ellett and Daniel Irimia**
BioMEMS Resource Center, Department of Surgery, Massachusetts General Hospital, Harvard Medical School, Boston, MA, United States

**Anne L. Robertson**
Boston Children's Hospital, Harvard Medical School, Boston, MA, United States

**Kevin M. Forrest, Kevin Judice, James M. Balkovec and Martin Springer**
Cidara Therapeutics, San Diego, CA, United States

**James F. Markmann**
BioMEMS Resource Center, Department of Surgery, Massachusetts General Hospital, Harvard Medical School, Boston, MA, United States
Division of Transplantation, Massachusetts General Hospital, Boston, MA, United States

**Jatin M. Vyas and H. Shaw Warren**
Division of Infectious Diseases, Massachusetts General Hospital, Harvard Medical School, Boston, MA, United States

**Karsten Jürchott**
Berlin-Brandenburg Center for Regenerative Therapies, Charité University Medicine Berlin, Berlin, Germany

**Mikalai Nienen**
Institute for Medical Immunology, Charité University Medicine Berlin, Berlin, Germany
Berlin-Brandenburg Center for Regenerative Therapies, Charité University Medicine Berlin, Berlin, Germany
Labor Berlin-Charité Vivantes GmbH, Berlin,Germany

**Ulrik Stervbo and Sviatlana Kaliszczyk**
Center for Translational Medicine, Immunology and Transplantation, Marien Hospital Herne, Ruhr University Bochum, Herne, Germany

**Felix Mölder and Sven Rahmann**
Genome Informatics, Institute of Human Genetics, University Hospital Essen, University of Duisburg-Essen, Essen, Germany

**Leon Kuchenbecker**
Applied Bioinformatics, Tübingen University, Tübingen, Germany

**Ludmila Gayova**
Bogomolets National Medical University, Kyiv, Ukraine

**Jochen Hecht**
Centre for Genomic Regulation (CRG), The Barcelona Institute of Science and Technology, Barcelona, Spain
Universitat Pompeu Fabra (UPF), Barcelona, Spain

**Avidan U. Neumann**
Institute of Environmental Medicine, German Research Center for Environmental Health, Helmholtz Zentrum München, Augsburg, Germany

**Brunhilde Schweiger**
Robert-Koch Institute, Berlin, Germany

**Filip Boyen and Freddy Haesebrouck**
Department of Pathology, Bacteriology and Avian Diseases, Faculty of Veterinary Medicine, Ghent University, Merelbeke, Belgium

**Petra Reinke**
Berlin-Brandenburg Center for Regenerative Therapies, Charité University Medicine Berlin, Berlin, Germany Department of Nephrology and Intensive Care, Charité University Medicine

**Cyril Le Nouën, Peter L. Collins and Ursula J. Buchholz**
RNA Viruses Section, LID, NIAID, NIH, Bethesda, MD, United States

**Andrés Pizzorno, Blandine Padey, Olivier Terrier and Manuel Rosa-Calatrava**
Virologie et Pathologie Humaine–VirPath Team, Centre International de Recherche en Infectiologie (CIRI), INSERM U1111, CNRS UMR5308, ENS Lyon, Université Claude Bernard Lyon 1, Université de Lyon, Lyon, France

**Anneleen M. F. Matthijs, Annelies Michiels and Dominiek Maes**
Department of Reproduction, Obstetrics and Herd Health, Faculty of Veterinary Medicine, Ghent University, Merelbeke, Belgium

**Gaël Auray, Obdulio García-Nicolás, Roman O. Braun and Artur Summerfield**
Institute of Virology and Immunology, Mittelhäusern, Switzerland
Department of Infectious Diseases and Pathobiology, Vetsuisse Faculty, University of Bern, Bern, Switzerland,

**Virginie Jakob, Nicolas Collin and Christophe Barnier-Quer**
Vaccine Formulation Laboratory, University of Lausanne, Epalinges, Switzerland

**Irene Keller**
Interfaculty Bioinformatics Unit, Swiss Institute of Bioinformatics, University of Bern, Bern, Switzerland Department of Biomedical Research, University of Bern, Bern, Switzerland

**Barbora Lajoie**
Laboratoire de Génie Chimique CNRS, INPT, UPS Université de Toulouse III, Faculté des Sciences Pharmaceutiques, Toulouse, France

**Rémy Bruggman**
Interfaculty Bioinformatics Unit, Swiss Institute of Bioinformatics, University of Bern, Bern, Switzerland

**Bert Devriendt**
Laboratory of Veterinary Immunology, Department of Virology, Parasitology and Immunology, Faculty of Veterinary Medicine, Ghent University, Merelbeke, Belgium

**Timm Westhoff**
Department of Internal Medicine, Marien Hospital Herne, Ruhr University Bochum, Herne, Germany

**Carlos A. Guzman**
Department of Vaccinology and Applied Microbiology, Helmholtz Centre for Infection Research, Brunswick, Germany

**Fusade-Boyer, Gabriel Dupré, Pierre Bessière, Stéphane Bertagnoli and Romain Volmer**
Université de Toulouse, ENVT, INRA, UMR 1225, Toulouse, France

**Samira Khiar and Frédéric Tangy**
Viral Genomics and Vaccination Unit, CNRS UMR-3569, Institut Pasteur, Paris, France

**Charlotte Quentin-Froignant**
Université de Toulouse, ENVT, INRA, UMR 1225, Toulouse, France
NeoVirTech SAS, Institute for Advanced Life Science Technology, Toulouse, France

**Cécile Beck and Sylvie Lecollinet**
UMR 1161 Virology, INRA, ANSES, Ecole Nationale Vétérinaire d'Alfort, ANSES Animal Health Laboratory, EURL for Equine Diseases, Maisons-Alfort, France

**Marie-Anne Rameix-Welti**
UMR INSERM U1173 2I, UFR des Sciences de la Santé Simone Veil—UVSQ, Montigny-le-Bretonneux, France AP-HP, Laboratoire de Microbiologie, Hôpital Ambroise Paré, Boulogne-Billancourt, France

**Jean-François Eléouët**
Unité de Virologie et Immunologie Moléculaires (UR892), INRA, Université Paris-Saclay, Jouy-en-Josas, France

**Pierre-Olivier Vidalain**
Laboratoire de Chimie et Biochimie Pharmacologiques et Toxicologiques, Equipe Chimie & Biologie, Modélisation et Immunologie pour la Thérapie, CNRS UMR 8601, Université Paris Descartes, Paris, France

**Laura Matarazzo, Fiordiligie Casilag, Rémi Porte, Frederic Wallet, Delphine Cayet, Christelle Faveeuw, Christophe Carnoy and Jean-Claude Sirard**
Univ. Lille, CNRS, Inserm, CHU Lille, Institut Pasteur de Lille, U1019 - UMR8204 - CIIL - Center for Infection and Immunity of Lille, Lille, France

**Franck Gallardo**
NeoVirTech SAS, Institute for Advanced Life Science Technology, Toulouse, France

# Index

Printed in the USA
CPSIA information can be obtained
at www.ICGtesting.com
JSHW060437061023
49754JS00014B/43

9 798887 404370